Road Dust in Urban and Industrial Environments: Sources, Pollutants, Impacts, and Management

Road Dust in Urban and Industrial Environments: Sources, Pollutants, Impacts, and Management

Editors

Dmitry Vlasov
Omar Ramírez
Ashok Luhar

MDPI • Basel • Beijing • Wuhan • Barcelona • Belgrade • Manchester • Tokyo • Cluj • Tianjin

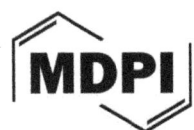

Editors

Dmitry Vlasov
Faculty of Geography,
Lomonosov Moscow State
University
Russia

Omar Ramírez
Faculty of Engineering,
Environmental Engineering,
Universidad Militar Nueva
Granada
Colombia

Ashok Luhar
Climate Science Centre,
CSIRO Oceans and
Atmosphere
Australia

Editorial Office
MDPI
St. Alban-Anlage 66
4052 Basel, Switzerland

This is a reprint of articles from the Special Issue published online in the open access journal *Atmosphere* (ISSN 2073-4433) (available at: https://www.mdpi.com/journal/atmosphere/special_issues/road_dust).

For citation purposes, cite each article independently as indicated on the article page online and as indicated below:

LastName, A.A.; LastName, B.B.; LastName, C.C. Article Title. *Journal Name* **Year**, *Volume Number*, Page Range.

ISBN 978-3-0365-3985-0 (Hbk)
ISBN 978-3-0365-3986-7 (PDF)

© 2022 by the authors. Articles in this book are Open Access and distributed under the Creative Commons Attribution (CC BY) license, which allows users to download, copy and build upon published articles, as long as the author and publisher are properly credited, which ensures maximum dissemination and a wider impact of our publications.

The book as a whole is distributed by MDPI under the terms and conditions of the Creative Commons license CC BY-NC-ND.

Contents

About the Editors ix

Dmitry Vlasov, Omar Ramírez and Ashok Luhar
Road Dust in Urban and Industrial Environments: Sources, Pollutants, Impacts, and Management
Reprinted from: *Atmosphere* **2022**, *13*, 607, doi:10.3390/atmos13040607 1

Yameli Aguilar, Francisco Bautista, Patricia Quintana, Daniel Aguilar, Rudy Trejo-Tzab, Avto Goguitchaichvili and Roberto Chan-Te
Color as a New Proxy Technique for the Identification of Road Dust Samples Contaminated with Potentially Toxic Elements: The Case of Mérida, Yucatán, México
Reprinted from: *Atmosphere* **2021**, *12*, 483, doi:10.3390/atmos12040483 11

Andrian Seleznev, Ekaterina Ilgasheva, Ilia Yarmoshenko and Georgy Malinovsky
Coarse Technogenic Material in Urban Surface Deposited Sediments (USDS)
Reprinted from: *Atmosphere* **2021**, *12*, 754, doi:10.3390/atmos12060754 25

Siyu Sun, Na Zheng, Sujing Wang, Yunyang Li, Shengnan Hou, Xue Song, Shanshan Du, Qirui An, Pengyang Li, Xiaoqian Li, Xiuyi Hua and Deming Dong
Source Analysis and Human Health Risk Assessment Based on Entropy Weight Method Modification of $PM_{2.5}$ Heavy Metal in an Industrial Area in the Northeast of China
Reprinted from: *Atmosphere* **2021**, *12*, 852, doi:10.3390/atmos12070852 43

Sebastián Vanegas, Erika M. Trejos, Beatriz H. Aristizábal, Guilherme M. Pereira, Julio M. Hernández, Jorge Herrera Murillo, Omar Ramírez, Fulvio Amato, Luis F. O. Silva, Néstor Y. Rojas, Carlos Zafra and Jorge E. Pachón
Spatial Distribution and Chemical Composition of Road Dust in Two High-Altitude Latin American Cities
Reprinted from: *Atmosphere* **2021**, *12*, 1109, doi:10.3390/atmos12091109 61

Dmitriy Moskovchenko, Roman Pozhitkov, Andrey Soromotin and Valeriy Tyurin
The Content and Sources of Potentially Toxic Elements in the Road Dust of Surgut (Russia)
Reprinted from: *Atmosphere* **2022**, *13*, 30, doi:10.3390/atmos13010030 79

Hyeryeong Jeong, Jin Young Choi, Jaesoo Lim and Kongtae Ra
Pollution Caused by Potentially Toxic Elements Present in Road Dust from Industrial Areas in Korea
Reprinted from: *Atmosphere* **2020**, *11*, 1366, doi:10.3390/atmos11121366 99

Min-Seob Kim, Jee-Young Kim, Jaeseon Park, Suk-Hee Yeon, Sunkyoung Shin and Jongwoo Choi
Assessment of Pollution Sources and Contribution in Urban Dust Using Metal Concentrations and Multi-Isotope Ratios (^{13}C, $^{207/206}Pb$) in a Complex Industrial Port Area, Korea
Reprinted from: *Atmosphere* **2021**, *12*, 840, doi:10.3390/atmos12070840 115

Van-Truc Nguyen, Nguyen Duy Dat, Thi-Dieu-Hien Vo, Duy-Hieu Nguyen, Thanh-Binh Nguyen, Ly-Sy Phu Nguyen, Xuan Cuong Nguyen, Viet-Cuong Dinh, Thi-Hong-Hanh Nguyen, Thi-Minh-Trang Huynh, Hong-Giang Hoang, Thi-Giang Huong Duong, Manh-Ha Bui and Xuan-Thanh Bui
Characteristics and Risk Assessment of 16 Metals in Street Dust Collected from a Highway in a Densely Populated Metropolitan Area of Vietnam
Reprinted from: *Atmosphere* **2021**, *12*, 1548, doi:10.3390/atmos12121548 137

Suzanne Beauchemin, Christine Levesque, Clare L. S. Wiseman and Pat E. Rasmussen
Quantification and Characterization of Metals in Ultrafine Road Dust Particles
Reprinted from: *Atmosphere* **2021**, *12*, 1564, doi:10.3390/atmos12121564 155

Muhammad Faisal, Zening Wu, Huiliang Wang, Zafar Hussain and Muhammad Imran Azam
Human Health Risk Assessment of Heavy Metals in the Urban Road Dust of Zhengzhou Metropolis, China
Reprinted from: *Atmosphere* **2021**, *12*, 1213, doi:10.3390/atmos12091213 173

Deepanjan Majumdar, Bratisha Biswas, Dipanjali Majumdar and Rupam Ray
Size-Segregated Elemental Profile and Associated Heath Risk Assessment of Road Dust along Major Traffic Corridors in Kolkata Mega City
Reprinted from: *Atmosphere* **2021**, *12*, 1677, doi:10.3390/atmos12121677 187

Mohamed Y. Hanfi, Ilia Yarmoshenko and Andrian A. Seleznev
Gross Alpha and Gross Beta Activity Concentrations in the Dust Fractions of Urban Surface-Deposited Sediment in Russian Cities
Reprinted from: *Atmosphere* **2021**, *12*, 571, doi:10.3390/ atmos12050571 207

Anahi Aguilera, Dorian Bautista-Hernández, Francisco Bautista, Avto Goguitchaichvili and Rubén Cejudo
Is the Urban Form a Driver of Heavy Metal Pollution in Road Dust? Evidence from Mexico City
Reprinted from: *Atmosphere* **2021**, *12*, 266, doi:10.3390/atmos12020266 215

Ilia Yarmoshenko, Georgy Malinovsky, Elena Baglaeva and Andrian Seleznev
A Landscape Study of Sediment Formation and Transport in the Urban Environment
Reprinted from: *Atmosphere* **2020**, *11*, 1320, doi:10.3390/atmos11121320 231

Dennis R. Fitz and Kurt Bumiller
SCAMPER Monitoring Platform to Measure PM_{10} Emission Rates from Unpaved Roads in Real-Time
Reprinted from: *Atmosphere* **2021**, *12*, 1301, doi:10.3390/atmos12101301 255

Dennis R. Fitz and Kurt Bumiller
Characterization of PM_{10} Emission Rates from Roadways in a Metropolitan Area Using the SCAMPER Mobile Monitoring Approach
Reprinted from: *Atmosphere* **2021**, *12*, 1332, doi:10.3390/atmos12101332 269

About the Editors

Dmitry Vlasov

Dmitry Vlasov is a senior researcher at the Department of Landscape Geochemistry and Soil Geography, Faculty of Geography, Lomonosov Moscow State University. His research interests lie in the areas of environmental geochemistry, aerosol and precipitation chemistry, road dust and other urban environments' interactions, and sustainable development. He has authored more than 80 publications in Russian and English and has served as an executor of more than 20 scientific projects funded by the Russian Science Foundation, Russian Foundation for Basic Research, Russian Geographical Society. He teaches courses in Lomonosov Moscow State University and its branch in Nur-Sultan (Kazakhstan), and in Shenzhen MSU-BIT University (China): urban geochemistry, environmental chemistry, aerosol and road dust geochemistry, soil science. He enjoys working with students to develop new approaches to assessing geochemical interactions and the pollution of urban environments.

Omar Ramírez

Omar Ramírez is a professor and researcher at the Environmental Engineering Program, Faculty of Engineering, Universidad Militar Nueva Granada in Colombia. He has a Ph.D. in Industrial and Environmental Science and Technology and several publications in international scientific journals. His research areas are air quality and atmospheric pollution, particularly physicochemical characterization of particulate matter, application of receptor models, aerosol geochemistry, identification of road dust components, health risk analysis, and urban pollution.

Ashok Luhar

Ashok Luhar is a principal research scientist at the Oceans and Atmosphere business unit of the Commonwealth Scientific and Industrial Research Organisation (CSIRO), Australia, and leads a research team in aerosol and chemistry modelling. His research interests include atmospheric flow, transport and air quality modelling, ranging from local to global scales and covering problems from air quality to climate change. He has authored several scientific papers, edited books and has been on the editorial board of international journals including *Atmospheric Environment*, *Journal of Air and Waste Management Association*, and *Atmosphere*.

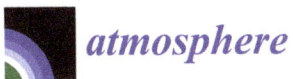

Editorial

Road Dust in Urban and Industrial Environments: Sources, Pollutants, Impacts, and Management

Dmitry Vlasov [1,*], Omar Ramírez [2,*] and Ashok Luhar [3,*]

1. Faculty of Geography, Lomonosov Moscow State University, 119991 Moscow, Russia
2. Faculty of Engineering, Environmental Engineering, Universidad Militar Nueva Granada, Cajicá 250247, Colombia
3. Climate Science Centre, CSIRO Oceans and Atmosphere, Aspendale, VIC 3195, Australia
* Correspondence: vlasov.msu@gmail.com (D.V.); omar.ramirez@unimilitar.edu.co (O.R.); ashok.luhar@csiro.au (A.L.)

Abstract: Road dust (RD) is one of the most important sources of particles in the atmosphere, especially in industrial areas and cities. In this special issue, we collected 16 original articles that describe field, experimental, and modeling studies related to RD and its various size fractions as a key issue in understanding the relationships between several urban and industrial environments and in the identification of pollution sources. Articles in the special issue focus primarily on the following main topics: (1) study of the chemical composition and speciation of RD and its source attribution; (2) assessment of RD and aerosol pollution levels (including express technique), environmental hazards and public health risks; (3) distribution of stable and radioactive isotopes in RD; (4) determination of factors affecting the level of dust accumulation on roads and the intensity of its pollution; and (5) study of the effect of RD on the atmosphere and other environments. Based on the results presented in this special issue, but not limited to, some of the current challenges in studying RD are formulated, including the need for further geographically wider and analytically deeper work on various aspects of the formation, transport pathways, and accumulation of RD in urban, industrial and other areas.

Keywords: air pollution; road dust and road pavement; particle size distribution; source apportionment; environmental interactions; toxic elements and compounds; nanoparticles and microplastic; spatial variation and modeling; health and ecological risks; mitigation strategies

Citation: Vlasov, D.; Ramírez, O.; Luhar, A. Road Dust in Urban and Industrial Environments: Sources, Pollutants, Impacts, and Management. *Atmosphere* **2022**, *13*, 607. https://doi.org/10.3390/atmos13040607

Received: 29 March 2022
Accepted: 8 April 2022
Published: 10 April 2022

Publisher's Note: MDPI stays neutral with regard to jurisdictional claims in published maps and institutional affiliations.

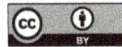

Copyright: © 2022 by the authors. Licensee MDPI, Basel, Switzerland. This article is an open access article distributed under the terms and conditions of the Creative Commons Attribution (CC BY) license (https://creativecommons.org/licenses/by/4.0/).

1. Introduction

Resuspended road dust (RD), enriched with toxic elements, polycyclic aromatic hydrocarbons (PAHs), black carbon, etc., is one of the most important sources of coarse, fine, and ultrafine particles in the atmosphere, which is especially true for industrial sites and cities with a high density of road network and large areas sealed under road pavements [1]. In turn, the chemical composition of RD is determined by the impact of a wide range of anthropogenic sources, as well as by the deflation and erosion by rainfall of roadside soils in summer (especially in the relatively dry climate), blowing out de-icing agents in winter and after snowmelt, transportation of particles with stormwater runoff, deposition of suspended atmospheric particles, and precipitation. The chemical and physical characterization of RD size fractions is a key issue in understanding the relationships between several urban and industrial environments and in the identification of pollution sources. However, in many cities and towns, there is a significant lack of knowledge of the composition of RD and its individual size fractions, dust loadings, the anthropogenic impact on the degree of RD pollution, and potential risks of RD to public health and ecosystems.

In this special issue, we collected 16 original articles that describe field, experimental, and modeling studies related to detailed analyses of RD and its various size fractions as a significant source of air pollution. Priority attention is paid to modern techniques, approaches, and methods for assessing the contribution of various sources to the chemical composition of RD size fractions (i.e., source apportionment) and the assessment of public health and ecological risks, as well as other related issues of particulate matter, including ultrafine particles.

The field data that formed the basis of the papers in this special issue were collected worldwide, which proves the considerable interest of researchers from the regions of North, Central and South America, Europe, Asia, and Africa in the study of RD, and countries including Brazil [2], Canada [3], Colombia [2], Costa Rica [2], Egypt [4], India [5], Mexico [6,7], Pakistan [8], People's Republic of China [8,9], Republic of Korea [10,11], Russian Federation [4,12–14], Spain [2], Taiwan (Republic of China) [15], the United States of America [16,17], and Vietnam [15]. The study areas included roads of various types and sizes within different land-use areas (commercial, residential, industrial, recreational, educational, etc.) in megacities [2,5,6,8,15], large [3,4,7,12,13] and medium-sized cities [2,12–14], industrial areas [9–11], paved and unpaved roads between cities and settlements [16,17]. In the literature, various terms are usually used to denote particles that accumulate on the roadway surfaces, such as "road dust(s)," "street dust(s)," "road-deposited sediments," "sweepsand", etc. The authors of the special issue predominantly used the term "road dust" [2,3,5–8,10,14], although terms such as "street dust" [15], "urban dust" [11], "road sediments" [2], "urban sediments" [12], "urban surface deposited sediments" [4,13] are also used.

Articles in the special issue focus primarily on the following main topics: (1) study of the chemical composition of dust and sources of various substances in it, (2) assessment of RD and aerosol pollution levels, environmental hazards and public health risks, (3) distribution of stable and radioactive isotopes in RD, (4) determination of factors affecting the level of dust accumulation on roads and the intensity of its pollution, and (5) study of the effect of dust on the atmosphere and other environments.

2. Chemical Composition and Source Apportionment

The study of the composition of RD and an assessment of their probable sources is one of the main topics of most work on RD worldwide, which was also reflected in our special issue. The largest number of papers in the special issue is devoted to the study of RD chemical elements, such as metals and heavy metals (HMs) [3,6,8,9,11,15], potentially toxic elements (PTEs) [7,10,14], major, mineral, minor, and trace elements [2,5,11,13], and ions [2]. Among the analytical methods, inductively coupled plasma mass spectrometry (ICP-MS) [2,3,8–10,14,15], inductively coupled plasma optical spectrometry (ICP-OES) [3,5,6,11], inductively coupled plasma atomic emission spectroscopy (ICP-AES) [14], X-ray fluorescence with dispersed energy (XRF-ED) [7], scanning electron microscope equipped with an energy-dispersive spectrometer (SEM-EDS) [7,13] are most frequently used. H. Jeong et al. [10] also measured the magnetic susceptibility of RD.

Several articles are devoted to studying the mineralogical composition and type of individual RD particles. For example, Y. Aguilar et al. [7] found that calcite, quartz, ankerite, anorthoclase, and albite are the main minerals of RD of the city of Mérida Yucatán, Mexico, and natural minerals such as hematite, goethite, boehmite, dikite, sanidine, tosidite, and yeelimite are found in smaller quantities; among the anthropogenic minerals, maghemite is the most common, which determines the highest magnetic signal to RD. A. Seleznev et al. [13] showed that 19% and 13% of particles in the urban surface-deposited sediments in the residential areas of ten Russian cities located in different economic, climatic, and geological zones are characterized as technogenic (e.g., plaster, car tires, household waste, glass, coal, paint, brick, silicate and iron microspheres, granulated and lithoid slag) in particle size fractions of 0.1–0.25 and 0.25–1 mm, respectively, and the rest of the particles is represented by the mineral and natural organic fragments. The results in this special issue prove the need for a detailed study of the mineralogy of RD and adjacent environments (such as soils, atmospheric depositions, and parent rocks), pavement condition, land use, etc. to obtain more accurate information about their mineral matrix and color variation features (see Section 3).

For source identification and apportionment of elements in RD and aerosols, a wide range of approaches and methods have been used, among which the most common are: enrichment factors (EFs) [2,5,11,14,15], Zn/Cu ratio to assess the contribution of traffic activities related to the abrasion of brake pads and tires [10], Cu/Sb ratio to evaluate the contribution of brake wear emissions in RD [2], as well as a hierarchical clustering analysis (HCA) [3,5,15], principal component analysis (PCA) [2,10,14,15], and positive matrix factorization receptor model (PMF) [9]. One of the EF calculation problems is the choice of the reference element [18]. In the special issue, Al and Fe are the most frequently used reference elements in the study of mineral environments [2,14,15]. However, Li was also used due to possible precipitation of Al and Fe hydroxides when the salinity is changed in an estuary environment [11], as well as Ti since it is a stable, non-reactive, and inert element with respect to the physicochemical parameters of the environment, and is negligibly added by anthropogenic activities [5].

In the work of S. Sun et al. [9], using data on the concentrations of HMs in atmospheric $PM_{2.5}$ in Huludao City, an industrial city in northeast China, and the results of PMF, it was shown that in the heating and non-heating periods the leading sources of pollutants are coal combustion (at Huagong Hospitals) and industrial emissions (Xinqu Park); the contribution of traffic emissions is 10–31%. S. Vanegas et al. [2], comparing the chemical composition of RD from two cities in Colombia, proved that volcanic ash could be an important source of SO_4^{2-}, Cl^-, and elements that form the mineral matrix of RD; while Cu, Pb, Cr, Ni, V, Sb, and Mo are mainly associated with exhaust and non-exhaust traffic emissions. D. Moskovchenko et al. [14] for Surgut, a rapidly developing city in Western Siberia, Russia, found that RD particles of size 100–250 μm originate from geogenic sources and abrasion processes caused by road traffic, while particles < 50 μm mainly originate from industrial emissions; the chemical composition of RD is mainly predetermined by contributions from sources associated with road traffic (the abrasion of car tires and brake pads), soil erosion, and solid waste incineration.

Articles of the special issue did not cover studying the chemical fractionation of elements in RD and its particles of various sizes, although this information is essential for understanding the potential sources of elements, their mobility, and environmental hazard [19].

3. Pollution Levels and Health Risks Assessment

The second central area of research in the special issue is the assessment of RD pollution levels, environmental hazards, and public health risks. The level of RD contamination with individual chemical elements was estimated using the enrichment factor, which was mentioned above, as well as the geo-accumulation index (Igeo) [8,10,15], pollution index (PI) or contamination factor (CF) [5,8,15], degree of contamination (Cdeg) [5], and global pollution index (PIr) [14]. Comprehensive assessment of contamination with several pollutants is carried out using pollution load index (PLI) [6,15], and total enrichment factor (Ze) [14]. To assess the environmental hazard of toxicants in RD, the potential ecological risk factor (Er) is calculated, and for the integral assessment, the comprehensive ecological risk (PER) is used [5,10,14,15].

H. Jeong et al. [10] showed that among PTEs in RD from nine industrial areas in the Republic of Korea, the potential ecological risk index is in the decreasing order of Cd > Pb > Hg > Cu > As > Zn > Ni > Cr, and the highest concentration of PTEs was at the Onsan Industrial Complex with many smelting facilities. M.-S. Kim et al. [11] found that the concentrations of Mn, Zn, Cd, and Pb in RD in a residential area near Donghae port, Republic of Korea, and in the port are approximately up to 112 times higher in comparison with the control area. S. Vanegas et al. [2] studied differences in the level of RD pollution in the Bogotá megacity and Manizales city, Colombia. In Bogotá, EFs show extremely high values for Mo and Sb, very high for Cu and Pb, high for Ni, Se, and Cr, while in Manizales, EFs are extremely high for Mo, Se, Sb, and Mn, very high for Cu and As, and high for Ni, Cr, and Pb; the results proved the need to study Se in RD of other cities due to its intense accumulation. A study of street dust from Ha Noi highway, Ho Chi Minh City, Vietnam, by V.T. Nguyen et al. [15], showed moderate contamination levels for Pb, Cd, Cu, Sn, Mo, and Zn (based on Igeo), moderate levels for Cd, Cu, Mo, and Sn and moderate–severe levels for Zn (based on EFs), while PER indicates a high potential ecological risk; also, Igeo levels for B close to the main pollutants were established, which can be helpful when choosing elements for ecological and geochemical monitoring of RD pollution. S. Beauchemin et al. [3] studied the chemical composition of ultrafine particle fraction (UFP) of RD in the City of Toronto, Canada, and showed up to 2 times higher concentrations of Cd, Cr, Zn, and V in UFP compared to the total dust, as well as higher levels of pollution (up to 2 times for Cd, Zn, and V and nine times for Cr) of UFP from arterial roads compared to local roads. The elevated concentrations of transition metals in UFP can cause oxidative stress in human lung cells.

Y. Aguilar et al. [7] developed a proxy methodology and innovative tool to identify RD samples contamination with PTEs using the RGB system and the Munsell color cards. This approach was verified by a discriminant analysis, which confirmed the identification of five groups of RD samples by colorimetric indices and PTE concentrations. Contamination level reaches high in "dark gray" (III) and "very dark gray" (V) samples, decreases to medium in "gray" (II) samples, and low in "greyish brown" (I) and "dark grayish brown" (IV) RD samples. At the same time, the "very dark gray" RD contains the highest concentrations of Pb, Cu, Zn, and Y; the redness and saturation rates showed high correlations with PTEs in "dark gray" and "very dark gray" RD. An important conclusion is that samples of "grayish brown" and "dark grayish brown" colors can be discarded from the chemical analysis when monitoring urban RD pollution.

Using U.S. EPA methodology, M. Faisal et al. [11] estimated non-carcinogenic and carcinogenic risks of Cr, Cu, Ni, Zn, Cd, As, Pb, and Hg in $PM_{2.5}$ portion of RD from five different land use areas of Zhengzhou, China. PI and Igeo show the extreme pollution of RD with Hg, Cd, and Zn. The most significant non-carcinogenic exposure to children is the exposure of Pb in commercial and industrial areas. Both children and adults in Zhengzhou's commercial, residential, and park areas are exposed to higher Cu, Pb, and Zn levels. However, the cancer risk value of Cr was more likely to be at the lower limit of the threshold value, particularly in the industrial area.

Using similar approaches, D. Majumdar et al. [5] assessed the health risks associated with pollution of RD by chemical elements at a few major commercial, traffic, and residential sites in the Kolkata megacity. They establish that Cd and Li have the highest enrichment level relative to the average composition of the earth's crust, among which only Cd posed significant ecological risk due to its high ecological toxicity. Although individual chemical elements do not form significant non-cancer health risks (except for Li for children), the cumulative non-cancer risk for children was almost four times higher than the acceptable level, being ingestion the primary exposure pathway. Lifetime exposure to carcinogenic elements at the current level may pose up to six times higher cancer risk in the adult population than the acceptable risk.

Using U.S. EPA methodology, D. Moskovchenko et al. [14] assessed the health risk to the population of Surgut (Russia) posed by RD contaminated with a large number of PTEs. EFs showed significant enrichment level of RD with Sb and Cu, and moderate enrichment with Zn, Pb, Mo, Ni, and W. Based on PIr and Ze, the RD was characterized by a low level of potential ecological risk, except for stretches of road subject to regular traffic jams, where a moderate ecological risk was identified. The greatest potential risks to human health were associated with the ingestion pathway. Children tend to be at higher risk than adults because of their relatively lower body weight. Sb, Ni, Cu, and As are generally the most harmful elements within Surgut, with additional health risks associated with Cd and Pb within some city areas. Despite the low Ni enrichment of RD, its health risk is high due to the high toxicity. However, both carcinogenic and non-carcinogenic risks of PTEs were generally acceptable or tolerable due to their low concentrations in the RD in Surgut.

S. Sun et al. [9] evaluated non-carcinogenic and carcinogenic risks for the population from HMs in atmospheric $PM_{2.5}$ using the U.S. EPA methodology and the entropy weight method (EWM) during heating and non-heating periods at two sites in Huludao City (China). $PM_{2.5}$ pollution with HMs is higher in the heating period than in the non-heating period. Human health risks are determined by differences in the contributions of HMs in $PM_{2.5}$ from various sources and differ significantly between children, adult men, and adult women. Children have the highest, and adult females have the lowest non-carcinogenic risk, whereas adult males have the highest and children have the lowest carcinogenic risk. In general, the traditional U.S. EPA and EWM methods give close estimates of health risks, but in cases where the differences are quite high, it is recommended to use EWM to estimate non-carcinogenic health risks due to the smaller dispersion of the result.

The special issue did not cover studies on environmentally hazardous chemical compounds and substances, which are both good indicators of pollution sources, such as black carbon and PAHs, environmentally persistent free radicals (EPFRs), organophosphate esters (OPEs) and other organic micro-pollutants [20], micro and nanoplastics [21], glass microspheres [22], platinum group elements (PGE) and rare earth elements (REE) [23], etc. In addition, no source-specific risk assessment nor characterization of bioaerosols in RD were conducted.

4. Isotopic Composition and Radioactivity of Road Dust

The isotopic composition of RD and its radioactivity remain rather poorly studied. However, these parameters can play a significant role in identifying and understanding the geochemical processes of sedimentation and migration of solid particles in urban and industrial areas. The special issue presents two studies to fill the gaps on this topic.

The first one, by M.Y. Hanfi et al. [4], is devoted to assessing gross alpha and gross beta activity in the road- and surface-deposited sediments in three Russian cities in different geographical zones (Ekaterinburg, Nizhny Novgorod, Rostov-on-Don). New methods dealing with low mass and low volume of dust-sized samples obtained after the size fractionation procedure were applied. Due to the presence of radionuclides transferred through natural and anthropogenic processes, the highest gross beta activity concentrations are in the 2–10 µm fraction size in Nizhny Novgorod and Rostov-On-Don and particles of 50–100 µm in Ekaterinburg. On the other hand, the highest gross alpha activity concentrations are characteristic of large particles of 50–100 µm compared to finer particles of 2–10 µm and 10–50 µm due to natural partitioning of the main minerals constituting the urban surface-deposited sediment and are found in Rostov-on-Don. In general, gross alpha and gross beta activity in the studied cities are associated with natural radionuclides, which are found in various cities regardless of climate, geographical location, and industrial development and whose primary sources are geological formations and natural building materials.

M.-S. Kim et al. [11] used isotopic compositions (^{13}C, $^{208/207}Pb$, $^{207/206}Pb$) of urban dust, topsoil, and PM_{10} samples from a residential area near Donghae port surrounded by various types of industrial factories and raw material stockpiled on empty land, and the Stable Isotope Analysis Bayesian mixing model within the R software to assess the contributions of the main pollution sources. It is shown that, depending on the influence of one or another source (cement, Zn ore, coal, coke, Mn ore, soil), isotopic values significantly change in the RD. The application of this method made it possible to prove a significant impact of wind-blown dust from raw material stockpiles near ports and factories, that is, port activities affect the air quality of residential areas in the city. The authors conclude that stable isotope compositions of metals can predict environmental changes and be used as a powerful tool to trace the present pollution and the history of contamination in complex contexts associated with peri-urban regions.

5. Factors of Road Dust Accumulation and Contamination

The chemical composition and particle-size distribution of RD and the amount of particles emitted during the movement of vehicles depend on meteorological, geochemical, anthropogenic, and other factors. Several articles of the special issue are devoted to this topic.

A. Aguilera et al. [6] studied the influence of various city parameters (namely, population density, job density, street intersections, road surface, distance to the airport, distance to the city center, manufacturing units, potentially polluting units, gray area, entropy index, vegetation, distance to vegetation, median strip area, and marginalization index) on Cr, Cu, Pb, Zn, and Ni accumulation in the RD of Mexico City using spatial autocorrelation (Global Moran's I) and applying ordinary least squares and spatial regression models. Low positive spatial autocorrelations in all HMs prove the greater relevance of the local aspects over regional processes as the determinants of the HM content in urban RD. Most variables, including the population density, street intersections, distance to the city center, a gray area, distance to vegetation, and marginalized areas, do not detect any relationship with HMs. The potentially polluting units positively impact the dust load, while vegetation, job density, and road surface significantly reduce the dust load. The median strip area in the roads has a weak but consistent positive relationship with Cr, Cu, Ni, Pb, and the PLI. The distance to the airport has a weak and inverse relationship with Pb. Manufacturing units are associated with an increase in Cu, while the entropy index is associated with an increase in Ni.

I. Yarmoshenko et al. [12] estimated natural and anthropogenic factors influencing the sedimentation processes in urbanized catchments in the residential areas of six large Russian cities based on field landscape surveys. The most significant impact on a high urban sediment formation potential in residential areas is formed by a low adaptation of infrastructure to a high density of automobiles, poor municipal services, and poor urban environmental management in the course of construction and earthworks. The significant impact of motor vehicles in the urban environment includes mechanical sediment transport that sharply increases the sediment connectivity within the urban landscape.

H. Jeong et al. [10] estimated the median total loading of RD in nine industrial sites in the Republic of Korea as 822 g/m^2, ranging from 334 to 1669 g/m^2, which is 2.1–6.5 and 15–16.4 times higher than that in the heavy traffic and urban (commercial and residential) areas, respectively. In Mexico City, the total loading of road dust particles of size < 250 μm ranges from 5.4 g/m^2 to 173.3 g/m^2, with a median value of 43 g/m^2 [6]. In Bogotá, the total loading of RD particles of <10 μm is within 1.8–45.7 mg/m^2 with an average of 11.8 mg/m^2, while in Manizales, it ranges between 0.8–26.7 mg/m^2 with an average of 5.7 mg/m^2; construction and demolition activities are identified as relevant emitters of RD [2]. According to M. Kim et al. [11], an important factor of RD contamination with Mn, Zn, Cd, and Pb is the distance to the source (port), with an increase in which the concentrations of pollutants decrease. Additionally, metal concentrations in ultrafine particles depend on the amount of traffic, the ratio of different types of transport (including light to heavy-duty vehicles), and the speed of transport [3]. Road dust pollution increases on sections of roads with traffic jams [14].

The special issue does not contain articles devoted to various aspects of RD management, assessment of the efficiency of various methods to reduce the amount of dust generated during traffic, methods of its disposal, etc., although these topics are very relevant [20]. Nevertheless, in some papers in the special issue, based on the results obtained, conclusions are drawn about the need for the urgent introduction of an efficient management strategy to reduce RD in industrial areas to protect the health of employees and residents around industrial complexes. In addition, to reduce coastal pollution induced by RD wash-off during rainfall events [10], to increase the coverage and frequency of cleaning roads from dust, especially in areas with possibilities of substantial human exposure and mainly using vacuum-assisted road sweeping machines to remove the most contaminated fine dust fractions [5], as well as the need for cleaning primary roads and areas with "dark gray-" and "very dark gray"-colored dust to more effectively reduce the risk to public health [7].

6. Resuspension of Road Dust and Relationships with Other Environments

Road dust is an essential source of particulate matter in the atmosphere [24], so many papers in the special issue are devoted to assessing the RD resuspension, highlighting the relationship between RD and the atmosphere.

D.R. Fitz and K. Bumiller using the SCAMPER method for measuring PM_{10} emission rates from roadways estimated mitigation methods for public unpaved sections of two different Arizona state highways and a treated mine haul road near the Cricket Mountains in Utah, USA [17], as well as for a wide variety of paved roads in the Phoenix metropolitan area, Arizona, USA, in March, June, September, and December [16]. The suppressant applied five months ago reduces PM_{10} emissions by five times, and applied a year ago reduces PM_{10} emissions by sixty times. The measured emission rates for unpaved roads are approximately seven times higher on a mass basis than those predicted by the AP-42 unpaved road equation. Loaded haul trucks blow almost twice as many PM_{10} particles as unloaded trucks. For paved roads in the Phoenix metropolitan area, the PM_{10} emission rates vary from 0 to 2000 μg per vehicle meter travelled (with an average of 79 μg per vehicle meter travelled) and are generally low unless the road is impacted with dust deposited by activities such as construction, sand and gravel operations, agriculture, and vehicles traveling on or near unpaved shoulders and roads. There is no significant difference in emission rates between seasons. There is a major drop in emission rates over a weekend, when dust generation activities such as construction are expected to be much reduced. By Monday, the PM_{10} emission rates had risen to the levels of the previous Friday, which indicates a rapid achievement of equilibrium in PM_{10} generating potential. The accuracy of the SCAMPER method is about 20% for unpaved sections of state highways and about 25% for paved roads in urban areas.

The efficiency of dust resuspension from the road surfaces, its hazard to public health and ecosystems, the ability to migrate over considerable distances, and the possibility of participation of its components in chemical reactions largely depend on the particle size distribution of dust. Therefore, in the special issue, studies are carried out on the particle size distribution of RD [3,5,10,13,14], as well as on the chemical composition of dust particles and aerosols of different sizes: 0.01–0.018 μm, 0.018–0.032 μm, 0.032–0.056 μm, 0.056–0.1 μm, 0.1–0.18 μm, 0.18–0.32 μm, 0.32–0.56 μm, 0.56–1.0 μm, 1.0–1.8 μm, 1.8–3.2 μm, 3.2–5.6 μm, 5.6–10 μm, and 10–21.1 μm [3], <2.5 μm [8,9], <10 μm [2,11,16,17], 2–10 μm, 10–50 μm, and 50–100 μm [4], <28 μm, 28–45 μm, 45–63 μm, and 63–106 μm [5], 100–250 μm, and 250–1000 μm [13], <149 μm [15], <250 μm [6], <500 μm [11], <1000 μm [10,14], <2000 μm [7]. D. Majumdar et al. [5] showed that with an increase in the particle size of RD, the concentrations of Cd, Cr, Co, Pb, Mn, Ni, Sr, Zn, Ti, and Cu decrease, while the concentrations of Li increase.

In our opinion, from the point of view of their health effects, it is crucial that many of the papers presented in the special issue are devoted to the study of fine and ultrafine particles, or size-segregated RD, which made it possible to obtain accurate information about the chemical composition of the most dangerous particles that blow within urban and industrial environments. Further researches are likely to be devoted to the thoracic fraction (<10 μm) [25–29], as well as fine, ultrafine particles and nanoparticles, which have been actively studied in recent years in various cities and industrial areas [30–33].

In addition to the links between RD and the atmosphere, the article by H. Jeong et al. [10] shows the RD as a potential pollution source for coastal environments: particles of <125 μm contribute up to 41% of the total load of suspended solids in stormwater runoff at intensive industrial areas of the Republic of Korea. However, the effect of RD on pollution of other environments (soils, surface waters, crops, suspended sediments, bottom sediments, etc.) has not been studied in detail in the special issue, although such an effect and the feedback of other environments on the chemical composition of RD may be significant [34,35].

7. Conclusions and Further Research Needs

The studies presented in this special issue are a snapshot of the RD investigations and, at the same time, point to the need for further geographically more extensive and analytically more profound studies of various aspects of the formation, migration, and accumulation of dust and its individual particles in urban, industrial, and other areas. Therefore, we formulate the following main directions for further research, which, in our opinion, will allow us to take a fresh look at the role of RD in the environment.

- More detailed studies of the distribution of black carbon, organic compounds, and their derivatives (PAHs, EPFRs, etc.) in RD are required to clarify the possibility of their use as indicators of individual sources of adverse impact in urban and industrial areas and combined use with chemical elements for source apportionment.
- It is necessary to include the determination of the content of cations and anions in the water extract in the list of routine indicators when studying the RD, as well as to expand the list of interests by B, P, Se, REE, PGE, which will improve the reproducibility of source apportionment results.
- Studies of radioactivity and stable isotope ratios can provide new insights into the relationship between resource and fuel consumption in industry and transport (burning specific fuel grades, consuming ore from certain locations with their typical isotope ratios, etc.) and isotopic "response" in RD and other environments.
- To improve the accuracy of assessments of environmental hazards and public health risks from contaminated RD, it will be useful to develop a methodology and make comprehensive observations in different cities to assess the ratio of the forms of chemical elements (geochemical fractionation) and determine the biological availability of elements, the distribution of pollutants in particle size fractions of RD (especially in fine particles and nanoparticles), conducting a source-specific risk assessment based on the results of the modern source apportionment methods (PMF and other receptor models), clarifying the risk assessment methodology (for example, using the EWM method, and also by taking into account data on the bioavailable fraction of pollutants instead of the total content) and assessing the intensity of RD resuspension into the atmosphere.
- From a methodological point of view, it will be helpful to unify dust sampling methods (sweeping, use of vacuum cleaners with dry sampling, wet vacuuming, etc.), methods for particle separation (air classification, dry and wet sieving, sedimentation with or without sonication and centrifugation, etc.), the choice of a more appropriate geochemical fractionation scheme (e.g., Tessier et al. scheme, BCR, etc.), to develop of a system of indices for assessing the intensity and hazard level of pollution (EF, Igeo, CF, PLI, NPI, etc.) with justification for the choice of comparison standards (background soils, atmospheric depositions, aerosols, the upper continental crust, etc.) and reference elements (Al, Sc, Ti, Fe, Rb, La, Ta, etc.) used for their calculations, as well as to introduce a methodology for the comprehensive analysis of RD and adjacent environments, such as atmospheric aerosols and precipitation, soils, stormwater, surface waters, bottom and suspended sediments.
- Considering the deleterious effects on human health of exposure to airborne microorganisms and the potential accumulation of bioaerosols in RD, research on the characterization of biological contaminants and the risks of exposure after resuspension of this material could be carried out.
- Quantification of the impact of RD to anthropogenic aerosol radiative forcing in climate change studies and potential feedbacks.

Of course, the list of problems of studying RD raised in the special issue is not exhaustive, but, in our opinion, this special issue makes a significant contribution to further research in various scientific areas, interacting with such an interesting and relatively challenging to study environmental object as road dust.

Author Contributions: Writing—original draft preparation, D.V. and O.R.; writing—review and editing, D.V., O.R. and A.L. All authors have read and agreed to the published version of the manuscript.

Funding: Future research needs were formulated with the financial support of the Russian Science Foundation (project no. 19-77-30004). Part of this material was prepared by Dmitry Vlasov according to the Development program of the Interdisciplinary Scientific and Educational School of Lomonosov Moscow State University "Future Planet and Global Environmental Change".

Institutional Review Board Statement: Not applicable.

Informed Consent Statement: Not applicable.

Data Availability Statement: Not applicable.

Acknowledgments: The editors would like to thank all authors for their contributions to this Special Issue. We are grateful to the reviewers for their helpful and constructive comments, which allowed us to comprehensively evaluate the submissions and significantly improve the quality of the accepted manuscripts presented in the special issue.

Conflicts of Interest: The authors declare no conflict of interest.

References

1. Semerjian, L.; Okaiyeto, K.; Ojemaye, M.O.; Ekundayo, T.C.; Igwaran, A.; Okoh, A.I. Global Systematic Mapping of Road Dust Research from 1906 to 2020: Research Gaps and Future Direction. *Sustainability* **2021**, *13*, 11516. [CrossRef]
2. Vanegas, S.; Trejos, E.M.; Aristizábal, B.H.; Pereira, G.M.; Hernández, J.M.; Murillo, J.H.; Ramírez, O.; Amato, F.; Silva, L.F.O.; Rojas, N.Y.; et al. Spatial Distribution and Chemical Composition of Road Dust in Two High-Altitude Latin American Cities. *Atmosphere* **2021**, *12*, 1109. [CrossRef]
3. Beauchemin, S.; Levesque, C.; Wiseman, C.L.S.; Rasmussen, P.E. Quantification and Characterization of Metals in Ultrafine Road Dust Particles. *Atmosphere* **2021**, *12*, 1564. [CrossRef]
4. Hanfi, M.Y.; Yarmoshenko, I.; Seleznev, A.A. Gross Alpha and Gross Beta Activity Concentrations in the Dust Fractions of Urban Surface-Deposited Sediment in Russian Cities. *Atmosphere* **2021**, *12*, 571. [CrossRef]
5. Majumdar, D.; Biswas, B.; Majumdar, D.; Ray, R. Size-Segregated Elemental Profile and Associated Heath Risk Assessment of Road Dust along Major Traffic Corridors in Kolkata Mega City. *Atmosphere* **2021**, *12*, 1677. [CrossRef]
6. Aguilera, A.; Bautista-Hernández, D.; Bautista, F.; Goguitchaichvili, A.; Cejudo, R. Is the Urban Form a Driver of Heavy Metal Pollution in Road Dust? Evidence from Mexico City. *Atmosphere* **2021**, *12*, 266. [CrossRef]
7. Aguilar, Y.; Bautista, F.; Quintana, P.; Aguilar, D.; Trejo-Tzab, R.; Goguitchaichvili, A.; Chan-Te, R. Color as a New Proxy Technique for the Identification of Road Dust Samples Contaminated with Potentially Toxic Elements: The Case of Mérida, Yucatán, México. *Atmosphere* **2021**, *12*, 483. [CrossRef]
8. Faisal, M.; Wu, Z.; Wang, H.; Hussain, Z.; Azam, M.I. Human Health Risk Assessment of Heavy Metals in the Urban Road Dust of Zhengzhou Metropolis, China. *Atmosphere* **2021**, *12*, 1213. [CrossRef]
9. Sun, S.; Zheng, N.; Wang, S.; Li, Y.; Hou, S.; Song, X.; Du, S.; An, Q.; Li, P.; Li, X.; et al. Source Analysis and Human Health Risk Assessment Based on Entropy Weight Method Modification of PM2.5 Heavy Metal in an Industrial Area in the Northeast of China. *Atmosphere* **2021**, *12*, 852. [CrossRef]
10. Jeong, H.; Choi, J.Y.; Lim, J.; Ra, K. Pollution Caused by Potentially Toxic Elements Present in Road Dust from Industrial Areas in Korea. *Atmosphere* **2020**, *11*, 1366. [CrossRef]
11. Kim, M.-S.; Kim, J.-Y.; Park, J.; Yeon, S.-H.; Shin, S.; Choi, J. Assessment of Pollution Sources and Contribution in Urban Dust Using Metal Concentrations and Multi-Isotope Ratios (13C, 207/206Pb) in a Complex Industrial Port Area, Korea. *Atmosphere* **2021**, *12*, 840. [CrossRef]
12. Yarmoshenko, I.; Malinovsky, G.; Baglaeva, E.; Seleznev, A. A Landscape Study of Sediment Formation and Transport in the Urban Environment. *Atmosphere* **2020**, *11*, 1320. [CrossRef]
13. Seleznev, A.; Ilgasheva, E.; Yarmoshenko, I.; Malinovsky, G. Coarse Technogenic Material in Urban Surface Deposited Sediments (USDS). *Atmosphere* **2021**, *12*, 754. [CrossRef]
14. Moskovchenko, D.; Pozhitkov, R.; Soromotin, A.; Tyurin, V. The Content and Sources of Potentially Toxic Elements in the Road Dust of Surgut (Russia). *Atmosphere* **2022**, *13*, 30. [CrossRef]
15. Nguyen, V.-T.; Duy Dat, N.; Vo, T.-D.-H.; Nguyen, D.-H.; Nguyen, T.-B.; Nguyen, L.-S.P.; Nguyen, X.C.; Dinh, V.-C.; Nguyen, T.-H.-H.; Huynh, T.-M.-T.; et al. Characteristics and Risk Assessment of 16 Metals in Street Dust Collected from a Highway in a Densely Populated Metropolitan Area of Vietnam. *Atmosphere* **2021**, *12*, 1548. [CrossRef]
16. Fitz, D.R.; Bumiller, K. Characterization of PM10 Emission Rates from Roadways in a Metropolitan Area Using the SCAMPER Mobile Monitoring Approach. *Atmosphere* **2021**, *12*, 1332. [CrossRef]
17. Fitz, D.R.; Bumiller, K. SCAMPER Monitoring Platform to Measure PM10 Emission Rates from Unpaved Roads in Real-Time. *Atmosphere* **2021**, *12*, 1301. [CrossRef]

18. Vodyanitskii, Y.; Vlasov, D. Integrated Assessment of Affinity to Chemical Fractions and Environmental Pollution with Heavy Metals: A New Approach Based on Sequential Extraction Results. *Int. J. Environ. Res. Public Health* **2021**, *18*, 8458. [CrossRef]
19. Jayarathne, A.; Egodawatta, P.; Ayoko, G.A.; Goonetilleke, A. Assessment of Ecological and Human Health Risks of Metals in Urban Road Dust Based on Geochemical Fractionation and Potential Bioavailability. *Sci. Total Environ.* **2018**, *635*, 1609–1619. [CrossRef]
20. Polukarova, M.; Markiewicz, A.; Björklund, K.; Strömvall, A.-M.; Galfi, H.; Andersson Sköld, Y.; Gustafsson, M.; Järlskog, I.; Aronsson, M. Organic Pollutants, Nano- and Microparticles in Street Sweeping Road Dust and Washwater. *Environ. Int.* **2020**, *135*, 105337. [CrossRef]
21. O'Brien, S.; Okoffo, E.D.; Rauert, C.; O'Brien, J.W.; Ribeiro, F.; Burrows, S.D.; Toapanta, T.; Wang, X.; Thomas, K.V. Quantification of Selected Microplastics in Australian Urban Road Dust. *J. Hazard. Mater.* **2021**, *416*, 125811. [CrossRef] [PubMed]
22. Migaszewski, Z.M.; Gałuszka, A.; Dołęgowska, S.; Michalik, A. Glass Microspheres in Road Dust of the City of Kielce (South-Central Poland) as Markers of Traffic-Related Pollution. *J. Hazard. Mater.* **2021**, *413*, 125355. [CrossRef] [PubMed]
23. Wiseman, C.L.S.; Hassan Pour, Z.; Zereini, F. Platinum Group Element and Cerium Concentrations in Roadside Environments in Toronto, Canada. *Chemosphere* **2016**, *145*, 61–67. [CrossRef] [PubMed]
24. Rienda, I.C.; Alves, C.A. Road Dust Resuspension: A Review. *Atmos. Res.* **2021**, *261*, 105740. [CrossRef]
25. Vlasov, D.; Kosheleva, N.; Kasimov, N. Spatial Distribution and Sources of Potentially Toxic Elements in Road Dust and Its PM10 Fraction of Moscow Megacity. *Sci. Total Environ.* **2021**, *761*, 143267. [CrossRef]
26. Ramírez, O.; Sánchez de la Campa, A.M.; Amato, F.; Moreno, T.; Silva, L.F.; de la Rosa, J.D. Physicochemical Characterization and Sources of the Thoracic Fraction of Road Dust in a Latin American Megacity. *Sci. Total Environ.* **2019**, *652*, 434–446. [CrossRef]
27. Alves, C.A.; Evtyugina, M.; Vicente, A.M.P.; Vicente, E.D.; Nunes, T.V.; Silva, P.M.A.; Duarte, M.A.C.; Pio, C.A.; Amato, F.; Querol, X. Chemical Profiling of PM10 from Urban Road Dust. *Sci. Total Environ.* **2018**, *634*, 41–51. [CrossRef]
28. Zhang, J.; Wu, L.; Zhang, Y.; Li, F.; Fang, X.; Mao, H. Elemental Composition and Risk Assessment of Heavy Metals in the PM10 Fractions of Road Dust and Roadside Soil. *Particuology* **2019**, *44*, 146–152. [CrossRef]
29. Bezberdaya, L.; Kosheleva, N.; Chernitsova, O.; Lychagin, M.; Kasimov, N. Pollution Level, Partition and Spatial Distribution of Benzo(a)Pyrene in Urban Soils, Road Dust and Their PM10 Fraction of Health-Resorts (Alushta, Yalta) and Industrial (Sebastopol) Cities of Crimea. *Water* **2022**, *14*, 561. [CrossRef]
30. Ramírez, O.; da Boit, K.; Blanco, E.; Silva, L.F.O. Hazardous Thoracic and Ultrafine Particles from Road Dust in a Caribbean Industrial City. *Urban Clim.* **2020**, *33*, 100655. [CrossRef]
31. Lanzerstorfer, C. Toward More Intercomparable Road Dust Studies. *Crit. Rev. Environ. Sci. Technol.* **2021**, *51*, 826–855. [CrossRef]
32. Ermolin, M.S.; Fedotov, P.S.; Ivaneev, A.I.; Karandashev, V.K.; Fedyunina, N.N.; Burmistrov, A.A. A Contribution of Nanoscale Particles of Road-Deposited Sediments to the Pollution of Urban Runoff by Heavy Metals. *Chemosphere* **2018**, *210*, 65–75. [CrossRef] [PubMed]
33. Kasimov, N.S.; Vlasov, D.V.; Kosheleva, N.E. Enrichment of Road Dust Particles and Adjacent Environments with Metals and Metalloids in Eastern Moscow. *Urban Clim.* **2020**, *32*, 100638. [CrossRef]
34. Gabarrón, M.; Faz, A.; Acosta, J.A. Soil or Dust for Health Risk Assessment Studies in Urban Environment. *Arch. Environ. Contam. Toxicol.* **2017**, *73*, 442–455. [CrossRef] [PubMed]
35. Vlasov, D.V.; Kukushkina, O.V.; Kosheleva, N.E.; Kasimov, N.S. Levels and Factors of the Accumulation of Metals and Metalloids in Roadside Soils, Road Dust and Their PM10 Fraction in the Western Okrug of Moscow. *Eurasian Soil Sci.* **2022**, *55*, 556–572. [CrossRef]

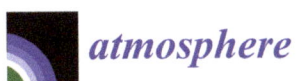

Article

Color as a New Proxy Technique for the Identification of Road Dust Samples Contaminated with Potentially Toxic Elements: The Case of Mérida, Yucatán, México

Yameli Aguilar [1], Francisco Bautista [2,*], Patricia Quintana [3], Daniel Aguilar [3], Rudy Trejo-Tzab [4], Avto Goguitchaichvili [2] and Roberto Chan-Te [2]

[1] Instituto Nacional de Investigaciones Forestales, Agrícolas y Pecuarias, Yucatán 91700, Mexico; aguilar.yameli@inifap.gob.mx
[2] Laboratorio Universitario de Geofísica Ambiental, Centro de Investigaciones en Geografía Ambiental e Instituto de Geofísica, Universidad Nacional Autónoma de México, Michoacán 58190, Mexico; avto@geofisica.unam.mx (A.G.); ctcarpediemr@gmail.com (R.C.-T.)
[3] Centro de Investigación y de Estudios Avanzados Unidad Mérida Yucatán, Mérida 97310, Mexico; pquint@cinvestav.mx (P.Q.); daniel.aguilar@cinvestav.mx (D.A.)
[4] Facultad de Ingeniería Química, Universidad Autónoma de Yucatán, Mérida 97000, Mexico; rudy.trejo@correo.uady.mx
* Correspondence: leptosol@ciga.unam.mx; Tel.: +52-443-322-3833

Citation: Aguilar, Y.; Bautista, F.; Quintana, P.; Aguilar, D.; Trejo-Tzab, R.; Goguitchaichvili, A.; Chan-Te, R. Color as a New Proxy Technique for the Identification of Road Dust Samples Contaminated with Potentially Toxic Elements: The Case of Mérida, Yucatán, México. *Atmosphere* **2021**, *12*, 483. https://doi.org/10.3390/atmos12040483

Academic Editor: Dmitry Vlasov

Received: 15 February 2021
Accepted: 7 April 2021
Published: 11 April 2021

Publisher's Note: MDPI stays neutral with regard to jurisdictional claims in published maps and institutional affiliations.

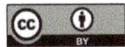

Copyright: © 2021 by the authors. Licensee MDPI, Basel, Switzerland. This article is an open access article distributed under the terms and conditions of the Creative Commons Attribution (CC BY) license (https://creativecommons.org/licenses/by/4.0/).

Abstract: The design of proxy techniques is an innovative tool to monitor the potentially toxic elements of pollution in road dust. This study evaluated the use of road dust color as a proxy methodology to identify samples contaminated with presumably contaminating elements. FRX determined the concentrations of Fe, Ti, Rb, Sr, Y, Cu, Zn, and Pb in eighty-five road dust samples. The appliance of the RGB system and the Munsell color cards identified five color groups of road dust samples. The discriminant analysis validated these groups by colorimetric indices and presumably contaminating elements. The "very dark gray" color of road dust contains the highest concentrations of Pb, Cu, Zn, and Y. The redness and saturation rates showed high correlations with presumably contaminating elements in "dark gray" and "very dark gray" color samples. The color of road dust, as a proxy technique, allows identifying samples contaminated with presumably contaminating elements.

Keywords: color indices; redness; hue; saturation; lead; pollution

1. Introduction

The World Health Organization [1] stated that around 6 million people living in cities die from environmental pollution, of which pollutants are presumably part of the problem because they can adhere to plant leaves and trees [2,3], on the soil [2,4,5], and in road dust [3,6].

Road dust is composed of fine particles with presumably contaminating elements; it is a mixture of natural soil; soil brought from other places for the refurbishment of green areas; cars' wear particles (combustion smoke, brakes, and oil, among others); and motor vehicles; and weathering particles of roads, mainly [7–10]. The prolonged exposure to particles with presumably contaminating elements and with sizes of 10 µm or smaller, can lead them to enter the respiratory system, deposit in the trachea and lungs, reach the bloodstream, and generate various health problems, including being precursors of cancer [11].

Potentially toxic elements pollution in road dust is an issue that affects the population health; however, its continuous monitoring is disregarded because of the expensive studies and prolonged analysis time. Then, in the last decade, proxy technologies (fast and low cost) have emerged for diagnosis. Among the proxy techniques, environmental magnetism [2,3,8,12]; and the color of the particles [6,13,14] stand out. In this sense, it will be of great help to have a type of proxy technology that allows the selection of tens and not hundreds or thousands of samples that could go to the laboratory to be analyzed.

Color is a physical property of particles that often correlates with chemical properties; for example, in soils, the color is related to organic matter [15,16], minerals [17–19], humidity, and drainage regime [20], among others. In road dust, the background on the subject is scarce, few authors have reported the relationship between road dust color and presumably contaminating elements [6,13,14].

Technological advances have allowed the measurement of color with the traditional alphanumeric system [21] to numerical measurements using the CIELab and RGB systems [20,22]. This fact has allowed the possibility of making mathematical relationships with the chemical properties of road dust [6,23].

On the other hand, for its exceptionally diverse components, each city is a particular case, because the color of road dust depends on the natural components (types of rock and soil), as well as on the types of the intensity of human activities and types of urban land use.

The objective of this study was to evaluate the use of color, a fast and low-cost proxy technique, as an indicator of potentially toxic element contamination in road dust samples from Mérida, México, as well as evaluating the concentration of potentially toxic elements by type of road.

2. Materials and Methods

2.1. Study Area

The city of Mérida Yucatán is located at coordinates 20°58'04" N 89°37'18" W, and is located on a structural karst plain with an average altitude of 9 m above sea level. The climate is warm subhumid (between 28–38 °C) with rains in summer Aw0 (i ') gw' 'is the driest subtype, with a thermal oscillation of 5 to 7 °C between the warmest month and the coldest month [24]. The dominant soils are from the Leptosol group with Nudilthic, Lithic, and Rendzic qualifiers [25].

Systematic sampling with homogeneously distributed samples was designed, 86 samples of road dust were taken on the streets, the sampling area was 1 m^2, and the geographical location of the sampling sites was taken. We select the place with the highest amount of road dust within a radius of 20 m around each sampling site, with the idea of having a sufficient amount of sample for chemical and mineralogical analyses (Figure 1).

The samples of the road dust were dried in the shade, ground with an agate mortar, and screened with ten mesh (2 mm).

2.2. Chemical and Physical Analyses of Road Dust

With the road dust samples, we prepared tablets with 0.4 g. The sample of road dust was placed in a die of 5 mm in diameter and compressed at 4000 psi pressure for 2 min, without any chemical or binder treatment. The tablets were placed on the sample holder and sealed using Mylar film. The road dust was analyzed using X-ray fluorescence with dispersed energy (FRX-ED), in a Jordan Valley spectrometer (EX-6600) equipped with a Si (Li) detector with an active area of 20 mm^2 and a resolution of 140 eV to 5.9 keV, operating at a maximum of 54 keV and 4800 µA; international reference patterns were utilized for rocks and soils [5,26,27].

As a quality control measure, the samples were analyzed five times. The calibration curve was made using the standards of the IGL series. The IGLsy-1 standard, which corresponds to a nepheline Syenite with a high content of Al and Si, was used as measurement control. The use of the XRF-DE technique is common and appropriate in pollution studies (soils and dust) in which the concentrations of potentially toxic elements are of the order of tenths and hundredths of mg/kg, as was the case with this study [5,27].

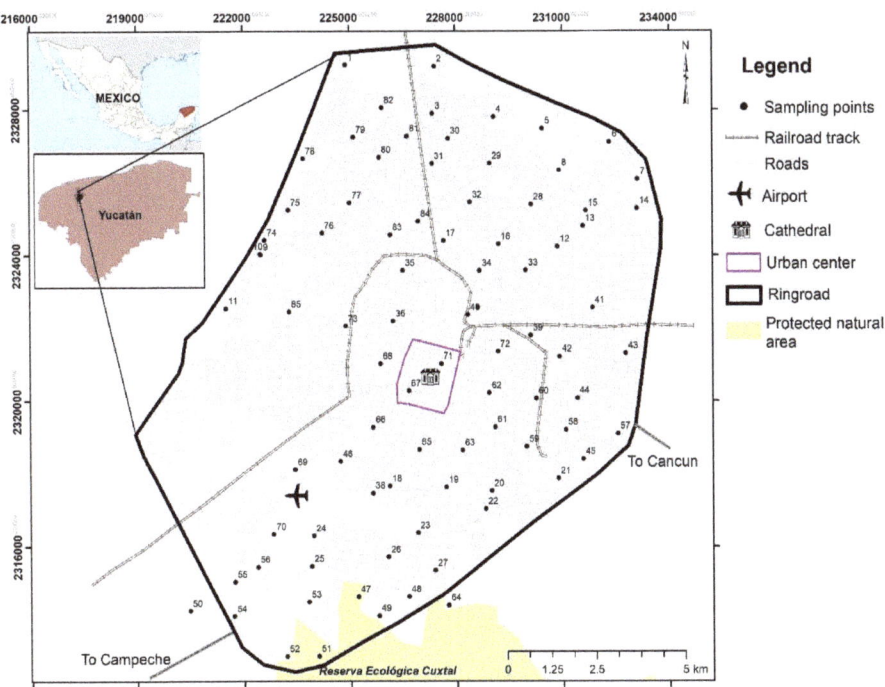

Figure 1. Geographical location of the road dust sampling sites.

The analyzed elements were those typically measured in contamination studies, such as copper (Cu), zinc (Zn), and lead (Pb). Those that come from the combustion of fossil fuels, such as iron oxides (Fe_2O_3) and titanium oxide (TiO_2). Three elements that are commonly found in the soils of the study area, such as strontium (Sr), yttrium (Y), and rubidium (Rb), and the following major elements: CaO, Na_2, K_2O, MgO, MnO, Al_2O_3, and SiO_2. The measurements were made in the National Laboratory of Nano and Biomaterials (LANNBIO), at CINVESTAV Mérida, Yucatán.

The samples of road dust were also analyzed using the Munsell table [21]. The color of the road dust was also measured using diffuse reflectance spectroscopy with an optical reflectance in a spectral range of 380–1100 nm using a UV/VIS fiber-optic spectrophotometer (AvaSpec HS2048 XL model) coupled to an integration sphere (AvaSphere-50-REFL model). The integration sphere minimizes the specular/diffuse reflectance ratio of the captured radiation [19]. In this configuration, a deuterium-halogen light source (AvaLight DH-S-BAL model) illuminates the sample, and the spectrometer receives the reflectance of the sample. Five measurements were done for each sample in order to obtain a representative value; the WS-2 standard (Avantes) was used as a blank standard. The results are generated in the color system X, Y, Z.

The X, Y, and Z color data were converted to the decimal RGB color system using the Color Slide Rule program, from this system, hue (HI), redness (RI), and saturation (SI) color indices were obtained. Color indices were obtained with the following equations, where R, G, and B, corresponding to red, green, and blue, respectively [28]:

$$HI = (2 \times R - G - B)/(G - B); \tag{1}$$

$$RI = R^2/(B \times G^3); SI = (R - B)/(R + B). \tag{2}$$

2.3. Mineralogy and Morphology of Road Dust Particles

XRD analyses were performed to identify minerals present in road dust. The particles were placed on a silicon sample holder coated with silicone grease suitable for XRD; subsequently, they were analyzed on a Siemens D-5000 diffractometer, Bragg-Brentano Mode, with a monochromatic Cu tube (l = 1.5418 Å), a step time of 3 s, step size 0.02 degrees, at 34 kV and 25 mA.

The shape, size, and composition of the particles were determined with a Philips ESEM XL30 scanning electron microscope coupled with EDAX GENESIS with SiLi detector, 10 L, 204 Bt (SEM-EDS). The particles were mounted on a double-sided (0.5 cm^2) carbon adhesive tape attached to a sample holder. Then, the micrographs were obtained to determine the size and the elemental composition of the particles by X-ray energy dispersion spectrometry (EDS). A total of 10 samples were analyzed by XRD and SEM-EDS.

2.4. Data Analyses

The color groups visually identified with the Munsell table were validated in two ways. The first using the color indices (HI, RI, and SI) as classification variables. The second validation was carried out using potentially toxic element concentrations as classification variables. For both, Statgraphic Plus 5.1 software was used [29].

The discriminant analysis was used to validate, or not, the formation of groups by color. This type of multivariate statistical analysis also identifies the number of correctly classified cases, as well as the variables that allow differentiating groups of objects. The groups of the road dust samples formed by color using the Munsell table were used as dependent variables or discriminant variables [6].

The medium concentrations of each potentially toxic element and major elements per road dust color group were compared using the Kruskal–Wallis test, considering statistically significant differences with $p < 0.05$, as it is the best method to compare populations where there is no Gaussian distribution of the data. This test evaluates the hypothesis that the medians of each group are equal, combines the data of all the groups, and orders them from least to greatest, then calculates the average range for the data of each group [30].

3. Results

3.1. Formation of the Grouping of Road Dust Samples by Color

Five groups of road dust colors were identified: I, GB, greyish brown; II, G, gray; III, DG, dark gray; IV, DGB, dark grayish brown; and V, VDG, very dark gray (Figure 2). Group I that corresponds to the greyish brown road dust had higher RGB values than the darkest color groups.

Groups	I	II	III	IV	V
Color samples					
Median values	GB Grayish brown	G Gray	DG Dark gray	DGB Dark grayish brown	VDG Very dark gray
R	52	38	30	30	22
G	55	44	39	32	34.5
B	45	37.5	34.5	27.5	31

Figure 2. Grouping of road dust samples by color using the Munsell chart and with the average values in RGB.

The comparison analysis of medians reveals that the formation of the five groups of the road dust samples by color, using the Munsell table, as a discriminant variable and the three-color indices (IH, IR, and IS) used as classification variables give a total of 93% of correctly assigned cases, which validates the formation of these five groups of road dust samples (Table 1).

Table 1. Congruence matrix between the color groups of road dust based on the Munsell color cards (discriminant variable) and those groups formed based on the color indices (classification variables).

Current Color (Groups)	n	Predicted Color				
		I	II	III	IV	V
I (GB)	17	16 94%	1 6%	0 0%	0 0%	0 0%
II (G)	32	1 3%	31 97%	0 0%	0 0%	0 0%
III (DG)	14	0 0%	0 0%	14 100%	0 0%	0 0%
IV (DGB)	12	0 0%	2 17%	1 8%	9 75%	0 0%
V (VDG)	8	0 0%	0 0%	0 0%	1 13%	7 88%

Percentage of correctly classified cases: 93%. I, GB, greyish brown; II, G, gray; III, DG, dark gray; IV, DGB, dark grayish brown; and V, VDG, very dark gray.

On the other hand, when presumably contaminating elements were used as dependent or classification variables, the discriminant analysis had 47% correctly classified cases. The very dark gray and greyish brown color samples reached 87.5% and 77.5% of correctly assigned cases, respectively (Table 2). On the contrary, gray colors obtained the lowest value of the percentage of correctly assigned cases. That is the formation of road dust groups by color, and considering the concentration of presumably contaminating elements makes sense only in the case of very dark gray and grayish brown groups.

Table 2. Congruence matrix between the color groups of road dust based (discriminant variables) and those groups formed based on the presumably contaminating elements (classification variables).

Current Color (Groups)	n	Predicted Color				
		I	II	III	IV	V
I (GB)	17	13 76%	1 6%	1 6%	2 12%	0 0%
II (G)	32	10 31%	8 25%	6 19%	5 16%	3 9%
III (DG)	14	0 0%	5 36%	6 43%	1 7%	2 14%
IV (DGB)	12	4 33%	2 17%	0 0%	5 42%	1 8%
V (VDG)	8	0 0%	0 0%	1 13%	0 0%	7 88%

Percentage of correctly classified cases: 47%. I, GB, greyish brown; II, G, gray; III, DG, dark gray; IV, DGB, dark grayish brown; and V, VDG, very dark gray.

3.2. Color Indices and Presumably Contaminating Elements by Color Groups of Road Dust Samples

Figure 3 shows significant differences ($p < 0.05$) in HI, SI, and RI. HI and SI values show a downward trend in groups I < II < III < V, only group IV does not follow the sequence. The trend ranges from the lightest to the darkest. The RI allows differentiating group IV, and it is the most blown group.

Potentially toxic element concentrations had significant differences with p values < 0.05), except for the Rb that had p values < 0.1 (Figure 4). There is a tendency to increase potentially toxic element concentrations (Y, Cu, Zn, Pb, TiO$_2$, and Fe$_2$O$_3$), according to the darkest color groups, that is, a sequence of I < II < III < V (Figure 4). Only in the case of Sr, road dust of group IV (dark grayish brown) reached the highest concentrations. This group of road dust samples is different from the other groups, probably with very different minerals.

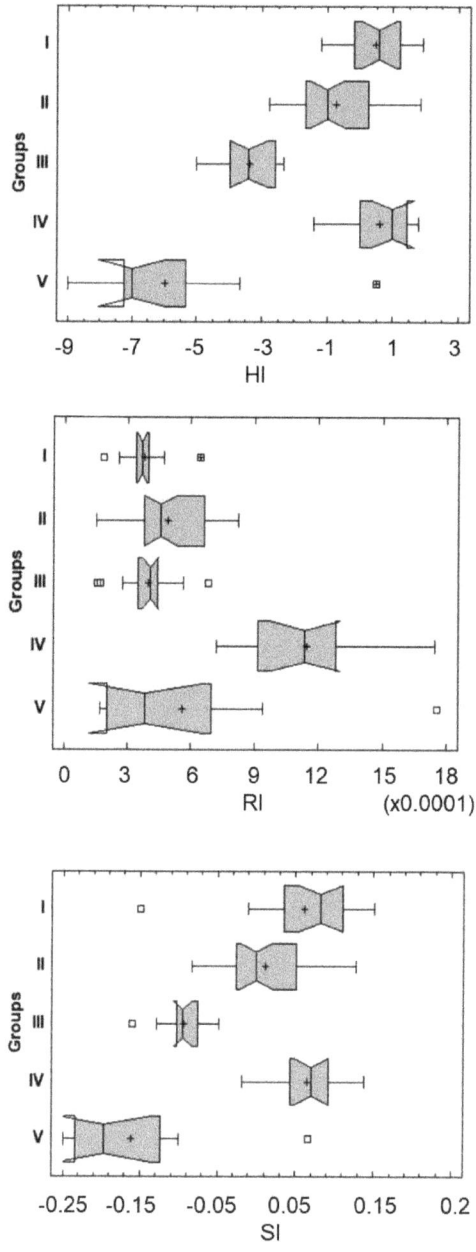

Figure 3. Comparison of medians of color indices (HI, RI, SI) by groups of road dust. I, GB, greyish brown; II, G, gray; III, DG, dark gray; IV, DGB, dark grayish brown; and V, VDG, very dark gray.

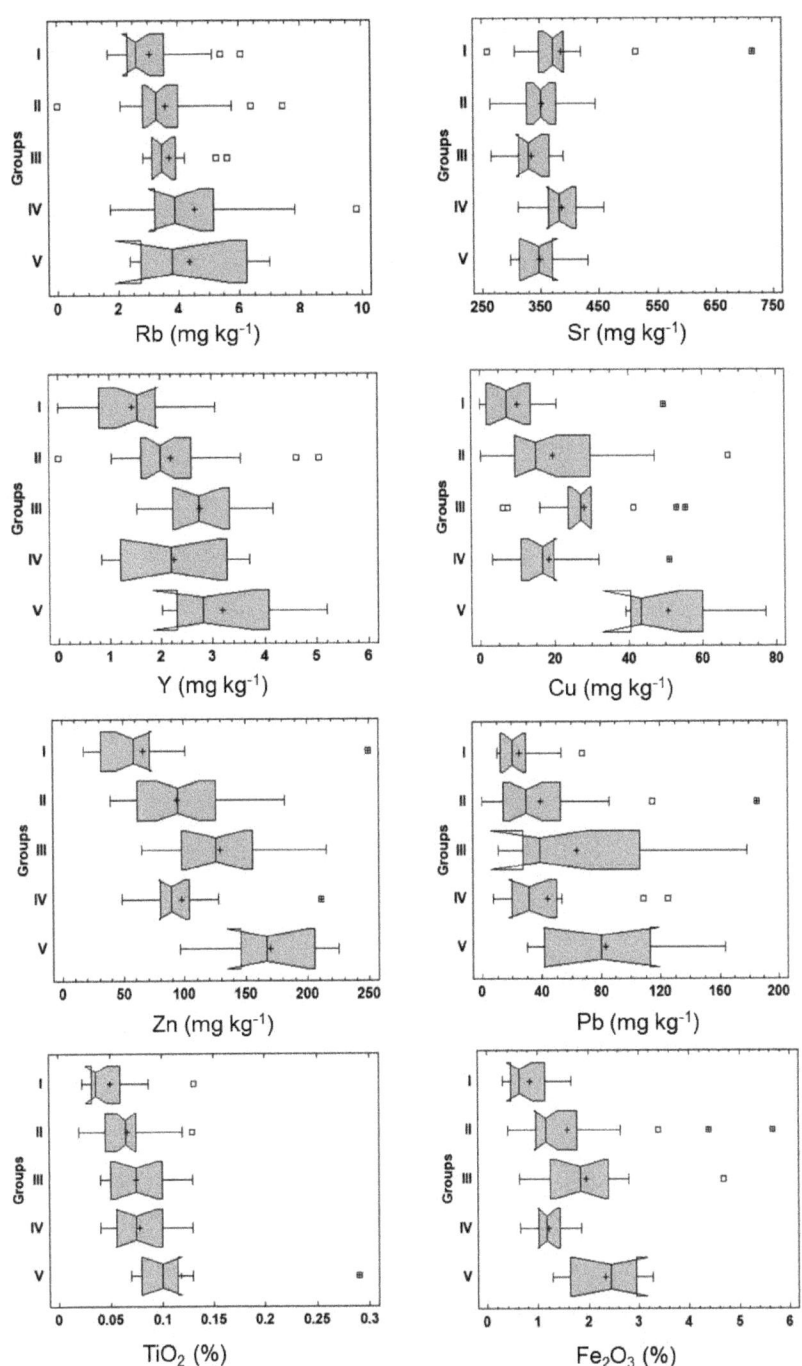

Figure 4. Comparison of medians of presumably contaminating elements and oxides by groups of road dust. I, GB, greyish brown; II, G, gray; III, DG, dark gray; IV, DGB, dark grayish brown; and V, VDG, very dark gray.

The primary roads had higher concentrations of Cu, Ni, Pb, and Zn in the road dust than the secondary and tertiary roads, as a consequence of the traffic of a greater number of cars (Figure 5). On the contrary, major elements such as CaO dominate on tertiary roads where fewer cars travel but where there is more dust of natural origin. Other elements as Na_2, K_2O, MgO, MnO, Al_2O_3, and SiO_2 did not show differences between types of roads.

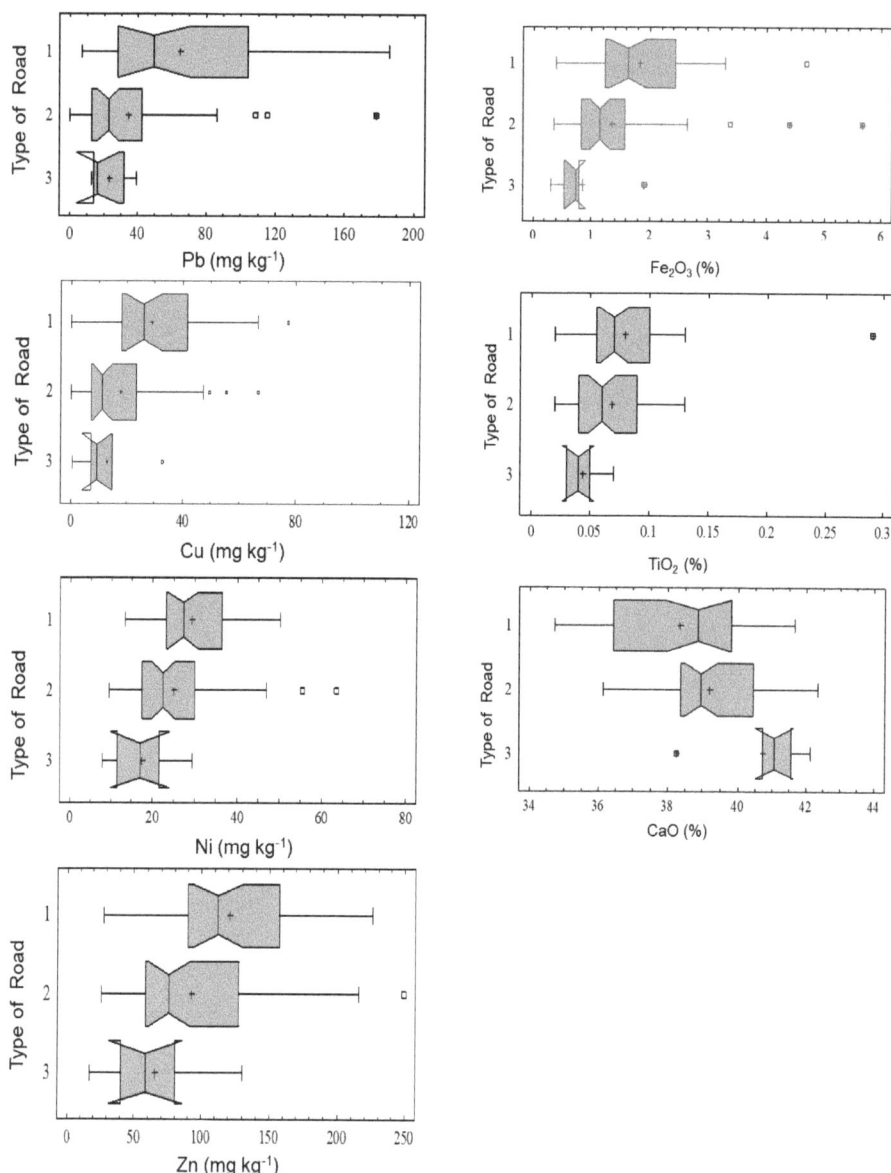

Figure 5. Comparison of medians of presumably contaminating elements and oxides by road dust. Primary road, 1; secondary roads, 2; tertiary roads, 3.

The percentages of Fe_2O_3 and TiO_2 in road dust were higher in primary roads because these elements come from the wear and tear of cars and are also found in combustion fumes.

Calcite, quartz, ankerite, anorthoclase, and albite were the main minerals of road dust (Figure 6). These minerals are generally white, colorless, and gray. In smaller quantities, natural minerals were found such as hematite (red), goethite (brown), boehmite (white), dikite (white), sanidine (white), tosidite (white, light yellow, light green), and yeelimite (colorless).

Maghemite (black, blackish-brown) is a mineral of anthropogenic origin in road dust [31–33] (Figure 6), it comes from car fumes, and which blackens dust. Maghemite is also the mineral that gives the highest magnetic signal to road dust, a property widely reported as a rapid diagnostic technique for heavy metals.

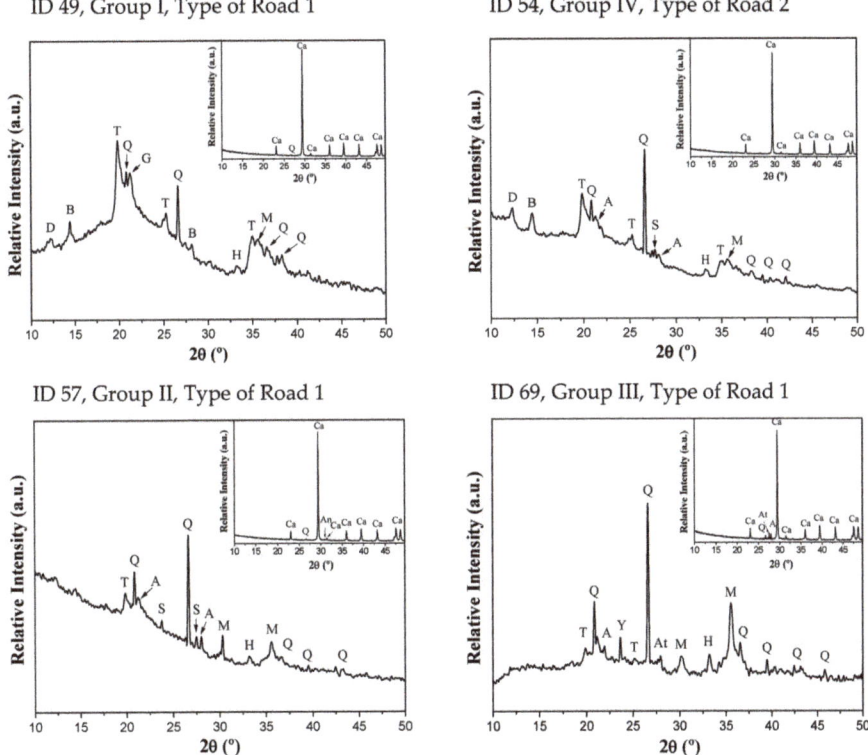

Figure 6. Major minerals in road dust with calcite and without calcite. A = albite, An = ankerite, At = anorthoclase, B = boehmite, Ca = calcite, D = dickite, G = goethite, H = hematite, M = maghemite, Q = quartz, S = sanidine, T = tosudite, Y = yeelimite.

Observations of the dust in the scanning electron microscope allowed the identification of spherical and laminar particles, both of anthropogenic origin. The spherical ones from the combustion of gasoline (Figure 7), and the laminar ones from car brakes.

The shape of the particles has been studied since the 1980s, to recognize the morphology of magnetic particles of anthropic origin [34]. For those studies, it has been concluded that spherical particles come from vehicle emissions, these are associated with the burning of gasoline [35].

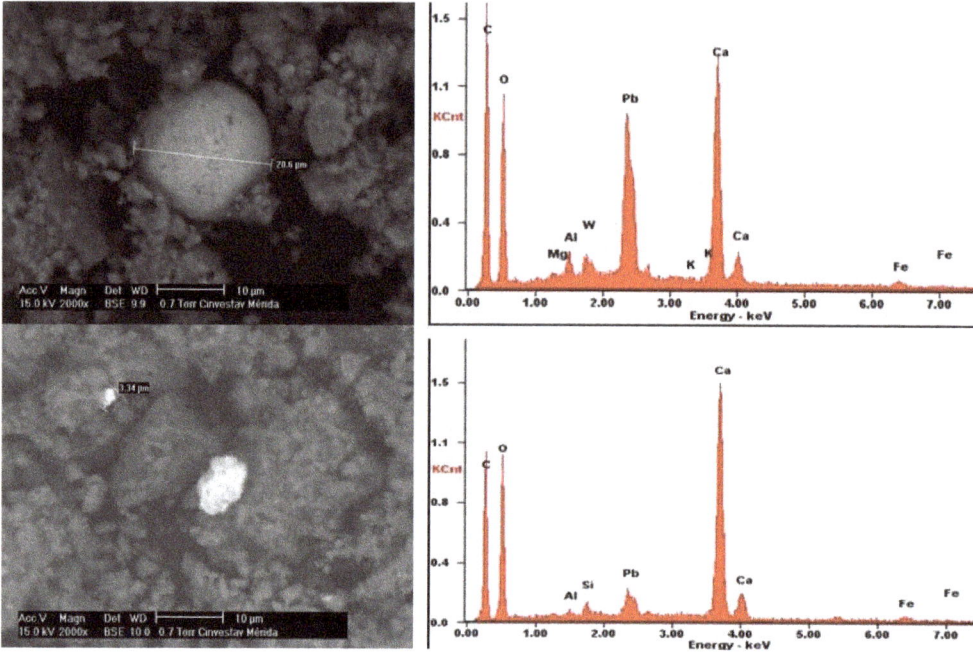

Figure 7. Anthropogenic particles in road dust.

4. Discussion

Previous studies conducted in Murcia, Spain [13] and Mexico City [14,36] reported that dark-colored samples were those with the highest concentrations of presumably contaminating elements; however, in a study conducted in the city of Ensenada, Mexico [6] it did not happen in the same way, in that case, the gray road dust was the most contaminated with presumably contaminating elements. In the same way, in this study, the road dust of groups IV and V were the darkest, but the dust of group IV was not the most contaminated.

The significant variability in the chemical and mineralogical properties of the soils of the city of Mérida with soils of red, brown, black, and gray [25] may be the cause of which not all dark soils in this study are the most contaminated with presumably contaminating elements.

Dark colors in road dust can occur naturally by mixing with soils with high organic matter content (fertilizers applied in gardens or with high humus contents) [25,37]. However, the dark color in road dust can also be acquired anthropically, by contamination with magnetite and maghemite products from the use of fossil fuels in industries, homes, and cars [36,38,39].

Smaller particles, such as carbon, magnetite, and maghemite nanoparticles produced in car smoke that are black, can have a profound effect on the color of road dust, despite not being the dominant particles in quantity or weight [40].

Rock magnetism techniques, such as magnetic susceptibility, have been used to discern whether the dark color is from anthropic contamination (high values) or due to natural causes (low values) resulting from organic matter [2,8,39–41].

On the other hand, with the idea of establishing a system for monitoring potentially toxic elements in road dust in the city of Mérida, it is recommended to make a color chart of road dust with the results of this work to be used in future road dust sampling. Although there are other more precise tools to measure the color of road dust, such as colorimeters in mobile equipment and digital cameras [6,28] and other color measurement systems [14,41–43], there will be nothing less expensive than a simple color chart especially designed for the road dust of each city.

With this technique of grouping road dust samples by color it will now be possible to implement a monitoring system in cities, many samples (hundreds or thousands) can be taken and then selected, by color, road dust samples to which will be analyzed presumably contaminating elements. In other words, it is necessary to go from the elaboration of isolated and punctual diagnoses to the instrumentation of a true monitoring system.

The measurement of color by comparison with a color chart of road dust made especially for each city would allow people to use it to assess the degree of potentially toxic element contamination of road dust inside their homes, and thus make decisions to reduce the risk of harm to health [44].

5. Conclusions

The five colors of road dust samples from the city of Mérida, Mexico, can be used as a guide to discard or select samples contaminated with presumably contaminating elements and oxides of Ti and Fe. That is, the color of road dust can be used as a proxy technique.

We conclude that there is low contamination by presumably contaminating elements, and oxides in both road dust samples of greyish brown (I) and dark grayish brown (IV) colors; medium contamination in gray (II) road dust samples; and high pollution in road dust samples with dark gray (III) and very dark gray (V) colors. Therefore, for monitoring the contamination of presumably contaminating elements in road dust, both samples of greyish brown and dark grayish brown colors can be discarded from the chemical analysis.

Munsell color charts and color indices (IH and IS) can be used as proxy indicators for samples of dust contaminated with metals such as lead, zinc, and copper.

The contamination is in descending order in the primary, secondary and tertiary roads. A strategy to avoid damage to health from road dust should begin by cleaning primary roads and areas with dark gray and very dark gray-colored dust.

Author Contributions: Y.A., participated in the design of the sampling, took the samples, and wrote the first version of the manuscript; F.B., was the project coordinator, designed the experiment, coordinated all project activities, and wrote the final version of the article; P.Q., performed the chemical analyses, and revised the text; D.A., assisted in the chemical analyses; R.T.-T., analyzed the color in the road dust samples; A.G., designed the experiment, and revised the text; R.C.-T., assisted in sampling, and observations of the particles in the SEM. All authors have read and agreed to the published version of the manuscript.

Funding: This study was financially supported by both the CONACYT project CB-2016-283135 and the project UNAM DGAPA-PAPIIT IN209218. The Laboratorio Nacional de Nano y Biomateriales, Cinvestav-IPN has been financed by FOMIX-Yucatán 2008-108160, CONACYT LAB-2009-01-123913, 292692, 294643, 188345 y 204822. Thanks to Ing. Emilio Corona for technical support.

Institutional Review Board Statement: Not applicable.

Informed Consent Statement: Not applicable.

Data Availability Statement: Not applicable.

Conflicts of Interest: The authors declare no conflict of interest.

References

1. World Health Organization. *Review of Evidence on Health Aspects of Air Pollution-REVIHAAPF*; Technical Report; WHO Regional Office for Europe: Copenhagen, Denmark, 2013.
2. Aguilar, B.; Bautista, F.; Goguitchaichvili, A.; Morton, O. Magnetic monitoring of top soils of Merida (Southern Mexico). *Stud. Geophys. Geod.* **2011**, *55*, 377–388.
3. Aguilar, R.B.; Bautista, F.; Goguitchaichvili, A.; Quintana, P.; Carvallo, C.; Battu, J. Rock-Magnetic properties of topsoils and urban dust from Morelia, México: Implications for anthropogenic pollution monitoring in medium-size cities. *Geofís. Int.* **2013**, *52*, 121–133.
4. Alcalá, J.; Sosa, M.; Moreno, M.; Rodríguez, J.C.; Quintana, C.; Terrazas, C.; Rivero, O. Metales pesados en suelo urbano como un indicador de la calidad ambiental: Ciudad de Chihuahua, México. *Multequina* **2009**, *18*, 53–69.

5. Ihl, T.; Bautista, F.; Cejudo, R.; Delgado, C.; Quintana, P.; Aguilar, D.; Goguitchaichvili, A. Concentration of toxic elements in topsoils of the metropolitan area of México City: A spatial analysis using ordinary Kriging and indicator Kriging. *Rev. Int. Contam. Ambie.* **2015**, *31*, 47–62.
6. Cortés, J.L.; Bautista, F.; Quintana, P.; Aguilar, D.; Goguichaishvili, A. The color of urban dust as an indicator of contamination by potentially toxic elements: The case of Ensenada, Baja California, Mexico. *RCHSCFA* **2015**, *21*, 255–266.
7. Bautista, F.; Cram, S.; Sommer, I.S. Técnicas de muestreo para el estudio del manejo de recursos naturales y el cuidado del ambiente. In *Editorial: Centro de Investigaciones en Geografía Ambiental*, 2nd ed.; Bautista, F., Palacio, J.L., Delfín, H., Eds.; Universidad Nacional Autónoma de México: Mexico City, Mexico, 2011; pp. 227–258.
8. Sánchez-Duque, A.; Bautista, F.; Goguichaishvili, A.; Cejudo-Ruiz, R.; Reyes-López, J.A.; Solís-Domínguez, F.A.; Morales-Contreras, J.J. Evaluación de la contaminación ambiental a partir del aumento magnético en polvos urbanos. Caso de estudio en la ciudad de Mexicali, México. *RMCG* **2015**, *32*, 501–513.
9. Jiang, L.; Guang, A.; Mu, Z.; Zhan, H.; Wu, Y. Contamination levels and human health risk assessment of toxic heavy metals in street dust in an industrial city in Northwest China. *Environ. Geochem. Health* **2018**, *40*, 2007–2020. [CrossRef]
10. Safiur, M.; Khan, M.D.H.; Jolly, Y.N.; Kabir, J.; Akter, S.; Salam, A. Assessing risk to human health for heavy metal contamination through street dust in the Southeast Asian Megacity: Dhaka, Bangladesh. *Sci. Total Environ.* **2019**, *660*, 1610–1622. [CrossRef]
11. Sabath, D.E.; Osorio, L.R. Medio ambiente y riñón: Nefrotoxicidad por metales pesados. Nefrología. *Publ. Soc. Esp. Nefrol.* **2012**, *32*, 279–286.
12. Wang, B.; Xia, D.; Yu, Y.; Jia, J.; Xu, S. Detection and differentiation of pollution in urban surface soils using magnetic properties in arid and semi-arid regions of northwestern China. *Environ. Poll.* **2014**, *184*, 335–346.
13. Marín, P.; Sánchez, A.; Díaz-Pereira, E.; Bautista, F.; Romero, M.; Delgado, M.J. Assessment of Heavy Metals and Color as Indicators of Contamination in Street Dust of a City in SE Spain: Influence of Traffic Intensity and Sampling Location. *Sustainability* **2018**, *10*, 4105.
14. García, R.; Delgado, C.; Cejudo, R.; Aguilera, A.; Gogichaishvili, A.; Bautista, F. The color of urban dust as an indicator of heavy metal pollution. *RCHSCFA* **2020**, *26*, 3–15.
15. Dobos, R.R.; Ciolkosz, E.J.; Waltman, W.J. The effect of organic carbon, temperature, time, and redox conditions on soil color. *Soil Sci.* **1990**, *150*, 506–512.
16. Schulze, D.G.; Nagel, J.L.; Van Scoyoc, G.E.; Henderson, T.L.; Baumgardner, M.F.; Stott, D.E. Significance of organic matter in determining soil colors. *Soil Color* **1993**, *31*, 71–90.
17. Schwertmann, U. Relations between iron oxides, soil color, and soil formation. *Soil Color* **1993**, *31*, 51–69.
18. Torrent, J.; Barrón, V. Laboratory measurement of soil color: Theory and practice. *Soil Color* **1993**, *31*, 21–33.
19. Quintana, P.; Tiesler, V.; Conde, M.; Trejo-Tzab, R.; Bolio, C.; Alvarado-Gil, J.J.; Aguilar, D. Spectrochemical characterization of red pigments used in classic period maya funerary practices. *Archaeometry* **2014**, *57*, 1045–1059.
20. Domínguez, J.M.; Román, A.D.; Prieto, F.; Acevedo, O. Sistema de Notación Munsell y CIELab como herramienta para evaluación de color en suelos. *Rev. Mex. Cienc. Agríc.* **2012**, *3*, 141–155.
21. Color, M. *Munsell Soil Color. Charts: Year 2000 Revised Washable Edition*; GretagMacbeth: New York, NY, USA, 2000.
22. Commision Internationale de l'Eclairage. *Technical Report: Colorimetry*, 2nd ed.; CIE: Vienna, Austria, 1986; pp. 1–68.
23. Viscarra, R.A.; Fouad, Y.; Walter, C. Using a digital camera to measure soil organic carbon and iron contents. *Biosyst. Eng.* **2008**, *100*, 149–159.
24. García, E. *Modificaciones al Sistema de Clasificación Climática de köppen*, 5th ed.; Universidad Nacional Autónoma de México: Urban, Mexico, 2004; p. 90.
25. Bautista, F.; Díaz-Garrido, S.; Castillo-González, M.; Zinck, J.A. Spatial heterogeneity of the soil cover in the Yucatán Karst: Comparison of Mayan, WRB and numerical classification. *Eurasian J. Soil Sci.* **2005**, *38*, 80–87.
26. Beckhoff, B.; Kanngießer, B.; Langhoff, N.; Wedell, R.; Wolff, H. *Handbook of Practical X-Ray Fluorescence Analysis*, 1st ed.; Springer: Berlin, Germany, 2006; pp. 1–410.
27. Lozano, R.; Bernal, J.P. Characterization of a new set of eight geochemical reference materials for XRF major and trace element analysis. *Rev. Mex. Cienc. Geol.* **2005**, *22*, 329–344.
28. Levin, N.; Ben-Dor, E.; Singer, A. A digital camera as a tool to measure color indices and related properties of sandy soils in semi-arid environments. *Int. J. Rem. Sens.* **2005**, *26*, 5475–5492.
29. Statgraphics. *Reference Manual, Manugistics*; Statgraphics Plus, Version 5.1; Statpoint Technologies, Inc.: Rockville, MD, USA, 1992.
30. Kruskal, W.H.; Wallis, W.A. Use of ranks in one-criterion variance analysis. *J. Am. Stat. Assoc.* **1952**, *47*, 583–621.
31. Magiera, T.; Jabłońska, M.; Strzyszcz, Z.; Rachwal, M. Morphological and Mineralogical Forms of Technogenic Magnetic Particles in Industrial Dusts. *Atmos. Environ.* **2011**, *45*, 4281–4290. [CrossRef]
32. Aguilera, A.; Armendariz, C.; Quintana, P.; García-Oliva, M.; Bautista, F. Influence of Land Use and Road Type on the Elemental Composition of Urban Dust in a Mexican Metropolitan Area. *Pol. J. Environ. Stud.* **2019**, *28*, 1535–1547. [CrossRef]
33. Aguilera, A.; Bautista, F.; Gutiérrez-Ruiz, M.; Ceniceros-Gómez, A.; Cejudo, R.; Goguitchaichvili, A. Heavy metal pollution of street dust in the largest city of Mexico, sources and health risk assessment. *Environ. Monit. Assess.* **2021**, *193*, 1–16. [CrossRef]
34. Liu, Q.; Roberts, A.; Larrasoaña, J.C.; Banerjee, S.K.; Guyodo, Y.; Tauxe, L.; Oldfield, F. Environmental Magnetism: Principles and Applications. *Rev. Geophys.* **2012**, *50*, RG4002. [CrossRef]

35. Aguilera, A.; Morales, J.J.; Goguitchaichvili, A.; García-Oliva, F.; Armendariz-Arnez, C.; Quintana, P.; Bautista, F. Spatial distribution of magnetic material in urban road dust classified by land use and type of road in San Luis Potosí, Mexico. *Air Qual. Atmos. Health* **2020**, *13*, 951–963. [CrossRef]
36. Bautista, F.; Gogichaishvili, A.; Delgado, C.; Quintana, P.; Aguilar, D.; Cejudo, R.; Cortés, J. El color como indicador de contaminación por metales pesados en suelos de la Ciudad de México. *Boletín de la Soc. Geológica Mex.* **2021**, *73*, A210920.
37. Bautista, F.; Frausto, O.; Ihl, T.; Aguilar, Y. Actualización del mapa de suelos de Yucatán utilizando un enfoque geomorfopedológico y WRB. *Ecosistemas y Recur. Agropecu.* **2015**, *2*, 303–315.
38. Maher, B.A.; Alekseev, A.; Alekseeva, T. Magnetic mineralogy of soils across the Russian Steppe: Climatic dependence of pedogenic magnetite formation. *Palaeo3* **2003**, *201*, 321–341.
39. Bautista, F.; Cejudo-Ruiz, R.; Aguilar-Reyes, B.; Gogichaishvili, A. El potencial del magnetismo en la clasificación de suelos: Una revisión. *Bol. Soc. Geol. Mex.* **2014**, *66*, 365–376.
40. Kumaravel, V.; Sangode, S.J.; Siddàiah, N.S.; Kumar, R. Interrelation of magnetic susceptibility, soil color, and elemental mobility in the Pliocene–Pleistocene Siwalik paleosol sequences of the NW Himalaya, India. *Geoderma* **2010**, *154*, 267–280.
41. Liu, J.G.; Moore, J.M. Hue image RGB colour composition. A simple technique to suppress shadow and enhance spectral signature. *Int. J. Remote Sens.* **1990**, *11*, 1521–1530.
42. Kirillova, N.P.; Vodyanitskii, Y.N.; Sileva, T.M. Conversion of soil color parameters from the Munsell system to the CIE-L*a*b* System, Genesis, and Geography of Soils. *Eurasian J. Soil Sci.* **2015**, *48*, 468–475.
43. Schwertmann, U. Relationships between iron oxides, soil color, and soil formation. In *Soil Color*; Special publication 31; Bigham, J.M., Ciolkosz, E.J., Eds.; Soil Science Society of America: Madison, WI, USA, 1993; pp. 51–69.
44. Aguilera, A.; Bautista, F.; Goguitchaichvili, A.; Garcia-Oliva, F. Health risk of heavy metals in street dust. *Front. Biosci (Landmark Ed.)* **2021**, *1*, 327–345.

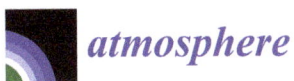

Article

Coarse Technogenic Material in Urban Surface Deposited Sediments (USDS)

Andrian Seleznev [1,2,*], Ekaterina Ilgasheva [1], Ilia Yarmoshenko [1] and Georgy Malinovsky [1]

1. Institute of Industrial Ecology, Ural Branch of the Russian Academy of Sciences, 20, S. Kovalevskoy Str., 620219 Ekaterinburg, Russia; boomo4ka@mail.ru (E.I.); ivy@ecko.uran.ru (I.Y.); georgy@ecko.uran.ru (G.M.)
2. Ural Federal University Named after the First President of Russia B.N. Yeltsin, 19, Mira Str., 620002 Ekaterinburg, Russia
* Correspondence: sandrian@rambler.ru

Citation: Seleznev, A.; Ilgasheva, E.; Yarmoshenko, I.; Malinovsky, G. Coarse Technogenic Material in Urban Surface Deposited Sediments (USDS). *Atmosphere* **2021**, *12*, 754. https://doi.org/10.3390/atmos12060754

Academic Editor: Rafael Borge

Received: 2 May 2021
Accepted: 8 June 2021
Published: 10 June 2021

Publisher's Note: MDPI stays neutral with regard to jurisdictional claims in published maps and institutional affiliations.

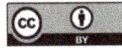

Copyright: © 2021 by the authors. Licensee MDPI, Basel, Switzerland. This article is an open access article distributed under the terms and conditions of the Creative Commons Attribution (CC BY) license (https://creativecommons.org/licenses/by/4.0/).

Abstract: In the current paper, the analysis of heavy mineral concentrate (Schlich analysis) was used to study the particles of technogenic origin in the samples of urban surface-deposited sediments (USDS). The USDS samples were collected in the residential areas of 10 Russian cities located in different economic, climatic, and geological zones: Ufa, Perm, Tyumen, Chelyabinsk, Nizhny Tagil, Magnitogorsk, Nizhny Novgorod, Rostov-on-Don, Murmansk, and Ekaterinburg. The number of technogenic particles was determined in the coarse particle size fractions of 0.1–0.25 and 0.25–1 mm. The types of technogenic particle were studied by scanning electron microscopy (SEM) analysis. The amount of technogenic material differed from city to city; the fraction of technogenic particles in the samples varied in the range from 0.01 to 0.43 with an average value of 0.18. The technogenic particles in USDS samples were represented by lithoid and granulated slag, iron and silicate microspheres, fragments of brick, paint, glass, plaster, and other household waste. Various types of technogenic particle differed in morphological characteristics as well as in chemical composition. The novelty and significance of the study comprises the following: it has been shown that technogenic particles are contained in a significant part of the USDS; the quantitative indicators of the accumulation of technogenic particles in the urban landscape have been determined; the contributions of various types of particles to the total amount of technogenic material were estimated for the urban landscape; the trends in the transformation of typomorphic elemental associations in the urban sediments associated with the material of technogenic origin were demonstrated; and the alteration trends in the USDS microelemental content were revealed, taking into account the impurities in the composition of technogenic particles.

Keywords: urban environment; residential area; urban surface deposited sediments; road dust; technogenic particles; slag; spherules; microplastic; plaster

1. Introduction

Sediment deposition in the urban area reduces the environmental quality, and affects health, aesthetics, economics, and other aspects of city life [1]. The constant sediment supply increases the costs of municipal services and cleaning the territories, as well as deteriorating urban infrastructure facilities [2–6]. The deposited loose sedimentary materials silt stormwater systems, compact urban soils, decrease the fertility of the topsoil, etc. [7–10]. The deposited solid matter on streets and sidewalks increases the wear and tear of vehicles [7–13]. Dust deposition in electrical equipment may cause outages on electricity lines [14].

Coarse sand material of road-deposited sediments is about 50% of road-deposited sediments mass [15]. The coarse particles of anthropogenic origin may contain toxic heavy metals [16–20]. The large size fraction material of road-deposited sediments (>100 μm) contains the mass of heavy metals within particulate matter similar to the fine fractions [21]. The coarse particles are involved in the transport of heavy metal pollution from roads to stormwater drains, and they absorb pollutants and may release them during rainy periods [6,15].

The local surface geochemical traps in an urban environment representing sediment of the depressed areas of microrelief (in other words, surface dirt sediment) were chosen as the main object of the study. This environmental component is deposited on various surfaces forming the upper part of the cultural layer on the territory of the city. The sediments participate in the processes of migration and accumulation of pollutants and particulate matter.

Sediments are formed as a result of the natural processes of the weathering of the material of building constructions, pavements, and roads under freezing and thawing in the presence of moisture, soil, and ground erosion under the influence of surface stormwater runoff, and atmospheric dust deposition. The material of the excavated ground, the products of road surface abrasion by passing parking cars, and household waste also contribute to the formation of the particulate materials of the urban sediment. The accumulation of sediments significantly increases under bad cleaning conditions and poor urban management and landscaping [1,16].

USDS (urban surface-deposited sediments) is a common term characterizing the various types of loose sediment formed as a result of weathering, erosion, and destruction of soils, pavements, and construction in the urban environment, which is deposited in depressed areas as a result of surface runoff of relief [22–24]. The solid material of the USDS is composed of the particles of soil, sand, peat, dust, and small debris [25]. The formation of sediments occurs within the urban area where the various surfaces and buildings are constructed in different years and decades [18,19]. The thickness of the sediments varies within the area of the quarter and landscape functional zones and is on average 5 cm. The content of pollutants in the sediments characterizes the pollution of the area from which the sediment was accumulated [25].

The sediment includes the particles of natural and anthropogenic origin. In the urban environment, about 60% of the sediment is represented by the material of bedrock, as well as organic material [26]. Many authors have shown that ash, slag, and metal particles of various shapes and composition, metal, wear products of vehicles and other mechanisms, small household waste, as well as microplastics can be found in the composition of various types of surface sediments in an urban environment [7,11,15–18,26–28]. Organic objects in the urban surface sediment may include bacteria and viruses [29]. The technogenic material produced by the road traffic and found along the roads mainly consists of magnetic particles, which can be the products of motor vehicles: angular and spherical iron-oxides, tungsten-rich particles, and sodium chloride, with a size of about 100 µm [30].

The studies of the technogenic phase in USDS and dust in the urban environment are mainly focused on the effect of traffic on the content of particles <100 microns in size [31], in particular smaller PM2–PM10 particles due to their greatest environmental hazard and the largest accession for wind transfer and inhalation by humans [21,32,33]. Larger particles are less studied, however, and they can also hold fine dust particles on their surfaces due to electrostatic charge. Solid material from non-exhaust emissions as well as coarse material from roadway destruction, pavement abrasion, and vehicle parts are less studied [31,34]. Such loose material may be as well transferred by the wind several tens of meters away from the roadway.

Particles are redistributed between the various landscape zones by stormwater runoff, may participate in the urban sedimentary cascade entering the water bodies, and form material of bottom sediments of lakes, rivers, and estuaries [35–39]. The particles may adsorb pollutants, bacteria, and viruses. Contemporary USDS in the city is a good collector of pollutants and material of different origins, including non-point sources of pollution.

Road traffic is one of the main sources of technogenic material [30,40,41] such as the particles of wear of tires, brake pads, and road abrasion products. Tire wear products contribute the most part of anthropogenic material in road dust, galley sediments, pavement dust, car park dust, and roadside soils and snow. Anthropogenic material from vehicles is represented by magnetic particles including spherules and slag, comprising the particles of about 100 μm size [30,32,42]. Smelters and coal-fired power plants also represent significant sources of anthropogenic solid material in cities, forming non-point sources of pollution, such as fly ash [17,43–45].

Thus, the identification of sources of anthropogenic material, the content of technogenic materials, and the assessment of the amount and types of anthropogenic particles in different parts of the landscape are among the significant environmental issues in an urban environment.

While the environmental role of the USDS in modern cities had been demonstrated in the previous studies involving such characteristics as pollution with the heavy metals [22,24,25,46] and the contribution of the dust fraction [23], this study has been focused on the technogenic particles in the urban environment. The objectives of the study were: (1) the identification of particles of the anthropogenic origin found in the urban environment compartments; (2) the classification and characterization of the morphological features of technogenic particles; (3) the assessment of the amount of technogenic material in urban surface deposited sediments; and (4) in an urban environment; and (5) the characterization of cities according to the amount of technogenic material in the contemporary urban surface sediments.

2. Materials and Methods

2.1. The Description of the Studied Cities

The USDS sample collection program was performed in 10 Russian cities located in different climatic and industrial zones, in the territories with different geological structure (Figure 1) [47]: Ufa, Perm, Tyumen, Chelyabinsk, Nizhny Tagil, Magnitogorsk, Nizhny Novgorod, Rostov-on-Don, Murmansk, and Ekaterinburg. The chosen cities have a high automobile traffic load, >250 cars per 1000 people, and high density of population.

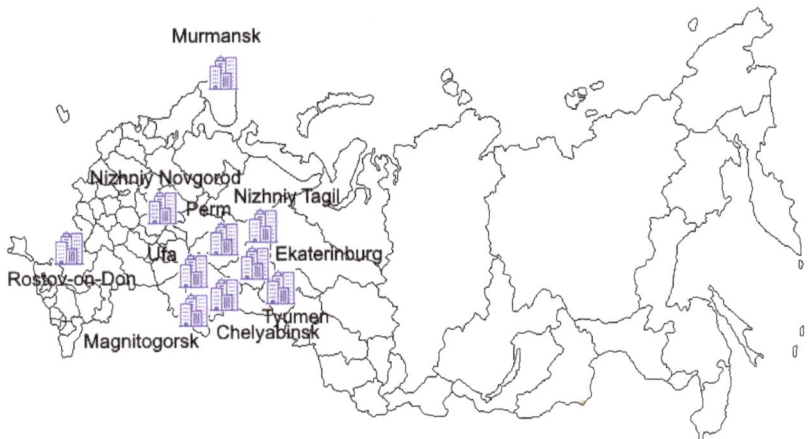

Figure 1. The location of the cities on the map of Russia where the collection of samples of urban surface deposited sediments was performed.

The significant development of urbanization in the cities occurred in the second half of the 20th century. The descriptions of the surveyed cities are represented in Table 1.

Table 1. The description of the surveyed cities.

City, Population, Million People/Cars per 1000 People/City Area (km^2)	Geographic and Climatic Zone, Average Temperature, °C, Jan/Jul	Geological Features [47]	Main Industries
Ufa, 1.1/278/707.9	Forest-steppe zone, temperate continental climate, −12.4/19.7	Volga-Ural Anteclise, Verkhnekamsk basin; gypsum, anhydrite, sandstone, marl, siltstone, dolomite, Pre-Jurassic limestones; alluvium, colluvium, diluvium, sandstones, sandy loams, loams, Upper Pliocene and Holocene clays.	Oil processing, oil chemical industry, machinery
Perm, 1.007/237/803	Forest zone, temperate continental climate, −12.8/18.6	East of the European part of Russia, banks of the Kama River. Pre-Ural geomorphological zone, Kungurian stage, Irvinskaya and Fillipovskaya formations of the Pre-Jurassic: gypsum, sandstone, limestones, dolomites, marls; clays, loam and sandy loam of Holocene alluvial, eluvial and diluvial sediments.	Electric power industry, oil and gas processing, machinery, chemistry and petrochemistry, woodworking.
Tyumen, 0.77/363/698.5	Western Siberia, forest taiga zone with waterlogged areas, temperate continental climate, −15/18.8	West Siberian plain, Tyumen downwarp; diorites and gabbros of the Pre-Jurassicformations; loams, clays, silts and lake-alluvium of the Upper Pliocene and Holocene.	Oil processing, gas-fired power plants
Chelyabinsk, 1.2/269/530	The South Urals, forest-steppe zone, temperate climate, −14.1/19.3	East Urals uplift and West Side of West Siberian plate; granites, diorites, coals, limestones, sandstones, dolomitic limestones of the Pre-Jurassic formations; sands, siltstones, loams, alluvial sediments of floodplain terraces, pebbles, gravels, and eluvial-diluvial sediments of the Upper Pliocene and Holocene.	Ferrous and non-ferrous metallurgy, chemical industry, machinery, coal-fired power plants
Nizhniy Tagil, 0.36/240/297.5	The Middle Urals, mountain-forest zone, temperate continental climate, −14.5/17.8	Middle Urals, Tagil megazone; harzburgites, serpentinites, basalts, green schists, mica-quartz and graphite-quartz schists, diorites, gabbros, andesites, dacites of the Pre-Jurassic formations; eluvial and diluvial sediments, clays, sandy loams, alluvial sediments of floodplain terraces, pebbles, sands, and loams of the Upper Pliocene and Holocene.	Ferrous and nonferous metallurgy, coking, machinery, chemical industry, production of building materials
Magnitogorsk, 0.42/297/392.4	The South Urals, steppe zone, harsh continental climate, −14.1/19.2	South Urals, West Magnitogorsk zone; trachibasalts, trachiriolites, basalts, andesites, rhyodacites, lavas, and clastolavas of the Prejurasic formations; alluvial sediments of floodplains, clays, sands, peat, diluvial sediments, eluvial-diluvial sediments, and limes of the Upper Pliocene and Holocene.	Ferrous metallurgy, metal processing, gas-fired power plant
Nizhniy Novgorod, 1.3/276/460	Broad-leaved forests, mixed forests and taiga zone, humid continental climate, −8.9/19.4	Volga-Ural Anteclise, Pre-Quarternary clays with interbeds of siltstone, sand with gravel of sedimentary rocks, siltstone, loam, marl, gypsum, limestones, and dolomites; alluvial sediments, sands with gravel, loam, clay, eluvial and solifluction formations, sand, eluvial and diluvial Holocene formations.	Machinery, river shipping
Rostov-on-Don, 1.1/285/354	Steppe zone, temperate continental climate, −3/23.4	East European plate, Rostov ledge; sands, clays, gravel, and pebbles of the Lower Pliocene;limestones, shells, siltstones, and marls of the Upper Miocene; alluvium floodplain terraces, sands, pebbles, loams, sandy loam, eluvial and proluvial sediments of the Upper Pliocene and Holocene.	Machinery, river shipping, food industry
Murmansk, 303.8/321/154.4	Arctic tundra zone, atlantic-arctic temperate climate, −10.1/12.8	Murmansk megablock represented by Archean granitoids. Pyroxene diorites, tonalites-plagiogranites, magmatite-plagiogranite amphibole, metamorphosed gabbros, diorites, granites, gneisses, biotite amphibolites, magnetite quartzites of the Pre-Jurassic. Declivial marine sediments: sandy silts, mixed-grained sands.	Machinery, shipping, metalworking, food industry, coal-fired power plant
Ekaterinburg, 1.387/302/486	The Middle Urals, forest zone, temperate continental climate, −12.6/19	Middle Urals, low mountains and hilly plains along the Iset River. Serpentinites, granites, gabbro, diorites, tuffs, tuff sandstones, siliceous and carbonaceous-siliceous shale, quartzite of the Pre-Jurassic; eluvial and diluvial sediments, clays, loams, alluvial sediments of floodplain terraces of the Holocene.	Metal processing, machinery, gas-fired power plant

2.2. Sample Collection

The USDS samples were collected on an irregular grid of at least 40 sampling sites in each city. The sampling site represents the courtyard area of the residential quarter with multi-story buildings. Each sample was taken from the local depressions of the microrelief from 3–5 localizations on the territory of the courtyard space of the quarter. The sample collection procedure was described in detail in previously published papers [22,25,46]. The sample mass was 1–1.5 kg. During the sample collection process, a questionnaire was filled for each sampling site containing information about the conditions of sediment formation, their thickness, the approximate area of the quarter, the proportion of landscaped functional zones, sidewalks, parking lots in the quarter, the quality of cleaning, carrying out construction work, and the approximate time of development of the territory.

2.3. Particle Size Analysis

Large roots, stones, debris, and foreign inclusions (glass, plastic, etc.) were removed from the samples. The samples were dried at room temperature. The dried sample was crushed manually using a rubber-tipped pestle, and thoroughly mixed. A representative subsample of about 200 g for particle size analysis was taken from each sample by quartering. To conduct particle size analysis, at least 5 samples were randomly chosen from 40 samples collected in each city.

The special separation procedure was used to determine the granulometric composition and to obtain the solid material of the various particle size fractions of the samples. The technique based on decantation and wet sieving of the material of subsample of 200 g was earlier described in detail by Seleznev and Rudakov [46]. The subsample of 200 g was fractionated into 6 granulometric subsamples with sizes: >1 mm, 0.25–1 mm, 0.1–0.25 mm, 0.05–0.1 mm, 0.01–0.05 mm, and 0.002–0.01 mm. The resulting granulometric subsamples were weighed. The mass fraction of each particle size fraction in the sediment sample was calculated.

2.4. Mineral Analysis

The analysis of the heavy mineral concentrate (Schlich analysis) of sediment was used to determine the particles of technogenic origin. Manual analysis was performed for 0.1–0.25 and 0.25–1 mm granulometric subsamples. The fraction of anthropogenic particles was calculated in 0.1–0.25 and 0.25–1 mm fractions. The analytical procedure is described below.

The solid material of the studied granulometric subsample was poured on paper and thoroughly mixed. Then a cone pile was formed from the poured loose material. After that, the material was flattened into a disk 1–2 mm thick. This disk was divided radially into quarters; two opposite quarters were taken for the further analysis of the subsample and the other two were discarded. Such a procedure of quartering and reducing the volume of the material of the granulometric subsample was repeated multiple times until the subsample of the desired weight or volume was obtained. The final volume of the quartered granulometric subsample was approximately 15 mL. Using a blade, the quartered granulometric subsample was distributed on the slide in three parallel lines. To identify and count particles, the lines were formed narrow and sparse. All manipulations with the grain mounts were conducted manually using the binocular microscope. Manipulation with the cone, disk, and the lines of particles, as well as quartering was performed using a wooden stick or copper needle.

The identification of the technogenic particles was carried out by morphology, structure, color, density, optical and physical properties (shape and crystal habitus, splinters, fracture, transparency, luster, elasticity, and hardness). Each particle was photographed using a Carl Zeiss Axioplan 2 optical microscope and binocular microscope equipped with an Olympus C-5060 camera. The size of particles was determined by a calibrated stage/objective micrometer (1 mm divided into 100 units) measurement scale of the optical microscope and its software.

All the particles of the quartered subsample were distributed by type; the fraction of particles of each type was counted.

After quartering and heavy mineral concentrate analysis 2–5 visually typical particles were selected from the part of granulometric subsample attributed to the technogenic phase. These particles were analyzed with a JEOLJSM-6390LV scanning electron microscope equipped with Oxford Instruments INCAEnergy 350 X-Max 50 energy-dispersive spectrometer. At least one image was obtained from the surface of each selected particle. The homogeneity of the chemical composition of the particle surface was identified visually by the color of the image. At least one spectrum of elemental composition was determined for a particle with a flat surface, characterizing its uniform composition. For particles with a concave or convex surface at least two spectra of elemental composition were taken from the surface (in the center of the surface and at its peripheral). For particles with visually different chemical compositions (different shades of gray in the image), at least one spectrum in each light area was taken. For particles with inclusions at least one spectrum was taken on each inclusion, and the linear size of the inclusion was measured. Similarly, at least one spectrum was taken on each area of the external contamination of particles (if it was present). Optical analysis, photography, and scanning electron microscopy (SEM) were carried out in the "Geoanalyst" Center for Collective Use at the Institute of Geology and Geochemistry of the Ural Branch of the Russian Academy of Sciences.

The origin of the particles (technogenic or natural) was finally determined according to the results of their visual analysis (color, luster, morphology, and size) and SEM investigations (surface morphology and chemical composition).

3. Results

The number of USDS samples collected in the cities and analyzed fortechnogenic phase is shown in Table 2. The analysis of heavy mineral concentrate was performed in 85 granulometric subsamples of 0.1–0.25 mm and 80 subsamples of 0.25–1 mm in size. For the particle size fraction of 0.1–0.25 mm, 11,985 particles were analyzed with the optical method, and 2306 of them were visually identified as technogenic. For subsamples of 0.25–1 mm in size, 10678 particles were inspected with a binocular microscope, of which 1409 particles were attributed to the technogenic phase.

Table 2. The number of urban surface-deposited sediment (USDS) samples collected in the cities and analyzed for technogenic phase.

City	Number of Samples for Particle Size Analysis	Number of Obtained Particle Size Subsamples, in Which Technogenic Particles Were Selected *	
		Fraction 0.1–0.25 mm	Fraction 0.25–1 mm
Ekaterinburg	6	5	6
Magnitogorsk	10	10	10
Murmansk	10	10	10
Nizhniy Novgorod	8	8	7
Nizhniy Tagil	11	11	11
Perm	5	5	3
Rostov-on-Don	9	7	9
Tyumen	7	7	5
Ufa	12	12	10
Chelyabinsk	10	10	9

* The subsample was quartered.

The statistical parameters of the fractional distribution of technogenic particles in the surveyed cities in particle size fractions of 0.1–0.25, 0.25–1, and combined fraction of 0.1–1 mm are shown in Figures 2 and 3.

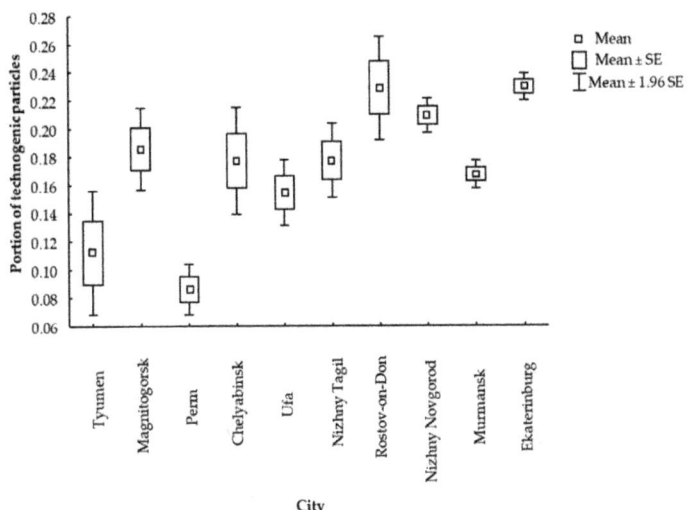

Figure 2. The proportion of technogenic particles in the cities in the particle size fraction of 0.1–1 mm (SE—standard error).

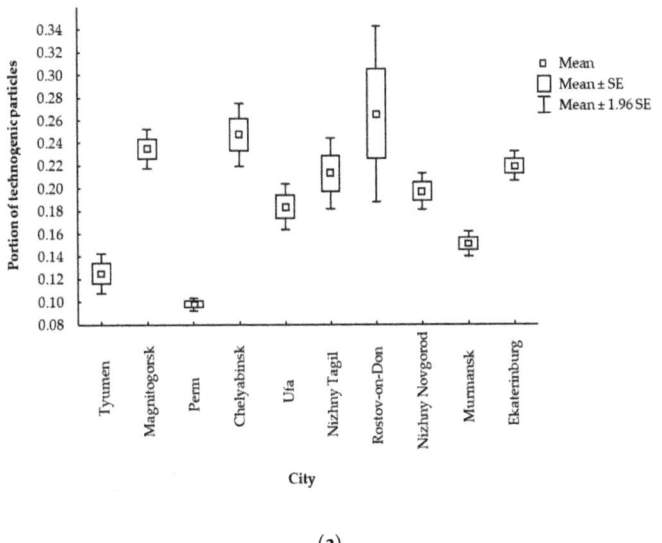

(a)

Figure 3. Cont.

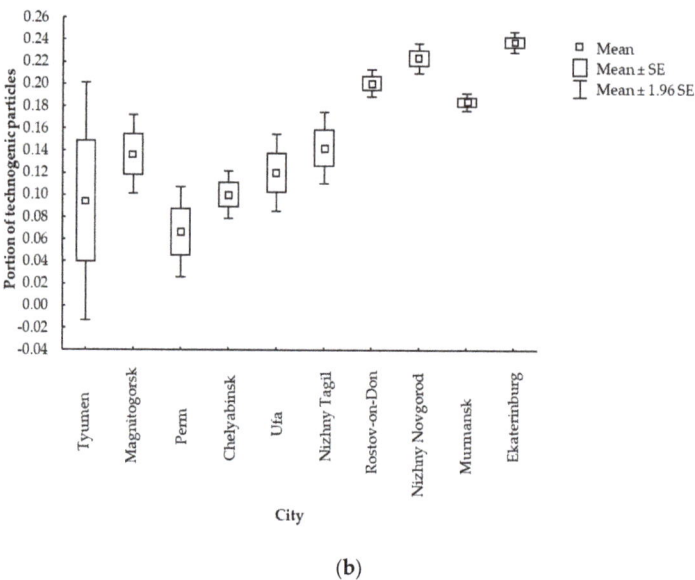

Figure 3. The proportion of technogenic particles in the cities: (**a**) in the particle size fraction of 0.1–0.25 mm, (**b**) in the particle size fraction of 0.25–1 mm (SE—standard error).

The additional parameters of distribution (kurtosis, skewness, and the coefficient of variation) of the proportion of technogenic particles in particle size fractions in cities are represented in Tables 3 and 4. The type of distribution of the proportion of technogenic particles in the samples for all cities and fractions is close to unimodal and lognormal. The proportion of technogenic fraction in the samples varies in the range from 0.01 to 0.43, the average value is 0.18. The average coefficient of variation (CV) of the portion of technogenic phase equal to 38% exhibits a wide range of data on the amount of technogenic phases in coarse particle size fraction of the USDS samples. The values of skewness are insignificant, and kurtosis is positive. The values of CV >20% were found in particle size fractions of 0.1–0.25, 0.25–1, and 0.1–1 mm in all cities besides Nizhny Novgorod, Murmansk, and Ekaterinburg.

When analyzing the individual particle size fractions of 0.1–0.25 and 0.25–1 mm (Table 3) and combined fraction of 0.1–1 mm by the cities (Table 4), the proportion of technogenic fraction exceeds 20% for all cities except Nizhny Novgorod, Murmansk and Ekaterinburg. The maximum proportion of the technogenic fraction equal to 0.43 is observed in Rostov-on-Don in the 0.1–0.25 mm fraction. The minimal portion was found in the 0.25–1 mm fraction in Tyumen. The amount of technogenic particles in granulometric fractions of 0.1–0.25 and 0.25–1 as well as in the combined fraction 0.1–1 mm varies significantly between different cities. The largest proportion of technogenic material was found in the USDS samples in Rostov-on-Don, Nizhniy Novgorod, and Ekaterinburg. The parameters of the distribution of portion of technogenic phase in urban areas in the combined particle size fraction of 0.1–1 mm are as follows: arithmetic mean 0.18, geometric mean 0.16, median 0.19, min–max 0.01–0.43, SD 0.07, CI (-/+) 0.06/0.08, CV 38.52 %, skewness 0.21, and kurtosis 1.23.

Table 3. The additional parameters of distribution of the proportion of technogenic particles in particle size fractions of 0.1–0.25 and 0.25–1 mm in cities.

City	Particle Size Fraction, mm	Kurtosis	Skewness	Coefficient of Variation, %	Min/Max
Tyumen	0.1–0.25	−0.79	−0.87	19.01	0.09/0.15
	0.25–1	4.51	2.09	129.91	0.01/0.31
Magnitogorsk	0.1–0.25	0.30	1.08	11.94	0.21/0.29
	0.25–1	−1.11	−0.62	41.88	0.04/0.2
Perm	0.1–0.25	0.90	0.97	6.61	0.09/0.11
	0.25–1	0.00	1.24	53.83	0.04/0.11
Chelyabinsk	0.1–0.25	5.41	2.10	18.12	0.2/0.36
	0.25–1	0.40	−0.72	32.88	0.04/0.14
Ufa	0.1–0.25	1.18	−0.94	19.11	0.1/0.23
	0.25–1	0.82	0.76	46.81	0.04/0.24
Nizhniy Tagil	0.1–0.25	0.04	0.93	24.75	0.15/0.31
	0.25–1	−1.23	−0.09	37.83	0.06/0.22
Rostov-on-Don	0.1–0.25	−0.80	1.22	39.36	0.19/0.43
	0.25–1	−1.19	0.29	9.33	0.17/0.23
Nizhniy Novgorod	0.1–0.25	1.12	−1.37	11.72	0.15/0.22
	0.25–1	0.80	−1.30	8.18	0.19/0.24
Murmansk	0.1–0.25	0.02	−0.62	11.66	0.12/0.18
	0.25–1	3.25	1.38	6.85	0.17/0.21
Ekaterinburg	0.1–0.25	−2.01	−0.40	6.75	0.2/0.24
	0.25–1	−2.52	0.15	4.82	0.23/0.25

Table 4. The additional parameters of distribution of the proportion of technogenic particles in particle size fraction of 0.1–1 mm in cities.

City	Curtosis	Skewness	Coefficient of Variation, %	Min/Max
Tyumen	3.40	1.40	69.04	0.01/0.31
Magnitogorsk	0.15	−0.78	35.91	0.04/0.29
Perm	0.67	−1.38	29.70	0.04/0.11
Chelyabinsk	−0.52	0.22	47.70	0.04/0.36
Ufa	−0.73	−0.41	35.72	0.04/0.24
Nizhniy Tagil	0.25	0.18	35.57	0.06/0.31
Rostov-on-Don	4.38	2.33	32.83	0.17/0.43
Nizhniy Novgorod	0.93	−0.97	11.65	0.15/0.24
Murmansk	0.37	−0.36	13.52	0.12/0.21
Ekaterinburg	−0.04	−0.43	6.94	0.2/0.25

According to SEM analysis, the studied technogenic particles were divided into types presented in Table 5.

Table 6 shows the morphological features of the various types of particles. Totally 464 particles were analyzed by SEM. The number of particles investigated by cities was: Ekaterinburg 151, Magnitogorsk 22, Murmansk 31, Nizhny Novgorod 127, Nizhny Tagil 30, Rostov-on-Don 71, Tyumen 22, Ufa 9, and Chelyabinsk 1. The chemical composition of the surfaces of various types of particles (without inclusions) is shown in Table 5 as well.

Table 5. The chemical composition of the surfaces of various types of particles without inclusions according to scanning electron microscopy (SEM) analysis.

Type of Particle	Elements	Composition, Mass Portion of Element, %
Lithoid slag	major	O (31%), Si (21%), C (15%), Fe (10%), Ca (9%), Al (6%),
	impurities	Mg (3%), Na (3%), K (2%)
Granulated slag	major	O (39%), Si (18%), Fe (15%), Ca (9%),
	impurities	Mg (4%), Al (4%), C (2%), Ti (1%), S (1%), K (1%)
Iron microsphere (magnetic)	major	Fe (69%), O (24%),
	impurities	Si (2%), Ca (1%)
Silicate microsphere	major	O (39%), Si (23%), Ca (12%), Fe (8%), Mg (5%),
	impurities	Al (4%), Na (2%), Cu (2%)
Brick	major	O (35%), Si (22%), Fe (17%), Ca (11%),
	impurities	K (3%), Al (3%), Na (2%), Ti (2%), C (2%)
Paint	major	O (39%), Ca (15%), Fe (14%), Si (13%), Pb (5%),
	impurities	Ti (4%), Mg (3%), Al (3%), K (1%), C (1%), Cr (1%)
Glass	major	O (35%), Si (28%), Fe (9%), Ca (8%),
	impurities	Al (4%), Cu (3%), Mg (2%), Na (2%), K (1%), Cr (1%)
Plaster fragment	major	O (36%), Ca (29%), Si (11%), Fe (6%), C (6%),
	impurities	Mg (3%), Al (3%), Na (1%), S (1%), K (1%), Cr (1%)
White-coated plaster	major	Ti (46%), O (18%), Ca (15%), Cu (11%),
	impurities	Ba (3%), Fe (1%), Al (1%), S (1%)
Paint coated plaster	major	Ca (55%), O (30%),
	impurities	Si (3%), Ti (3%), C (3%), Fe (2%), Al (1%), Pb (1%)

Table 6. Morphological features of types of technogenic particles in the studied cities.

Type of Particle	Morphological Features	Size, mm	Possible Origin
Granulated slag	Glassy structure, shell-like breakage, poorly rounded, black, dark brown, dark green, grey, light yellow or colorless, transparent or translucent	0.3–1	Metallurgy
Lithoid (stone-like) slag	Stone-shaped particles, with a porous structure, crystallized, medium rounded, grey, dark brown, dark green, translucent or opaque	0.3–1	Metallurgy
Iron microsphere (magnetic)	Spheres, with a smooth or polygonal textured surface, steel-grey, often with thin films of iron oxides, opaque	0.1–1	Metallurgy
Silicate microsphere	Spheres, sometimes slightly flattened or deformed; the surface is corroded, with cavities and visible cracks; black, dark brown; opaque or colorless translucent with a strong glassy luster	0.45–1	Combustion of high ash raw material
Brick	Well or completely rounded debris (quartz, clay material, whitewash); red-brown, dark red with inclusions, opaque	0.5–1	Construction materials
Plaster	Thin, flattened particles, highly fragile; light grey, white, opaque, matt	0.5–0.8	Construction materials
Glass	Glassy, poorly or perfectly rounded; colorless, yellow, blue, green, transparent	0.5–1	Household waste
Paint	Thin, flattened, elastic particles; yellow, red, blue, green, with a matt or shiny surface	0.25–1	Construction materials
Car tires	Smooth particles, high elasticity; black, opaque, matt	200–1000	Automobile nonexhaust emissions

The distribution of different types of technogenic particle in urban areas in the 0.1–1 mm grain size fraction and 0.1–0.25 and 0.25–1 mm fractions are shown in Figures 4–6.

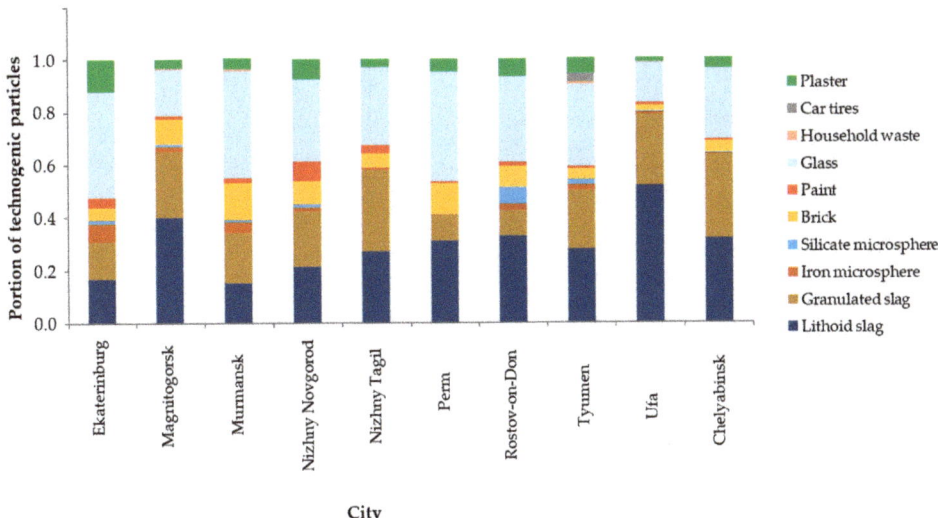

Figure 4. Distribution of the amount of different types of technogenic particle in the cities in the granulometric fraction of 0.1–1 mm.

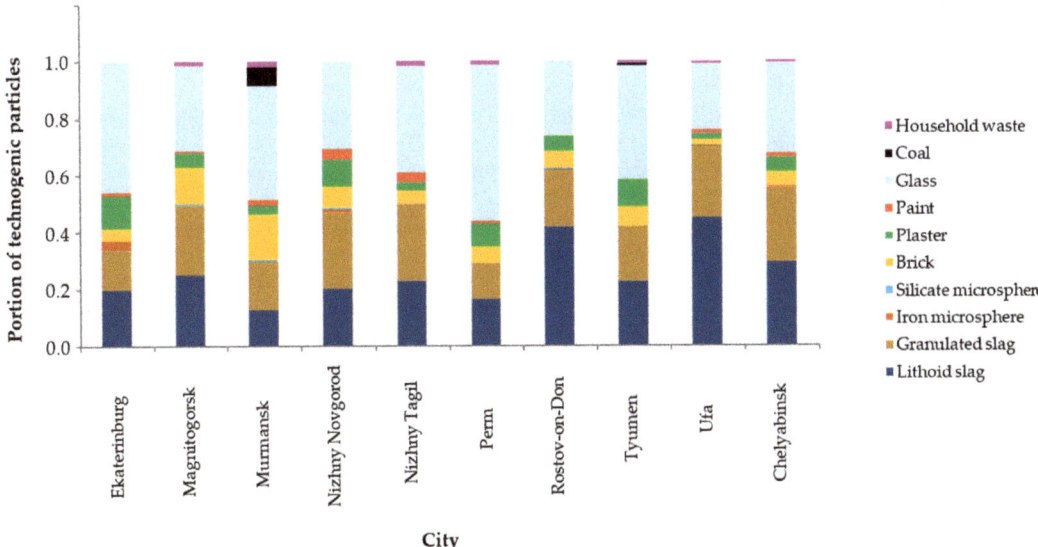

Figure 5. Distribution of the amount of different types of technogenic particle in the cities in the granulometric fraction of 0.1–0.25 mm.

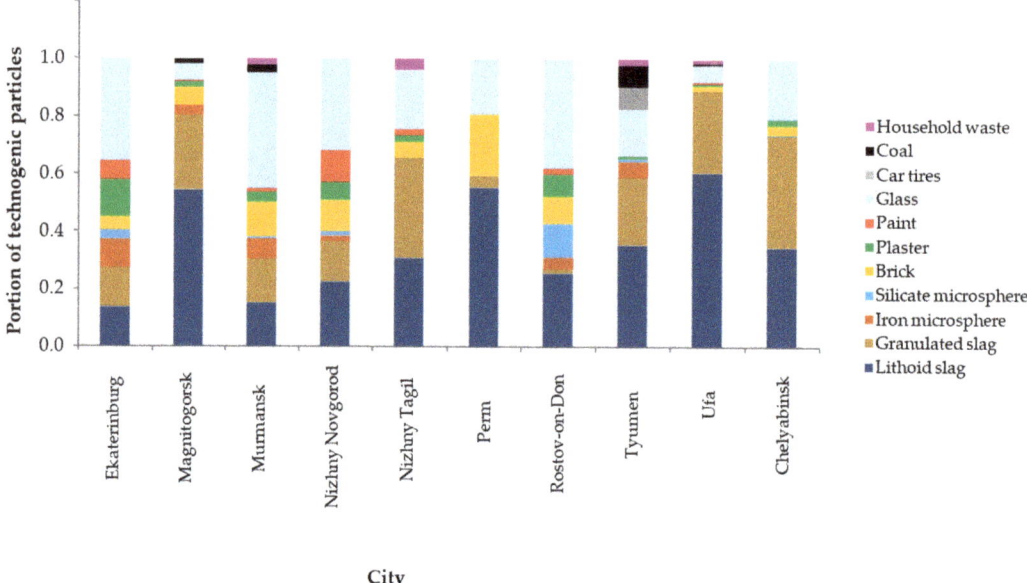

Figure 6. Distribution of the amount of different types of technogenic particle in the cities in the granulometric fraction of 0.25–1 mm.

4. Discussion

The USDS samples were collected in 10 large cities located in different geographic and climatic zones, and in territories with different geological setting, anthropogenic pressure, and economy. The research was carried out according to the uniform methodology in all the studied cities. A part of the obtained particle size subsamples of 0.1–0.25 mm and 0.25–1 mm in size did not have enough material to conduct the analysis of heavy mineral concentrate, thus these subsamples were rejected from the technogenic particle investigations. In the cities of Perm, Ekaterinburg, and Tyumen a smaller number of USDS samples were collected, thus a correspondingly smaller number of subsamples for the analysis of heavy mineral concentrate were selected. Such a homogeneous distribution of the USDS sample amount and particle size subsamples did not affect the results of the analysis of heavy mineral concentrate and was suitable for the current study.

The total number of the studied samples is sufficient to assess the contribution of the technogenic component to the USDS solid coarse fractions of 0.1–0.25 and 0.25–1 mm in size. According to the visual mineral analysis, 19% and 13% of particles were characterized as technogenic in particle size fractions of 0.1–0.25 and 0.25–1 mm, respectively. The rest of the particles is represented by the mineral and natural organic fragments.

The proportion of technogenic particles differs from city to city. The largest portion of anthropogenic particles in the USDS coarse fraction was found in Rostov-on-Don, Ekaterinburg, Nizhny Novgorod, Nizhny Tagil, and Magnitogorsk. The high proportion of technogenic particles in these four cities is apparently related to the ferrous metallurgy and mechanical engineering industries. The city of Rostov-on-Don is the most southern of the surveyed cities. According to previous studies, the city has the highest accumulation of dust and USDS due to the arid climate and bad cleaning and management of the urban environment [1,22]. The lower amount of the anthropogenic coarse material was found in Perm and Tyumen. Tyumen is one of the least-polluted cities in Russia, although it has a slightly large number of cars per capita in comparison with other cities [22]. It should be noted that for all cities the proportion of technogenic phase in the combined fraction of 0.1–1 mm will be consistent with the proportions of the anthropogenic material in the separate fractions of 0.1–0.25 and 0.25–1 mm (Figure 4).

The ratio between the number of technogenic particles visually identified and the total amount of particles in the granulometric subsamples may be used to roughly estimate an error in determining the number of technogenic particles by visual inspection (for subsamples of 0.1–0.25 and 0.25–1 mm, 19% and 13%, respectively).

The SEM-EDS (energy-dispersive spectroscopy) technique allows us to analyze the surface of the particle and determine its chemical composition. Thus this method of analysis is more reliable for the determination of particle type than visual diagnostics. Visual inspection depends on the qualification, physical abilities, and experience of the operator. Therefore, optical methods of research do not fully guarantee the reliability of determination of the particle type. Fully reliable determination of the particle type by its visual features is unattainable and is not required. However, the combination of methods of analysis of heavy mineral concentrate and visual diagnostics is a suitable and easy technically realized procedure to discriminate technogenic particles in comparison with SEM-EDS analysis that requires the investigator to have skills in electron microscopy. At the same time, the analysis of heavy mineral concentrate provides the search of the required particles among the big amount of the similar objects and a rough estimation of the quantity of the objects of interest.

Various types of technogenic particles differ in shape and physical characteristics as well as in chemical composition. The major elements forming the composition of the particle core were O, Si, Fe, Al, Ca, Ti, etc. The minor elements found on the surfaces of the particles and forming the impurities were Mg, K, Cu, Na, etc. In many cases, impurity elements contribute to the environmental pollution, in particular, the composition of various particles of plaster coated with paint and whitewash includes Pb, Cu, and Cr.

The separate group of the cities of the Ural region with a metallurgical industry (Nizhny Tagil, Chelyabinsk, and Magnitogorsk) can be distinguished among the studied cities. Each city in this group has a large metallurgical plant, coking, and coal power plants. The number of technogenic particles does not differ significantly both in fractions of 0.1–0.25 and 0.25–1 mm separately and in the combined particle size fraction of 0.1–1 mm in these cities. According to the results of previous studies [46], the anthropogenic material in the form of slag is used in such cities as a building material, for example, instead of sand and stone in pavement and road construction in residential areas. There is also a coal power plant in Murmansk. It can be assumed that in the group of four cities, technogenic particles, in particular slag, can enter the USDS material with emissions from power plants and smelters.

All the studied cities have a high automobile traffic network, as well as road construction works being underway. The technogenic components (especially fly ash) are often used as construction materials or backfill materials on pavements. Such material can be transferred into the USDS by the wheels of vehicles in the residential area. In general, the amount of technogenic material is comparable to the data obtained for other cities [15].

The distribution of the proportion of technogenic particles in the samples deviates from the normal and is close to lognormal and asymmetric. Several studies conclude that the lognormal distribution of elemental concentrations in environmental compartments or close to it relates to additional anthropogenic input of the elements [48–50]. In our study, the conclusion about the distribution of the proportion of anthropogenic particles in the studied samples close to lognormal was expected; however, it is important to take into account the uncertainty of information about the source of technogenic particles in the urban environment. The coefficient of variation of the portion of anthropogenic particles also confirms the fact of the heterogeneity of the sample populations in the studied cities.

The analysis of the technogenic phase composition of USDS samples in the combined fraction of 0.1–1 mm shows that slag particles predominate in all cities and, besides, a large amount of domestic wastes (glass), the particles of construction materials (plaster and brick), and to a lesser extent paint particles, are observed. The analysis of the distribution of the number of technogenic particles in fractions of 0.25–1 and 0.1–0.25 in combination with the results of analysis of heavy mineral concentrate allows concluding that technogenic particles in finer fraction of 0.1–0.25 mm may be the result of the destruction of larger particles from particle size fraction of 0.25–1 mm.

The individual particle size subsamples reveal the features of the cities that may be related to the contribution of the studied types of technogenic particle to the city pollution. For example, the granulometric fraction of 0.25–1 mm in Tyumen contains about 10% of coal, which indicates the presence of local coal-fired boilers in addition to the main stationary gas-fired power plants in the city. Moreover, the residential neighborhoods with multi-story buildings in Tyumen are adjacent to low-rise wooden buildings, where heating is provided from coal combustion [51]. Tyumen also has approximately 8% of tire material in fraction of 0.25–1 mm, indicating a high number of cars per capita (higher than in other cities). In Murmansk, with a coal cargo port located within the city center, about 7% of coal is found in particle size fraction of 0.1–0.25 mm.

The elemental composition of technogenic particles is formed by different elements depending on the particle origin. Major elements may include the same elements that form the mineral component of the urban sediment: Si, Al, Ca, Fe, Mg, etc. [23]. However, each type of anthropogenic particle relates to some source of environmental pollution and to a related potentially harmful elements. In the current study, the granulometric subsamples were obtained after washing the samples with distilled water and, therefore, minor element content in the studied technogenic particles refers to trace elements rather than to material adsorbed on the particle surfaces. The accumulation of paint particles and colored plaster debris in the USDS contributes to the pollution of the urban environment with potentially toxic elements. The technogenic particles in the USDS samples tend to the formation of the geochemical anomalies in the urban area and increased concentrations of heavy metals in contemporary surface sediments.

The uncertainties in this study are related to the following factors:
- the errors of the operator in identifying the particle type;
- particle loss in particle size analysis under water washing and decantation;
- counting errors in the analysis of heavy mineral concentrate;
- the location of sampling sites in residential blocks far from roads, etc.

Taking into account the sources of uncertainty, the obtained results satisfactory characterize the anthropogenic component of the surface sediments in residential areas in large Russian cities.

The total amount of the USDS estimated for several Russian cities varies in the range from 1.8 to 3.2 kg/m^2 including approx. 65% of fraction >100 µm [23,24]. Thus, the amount of anthropogenic material in Russian cities varies from 0.21 to 0.37 kg/m^2. This result shows a quite large accumulation of technogenic material in the urban environment.

The preliminary analysis of microplastic particles in the USDS samples in Russian cities allowed the amount of microplastic particles <1 mm to be considered insignificant in this environmental compartment [28]. The results of the assessment of the number of microplastics are not presented in the current paper; however, further studies may use the methodological approaches represented in the paper to search for plastic microparticles and estimate their amount.

5. Conclusions

The combined approach was applied to assess the number of technogenic components in loose coarse sedimentary material in an urban environment. When determining the types of technogenic particle, the shape of the particles as well as their color and surface morphology are of great importance. The approach was based on the methods of quantitative and quantitative mineral, SEM-EDS, and environmental analysis. This approach can be implemented in other environmental studies for similar purposes.

The study of technogenic particles in the contemporary anthropogenic sediments allows important information about the sources of pollution to be obtained, especially about local non-point sources of pollution and their characteristics in an urban area. According to revealed quantitative indicators, it has been shown that the USDS in Russian cities contain a significant part of technogenic particles. Surveyed cities are differentiated by the amount and types of the technogenic particles preferably presented in the local USDS in residential area. Techogenic material may impact the transformation of typomorphic element associations in the urban environmental compartments. The trace elements found among the technogenic particles as impurities may change the microelement composition within the components of the urban sediment cascade.

Author Contributions: Conceptualization, methodology, formal analysis, data curation, writing—Original draft preparation, supervision, review and editing, visualization, project administration, funding acquisition, planning of laboratory analysis, A.S.; laboratory analysis, E.I.; field study, writing—Original draft preparation, review and editing, I.Y.; field study, review and editing, G.M. All authors have read and agreed to the published version of the manuscript.

Funding: The reported study was funded by Russian Science Foundation, project number № 18-77-10024.

Institutional Review Board Statement: Not applicable.

Informed Consent Statement: Not applicable.

Data Availability Statement: Not applicable.

Acknowledgments: The optical, mineral, and SEM-EDS analyses were conducted in the Common Use Center "Geoanalyst" in IGG UB RAS.

Conflicts of Interest: The authors declare no conflict of interest.

References

1. Yarmoshenko, I.; Malinovsky, G.; Baglaeva, E.; Seleznev, A. A Landscape Study of Sediment Formation and Transport in the Urban Environment. *Atmosphere* **2020**, *11*, 1320. [CrossRef]
2. Taylor, K. Urban environments. In *Environmental Sedimentology*; Perry, C., Taylor, K., Eds.; Wiley-Blackwell: Hoboken, NJ, USA, 2007; pp. 190–222.
3. Sevilla, A.; Rodríguez, M.L.; García-Maraver, Á.; Zamorano, M. An Index to Quantify Street Cleanliness: The Case of Granada (Spain). *Waste Manag.* **2013**, *33*, 1037–1046. [CrossRef] [PubMed]
4. Bartolozzi, I.; Baldereschi, E.; Daddi, T.; Iraldo, F. The Application of Life Cycle Assessment (LCA) in Municipal Solid Waste Management: A Comparative Study on Street Sweeping Services. *J. Clean. Prod.* **2018**, *182*, 455–465. [CrossRef]
5. Russell, K.L.; Vietz, G.J.; Fletcher, T.D. A Suburban Sediment Budget: Coarse-grained Sediment Flux through Hillslopes, Stormwater Systems and Streams. *Earth Surf. Process. Landf.* **2019**, *44*, 2600–2614. [CrossRef]
6. Polukarova, M.; Markiewicz, A.; Björklund, K.; Strömvall, A.-M.; Galfi, H.; AnderssonSköld, Y.; Gustafsson, M.; Järlskog, I.; Aronsson, M. Organic Pollutants, Nano- and Microparticles in Street Sweeping Road Dust and Washwater. *Environ. Int.* **2020**, *135*, 105377. [CrossRef] [PubMed]
7. Muthusamy, M.; Tait, S.; Schellart, A.; Beg, M.N.A.; Carvalho, R.F.; de Lima, J.L.M.P. Improving Understanding of the Underlying Physical Process of Sediment Wash-off from Urban Road Surfaces. *J. Hydrol.* **2018**, *557*, 426–433. [CrossRef]
8. Butler, D.; Davies, J.W. *Urban. Drainage*, 3rd ed.; Spon Press: London, UK, 2011.
9. Murakami, M.; Fujita, M.; Furumai, H.; Kasuga, I.; Kurisu, F. Sorption Behavior of Heavy Metal Species by Soakaway Sediment Receiving Urban Road Runoff from Residential and Heavily Trafficked Areas. *J. Hazard. Mater.* **2009**, *164*, 707–712. [CrossRef] [PubMed]
10. Grant, S. *A Review of the Contaminants and Toxicity Associated with Particles in Stormwater Runoff*; California Department of Transportation: Sacramento, CA, USA, 2015. [CrossRef]
11. Knox, E.G.; Bouchard, C.E.; Barrett, J.G.; Brown, R.B.; Huddleston, J.H.; Anderson, J.L. Erosion and Sedimentation in Urban Areas. *Agronomy Monographs* **2015**, 179–197. [CrossRef]
12. Hewett, C.J.M.; Simpson, C.; Wainwright, J.; Hudson, S. Communicating risks to infrastructure due to soil erosion: A bottom-up approach. *Land Degrad. Dev.* **2018**, *29*, 1282–1294. [CrossRef]
13. Vlasov, D.; Kasimov, N.; Eremina, I.; Shinkareva, G.; Chubarova, N. Partitioning and solubilities of metals and metalloids in spring rains in Moscow megacity. *Atmospheric Pollut. Res.* **2021**, *12*, 255–271. [CrossRef]
14. Volpov, E.; Kishcha, P. An advanced technique for outdoor insulation pollution mapping in the israel electric company power grid. *IEEE Trans. Dielectr. Electr. Insul.* **2017**, *24*, 3539–3548. [CrossRef]

15. Breault, R.F.; Smith, K.P.; Sorenson, J.R. Residential street-dirt accumulation rates and chemical composition, and removal efficiencies by mechanical-and vacuum-type sweepers, New Bedford, Massachusetts, 2003–2004. *Sci. Investig. Rep.* **2005**, *27*. [CrossRef]
16. Nawrot, N.; Wojciechowska, E.; Rezania, S.; Walkusz-Miotk, J.; Pazdro, K. The effects of urban vehicle traffic on heavy metal contamination in road sweeping waste and bottom sediments of retention tanks. *Sci. Total. Environ.* **2020**, *749*, 141511. [CrossRef] [PubMed]
17. Golokhvast, K.S.; Soboleva, E.V.; Borisovsky, A.O.; Khristoforova, N.K. Composition of atmospheric suspensions of Ussuriisk City according to snow pollution. In Proceedings of the 20th International Symposium on Atmospheric and Ocean Optics: Atmospheric Physics, Novosibirsk, Russia, 23–27 June 2014; Volume 9292, p. 929242.
18. Hwang, H.-M.; Fiala, M.J.; Park, D.; Wade, T.L. Review of pollutants in urban road dust and stormwater runoff: Part 1. Heavy metals released from vehicles. *Int. J. Urban. Sci.* **2016**, *20*, 334–360. [CrossRef]
19. Yu, B.; Lu, X.; Fan, X.; Fan, P.; Zuo, L.; Yang, Y.; Wang, L. Analyzing environmental risk, source and spatial distribution of potentially toxic elements in dust of residential area in Xi'an urban area, China. *Ecotoxicol. Environ. Saf.* **2021**, *208*, 111679. [CrossRef] [PubMed]
20. Chang, X.; Li, Y.-X. Lead distribution in urban street dust and the relationship with mining, gross domestic product GDP and transportation and health risk assessment. *Environ. Pollut.* **2020**, *262*, 114307. [CrossRef] [PubMed]
21. Lanzerstorfer, C. Heavy metals in the finest size fractions of road-deposited sediments. *Environ. Pollut.* **2018**, *239*, 522–531. [CrossRef]
22. Seleznev, A.A.; Yarmoshenko, I.V.; Malinovsky, G.P. Urban geochemical changes and pollution with potentially harmful elements in seven Russian cities. *Sci. Rep.* **2020**, *10*, 1–16. [CrossRef]
23. Seleznev, A.; Yarmoshenko, I.; Malinovsky, G.; Ilgasheva, E.; Baglaeva, E.; Ryanskaya, A.; Kiseleva, D.; Gulyaeva, T. Snow-dirt sludge as an indicator of environmental and sedimentation processes in the urban environment. *Sci. Rep.* **2019**, *9*, 1–12. [CrossRef]
24. Seleznev, A.A.; Yarmoshenko, I.V.; Malinovsky, G.P. Assessment of Total Amount of Surface Sediment in Urban Environment Using Data on Solid Matter Content in Snow-Dirt Sludge. *Environ. Process.* **2019**, *6*, 581–595. [CrossRef]
25. Seleznev, A.A.; Yarmoshenko, I.V. Study of urban puddle sediments for understanding heavy metal pollution in an urban environment. *Environ. Technol. Innov.* **2014**, *1–2*, 1–7. [CrossRef]
26. Gunawardana, C.; Goonetilleke, A.; Egodawatta, P.; Dawes, L.; Kokot, S. Source characterisation of road dust based on chemical and mineralogical composition. *Chemosphere* **2012**, *87*, 163–170. [CrossRef] [PubMed]
27. Magiera, T.; Górka-Kostrubiec, B.; Szumiata, T.; Wawer, M. Technogenic magnetic particles from steel metallurgy and iron mining in topsoil: Indicative characteristic by magnetic parameters and Mössbauer spectra. *Sci. Total. Environ.* **2021**, *775*, 145605. [CrossRef] [PubMed]
28. Seleznev, A.; Pankrushina, E.; Ilgasheva, E. Do the contemporary urban surface sediments contain particles of microplastic? In Proceedings of the VII International Young Researchers' Conference Physics, Technology, Innovations (PTI-2020), Ekaterinburg, Russia, 8–22 May 2020; Volume 2313, p. 060040.
29. Hui, N.; Parajuli, A.; Puhakka, R.; Grönroos, M.; Roslund, M.I.; Vari, H.K.; Selonen, V.A.; Yan, G.; Siter, N.; Nurminen, N.; et al. Temporal variation in indoor transfer of dirt-associated environmental bacteria in agricultural and urban areas. *Environ. Int.* **2019**, *132*, 105069. [CrossRef]
30. Bućko, M.S.; Mattila, O.-P.; Chrobak, A.; Ziółkowski, G.; Johanson, B.; Čuda, J.; Filip, J.; Zbořil, R.; Pesonen, L.J.; Leppäranta, M. Distribution of magnetic particulates in a roadside snowpack based on magnetic, microstructural and mineralogical analyses. *Geophys. J. Int.* **2013**, *195*, 159–175. [CrossRef]
31. Pant, P.; Harrison, R.M. Estimation of the contribution of road traffic emissions to particulate matter concentrations from field measurements: A review. *Atmos. Environ.* **2013**, *77*, 78–97. [CrossRef]
32. Chen, L.-W.A.; Watson, J.G.; Chow, J.C.; Green, M.C.; Inouye, D.; Dick, K. Wintertime particulate pollution episodes in an urban valley of the Western US: A case study. *Atmos. Chem. Phys. Discuss.* **2012**, *12*, 10051–10064. [CrossRef]
33. Lim, S.S.; Vos, T.; Flaxman, A.D.; Danaei, G.; Shibuya, K.; Adair-Rohani, H.; A AlMazroa, M.; Amann, M.; Anderson, H.R.; Andrews, K.G.; et al. A comparative risk assessment of burden of disease and injury attributable to 67 risk factors and risk factor clusters in 21 regions, 1990–2010: A systematic analysis for the Global Burden of Disease Study 2010. *Lancet* **2012**, *380*, 2224–2260. [CrossRef]
34. Shi, X.; Jungwirth, S.; Akin, M.; Wright, R.; Fay, L.; Veneziano, D.A.; Zhang, Y.; Gong, J.; Ye, Z. Evaluating Snow and Ice Control Chemicals for Environmentally Sustainable Highway Maintenance Operations. *J. Transp. Eng.* **2014**, *140*, 05014005. [CrossRef]
35. Unice, K.M.; Kreider, M.L.; Panko, J.M.; Unice, K. Comparison of Tire and Road Wear Particle Concentrations in Sediment for Watersheds in France, Japan, and the United States by Quantitative Pyrolysis GC/MS Analysis. *Environ. Sci. Technol.* **2013**, 130710100101002. [CrossRef]
36. Knox, E.G.; Bouchard, C.E.; Barrett, J.G. Erosion and Sedimentation in Urban Areas. In *Agronomy Monographs*; American Society of Agronomy; Crop Science Society of America; Soil Science Society of America: Madison, WI, USA, 2015; pp. 179–197.
37. Taylor, K.G.; Owens, P. Sediments in urban river basins: A review of sediment–contaminant dynamics in an environmental system conditioned by human activities. *J. Soils Sediments* **2009**, *9*, 281–303. [CrossRef]

38. Piazzolla, D.; Cafaro, V.; de Lucia, G.A.; Mancini, E.; Scanu, S.; Bonamano, S.; Piermattei, V.; Vianello, A.; Della Ventura, G.; Marcelli, M. Microlitter pollution in coastal sediments of the northern Tyrrhenian Sea, Italy: Microplastics and fly-ash occurrence and distribution. *Estuarine Coast. Shelf Sci.* **2020**, *241*, 106819. [CrossRef]
39. Blair, R.M.; Waldron, S.; Phoenix, V.R.; Gauchotte-Lindsay, C. Microscopy and elemental analysis characterisation of microplastics in sediment of a freshwater urban river in Scotland, UK. *Environ. Sci. Pollut. Res.* **2019**, *26*, 12491–12504. [CrossRef] [PubMed]
40. Walraven, N.; van Os, B.; Klaver, G.; Middelburg, J.; Davies, G. The lead (Pb) isotope signature, behaviour and fate of traffic-related lead pollution in roadside soils in The Netherlands. *Sci. Total. Environ.* **2014**, *472*, 888–900. [CrossRef]
41. Adamiec, E.; Wieszała, R.; Strzebońska, M.; Jarosz-Krzemińska, E. An attempt to identify traffic related elements in snow. *Geol. Geophys. Environ.* **2013**, *39*, 317. [CrossRef]
42. Apeagyei, E.; Bank, M.S.; Spengler, J.D. Distribution of heavy metals in road dust along an urban-rural gradient in Massachusetts. *Atmos. Environ.* **2011**, *45*, 2310–2323. [CrossRef]
43. Chen, L.; Zhi, X.; Shen, Z.; Dai, Y.; Aini, G. Comparison between snowmelt-runoff and rainfall-runoff nonpoint source pollution in a typical urban catchment in Beijing, China. *Environ. Sci. Pollut. Res.* **2017**, *25*, 2377–2388. [CrossRef]
44. Anshits, N.N.; Fedorchak, M.A.; Fomenko, E.V.; Mazurova, E.V.; Anshits, A.G. Composition, Structure, and Formation Routes of Blocklike Ferrospheres Separated from Coal and Lignite Fly Ashes. *Energy Fuels* **2020**, *34*, 3743–3754. [CrossRef]
45. Danish, A.; Mosaberpanah, M.A. Formation mechanism and applications of cenospheres: A review. *J. Mater. Sci.* **2020**, *55*, 4539–4557. [CrossRef]
46. Seleznev, A.; Rudakov, M. some geochemical characteristics of puddle sediments from cities located in various geological, geographic, climatic and industrial zones. *Carpathian J. Earth Environ. Sci.* **2018**, *14*, 95–106. [CrossRef]
47. State Geological Map of Russia. Available online: http://vsegei.com/ru/info/ggk/ (accessed on 2 May 2021).
48. Matschullat, J.; Ottenstein, R.; Reimann, C. Geochemical background-can we calculate it? *Environ. Earth Sci.* **2000**, *39*, 990–1000. [CrossRef]
49. Reimann, C.; Garrett, R.G. Geochemical background—concept and reality. *Sci. Total. Environ.* **2005**, *350*, 12–27. [CrossRef]
50. Reimann, C.; Filzmoser, P.; Garrett, R.G. Background and threshold: Critical comparison of methods of determination. *Sci. Total Environ.* **2005**, *346*, 1–16. [CrossRef]
51. Yarmoshenko, I.; Malinovsky, G.; Vasilyev, A.; Onischenko, A.; Seleznev, A. Geogenic and anthropogenic impacts on indoor radon in the Techa River region. *Sci. Total. Environ.* **2016**, *571*, 1298–1303. [CrossRef]

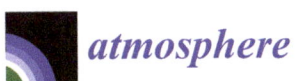

Article

Source Analysis and Human Health Risk Assessment Based on Entropy Weight Method Modification of PM$_{2.5}$ Heavy Metal in an Industrial Area in the Northeast of China

Siyu Sun [1], Na Zheng [1,2,*], Sujing Wang [1], Yunyang Li [2,3], Shengnan Hou [2,3], Xue Song [2], Shanshan Du [1], Qirui An [1], Pengyang Li [1], Xiaoqian Li [1], Xiuyi Hua [1] and Deming Dong [1]

[1] Key Laboratory of Groundwater Resources and Environment of the Ministry of Education, College of New Energy and Environment, Jilin University, Changchun 130012, China; ssy19@mails.jlu.edu.cn (S.S.); sjw20@mails.jlu.edu.cn (S.W.); Dss18@mails.jlu.edu.cn (S.D.); anqr19@mails.jlu.edu.cn (Q.A.); pyli19@mails.jlu.edu.cn (P.L.); xqli20@mails.jlu.edu.cn (X.L.); huaxy@jlu.edu.cn (X.H.); dmdong@jlu.edu.cn (D.D.)

[2] Northeast Institute of Geography and Agricultural Ecology, Chinese Academy of Sciences, Changchun 130102, China; liyunyang@iga.ac.cn (Y.L.); houshengnan@iga.ac.cn (S.H.); songxue0608@163.com (X.S.)

[3] Graduate University of Chinese Academy of Sciences, Beijing 100049, China

* Correspondence: zhengnalzz@neigae.ac.cn or zhengnalzz@jlu.edu.cn; Tel.: +86-431-85542265; Fax: +86-431-85542298

Citation: Sun, S.; Zheng, N.; Wang, S.; Li, Y.; Hou, S.; Song, X.; Du, S.; An, Q.; Li, P.; Li, X.; et al. Source Analysis and Human Health Risk Assessment Based on Entropy Weight Method Modification of PM$_{2.5}$ Heavy Metal in an Industrial Area in the Northeast of China. *Atmosphere* **2021**, *12*, 852. https://doi.org/10.3390/atmos12070852

Academic Editors: Ashok Luhar, Omar Ramírez Hernández and Dmitry Vlasov

Received: 26 May 2021
Accepted: 28 June 2021
Published: 30 June 2021

Publisher's Note: MDPI stays neutral with regard to jurisdictional claims in published maps and institutional affiliations.

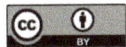

Copyright: © 2021 by the authors. Licensee MDPI, Basel, Switzerland. This article is an open access article distributed under the terms and conditions of the Creative Commons Attribution (CC BY) license (https://creativecommons.org/licenses/by/4.0/).

Abstract: In this study, PM$_{2.5}$ was analyzed for heavy metals at two sites in industrial northeast China to determine their sources and human health risks during heating and non-heating periods. A positive matrix factorization (PMF) model determined sources, and US Environmental Protection Agency (USEPA) and entropy weight methods were used to assess human health risk. PM$_{2.5}$ heavy metal concentrations were higher in the heating period than in the non-heating period. In the heating period, coal combustion (59.64%) was the primary heavy metal source at Huagong Hospitals, and the contribution rates of industrial emissions and traffic emissions were 21.06% and 19.30%, respectively. Industrial emissions (42.14%) were the primary source at Xinqu Park, and the contribution rates of coal combustion and traffic emissions were 34.03% and 23.83%, respectively. During the non-heating period, coal combustion (45.29%) and industrial emissions 45.29% and 44.59%, respectively, were the primary sources at Huagong Hospital, and the traffic emissions were 10.12%. Industrial emissions (43.64%) were the primary sources at Xinqu Park, where the coal combustion and traffic emissions were 25.35% and 31.00%, respectively. In the heating period, PM$_{2.5}$ heavy metals at Xinqu Park had noncarcinogenic and carcinogenic risks, and the hazard index of children (5.74) was higher than that of adult males (5.28) and females (4.49). However, adult males and females had the highest lifetime carcinogenic risk (1.38×10^{-3} and 1.17×10^{-3}) than children (3.00×10^{-4}). The traditional USEPA and entropy weight methods both produced reasonable results. However, when there is a difference between the two methods, the entropy weight method is recommended to assess noncarcinogenic health risks.

Keywords: particulate matter; source apportionment analysis; health risk assessment; Huludao

1. Introduction

According to the latest results of the Global Burden of Disease Study, particulate matter (PM) has become the sixth leading cause of death [1,2], and air pollution is responsible for 1.5% of the total mortality worldwide [3]. Many epidemiological studies demonstrate that when inhaled and deposited in the lungs, PM$_{2.5}$ (particle diameter less than 2.5 μm) can cause respiratory and cardiovascular disease in humans [4–6]. Thus, exposure to high concentrations of PM$_{2.5}$ leads to increases in morbidity and mortality. There are many sources of PM$_{2.5}$, including industrial emissions, coal combustion, traffic emissions, rocks, and soil weathering [7–9]. The contributions to $PM_{2.5}$ from different sources depend on geographic location, climatic conditions, economic structure, and populations [10,11]. When industrial production is reduced, $PM_{2.5}$ pollution is also reduced in many cities in China. However, industrial emissions and associated $PM_{2.5}$ levels remain a cause for concern in China [10]. The increased burning of coal and biomass in the winter, particularly in northern China, is the main source of $PM_{2.5}$ [12,13], in contrast to southern China [14,15]. In industrial cities in northern China, the dual effects of emissions from industry and coal combustion need to be monitored and evaluated. Heavy metals in $PM_{2.5}$ can harm multiple human physiological systems and organs, and therefore, effects on human health are a concern [16–18]. Moreover, the characteristics of heavy metals in atmospheric particulates vary depending on the source [19–21]. Studies have shown that the concentration of $PM_{2.5}$ in Zibo, which is dominated by petrochemical industry, is relatively high in the spring, with K^+ and Mg^{2+} mainly representing the source of fugitive dust; in winter, the concentration of F^- and NO_3^- is relatively high, which represents coal burning; Cd and Ni, the elements of industrial emissions, do not change significantly throughout the year; research on industrial cities such as Baoding and the plateau city of Kunming also shows that the concentration of As and Hg, the elements of coal combustion, is higher in winter; Cd and Pb produced by zinc smelting are important sources of pollution in Huludao City [8,22–24].

To assess the impact of $PM_{2.5}$ on human health, the human health risk assessment method of the US Environmental Protection Agency (USEPA) is often selected [25–29]. Most analyses of $PM_{2.5}$ sources and human health risk assessment calculate human health risk without considering the effects of different sources, and the default parameters of models assume that factors do not interact or that interactions can be ignored [27,30,31]. However, because of factors such as humidity, wind speed and direction, temperature, and human activity, there may be different combinations of pollution sources with different levels of contribution and concentrations [32]. The USEPA method can be improved by coupling the source of the pollution analysis model with the human health risk assessment model; however, such models only analyze data for a specific time [33], and there is no approach for comprehensive analysis of long time series data. Heavy metals may bioaccumulate, and animal models indicate that the concentrations of heavy metals and the extent of their effects are nonlinear [34]. Moreover, the cellular toxicity of multiple heavy metals is not merely the sum of the toxicity of single heavy metals, and combinations of different heavy metals can produce synergistic or antagonistic effects [35,36]. Therefore, the health risks of different heavy metals to a population should not be simply determined by the addition of effects. To determine the effects of different combinations of pollution sources on human health risk in a long time series, the possible compound effects of multiple heavy metals on human health need to be considered. In this article, multiple heavy metals were regarded as a system, and the entropy weight method was introduced to supplement human health risk assessment.

Entropy was proposed by the German physicist Clausius to describe random thermal motion in thermodynamics [37]. Thereafter, Boltzmann developed entropy theory and applied it to information theory, in which entropy is defined as a random variable [37] and the acquisition of entropy indicates a loss of information. Therefore, with an increase in the entropy value, less information is provided by a factor, and it is less important in a comprehensive evaluation [38]. To reduce the uncertainty of factors in an evaluation model, the information entropy model was established, which calculates a factor's entropy weight [37,39]. The biggest advantage of the entropy method is to use the data itself to calculate the weight index instead of human factors, thereby improving the objectivity of the comprehensive evaluation results [40]. The entropy weight method has been validated in many types of assessments, including environmental pollution assessment, vulnerability distribution in coastal aquifers, ecological risk assessment, and comprehensive water quality assessment [39,41,42]. In such studies, the weightings between the indicators in the index and the weightings of the subsystems in the evaluation system are applied reasonably, demonstrating the suitability of the weighting method in evaluation systems. Thus, this approach should also be applicable to human health risk assessment of atmospheric PM.

To assess heavy metal pollution in Huludao City, Liaoning Province, China, environmental pollution study has focused on soils, indoor and outdoor dust, sediments, fresh water, insects, and food, and has included heavy metal accumulation, distribution, and degree of pollution, as well as human health risk assessment [22,43–46]. In this research, the concentrations of heavy metals in atmospheric $PM_{2.5}$ were determined, and the health risks were assessed at two sites in Huludao City. To assess human health risk, the entropy weight method was compared with the traditional USEPA method. The objectives of the study were the following: (1) to identify changes in $PM_{2.5}$ and the heavy metal concentrations during heating and non-heating periods; (2) to determine the main sources of heavy metals and their contributions in the different periods; (3) to assess the human health risks of heavy metals in $PM_{2.5}$ (carcinogenic and noncarcinogenic risks); and (4) to compare different methods that estimate the human health risk over the long-term.

2. Materials and Methods

2.1. Study Area

The research was conducted at two sites in Huludao City, an industrial city in northeast China. The city is in the southwestern part of Liaoning Province adjacent to the Liaodong Gulf of the Bohai Sea (Figure 1). The region has a north temperate continental monsoon climate. The west monsoon is dominant in winter, and the east monsoon prevails in summer. The average annual wind speed is 3 m/s. The main industries in Huludao City are petrochemicals, nonferrous metals, mechanical shipbuilding, and energy and power. The city has the largest zinc smelter in Asia, the Huludao Zinc Plant (HZP). As a result of the smelting operations, heavy metals are discharged into the environment and pollute the atmosphere, soil, and rivers [22,43]. Industrial activities and coal combustion are responsible for an approximate twofold increase in pollution in the study area. One sampling site was at Huagong Hospital, which is in the Lianshan District of Huludao City. Metal mining is the main industry in the region, and the city has a large proportion of secondary and tertiary industries. The other sampling site was at Xinqu Park, which is in the Longgang District of Huludao City. The forested land in this area accounted for 50.6% of the total land area, and it is a relatively new urban area dominated by secondary and tertiary industries.

2.2. Sample Collection and Preparation

The distribution of sampling sites is shown in Figure 1. At the Huagong Hospital site, the $PM_{2.5}$ mass concentrations and the atmospheric particle samples were collected and measured continuously using an atmospheric particulate monitor (APM; Dasibi 7201, Beijing Zhongshengtyco Environmental Science and Technology Development Co. Ltd., Beijing, China). The duration of sample collection was 1 h, and the airflow was 16.7 L min^{-1}. At the Xinqu Park site, the $PM_{2.5}$ mass concentrations and the atmospheric particulate samples were collected separately by using two APM systems (i-5030 and i-FH62C14, Thermo Fisher, Franklin, MA, USA). The duration for both sample collections was 6 h, and the airflow was 16.7 L min^{-1}. The $PM_{2.5}$ was sampled in the study areas from April 2015 to March 2016. According to the "Huludao City Heating Management Measures" (2011), November to March is the heating period, and April to October is the non-heating period [47]. The $PM_{2.5}$ was sampled at two points in both Huagong Hospital and Xinqu Park, and a total of 96 valid samples were collected.

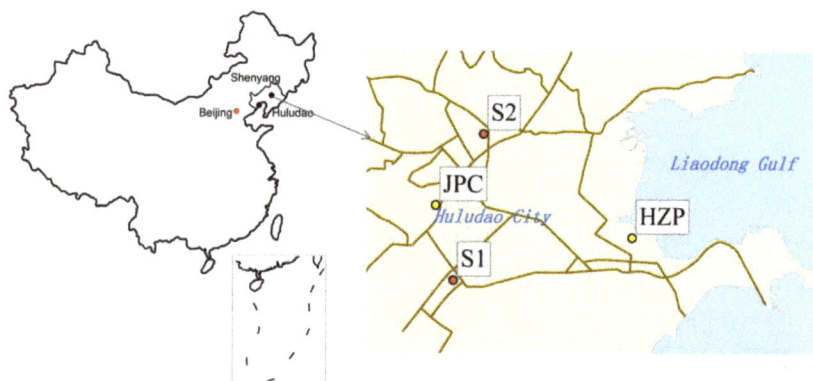

Figure 1. Study area. S1: Xinqu Park sampling area; S2: Huagong Hospital sampling area.

2.3. Chemical Analyses

The $PM_{2.5}$ samples were collected on 47 mm diameter quartz fiber filters. A sample was weighed after constant temperature (25 °C) and relative humidity (30%) for 24 h, the filter membrane was cut in half and transferred to a Teflon digestion vessel. Then, HNO_3, HF, and $HClO_4$ (1:1:5) were added to the vessel. The sample mixture was heated for 3 h at 200 °C [48]. After digestion, the sample was cooled to room temperature, and the solution was quantitatively transferred to a 50 mL volumetric flask, which was filled to the mark. The sample digests were analyzed using inductively coupled plasma mass spectrometry (Thermo Fisher, Germany) to determine the concentrations of nickel (Ni), cadmium (Cd), lead (Pb), copper (Cu), and arsenic (As) on the filters [31].

For quality assurance/quality control, 10 blank filters and river sediment standard (Fluvial sediments: GBW08301) were digested and analyzed as described above to determine heavy metal detection limits and recovery rates. The average concentrations in the blank filters were the following (µg m^{-3}): 0.021 ± 0.006 Ni; 0.088 ± 0.006 Cu; 0.249 ± 0.034 As; 0.003 ± 0.002 Cd; and 0.037 ± 0.020 Pb. The detection limits were the following (µg m^{-3}): 0.016 Ni, 0.018 Cu, 0.098 As, 0.006 Cd, and 0.057 Pb. According to the river sediment tests, the average recovery rates of heavy metals ranged from 89.83% to 115.15%. The calculated values of the atmospheric $PM_{2.5}$ samples used in this article were obtained by subtracting the blank filter value from the test value.

2.4. Positive Matrix Factorization Model (PMF)

A positive matrix factorization (PMF) model allocates sources based on internal correlation of the data and determines the main contributing factors according to the size of the contribution and the actual local conditions [19,49]. The eigenvalues of each component are analyzed, and the source type represented by each factor is determined [19,49]. The PMF model has been widely used in the analysis of sources of heavy metals, aerosols, and organic matter in atmospheric PM and has performed well in separating different combustion sources [19,20,50]. The goal of PMF is to solve the chemical mass balance between the measured species concentrations and the source profiles [19,49]. In addition, minimization of the objective function of the PMF model enables derivation of the factor contributions and the profiles. The species method-specific limit of detection limit (MDL) is calculated to determine the uncertainty of an element [50–52]. In this study, the PMF model used 96 samples as the input items. For the model, the MDL was 2.82 times the standard deviation of the 10 blank filters. The uncertainty was calculated according to Equations (1) and (2). When the concentration was lower than the MDL, Equation (1) was used to calculate the uncertainty, and when the concentration was higher than the MDL, Equation (2) was used, with the error function the relative standard deviation. According to the PMF5.0 user guide, a signal-to-noise ratio lower than 0.5 is defined as "Bad", a ratio higher than 0.5 and lower than 1 is "Weak", and a ratio higher than 1 is "Strong". According to the running result of the model objective function, the residual result between −3 and +3 was selected, and the minimum objective function was the output result [53,54].

$$Unc = \frac{5}{6} \times MDL \quad (1)$$

$$Unc = \sqrt{(Error\ Fraction \times concentration)^2 + (0.5 \times MDL)^2} \quad (2)$$

2.5. Health Risk Assessment

Heavy metals are readily accumulated in human organs such as the liver and kidney and are difficult to degrade and excrete from the body [55]. Heavy metals in atmospheric particulates will enter the human body via respiration, skin absorption, and oral intake, and pose risks to human health [56,57]. Currently, the USEPA's human health risk assessment model is widely used to estimate heavy metal exposure levels. The model is based on the exposure mode, exposure time, concentration factor, and the average daily inhaled dose of non-carcinogenic metal (ADD_{inh}, mg·kg^{-1}·day^{-1}) and the average daily inhaled dose of metal carcinogen for lifetime exposure ($LADD_{inh}$, mg·kg^{-1}·day^{-1}) in order to calculate the risk index for the human health, as given by Equations (3)–(5) [29,58]. In this study, a risk assessment for heavy metal (Ni, Cu, As, Cd, and Pb) exposure based on intake of PM$_{2.5}$ was carried out. The metals were divided into two categories, in which all the heavy metals were considered non-carcinogenic, and Ni, As, and Cd were considered carcinogenic [59].

The basic statistical data and abbreviations used in the study are as follows:

$$ADD_{inh\ i}(LADD_{inh\ i}) = C \times \frac{InhR \times EF \times ED}{BW \times AT_n(AT_c)} \quad (3)$$

C: concentration of heavy metals in PM$_{2.5}$, mg/m^3. *InhR*: inhalation rate, 19.20 m^3/day for adult males, 14.17 m^3/day for adult females, 5.00 m^3/day for children [29,58]. *EF*: exposure frequency, 350 day/year in this study [56]. *ED*: exposure duration, 30 years for adults, and 6 years for children [29,58]. *BW*: average body weight, 62.70 kg for adult males, 54.40 kg for adult females, 15.00 kg for children [30,60]. ATn: averaging time for non-carcinogens, $ED \times 365$ days [30,60]. ATc: averaging time for carcinogens, 70×365 days [29,58]. Age of children, 0–16 years; adults, 17–70 years [56].

The hazard quotient (*HQ*) represents the risk due to non-carcinogens, and the incremental lifetime cancer risk (*ILCR*) for carcinogens was calculated using the following equations [22,29,56,58]:

$$HQ_i = \frac{ADD_{inh\ i}}{RfD_i} \quad (4)$$

$$ILCR_i = LADD_{inh\ i} \times CSF_i \quad (5)$$

RfD: reference dose; Ni 2.00×10^{-2} mg·kg^{-1}·day^{-1}; Cu 4.00×10^{-2} mg·kg^{-1}·day^{-1}; As 3.00×10^{-4} mg·kg^{-1}·day^{-1}; Cd 1.00×10^{-3} mg·kg^{-1}·day^{-1}; Pb 3.50×10^{-3} mg·kg^{-1}·day^{-1} [29,58]. *CSF*: carcinogens slope factor; Ni 0.84 mg·kg^{-1}·day^{-1}; As 1.51 mg·kg^{-1}·day^{-1}; Cd 6.30 mg·kg^{-1}·day^{-1} [29,58].

As in previous studies [8,29,54], and without considering the interaction between heavy metals, the hazard index (*HI*) was calculated by superimposing the HQ value of each heavy metal, and the *ILCR*$_{total}$ was calculated by superimposing the ILCR value of each heavy metal, as shown in Equations (6) and (7).

$$HI = \sum_i HQ_i \quad (6)$$

$$ILCR_{total} = \sum_i ILCR_i \quad (7)$$

The human health risk index, however, calculated by the above method does not take into account the impact of different pollution sources. Although the ME2 model can also calculate health risks from different sources, it does not consider the long-term effects of the factors on the population, especially heavy metal pollutants [33,61]. Therefore, this study introduces the entropy weight method into the human health risk assessment to evaluate the impact of factors which pose a long-term effect. First, we establish relevant feature matrices based on the samples and the evaluation parameters:

$$A = \begin{bmatrix} a_{11} & a_{12} & \cdots & a_{1n} \\ a_{21} & a_{22} & \cdots & a_{2n} \\ \vdots & \vdots & \vdots & \vdots \\ a_{m1} & a_{m2} & \cdots & a_{mn} \end{bmatrix} \quad (8)$$

where A represents the relevant feature matrices, m is the number of considered features (in this paper m is the number of heavy metals), and n is the number of samples [39,62]. The parameter index amount, j, in sample i is subsequently (y_{ij}) calculated by Equation (9); the information entropy (H_i) is calculated by Equation (10); and the entropy weight, E_i, is calculated by Equation (11) [62].

$$y_{ij} = a_{ij} / \sum_{i=1}^{m} a_{ij} \quad i = 1, 2, \cdots, m; j = 1, 2, \cdots, n. \quad (9)$$

$$H_i = -\frac{1}{\ln n} \sum_{j=1}^{n} y_{ij} \ln y_{ij} \quad i = 1, 2, \cdots, m; j = 1, 2, \cdots, n \quad (10)$$

$$E_i = \frac{1 - H_i}{m - \sum_{i=1}^{m} H_i} i = 1, 2, \cdots, m. \quad (11)$$

To show the impact of different pollution sources on the human health risk, the entropy weight method was used to calculate the weight value of the HQ value and the ILCR for each heavy metal, and the weighted correction of the HI' value and the $ILCR_{total}$' for human health risk, as shown in Equations (12) and (13):

$$HI' = \sum_i HQ_i \cdot E_i \quad (12)$$

$$ILCR'_{total} = \sum_i ILCR_i \cdot E_i \quad (13)$$

where E_i represents the weight of different heavy metal HQ values or ILCR values in the method for calculation (see Equations (9)–(11)). If HQ and HI exceed 1 or if ILCR and $ILCR_{total}$ exceed 10^{-4}, then there is a chance that non-carcinogenic or carcinogenic effects might occur. If the ILCR and $ILCR_{total}$ values exceed 10^{-6}, but do not exceed 10^{-4}, there is a potential carcinogenic risk for the heavy metals [22,55].

2.6. Data Analysis

SPSS Statistics 25 was used for statistical analysis and Origin 2017 for plotting. Excel in office 2016 calculates the coefficient of variation (CV).

3. Results and Discussion

3.1. Particulate Matter Concentrations

The average $PM_{2.5}$ concentrations were 45.31 µg m^{-3} in Xinqu Park and 57.36 µg m^{-3} in Huagong Hospital. The concentrations were higher during the heating period (62.63 µg m^{-3} in Xinqu Park; 68.36 µg m^{-3} in Huagong Hospital) than in the non-heating period (33.91 µg m^{-3} in Xinqu Park; 52.05 µg m^{-3} in Huagong Hospital). This finding is consistent with the results of several studies [48,63]. The concentrations in the study area were relatively low compared with those in Beijing (89.60 to 196.3 µg m^{-3}) [48], Shanghai (103.1 µg m^{-3}) [63], and other large cities.

In addition, the concentrations in Chengdu (41.45 to 115.4 µg m^{-3}) [64], a city of greater size and population density than Huludao, were generally higher. The highest PM$_{2.5}$ concentrations in Huludao were similar to those in the tourist city of Tai'an (63.00 µg m^{-3}) [65] but were lower than those in the industrial city of Zhuzhou (81.00 to 201.3 µg m^{-3}) [27]. Existing studies have shown that only considering the level of social and economic development, when the share of urban secondary industry is low, PM$_{2.5}$ pollution is lighter, and the polycentric and scattered population distribution will increase the concentration of PM$_{2.5}$ in Chinese cities [10,11].

The concentration of PM$_{2.5}$ at Huagong Hospital was higher than that at Xinqu Park. However, the PM$_{2.5}$ concentration (33.91 µg m^{-3}) at Xinqu Park only met the ambient air quality standards (35.00 µg m^{-3}) during the non-heating period. High concentrations of PM$_{2.5}$ may increase human health risks [60]. A nonparametric test indicated the PM$_{2.5}$ concentration in Huagong Hospital and Xinqu Park was significantly different ($p < 0.05$). The concentration was also significantly different between the two sampling sites during the heating and the non-heating periods ($p < 0.05$). These results indicated that the main sources of PM$_{2.5}$ at the two sampling sites were different. This difference might be because Xinqu Park is downwind of the HZP, whereas Huagong Hospital is in the old part of the city northwest of the HZP and is relatively less affected by plant emissions.

3.2. Heavy Metal Content of PM$_{2.5}$

Figure 2 shows heavy metal concentrations in PM$_{2.5}$ in the study area. Except for As and Pb at Huagong Hospital, the concentration of heavy metals in the heating period was higher than that in the non-heating period. The concentration of heavy metals in PM$_{2.5}$ at Xinqu Park was higher than that at Huagong Hospital during the heating period, and the concentrations of Ni and Cd at Xinqu Park were higher than those at Huagong Hospital during the non-heating period. Differences in the locations and sources of the two sampling sites might have affected the concentrations of heavy metals. In previous studies, the concentration of heavy metals is highest in winter and lowest in summer [13,64]. The heavy metal content of PM$_{2.5}$ in the industrial city of Changzhou in southern China in autumn and winter was higher than that in the present study. In Changzhou, traffic and industrial emissions are the main sources of pollution, with coal combustion sources the smallest contributor [30]. By contrast, in Chifeng City in northern China, the main sources of heavy metal pollution are coal combustion and vehicle emissions [66]. The heavy metal concentrations of PM$_{2.5}$ in Chifeng City are slightly lower than those in the present study, and the highest concentrations occur in winter and the lowest concentrations occur in summer [66].

Nonparametric tests on the heavy metal concentrations in the different sampling periods detected differences between heavy metals ($p < 0.05$), suggesting there were multiple sources of heavy metals. During the heating period, the concentrations of As, Pb, and Cu were relatively high. Arsenic is an important indicator of coal combustion, and Pb is an important pollutant from zinc smelting and may also be a product of coal combustion [64,67]. Therefore, during the heating period, heavy metal concentrations in PM$_{2.5}$ might be most affected by coal combustion and industrial production. In the non-heating period, the concentrations of As, Pb, and Cu were higher at Huagong Hospital than at Xinqu Park, whereas the concentrations of Ni and Pb were higher at Xinqu Park than at Huagong Hospital. Nickel is primarily derived from the burning of fossil fuels, the wear of auto parts, and ship emissions [64,67,68]. Therefore, during the non-heating period, the differences in the concentrations of heavy metals between the two sampling points might be due to the different locations and sources.

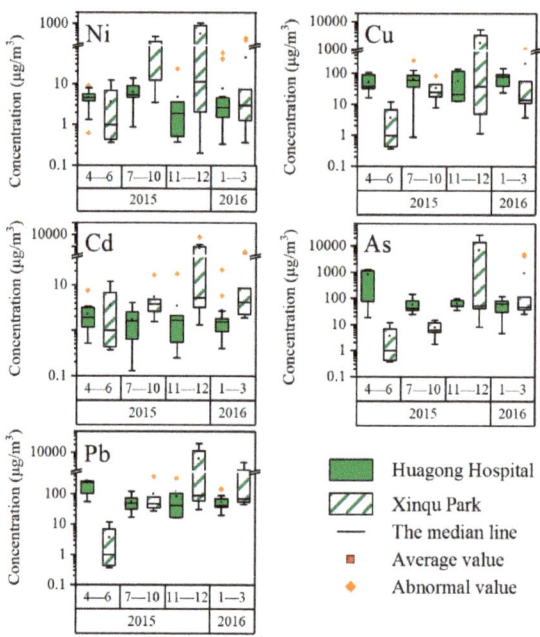

Figure 2. Heavy metal concentrations of PM$_{2.5}$ in Huagong Hospital and Xinqu Park. Note: (**a**) represents April to June; (**b**) represents July to September; (**c**) represents October to De-cember; (**d**) represents January to March.

3.3. Source Apportionment Analysis

3.3.1. Identification of Factors

The USEPA PMF5.0 model was used to classify the sources of heavy metals in PM$_{2.5}$ at Huagong Hospital and Xinqu Park. Figure 3 shows the major air pollution sources and their contributions. The first factor had high concentrations of As (44.30–84.53%), Pb (36.61–47.86%), and Cd (6.50–66.20%). Many studies show that As and Pb are important indicators of coal combustion, especially As [64,69,70]. The combustion of coal also releases many trace elements, including Pb and Cd [58,71], and thus, those metals in PM$_{2.5}$ indicated that coal combustion might be the source. The second factor had high concentrations of Cd (22.53–57.46%), Pb (33.95–50.60%), and Cu (13.87–74.23%). The metals Cd, Cu, and Pb are typically associated with smelting and nonferrous metal industries [64,72–74], Cd and Pb are important pollution signs in zinc smelting [40–42], and therefore, the emission signature was attributed to industrial emissions. The third factor had relatively high concentrations of Ni (12.41–79.05%), Cd (11.27–36.04%), and Pb (12.79–22.62%). Nickel is primarily derived from the combustion of fossil fuels but is also an important indicator of ship emissions and is closely linked with road dust derived from worn vehicle components (e.g., brake linings and tire wear) and vehicle exhaust (oil, diesel combustion) [66,68,75]. The study area is adjacent to Liaodong Bay, and ship emissions might be a source of heavy metals in PM$_{2.5}$, which were classified as traffic emissions. In this article, the traffic emissions are the total emissions generated by vehicle and ship emissions. The study area is in northeast China and is a typical metallurgical processing area. The HZP produces 3.3×10^5 tonnes of zinc per year, as well as Cd [46] and a variety of heavy metals [76]. Thus, industrial emissions and coal combustion were the main sources of PM$_{2.5}$ in the study area.

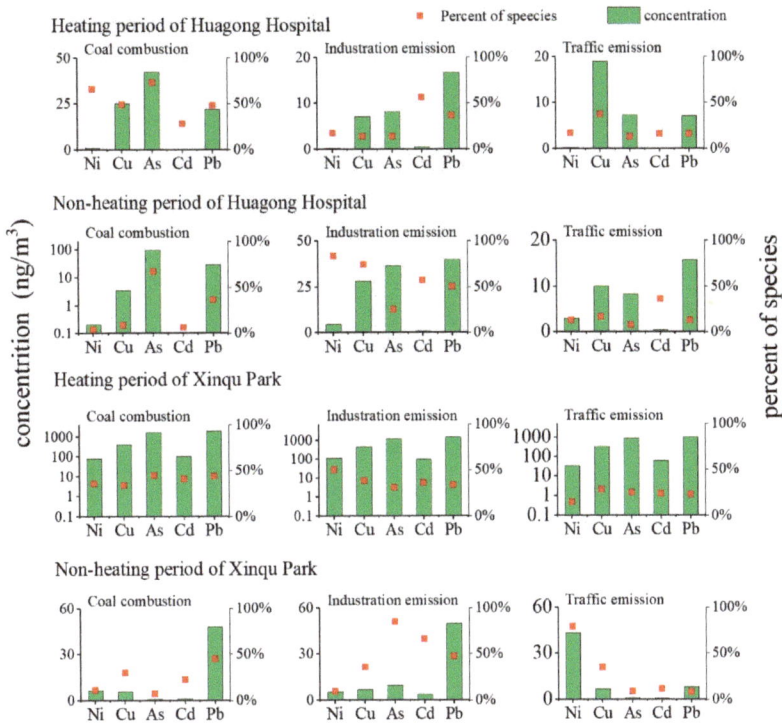

Figure 3. Source profiles and percentage contributions of heavy metals in PM$_{2.5}$ by PMF.

3.3.2. Source Apportionment for the Non-Heating Period

Figure 4 shows the source contributions from the PMF model. In the non-heating period, the main source of heavy metals in PM$_{2.5}$ at Huagong Hospital was industrial emissions (45.29%), followed by coal combustion (44.59%) and traffic emissions (10.12%). At Xinqu Park, the main source was industrial emissions (43.64%), followed by traffic emissions (31.00%) and coal combustion (25.35%). According to the model results, industrial emissions were the main source of PM$_{2.5}$ in the study area. The different secondary sources for the two sampling points might be related to their locations and meteorological factors. During the non-heating period, the study area is dominated by southerly and southwesterly winds. Therefore, the sampling points in Xinqu Park were likely affected by emissions from ships in Liaodong Bay, and the contribution from traffic emissions was relatively high. The results in this study are consistent with those for Chengdu and Tai'an in southern China [64,65]. However, industrial emissions had a relatively high contribution in the study area, likely because zinc smelting was the dominant industry. Chengdu is a provincial capital city, and Tai'an is a tourist destination [64,65]. The contribution of industrial emissions during the non-heating period (summer) was higher than that of coal burning, which is in contrast to results from the industrial city of Chifeng in northern China [66]. The contrast may be due to coal-fired power generation and coke plants in Chifeng City, which increase the contribution of coal combustion during the non-heating period [66], compared with that in the study area.

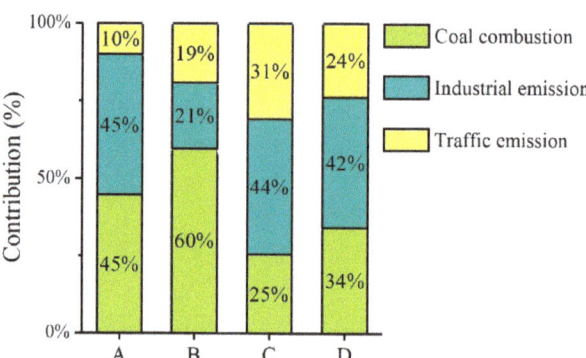

Figure 4. Contribution of PM$_{2.5}$ heavy metals from different source. Note: (**A**) represents non-heating period of Huagong Hospital in 2015; (**B**) represents heating period of Huagong Hospital in 2015; (**C**) represents non-heating period of Xinqu Park in 2015; (**D**) represents heating period of Xinqu Park in 2015.

3.3.3. Source Apportionment for the Heating Period

The PMF model identified the main sources of PM$_{2.5}$ in the study area (Figure 4). During the heating period, the main source of heavy metals in PM$_{2.5}$ at Huagong Hospital was coal combustion (59.64%), followed by industrial emissions (21.06%) and traffic emissions (19.30%), whereas at Xinqu Park, industrial emissions (42.14%) dominated, followed by coal combustion (34.03%) and traffic emissions (23.83%). Thus, there were differences in the main sources of PM$_{2.5}$ heavy metals at the two sampling sites. The differences might be because Huagong Hospital is in the old urban area of the city where the population is relatively dense. Coal-fired heating might also affect the site, in addition to industrial production, particularly considering the wind direction. During the heating period, the wind direction is mainly northerly and southwesterly, and because of the dilution/dispersal effect, the wind direction might have had a disproportionate effect on pollutant dispersal [77]. Coal-fired heating might have had less effect on Xinqu Park. In Liaoning Province, for example, coal consumption for industrial processes reached 175 million tonnes in 2015, including the burning of 140 million tonnes of coal for fuel [78]. In Chengdu, air conditioners are heavily used in the cold period, and that usage creates an increased demand for coal in thermal power generation; hence, the contribution of PM$_{2.5}$ associated with coal combustion increases in winter [64].

Overall, industrial emissions were the main source of PM$_{2.5}$ in the study area, followed by coal combustion and then traffic emissions. These results are the same as those for Tai'an and Chengdu [64,65], whereas the differences between Chifeng City and the present study are only because the research area is an industrial city dominated by zinc smelting [66]. At Huagong Hospital, coal-fired heating increased the contribution of coal combustion to heavy metals in PM$_{2.5}$. A similar conclusion was also reached in a PM$_{10}$ source analysis in northeast China [79]. According to the data of the Department of Ecology and Environment of Liaoning Province (2015), the contributions to PM$_{2.5}$ from industrial emissions are much higher than those from traffic emissions. Because contributions from pollution sources change in time and space, there are different combinations of pollutants, and they likely have different health risks to populations.

3.4. Health Risk Assessment

The human health risk assessment index only represents the assessment results for a particular period. However, because of the bioaccumulation of heavy metals, the assessment results of individual sampling periods cannot fully represent the human health risks in a study area. Therefore, in this paper, the average value of heavy metal concentrations during the sampling period was used to represent the human health risk associated with heavy metals in PM$_{2.5}$. In this study, HQ was used to evaluate the noncarcinogenic risk, and the ILCR was used to evaluate the carcinogenic risk. The different types of risk were analyzed separately for the heating and non-heating periods. The total carcinogenic risk and the total noncarcinogenic risk were calculated by the traditional USEPA method and the entropy weight method; the calculation results are shown in Figure 5.

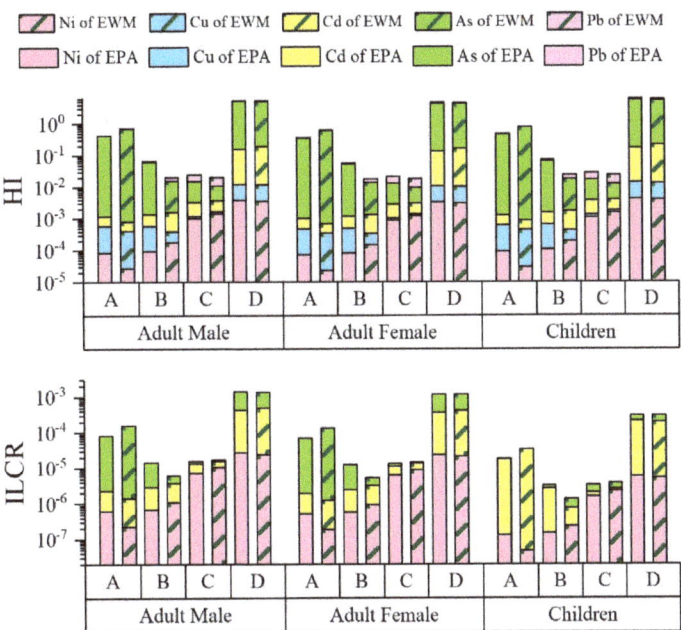

Figure 5. Risk indices of the two methods. Note: (**A**) represents non-heating period in Huagong Hospital; (**B**) represents heating period in Huagong Hospital; (**C**) represents non-heating period in Xinqu Park; (**D**) represents heating period in Xinqu Park. Children: 0–16 years; males: 17–70 years; females: 17–70 years. EWM: entropy weight method.

3.4.1. Non-Carcinogenic Risk Assessment

The lowest noncarcinogenic risk index in the non-heating period was for adult women at Xinqu Park (2.14×10^{-2} (USEPA) and 1.78×10^{-2} (entropy weight method)), whereas the highest noncarcinogenic risk index was for children at Huagong Hospital (0.469 (USEPA) and 0.788 (entropy weight method)) (Figure 5). In the non-heating period, the hazard index was less than 1, indicating that heavy metals in $PM_{2.5}$ in the study area did not pose a noncarcinogenic human health risk. During the heating period, adult women at Huagong Hospital had the lowest noncarcinogenic risk (5.67×10^{-2} (USEPA) and 1.79×10^{-2} (entropy weight method)), whereas children at Xinqu Park had the highest noncarcinogenic risk index (5.90 (USEPA) and 5.74 (entropy weight method)). The HI value of Xinqu Park was greater than 1, indicating that heavy metals posed a noncarcinogenic risk to human health in the area. Similar results are also reported for Tianjin City and Sistan in Iran [80,81]. Increased human health risks associated with increased heavy metal concentrations have been reported previously [16,82]. For the different populations at the two sampling locations within the same sampling period, the noncarcinogenic risk index was ranked as children > adult males > adult females. Thus, children likely faced the greatest noncarcinogenic risk from heavy metal pollution. This finding is consistent with studies in which the noncarcinogenic risk for children is higher than that for adults. In addition, the exposure parameters of weight and breathing rate, among others, are higher for adult males than for adult females [8,11,31]. A nonparametric test of the population HI determined by the two methods in the different periods showed that the results were significantly different at Huagong Hospital ($p < 0.05$). However, there was no significant difference between the results of the two methods at Xinqu Park ($p > 0.05$). This difference might be because the main sources of heavy metals in $PM_{2.5}$ in the heating and non-heating periods at Huagong Hospital were different, as were the main contributing heavy metals. Therefore, the weight of the HQ value of each heavy metal calculated by the entropy weight method was different. To compare the difference in the results of the two methods, the coefficient of variation (CV) of the HI value during the period was calculated. At Huagong Hospital, the CV values of the entropy weight method were slightly higher (1.185 for the non-heating period and 0.524 for the heating period) than those of the USEPA method (1.182 for the non-heating period and 0.453 for the heating period). At Xinqu Park, the CV values of the entropy weight method were lower (0.561 for the non-heating period and 1.419 for the heating period) than those of the USEPA method (0.563 for the non-heating period and 1.437 for the heating period). Thus, there was little difference between the results of the two methods at Xinqu Park, and the values calculated by the entropy weight method had a lower degree of dispersion. In evaluating the effects of long-term changes in heavy metal concentrations in $PM_{2.5}$ on human health risks, the calculation results of entropy weight method might be more representative.

3.4.2. Carcinogenic Risk Assessment

Figure 5 shows the carcinogenic risk assessment results for the study area. The lowest carcinogenic risk index for the non-heating period was for children at Xinqu Park (3.31×10^{-6} (USEPA) and 3.73×10^{-6} (entropy weight method)), whereas the highest carcinogenic risk index was for adult males at Huagong Hospital (8.30×10^{-5} (USEPA) and 1.55×10^{-4} (entropy weight method)). Therefore, according to the entropy weight method, the heavy metals in $PM_{2.5}$ in the non-heating period were a potential carcinogenic risk in the study area or a carcinogenic risk to adults at Huagong Hospital (1.55×10^{-4} for males and 1.32×10^{-4} for females). The lowest carcinogenic risk index for the heating period was for children at Huagong Hospital (3.17×10^{-6} (USEPA) and 1.33×10^{-6} (entropy weight method)), whereas the highest carcinogenic risk index was for adult males at Xinqu Park (1.38×10^{-3} (USEPA) and 1.37×10^{-3} (entropy weight method)). During the heating period, the heavy metals in $PM_{2.5}$ were a potential carcinogenic risk to people at Huagong Hospital and a carcinogenic risk to people at Xinqu Park. A nonparametric test of the population HI of the two methods in different periods showed that the two methods produced different results at Huagong Hospital ($p < 0.05$) but not at Xinqu Park ($p > 0.05$). At Huagong Hospital, the CV values of the entropy weight method were slightly higher (1.185 for the non-heating period and 0.889 for the heating period) than those of the USEPA method (1.160 for the non-heating period and 0.518 for the heating period). At Xinqu Park, the CV values of the entropy weight method were lower (0.742 for the non-heating period and 1.396 for the heating period) than those of the USEPA method (0.607 for the non-heating period and 1.396 for the heating period). The results of the two methods at Xinqu Park were similar, although the result of the USEPA method had a smaller degree of dispersion. For ILCR, the traditional USEPA method might be more applicable. At Xinqu Park, the carcinogenic risk during the heating period was higher than that in the non-heating period, a conclusion also reached in a recent study [8]. However, at Huagong Hospital, the risk of carcinogenesis was high during the non-heating period. For the different population groups, the risk of carcinogenesis was higher in adults than that in children, and the health risks of adult males were higher than those of adult females. Studies of the Pearl River delta region and Baoding City reached conclusions consistent with those of this study [8,83]. With respect to the study area, industrial emissions and coal combustion were the main sources of carcinogenic risk for the population, and heavy metals caused the highest carcinogenic risk to adult males and the lowest carcinogenic risk to children.

4. Conclusions

In this study, $PM_{2.5}$ concentrations were quantified, the sources were identified, and health risks were assessed in an industrial area of northeast China. The concentrations of $PM_{2.5}$ in the heating period were higher than those in the non-heating period. In addition, the $PM_{2.5}$ concentrations in the old city at Huagong Hospital were higher than those at Xinqu Park. The $PM_{2.5}$ concentrations of various metals differed. In general, the heavy metal concentrations in the heating period were higher than those in the non-heating period. Nonparametric tests detected differences between concentrations of heavy metals in $PM_{2.5}$, indicating there were different sources of heavy metals in the study area. The PMF model identified industrial emissions as the main source of heavy metals in $PM_{2.5}$, followed by coal combustion and then traffic emissions. Compared with the sources of emissions at Xinqu Park, an increased demand for coal combustion for heating during the winter led to elevated concentrations of heavy metals in $PM_{2.5}$ at Huagong Hospital, demonstrating coal combustion was the most important source of pollution. In the heating period, coal combustion (59.64%) was primary heavy metal source at Huagong Hospitals, and the contribution rates of industrial emissions and traffic emissions were 21.06% and 19.30%, respectively. Industrial emissions (42.14%) were the primary source at Xinqu Park, and the contribution rates of coal combustion and traffic emissions were 34.03% and 23.83%, respectively. During the non-heating period, coal combustion (45.29%) and industrial emissions (44.59%) were the primary sources at Huagong Hospital, and the traffic emissions were 10.12%. Industrial emissions (43.64%) were the primary sources at Xinqu Park, the coal combustion and traffic emissions were 25.35% and 31.00%, respectively. Differences in the contributions of heavy metals in $PM_{2.5}$ from different pollution sources affected the risks to human health. Children had the highest noncarcinogenic risk and adult females had the lowest noncarcinogenic risk, whereas adult males had the highest carcinogenic risk and children had the lowest carcinogenic risk. Furthermore, during the heating period, there were noncarcinogenic and carcinogenic risks to the public only at Xinqu Park, whereas during the non-heating period, there was potential carcinogenic risk for people in Huagong Hospitals and Xinqu Park. Compared with the traditional USEPA method, the results of the entropy weight method were also reasonable. However, when there is a difference between the two methods, the entropy weight method is recommended to assess noncarcinogenic health risks, because the result has smaller dispersion and is more representative. In contrast, the USEPA method is recommended for ILCR.

Author Contributions: Conceptualization, S.S., N.Z., S.W., X.S., D.D.; Methodology, S.S., S.W., Y.L., S.H., S.D., Q.A., P.L., X.L.; Software, S.S., N.Z., X.H.; Formal analysis, S.S., Y.L., S.D., P.L.; Investigation, S.S., S.W., Q.A.; Writing—original draft preparation, S.S., Y.L., X.L.; Writing—review and editing, S.S., N.Z., S.W., S.H., X.S., Q.A., X.L.; Visualization, S.S., X.S., Q.A., P.L., X.L., D.D.; Resources, N.Z., Y.L., S.H., X.S., Q.A., X.H.; Supervision, N.Z., S.D., P.L., X.H., D.D.; Project administration, N.Z., X.H., D.D.; Funding acquisition, N.Z.; Data curation, S.W., Y.L., S.D., P.L.; Validation, Y.L., S.H., X.L., D.D. All authors have read and agreed to the published version of the manuscript.

Funding: This work was supported by the National Natural Science Foundation of China (Grant Nos. 41722110 and 41571474), Leading Talents and Team Project of Scientific and Technological Innovation for Young and Middle-aged Groups of Jilin Province (20200301015RQ), and Major Special Program of Scientific and Technological of Jilin Province (20200503003SF).

Institutional Review Board Statement: Not applicable.

Informed Consent Statement: Not applicable.

Data Availability Statement: Not applicable.

Acknowledgments: We want to thank the editor and anonymous reviewers for their valuable comments and suggestions to this paper.

Conflicts of Interest: The authors declare no conflict of interest.

References

1. Quan, J.; Tie, X.; Zhang, Q.; Liu, Q.; Li, X.; Gao, Y.; Zhao, D. Characteristics of heavy aerosol pollution during the 2012–2013 winter in Beijing, China. *Atmos. Environ.* **2014**, *88*, 83–89. [CrossRef]
2. Stafoggia, M.; Bellander, T.; Bucci, S.; Davoli, M.; De Hoogh, K.; De'Donato, F.; Gariazzo, C.; Lyapustin, A.; Michelozzi, P.; Renzi, M.; et al. Estimation of daily PM_{10} and $PM_{2.5}$ concentrations in Italy, 2013–2015, using a spatiotemporal land-use random-forest model. *Environ. Int.* **2019**, *124*, 170–179. [CrossRef] [PubMed]
3. Al-Hemoud, A.; Gasana, J.; Al-Dabbous, A.; Alajeel, A.; Al-Shatti, A.; Behbehani, W.; Malak, M. Exposure levels of air pollution ($PM_{2.5}$) and associated health risk in Kuwait. *Environ. Res.* **2019**, *179*, 108730. [CrossRef] [PubMed]
4. Makkonen, U.; Hellén, H.; Anttila, P.; Ferm, M. Size distribution and chemical composition of airborne particles in south-eastern Finland during different seasons and wildfire episodes in 2006. *Sci. Total Environ.* **2010**, *408*, 644–651. [CrossRef]
5. Fang, D.; Wang, Q.; Li, H.; Yu, Y.; Lu, Y.; Qian, X. Mortality effects assessment of ambient $PM_{2.5}$ pollution in the 74 leading cities of China. *Sci. Total Environ.* **2016**, *569–570*, 1545–1552. [CrossRef]
6. Kan, H.; Chen, R.; Tong, S. Ambient air pollution, climate change, and population health in China. *Environ. Int.* **2012**, *42*, 10–19. [CrossRef]
7. Sulong, N.A.; Latif, M.T.; Khan, F.; Amil, N.; Ashfold, M.J.; Wahab, M.I.A.; Chan, K.M.; Sahani, M. Source apportionment and health risk assessment among specific age groups during haze and non-haze episodes in Kuala Lumpur, Malaysia. *Sci. Total Environ.* **2017**, *601–602*, 556–570. [CrossRef]
8. Liang, B.; Li, X.-L.; Ma, K.; Liang, S.-X. Pollution characteristics of metal pollutants in $PM_{2.5}$ and comparison of risk on human health in heating and non-heating seasons in Baoding, China. *Ecotoxicol. Environ. Saf.* **2019**, *170*, 166–171. [CrossRef]
9. Schwarz, J.; Pokorná, P.; Rychlík, Š.; Škáchová, H.; Vlček, O.; Smolík, J.; Ždímal, V.; Hůnová, I. Assessment of air pollution origin based on year-long parallel measurement of $PM_{2.5}$ and PM_{10} at two suburban sites in Prague, Czech Republic. *Sci. Total Environ.* **2019**, *664*, 1107–1116. [CrossRef]
10. Li, Y.; Zhu, K.; Wang, S. Polycentric and dispersed population distribution increases $PM_{2.5}$ concentrations: Evidence from 286 Chinese cities, 2001–2016. *J. Clean. Prod.* **2020**, *248*, 119202. [CrossRef]
11. Liang, D.; Wang, Y.-Q.; Wang, Y.-J.; Ma, C. National air pollution distribution in China and related geographic, gaseous pollutant, and socio-economic factors. *Environ. Pollut.* **2019**, *250*, 998–1009. [CrossRef]
12. Ma, B.; Wang, L.; Tao, W.; Liu, M.; Zhang, P.; Zhang, S.; Li, X.; Lu, X. Phthalate esters in atmospheric $PM_{2.5}$ and PM_{10} in the semi-arid city of Xi'an, Northwest China: Pollution characteristics, sources, health risks, and relationships with meteorological factors. *Chemosphere* **2020**, *242*, 125226. [CrossRef]
13. Li, X.; Jiang, L.; Bai, Y.; Yang, Y.; Liu, S.; Chen, X.; Xu, J.; Liu, Y.; Wang, Y.; Guo, X.; et al. Wintertime aerosol chemistry in Beijing during haze period: Significant contribution from secondary formation and biomass burning emission. *Atmos. Res.* **2019**, *218*, 25–33. [CrossRef]
14. Xu, G.; Ren, X.; Xiong, K.; Li, L.; Bi, X.; Wu, Q. Analysis of the driving factors of $PM_{2.5}$ concentration in the air: A case study of the Yangtze River Delta, China. *Ecol. Indic.* **2020**, *110*, 105889. [CrossRef]
15. Luo, J.; Zhang, J.; Huang, X.; Liu, Q.; Luo, B.; Zhang, W.; Rao, Z.; Yu, Y. Characteristics, evolution, and regional differences of biomass burning particles in the Sichuan Basin, China. *J. Environ. Sci.* **2020**, *89*, 35–46. [CrossRef]
16. Liang, L.; Wang, Z.; Li, J. The effect of urbanization on environmental pollution in rapidly developing urban agglomerations. *J. Clean. Prod.* **2019**, *237*, 117649. [CrossRef]
17. Ledoux, F.; Kfoury, A.; Delmaire, G.; Roussel, G.; El Zein, A.; Courcot, D. Contributions of local and regional anthropogenic sources of metals in $PM_{2.5}$ at an urban site in northern France. *Chemosphere* **2017**, *181*, 713–724. [CrossRef]
18. Vannini, A.; Paoli, L.; Russo, A.; Loppi, S. Contribution of submicronic (PM1) and coarse (PM > 1) particulate matter deposition to the heavy metal load of lichens transplanted along a busy road. *Chemosphere* **2019**, *231*, 121–125. [CrossRef]
19. Bergthorson, J.; Goroshin, S.; Soo, M.; Julien, P.; Palecka, J.; Frost, D.; Jarvis, D. Direct combustion of recyclable metal fuels for zero-carbon heat and power. *Appl. Energy* **2015**, *160*, 368–382. [CrossRef]
20. Men, C.; Liu, R.; Xu, F.; Wang, Q.; Guo, L.; Shen, Z. Pollution characteristics, risk assessment, and source apportionment of heavy metals in road dust in Beijing, China. *Sci. Total Environ.* **2018**, *612*, 138–147. [CrossRef]
21. Wang, W.; Yu, J.; Cui, Y.; He, J.; Xue, P.; Cao, W.; Ying, H.; Gao, W.; Yan, Y.; Hu, B.; et al. Characteristics of fine particulate matter and its sources in an industrialized coastal city, Ningbo, Yangtze River Delta, China. *Atmos. Res.* **2018**, *203*, 105–117. [CrossRef]
22. Zheng, N.; Liu, J.; Wang, Q.; Liang, Z. Health risk assessment of heavy metal exposure to street dust in the zinc smelting district, Northeast of China. *Sci. Total Environ.* **2010**, *408*, 726–733. [CrossRef]
23. Luo, Y.; Zhou, X.; Zhang, J.; Xiao, Y.; Wang, Z.; Zhou, Y.; Wang, W. $PM_{2.5}$ pollution in a petrochemical industry city of northern China: Seasonal variation and source apportionment. *Atmos. Res.* **2018**, *212*, 285–295. [CrossRef]
24. Guo, W.; Zhang, Z.; Zheng, N.; Luo, L.; Xiao, H.; Xiao, H. Chemical characterization and source analysis of water-soluble inorganic ions in $PM_{2.5}$ from a plateau city of Kunming at different seasons. *Atmos. Res.* **2020**, *234*, 104687. [CrossRef]
25. Tang, Z.; Zhang, L.; Huang, Q.; Yang, Y.; Nie, Z.; Cheng, J.; Yang, J.; Wang, Y.; Chai, M. Contamination and risk of heavy metals in soils and sediments from a typical plastic waste recycling area in North China. *Ecotoxicol. Environ. Saf.* **2015**, *122*, 343–351. [CrossRef]
26. Hou, S.; Zheng, N.; Tang, L.; Ji, X.; Li, Y.; Hua, X. Pollution characteristics, sources, and health risk assessment of human exposure to Cu, Zn, Cd and Pb pollution in urban street dust across China between 2009 and 2018. *Environ. Int.* **2019**, *128*, 430–437. [CrossRef]

27. Zhang, X.; Zhang, K.; Lv, W.; Liu, B.; Aikawa, M.; Wang, J. Characteristics and risk assessments of heavy metals in fine and coarse particles in an industrial area of central China. *Ecotoxicol. Environ. Saf.* **2019**, *179*, 1–8. [CrossRef]
28. Perez, P.; Gramsch, E. Forecasting hourly PM$_{2.5}$ in Santiago de Chile with emphasis on night episodes. *Atmos. Environ.* **2016**, *124*, 22–27. [CrossRef]
29. U.S. EPA. *Risk Assessment Guidance for Superfund, Volume I: Human Health Evaluation Manual*; EPA/540/1-89/002; Office of Solid Waste and Emergency Response: Washington, DC, USA, 1989. Available online: https://www.epa.gov/risk/risk-assessment-guidance-superfund-volume-i-human-health-evaluation-manual-supplemental (accessed on 30 June 2021).
30. Bi, C.; Chen, Y.; Zhao, Z.; Li, Q.; Zhou, Q.; Ye, Z.; Ge, X. Characteristics, sources and health risks of toxic species (PCDD/Fs, PAHs and heavy metals) in PM$_{2.5}$ during fall and winter in an industrial area. *Chemosphere* **2020**, *238*, 124620. [CrossRef] [PubMed]
31. Agarwal, A.; Mangal, A.; Satsangi, A.; Lakhani, A.; Kumari, K.M. Characterization, sources and health risk analysis of PM$_{2.5}$ bound metals during foggy and non-foggy days in sub-urban atmosphere of Agra. *Atmos. Res.* **2017**, *197*, 121–131. [CrossRef]
32. Gui, K.; Che, H.; Wang, Y.; Wang, H.; Zhang, L.; Zhao, H.; Zheng, Y.; Sun, T.; Zhang, X. Satellite-derived PM$_{2.5}$ concentration trends over Eastern China from 1998 to 2016: Relationships to emissions and meteorological parameters. *Environ. Pollut.* **2019**, *247*, 1125–1133. [CrossRef]
33. Peng, X.; Shi, G.; Liu, G.; Xu, J.; Tian, Y.; Zhang, Y.; Feng, Y.; Russell, A.G. Source apportionment and heavy metal health risk (HMHR) quantification from sources in a southern city in China, using an ME2-HMHR model. *Environ. Pollut.* **2017**, *221*, 335–342. [CrossRef]
34. Gao, Y.; Zhang, Y.; Feng, J.; Zhu, L. Toxicokinetic-toxicodynamic modeling of cadmium and lead toxicity to larvae and adult zebrafish. *Environ. Pollut.* **2019**, *251*, 221–229. [CrossRef]
35. Eze, C.T.; Michelangeli, F.; Otitoloju, A.A. In vitro cyto-toxic assessment of heavy metals and their binary mixtures on mast cell-like, rat basophilic leukemia (RBL-2H3) cells. *Chemosphere* **2019**, *223*, 686–693. [CrossRef]
36. Yuan, Y.; Wu, Y.; Ge, X.; Nie, D.; Wang, M.; Zhou, H.; Chen, M. In vitro toxicity evaluation of heavy metals in urban air particulate matter on human lung epithelial cells. *Sci. Total Environ.* **2019**, *678*, 301–308. [CrossRef]
37. He, Y.; Guo, H.; Jin, M.; Ren, P. A linguistic entropy weight method and its application in linguistic multi-attribute group decision making. *Nonlinear Dyn.* **2016**, *84*, 399–404. [CrossRef]
38. Chaji, A. Analytic approach on maximum Bayesian entropy ordered weighted averaging operators. *Comput. Ind. Eng.* **2017**, *105*, 260–264. [CrossRef]
39. Bordbar, M.; Neshat, A.; Javadi, S. Modification of the GALDIT framework using statistical and entropy models to assess coastal aquifer vulnerability. *Hydrol. Sci. J.* **2019**, *64*, 1117–1128. [CrossRef]
40. Zhu, Y.; Tian, D.; Yan, F. Effectiveness of Entropy Weight Method in Decision-Making. *Math. Probl. Eng.* **2020**, *2020*, 3564835. [CrossRef]
41. Yang, J.Y.; Zhang, L.L. Fuzzy Comprehensive Evaluation Method on Water Environmental Quality Based on Entropy Weight with Consideration of Toxicology of Evaluation Factors. *Adv. Mater. Res.* **2011**, *356–360*, 2383–2388. [CrossRef]
42. Zhang, X.; Wang, C.; Li, E.; Xu, C. Assessment Model of Ecoenvironmental Vulnerability Based on Improved Entropy Weight Method. *Sci. World J.* **2014**, *2014*, 797814. [CrossRef]
43. Zheng, N.; Wang, Q.; Zhang, X.; Zheng, D.; Zhang, Z.; Zhang, S. Population health risk due to dietary intake of heavy metals in the industrial area of Huludao city, China. *Sci. Total Environ.* **2007**, *387*, 96–104. [CrossRef]
44. Zheng, N.; Wang, Q.; Zheng, D. Health risk of Hg, Pb, Cd, Zn, and Cu to the inhabitants around Huludao Zinc Plant in China via consumption of vegetables. *Sci. Total Environ.* **2007**, *383*, 81–89. [CrossRef]
45. Zheng, N.; Wang, Q.; Liang, Z.; Zheng, D. Characterization of heavy metal concentrations in the sediments of three freshwater rivers in Huludao City, Northeast China. *Environ. Pollut.* **2008**, *154*, 135–142. [CrossRef]
46. Lu, C.; Zhang, J.; Jiang, H.; Yang, J.; Zhang, J.; Wang, J.; Shan, H. Assessment of soil contamination with Cd, Pb and Zn and source identification in the area around the Huludao Zinc Plant. *J. Hazard. Mater.* **2010**, *182*, 743–748. [CrossRef]
47. Huludao City Heating Management Measures. 2011. Available online: http://www.hld.gov.cn/zwgk/zc/zfl/201110/t20111021_457584.html (accessed on 30 June 2021).
48. Yang, H.; Chen, J.; Wen, J.; Tian, H.; Liu, X. Composition and sources of PM$_{2.5}$ around the heating periods of 2013 and 2014 in Beijing: Implications for efficient mitigation measures. *Atmos. Environ.* **2016**, *124*, 378–386. [CrossRef]
49. Paatero, P.; Eberly, S.; Brown, S.G.; Norris, G.A. Methods for estimating uncertainty in factor analytic solutions. *Atmos. Meas. Tech.* **2014**, *7*, 781–797. [CrossRef]
50. Deng, J.; Zhang, Y.; Qiu, Y.; Zhang, H.; Du, W.; Xu, L.; Hong, Y.; Chen, Y.; Chen, J. Source apportionment of PM$_{2.5}$ at the Lin'an regional background site in China with three receptor models. *Atmos. Res.* **2018**, *202*, 23–32. [CrossRef]
51. Tan, J.; Duan, J.-C.; Ma, Y.-L.; Yang, F.-M.; Cheng, Y.; He, K.-B.; Yu, Y.-C.; Wang, J.-W. Source of atmospheric heavy metals in winter in Foshan, China. *Sci. Total Environ.* **2014**, *493*, 262–270. [CrossRef]
52. Chen, X.; Lu, X. Contamination characteristics and source apportionment of heavy metals in topsoil from an area in Xi'an city, China. *Ecotoxicol. Environ. Saf.* **2018**, *151*, 153–160. [CrossRef]
53. Callén, M.S.; Iturmendi, A.; López, J.M. Source apportionment of atmospheric PM$_{2.5}$-bound polycyclic aromatic hydrocarbons by a PMF receptor model. Assessment of potential risk for human health. *Environ. Pollut.* **2014**, *195*, 167–177. [CrossRef]

54. Lu, Z.; Liu, Q.; Xiong, Y.; Huang, F.; Zhou, J.; Schauer, J.J. A hybrid source apportionment strategy using positive matrix factorization (PMF) and molecular marker chemical mass balance (MM-CMB) models. *Environ. Pollut.* **2018**, *238*, 39–51. [CrossRef] [PubMed]
55. Gao, P.; Guo, H.; Zhang, Z.; Ou, C.; Hang, J.; Fan, Q.; He, C.; Wu, B.; Feng, Y.; Xing, B. Bioaccessibility and exposure assessment of trace metals from urban airborne particulate matter (PM_{10} and $PM_{2.5}$) in simulated digestive fluid. *Environ. Pollut.* **2018**, *242*, 1669–1677. [CrossRef] [PubMed]
56. Gao, Y.; Guo, X.; Ji, H.; Li, C.; Ding, H.; Briki, M.; Tang, L.; Zhang, Y. Potential threat of heavy metals and PAHs in $PM_{2.5}$ in different urban functional areas of Beijing. *Atmos. Res.* **2016**, *178–179*, 6–16. [CrossRef]
57. Gao, Y.; Guo, X.; Li, C.; Ding, H.; Tang, L.; Ji, H. Characteristics of $PM_{2.5}$ in Miyun, the northeastern suburb of Beijing: Chemical composition and evaluation of health risk. *Environ. Sci. Pollut. Res.* **2015**, *22*, 16688–16699. [CrossRef] [PubMed]
58. U.S. EPA. *Exposure Factors Handbook 2011 Edition (Final)*; EPA/600/R-09/052F; U.S. Environmental Protection Agency: Washington, DC, USA, 2011. Available online: https://cfpub.epa.gov/si/si_public_record_report.cfm?Lab=NCEA&count=10000&dirEntryId=236252&searchall=&showcriteria=2&simplesearch=0&timstype= (accessed on 30 June 2021).
59. Di Vaio, P.; Magli, E.; Caliendo, G.; Corvino, A.; Fiorino, F.; Frecentese, F.; Saccone, I.; Santagada, V.; Severino, B.; Onorati, G.; et al. Heavy Metals Size Distribution in PM_{10} and Environmental-Sanitary Risk Analysis in Acerra (Italy). *Atmosphere* **2018**, *9*, 58. [CrossRef]
60. Sulaymon, I.D.; Mei, X.; Yang, S.; Chen, S.; Zhang, Y.; Hopke, P.K.; Schauer, J.J.; Zhang, Y. $PM_{2.5}$ in Abuja, Nigeria: Chemical characterization, source apportionment, temporal variations, transport pathways and the health risks assessment. *Atmos. Res.* **2020**, *237*, 104833. [CrossRef]
61. Salameh, D.; Pey, J.; Bozzetti, C.; El Haddad, I.; Detournay, A.; Sylvestre, A.; Canonaco, F.; Armengaud, A.; Piga, D.; Robin, D.; et al. Sources of $PM_{2.5}$ at an urban-industrial Mediterranean city, Marseille (France): Application of the ME-2 solver to inorganic and organic markers. *Atmos. Res.* **2018**, *214*, 263–274. [CrossRef]
62. Harte, J.; Newman, E. Maximum information entropy: A foundation for ecological theory. *Trends Ecol. Evol.* **2014**, *29*, 384–389. [CrossRef]
63. Wang, J.; Hu, Z.; Chen, Y.; Chen, Z.; Xu, S. Contamination characteristics and possible sources of PM_{10} and $PM_{2.5}$ in different functional areas of Shanghai, China. *Atmos. Environ.* **2013**, *68*, 221–229. [CrossRef]
64. Kong, L.; Tan, Q.; Feng, M.; Qu, Y.; An, J.; Liu, X.; Cheng, N.; Deng, Y.; Zhai, R.; Wang, Z. Investigating the characteristics and source analyses of $PM_{2.5}$ seasonal variations in Chengdu, Southwest China. *Chemosphere* **2020**, *243*, 125267. [CrossRef]
65. Liu, B.; Song, N.; Dai, Q.; Mei, R.; Sui, B.; Bi, X.; Feng, Y. Chemical composition and source apportionment of ambient $PM_{2.5}$ during the non-heating period in Taian, China. *Atmos. Res.* **2016**, *170*, 23–33. [CrossRef]
66. Hao, Y.; Meng, X.; Yu, X.; Lei, M.; Li, W.; Yang, W.; Shi, F.; Xie, S. Quantification of primary and secondary sources to $PM_{2.5}$ using an improved source regional apportionment method in an industrial city, China. *Sci. Total Environ.* **2020**, *706*, 135715. [CrossRef]
67. Olawoyin, R.; Schweitzer, L.; Zhang, K.; Okareh, O.; Slates, K. Index analysis and human health risk model application for evaluating ambient air-heavy metal contamination in Chemical Valley Sarnia. *Ecotoxicol. Environ. Saf.* **2018**, *148*, 72–81. [CrossRef]
68. Tao, J.; Zhang, L.; Cao, J.; Zhong, L.; Chen, D.; Yang, Y.; Chen, D.; Chen, L.; Zhang, Z.; Wu, Y.; et al. Source apportionment of $PM_{2.5}$ at urban and suburban areas of the Pearl River Delta region, south China—With emphasis on ship emissions. *Sci. Total Environ.* **2017**, *574*, 1559–1570. [CrossRef]
69. Chen, Y.-C.; Hsu, C.-Y.; Lin, S.-L.; Chang-Chien, G.-P.; Chen, M.-J.; Fang, G.-C.; Chiang, H.-C. Characteristics of Concentrations and Metal Compositions for $PM_{2.5}$ and $PM_{2.5-10}$ in Yunlin County, Taiwan during Air Quality Deterioration. *Aerosol Air Qual. Res.* **2015**, *15*, 2571–2583. [CrossRef]
70. Gupta, T.; Mandariya, A. Sources of submicron aerosol during fog-dominated wintertime at Kanpur. *Environ. Sci. Pollut. Res.* **2013**, *20*, 5615–5629. [CrossRef]
71. Liu, X.; Ouyang, W.; Shu, Y.; Tian, Y.; Feng, Y.; Zhang, T.; Chen, W. Incorporating bioaccessibility into health risk assessment of heavy metals in particulate matter originated from different sources of atmospheric pollution. *Environ. Pollut.* **2019**, *254*, 113113. [CrossRef]
72. Mohanraj, R.; Azeez, P.A.; Priscilla, T. Heavy Metals in Airborne Particulate Matter of Urban Coimbatore. *Arch. Environ. Contam. Toxicol.* **2004**, *47*, 162–167. [CrossRef]
73. Gioda, A.; Pérez, U.; Rosa, Z.; Jimenez-Velez, B.D. Concentration of Trace Elements in Airborne PM_{10} from Jobos Bay National Estuary, Puerto Rico. *Water Air Soil Pollut.* **2006**, *174*, 141–159. [CrossRef]
74. Duan, J.; Tan, J. Atmospheric heavy metals and Arsenic in China: Situation, sources and control policies. *Atmos. Environ.* **2013**, *74*, 93–101. [CrossRef]
75. Khillare, P.S.; Sarkar, S. Airborne inhalable metals in residential areas of Delhi, India: Distribution, source apportionment and health risks. *Atmos. Pollut. Res.* **2012**, *3*, 46–54. [CrossRef]
76. Li, Y.; Yu, Y.; Zheng, N.; Hou, S.; Song, X.; Dong, W. Metallic elements in human hair from residents in smelting districts in northeast China: Environmental factors and differences in ingestion media. *Environ. Res.* **2020**, *182*, 108914. [CrossRef] [PubMed]
77. Kuerban, M.; Waili, Y.; Fan, F.; Liu, Y.; Qin, W.; Dore, A.J.; Peng, J.; Xu, W.; Zhang, F. Spatio-temporal patterns of air pollution in China from 2015 to 2018 and implications for health risks. *Environ. Pollut.* **2020**, *258*, 113659. [CrossRef]
78. Department of Ecology and Environment of Liaoning Province. 2015 Annual Environmental Statistics of Liaoning Province. 2017. Available online: http://sthj.ln.gov.cn/xxgk/zwgk/hjcjnb/201711/t20171106_88215.html (accessed on 30 June 2021).

79. Ni, T.; Han, B.; Bai, Z. Source Apportionment of PM_{10} in Four Cities of Northeastern China. *Aerosol Air Qual. Res.* **2012**, *12*, 571–582. [CrossRef]
80. Behrooz, R.D.; Kaskaoutis, D.; Grivas, G.; Mihalopoulos, N. Human health risk assessment for toxic elements in the extreme ambient dust conditions observed in Sistan, Iran. *Chemosphere* **2021**, *262*, 127835. [CrossRef]
81. Han, W.; Gao, G.; Geng, J.; Li, Y.; Wang, Y. Ecological and health risks assessment and spatial distribution of residual heavy metals in the soil of an e-waste circular economy park in Tianjin, China. *Chemosphere* **2018**, *197*, 325–335. [CrossRef]
82. Wu, Y.; Li, G.; Yang, Y.; An, T. Pollution evaluation and health risk assessment of airborne toxic metals in both indoors and outdoors of the Pearl River Delta, China. *Environ. Res.* **2019**, *179*, 108793. [CrossRef]
83. Hime, N.J.; Marks, G.B.; Cowie, C.T. A Comparison of the Health Effects of Ambient Particulate Matter Air Pollution from Five Emission Sources. *Int. J. Environ. Res. Public Health* **2018**, *15*, 1206. [CrossRef]

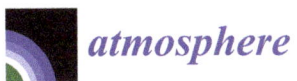

Article

Spatial Distribution and Chemical Composition of Road Dust in Two High-Altitude Latin American Cities †

Sebastián Vanegas [1], Erika M. Trejos [2], Beatriz H. Aristizábal [2], Guilherme M. Pereira [3], Julio M. Hernández [4], Jorge Herrera Murillo [4], Omar Ramírez [5,*], Fulvio Amato [6], Luis F. O. Silva [7], Néstor Y. Rojas [1], Carlos Zafra [8] and Jorge E. Pachón [9,*]

1. Department of Chemical and Environmental Engineering, Universidad Nacional de Colombia—Sede Bogotá, Bogotá 111321, Colombia; jovanegasg@unal.edu.co (S.V.); nyrojasr@unal.edu.co (N.Y.R.)
2. Hydraulic Engineering and Environmental Research Group, Universidad Nacional de Colombia—Sede Manizales, Manizales 170004, Colombia; emtrejosz@unal.edu.co (E.M.T.); bharistizabalz@unal.edu.co (B.H.A.)
3. Institute of Chemistry, Universidade de São Paulo, São Paulo 05580-000, Brazil; guilherme.martins.pereira@usp.br
4. Environmental Analysis Laboratory, Environmental Sciences School, Universidad Nacional de Costa Rica, Heredia 40101, Costa Rica; jucemuhe@gmail.com (J.M.H.); jorge.herrera.murillo@una.cr (J.H.M.)
5. Environmental Engineering Program, Universidad Militar Nueva Granada, Cajicá-Zipaquirá 250247, Colombia
6. Institute for Environmental Assessment and Water Research (IDÆA), Spanish National Research Council (CSIC), 08034 Barcelona, Spain; fulvio.amato@idaea.csic.es
7. Department of Civil and Environmental Engineering, Universidad de la Costa, Barranquilla 080002, Colombia; lsilva8@cuc.edu.co
8. Environmental Engineering Research Group—GIIAUD, Universidad Distrital Francisco José de Caldas, Bogotá 110321, Colombia; czafra@udistrital.edu.co
9. Centro Lasallista de Investigación y Modelación Ambiental—CLIMA, Universidad de La Salle, Bogotá 111711, Colombia
* Correspondence: omar.ramirez@unimilitar.edu.co (O.R.); jpachon@unisalle.edu.co (J.E.P.); Tel.: +57-301-2414281 (O.R.); +57-310-3173756 (J.E.P.)
† This paper is dedicated to the memory of Professor Beatriz H. Aristizábal.

Abstract: Road dust (RD) resuspension is one of the main sources of particulate matter in cities with adverse impacts on air quality, health, and climate. Studies on the variability of the deposited PM_{10} fraction of RD (RD_{10}) have been limited in Latin America, whereby our understanding of the central factors that control this pollutant remains incomplete. In this study, forty-one RD_{10} samples were collected in two Andean cities (Bogotá and Manizales) and analyzed for ions, minerals, and trace elements. RD_{10} levels varied between 1.8–45.7 mg/m^2, with an average of 11.8 mg/m^2, in Bogotá and between 0.8–26.7 mg/m^2, with an average of 5.7 mg/m^2, in Manizales. Minerals were the most abundant species in both cities, with a fraction significantly larger in Manizales (38%) than Bogotá (9%). The difference could be explained mainly by the complex topography and the composition of soil derived from volcanic ash in Manizales. The volcanic activity was also associated with SO_4^{-2} and Cl^-. Enrichment factors and principal component analysis were conducted to explore potential factors associated to sources of RD_{10}. Elements such as Cu, Pb, Cr, Ni, V, Sb, and Mo were mainly associated with exhaust and non-exhaust traffic emissions.

Keywords: PM_{10}; dust resuspension; sediment load; non-exhaust emissions; chemical profile; enrichment factors; Colombia

1. Introduction

Particulate matter (PM) emitted by road transport can be released both from the exhaust pipe, as a result of incomplete fuel combustion, and from non-exhaust processes [1]. Exhaust particles have shown a trend of decreasing emissions due to stringent tailpipe standards, better fuel quality, and migration towards zero- or low-emission vehicles in recent decades [2]. However, detailed information concerning non-exhaust PM emissions is still relatively limited in developing countries, particularly in Latin America, where there is not enough knowledge regarding physicochemical characteristics of PM, its spatial distribution, and associated adverse health effects, among other variables.

Non-exhaust emissions have been identified as one of the most significant sources of air pollution in urban environments due to their contribution of coarse, fine, and ultrafine particles [1,3–6]. These emissions are constituted by direct releases of particles due to abrasion processes, including tire, brake, clutch, and road wear [7–9]. They also include the resuspension of road dust, namely PM emitted from natural and anthropogenic sources, deposited on the road surface, and resuspended as a result of vehicular turbulence and the action of the wind [2].

Road dust is composed mainly of crustal dust and soil material, but also of particles derived from several anthropogenic sources, such as traffic, industrial emissions, quarries, and construction activities, among others [6,10,11]. Therefore, the chemical composition of road dust is variable and is associated with the characteristics of the emission sources. This includes abundant crust elements, such as Al, Fe, Mg, Na, P, and Ti, among others, but also hazardous components such as Pb, V, Cd, Cu, Sb, and polycyclic aromatic hydrocarbons (PAHs). The latter ones generate adverse effects on human health, especially on the cardiorespiratory system [12]. Road dust loadings, as well as their chemical speciation, vary geographically depending on parameters such as meteorology, geology of the region, and even the type of pavement sampled [13,14].

Some studies have investigated the association of road dust particles and mortality from cardiorespiratory diseases and other causes. Researchers have found that an incremental increase of particles related to road dust resuspension can increase mortality risk by 4.0%, higher than the observed for vehicle exhaust [15]. Other studies have reported a significant daily mortality because of an increase of 10 $\mu g/m^3$ of particles related to road dust in Stockholm [16]. Lastly, chemical species associated with road dust and mineral resuspension, such as SiO_2, Ca, Fe, and Ti, have shown deleterious health effects [17,18]. Consequently, studying the loadings and the chemical composition of road dust, as well as its spatial variability, is crucial to identify the origin of the PM, to formulate mitigation measures and to identify potential adverse effects on the population.

Studies on loadings and chemical characterization of particles below 10 μm from road dust (PM_{10} but termed RD_{10} in this study) have been carried out in several cities. For example, Alves et al. [7] used a portable resuspension chamber to collect road dust from five main roads in Oporto and an urban tunnel in Braga, Portugal. Researchers reported dust loadings of 0.48 ± 0.39 mg PM_{10}/m^2 for asphalt paved roads. Furthermore, they found that crustal and anthropogenic elements, associated with tire and brake wear, dominated the inorganic fraction. Vlasov et al. [19] analyzed potentially toxic elements (PTEs) in road dust in Moscow, finding that the main pollutants of the PM_{10} fraction included Sb, Zn, W, Sn, Bi, Cd, Cu, Pb, and Mo. They concluded that particles were most contaminated in the central part of the city due to the large number of cars and traffic congestions. Zhang et al. [20] analyzed a total of 64 dust samples collected from five urban roads and four parks in Tianjin, China to determine the size distribution and elemental composition of the PM_{10} fraction. The researchers found that crustal elements accounted for 30.14% of the PM_{10} fractions and the most abundant trace elements were Zn, Mn, and Cu (range, 277 to 874 mg/kg). Pant et al. [21] obtained road dust samples collected at two sites in Birmingham, UK and one site in New Delhi, India. They found that dust loadings were found to be much higher for New Delhi (72.9 ± 24.3 mg/m^2) compared to Birmingham (range, 9.34 ± 5.56 to 12.1 ± 9.3 mg/m^2). In addition, Cu was found to be a factor significantly associated with oxidative potential in the PM_{10} fraction.

Although some emission inventories have recognized resuspended road dust as one of the most significant sources of PM in urban centers [22], research on RD_{10} conducted in Latin American countries has been scarce. Pachón et al. [23] studied influencing factors of road dust in Bogotá, finding that meteorology, land use, traffic characteristics, and road conditions determine RD_{10} levels in the city. Ramírez et al. [24] characterized inorganic compounds (water-soluble ions, major and trace elements, organic and elemental carbon) and estimated source contributions to the PM_{10} fraction of road dust sampled in Bogotá, the capital of Colombia. Crustal elements were the most abundant species, accounting for 49–62% of the PM_{10} fraction, followed by OC (13–29%), water-soluble ions (1.4–3.8%), EC (0.8–1.9%), and trace elements (0.2–0.5%). On the other hand, Ramírez et al. [25] evaluated road dust in Barranquilla, a major industrial city in the Caribbean region, finding that the major elements, including Al, Ca, Fe, K, Mg, Na, and S, were the most abundant species, accounting for 23% ± 18% of the mass of thoracic particles.

The objective of this paper was to show an analysis of the spatial distribution and chemical composition of road dust in two high-altitude Latin American cities. This study was conducted in two cities in Colombia (Bogotá and Manizales), located in the Andean mountains at 2000 m above sea level (m.a.s.l.). The cities were selected for presenting different demographic conditions, transportation patterns, industrial dynamics, and pollution levels. The aims of the research were (i) to determine the RD_{10} load in each city according to land use, (ii) to evaluate the spatial distribution and the chemical composition of RD_{10} in Bogota and Manizales, and (iii) to explore potential factors associated to sources of RD_{10} for the two cities mentioned.

2. Materials and Methods

2.1. Sampling Locations

Bogotá is the capital of Colombia and the largest city in the country (population of 8.1 million), located in the South America Andes Cordillera at an altitude of 2640 m.a.s.l. (Figure 1). The urban region has an approximate area of 420 km² and a high population density, ~17,700 inhabitants per km² [24]. Meteorological conditions in Bogotá are characterized by having an average temperature of 15 °C and average annual precipitation of 844 mm. Winds from NE–E and SE–E predominate, with average speeds of 1.5–3.5 m/s. The trade winds reach the city between June and August, favoring pollutant dispersion. The city has a high motorization rate, 313 vehicles per 1000 inhabitants in the year of 2018 [26]. The city's vehicle fleet in 2018 was composed of 2.4 million vehicles, in which 47% were passenger cars, 25% pick-up trucks, 22% motorcycles, 3% heavy-duty cargo fleet, 2% taxis, and 1.9% collective transport buses [27]. Private vehicles and motorcycles use mainly gasoline, taxis use gasoline and vehicular natural gas (NG), buses use diesel and NG, and heavy vehicles use predominantly diesel as fuel.

Bogotá has a mix of industries, such as manufacturing, chemical, plastics, food and beverages, metallurgy, exploitation of quarries, and mining (nonmetallic) areas, among others. This sector has an intensive use of fossil fuels for goods production and transportation. The industries are located both within the urban area and at nearby municipalities, generating land-use and environmental conflicts [28]. Frequently, PM exceeds national air quality standards in the southern and western areas of the city, given the emission sources, and local and meteorological conditions [24].

Manizales is a medium-sized Andean city (population of 434,403 inhabitants) [29], located in the central-west of Colombia on the western slope of the Cordillera Central at an altitude of 2150 m.a.s.l. [30] (Figure 1). The urban region has an approximate area of 54 km² [29] and high population density (~7504 inhabitants per km² in the urban area). Meteorological conditions in Manizales are characterized by a high annual precipitation (1670 mm) with a high spatial variability. The diurnal temperature profile ranges between 12–24 °C, high relative humidity between 69–86%, and low wind speeds (≤2 m/s). These meteorological conditions enhance minimum dispersion of pollutants in the urban area [31,32]. Local atmospheric chemistry is influenced by proximity to the Nevado del Ruiz volcano (located approximately 28 km from the southeast of Manizales and 140 km from the northwest of Bogotá), one of the most active in Latin America, registering significant activity since 2010 with daily SO_2 and ash emission episodes [33]. Valley–mountain wind circulation patterns in the city are characterized as ascending by day and descending by night [30,31], with possible transport of volcanic emissions during downslope wind.

Manizales has a high motorization rate, 455.2 vehicles per 1000 inhabitants in the year of 2018 [31,34]. The city's vehicle fleet in 2017 was composed of 169,142 vehicles, in which 48.3% were passenger cars, 47.1% motorcycles, 1.4% taxis, 1.5% collective transport buses, and 1.7% pick-up trucks. Private vehicles and motorcycles use gasoline, taxis use gasoline and NG, and buses and heavy vehicles use diesel as fuel. Manizales has a diverse industrial sector of food and beverages, chemical, plastics, metallurgy, foundry, and minerals, among others. These industries use natural gas, coal, and diesel as fuels [32].

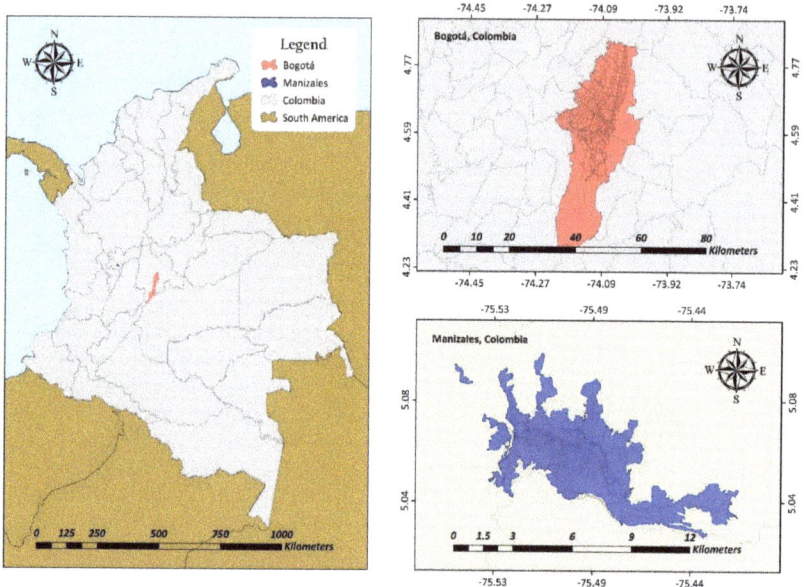

Figure 1. Location of the study cities—Bogotá and Manizales, Colombia.

2.2. Road Dust Samplings

A total of 41 samples were obtained from the two cities, 20 samplings were carried out in Bogotá and 21 in Manizales. Road dust sampling was conducted in dry weather and at least 48 h after a precipitation event. This condition guarantees that particles are mobilized and not retained by the surface humidity [35]. Field campaigns were carried out between December 2017 and March 2018 in Bogotá, and between July and September 2019 in Manizales (Table 1). As a result of the closeness with the equator (latitudes between 4.5 and 5.1 degrees north for Bogotá and Manizales, respectively), the seasonal variations of temperature and solar radiation between these two cities in question are small, and even negligible if the length of the day is considered. Of all samples, 23 were collected in areas of the cities where commercial activities predominate (average conditions typical of each city)—7 in Bogotá and 16 in Manizales; nine samples were taken in sites of interest such as industrial areas—6 in Bogotá and 3 in Manizales; nine samples were taken in sites of interest with little activity, such as residential areas—7 in Bogotá and 2 in Manizales.

Table 1. Average loading of RD_{10} at each location.

ID Point	Length	Latitude	Sampling Date	Classification	RD_{10} (mg/m^2)
			Bogotá		
1	74°03′59.07″ W	4°45′34.48″ N	19 December 2017	Commercial Land Use	3.26
2	74°01′28.05″ W	4°45′21.12″ N	19 December 2017	Residential Land Use	7.04
3	74°01′56.41″ W	4°43′12.28″ N	20 December 2017	Residential Land Use	14.31
4	74°02′50.84″ W	4°41′14.78″ N	20 December 2017	Residential Land Use	18.92
5	74°03′58.63″ W	4°38′22.69″ N	22 December 2017	Commercial Land Use	7.06
6	74°04′14.20″ W	4°39′26.73″ N	27 January 2018	Commercial Land Use	10.33
7	74°05′38.62″ W	4°41′18.01″ N	26 January 2018	Commercial Land Use	4.60
8	74°07′25.07″ W	4°43′27.55″ N	26 March 2018	Commercial Land Use	45.75
9	74°09′11.51″ W	4°40′31.39″ N	26 January 2018	Industrial Land Use	1.82
10	74°07′25.32″ W	4°39′07.38″ N	26 January 2018	Industrial Land Use	2.41
11	74°07′11.76″ W	4°38′07.65″ N	24 January 2018	Industrial Land Use	7.08
12	74°05′52.42″ W	4°37′33.33″ N	24 January 2018	Industrial Land Use	8.35
13	74°04′36.13″ W	4°36′29.91″ N	22 December 2017	Commercial Land Use	12.07
14	74°06′01.31″ W	4°36′11.21″ N	21 December 2017	Residential Land Use	9.40
15	74°08′13.84″ W	4°35′48.87″ N	23 January 2018	Industrial Land Use	23.14
16	74°10′06.66″ W	4°37′47.06″ N	3 March 2018	Residential Land Use	21.15
17	74°10′38.49″ W	4°35′51.84″ N	27 January 2018	Industrial Land Use	6.05
18	74°07′33.38″ W	4°34′09.98″ N	25 January 2018	Commercial Land Use	10.65
19	74°05′14.33″ W	4°34′11.51″ N	25 January 2018	Residential Land Use	16.71
20	74°07′02.07″ W	4°31′00.78″ N	27 March 2018	Residential Land Use	6.04
			Manizales		
1	75°27′05.00″ W	5°01′40.58″ N	2 September 2019	Industrial Land Use	26.75
2	75°27′04.86″ W	5°01′58.84″ N	20 August 2019	Industrial Land Use	11.72
3	75°27′41.15″ W	5°02′10.10″ N	2 September 2019	Industrial Land Use	0.77
4	75°27′56.27″ W	5°01′55.02″ N	31 July 2019	Mixed Land Use	8.54
5	75°27′59.94″ W	5°02′02.87″ N	30 August 2019	Residential Land Use	2.52
6	75°28′52.54″ W	5°02′01.90″ N	28 August 2019	Mixed Land Use	1.74
7	75°29′01.39″ W	5°02′49.34″ N	9 August 2019	Mixed Land Use	1.96
8	75°28′54.88″ W	5°03′05.36″ N	8 August 2019	Mixed Land Use	7.19
9	75°29′24.04″ W	5°03′07.42″ N	28 August 2019	Residential Land Use	2.22
10	75°29′12.30″ W	5°03′27.14″ N	9 August 2019	Mixed Land Use	2.72
11	75°29′38.04″ W	5°03′35.71″ N	30 August 2019	Mixed Land Use	3.17
12	75°30′06.37″ W	5°03′50.11″ N	20 August 2019	Mixed Land Use	2.73
13	75°29′55.54″ W	5°04′12.86″ N	22 August 2019	Mixed Land Use	3.57
14	75°30′20.88″ W	5°03′57.53″ N	6 August 2019	Mixed Land Use	6.46
15	75°30′38.84″ W	5°04′04.84″ N	22 August 2019	Mixed Land Use	1.43
16	75°30′55.37″ W	5°04′04.19″ N	1 August 2019	Mixed Land Use	7.14
17	75°30′54.04″ W	5°04′13.44″ N	28 August 2019	Mixed Land Use	4.16
18	75°31′00.55″ W	5°04′08.76″ N	6 August 2019	Mixed Land Use	5.92
19	75°30′20.88″ W	5°04′07.18″ N	8 August 2019	Mixed Land Use	6.52
20	75°31′29.75″ W	5°04′17.44″ N	1 August 2019	Mixed Land Use	7.53
21	75°31′51.10″ W	5°03′21.28″ N	6 August 2019	Mixed Land Use	5.03

A dry dust sampler designed at the Spanish National Research Council (CSIC) was used in the field campaigns. A description of the instrument is available elsewhere [8,35]. Briefly, the instrument consists of a PVC deposition chamber followed by a stainless steel elutriation filter designed to allow passage to only PM_{10}-grade material [23]. Road sediments from the pavement of the active traffic lanes were sampled by suction (in a total area of 3.0 m^2 divided into three sections of 1.0 m^2 each), using a vacuum pump (a 30 min sampling was performed at each section with an air flow of 25 ± 2.5 L/min) powered by a field generator (located at some distance downwind with respect to the sampling area). These sediments were immediately resuspended in the deposition chamber. The particles that were small and/or light enough to be carried by the air current continued their journey through the system and entered the stainless steel elutriation filter. Finally, the particles able to penetrate this barrier (PM_{10}) were collected on 47 mm filters made of quartz fiber (in Bogotá) and glass fiber (in Manizales). PM_{10} losses by sedimentation in the deposition chamber have been shown to be negligible (on average only 0.6% and 0.1% (in volume) of samples sieved at 250 μm and 63 μm, respectively) [35]. The surroundings to the sampling point were observed for safety, traffic characteristics, road condition, and land-use types [23,36].

Filters were baked at 500 °C for 12 h before sampling and then conditioned for 48 h at a constant temperature and relative humidity (20 ± 2 °C and RH 50% ± 5%). The weight of each filter was determined with a microbalance every 24 h. The mass fraction of road dust per m^2 (RD_{10}) was calculated at each location by averaging the mass collected at the three sampling points.

2.3. Chemical Analysis

After sampling, filters were kept refrigerated in the laboratory in a sealed bag protected from light until analysis. The road dust mass fraction per m^2 (RD_{10} load) at each site was calculated by difference in filter weights before and after sample collection, and averaging the mass collected after weighing three times (mg/m^2). After the sample weights were established, the filters were sent for destructive analysis at the "Laboratorio de Análisis Ambiental de la Universidad Nacional de Costa Rica" (Heredia, Costa Rica). Each filter was divided into small parts for the analysis of ions (3.5 cm^2 approximately for ion chromatography, IC), minerals, and trace elements (6.25 cm^2 approximately for inductively coupled plasma mass spectrometry, ICP-MS).

For mineral and trace elements, a portion of the impacted filter was acid-digested using 10 mL of a mixture of HNO_3 (5.55% v/v) and HCl (16.75% v/v) with deionized water. Microwave heating for 15 min was used by temperature ramps that reached 200 °C. After achieving 200 °C, the temperature was maintained for another 15 min. Then, this solution was filtered through a quantitative filter and diluted with deionized water in a 25 mL volumetric flask. A 15 mL aliquot was transferred to the sampler tubes of the spectroscope. The digested samples were injected to the ICP-MS by a peristaltic pump to the nebulizer system, where it was transformed into an aerosol due to the action of argon gas. The ions that originated in the argon plasma were injected into the mass spectrometer, mass/charge ratio was used for the identification.

Another portion of the filter was leached into 30 mL of deionized water in an ultrasonic bath for 45 min for the extraction of water-soluble ions. The residual liquid was then filtered through a membrane filter and diluted with deionized water in a 50 mL volumetric flask. A portion of the liquid was taken then for further analysis by IC. Sulphate, nitrate, and chloride ions were analyzed [37]. The blanks were submitted to the same chain of custody and treatment as the samples. The Supplementary Materials Table S1 shows the calculations made for the determination of charges for each chemical species.

2.4. Enrichment Factors

Enrichment factors (EFs) were calculated for the fraction of road dust using Equation (1). EFs have generally been used to determine the degree of enrichment from anthropogenic sources in road dust [24].

$$EF_{Element} = \frac{(Element\ RD_{10}/Reference\ RD_{10})}{(Element\ Crust/Reference\ Crust)} \quad (1)$$

where element is the concentration of the element under consideration and reference is the concentration of the chosen referenced element. Subscripts indicate to which source the concentration refers, sample (RD_{10}) or the earth's crust (Crust). EF values were calculated based on the upper continental crust composition (see Supplementary Materials Table S2) using aluminum as the reference element [38]. Aluminum was selected because it is one of the most abundant elements in the earth's crust, and it has been the most used normalizing element in the geochemical literature [38,39]. The enrichment values of elements from anthropogenic sources are classified according to the following ranges: minimal (EF = 1–2), moderate (EF = 2–5), significant (EF = 5–20), very high (EF = 20–40), and extremely high (EF > 40) [40].

2.5. Principal Component Analysis (PCA)

A PCA was carried out to explore qualitative contributions to the chemical composition of RD_{10} from different factors associated with sources such as brake wear, tire wear, fugitive dust, industrial emissions, and natural emissions, among others. The factors identified by PCA can be associated with emissions sources, but they do not represent the actual sources. The application of a more refined receptor model was not possible due to the lower number of samples. PCA was performed for the dataset recorded in Bogotá and Manizales, and a varimax rotation (with Kaiser normalization) was applied to facilitate the interpretation of the results. In general, this method of rotation maximizes the sum of the variance of the squared loadings, where 'loadings' means correlations between variables and factors. This usually results in high factor loadings for a smaller number of variables and low factor loadings for the rest. The remaining components all have eigenvalues of more than one. In simple terms, the result is that a small number of important variables are highlighted, which makes it easier to interpret the principal component analysis [41].

3. Results and Discussion

3.1. RD_{10} Levels

The RD_{10} loadings observed in Bogotá (average 11.8 mg/m^2, interquartile range between 6.0–16.1 mg/m^2) and Manizales (average 5.7 mg/m^2, interquartile range between 2.4–7.2 mg/m^2) were comparable to those reported for European cities such as Barcelona (3.0–80.0 mg/m^2), Birmingham (3.8–42.7 mg/m^2), the Andalusia region (2.0–22.0 mg/m^2), and Turin (0.8–42.7 mg/m^2), but they were higher than Girona (1.3–7.1 mg/m^2), Porto (0.1–0.9 mg/m^2), Paris (0.7–2.2 mg/m^2), and Zürich (0.2–1.3 mg/m^2). However, RD_{10} values in Bogotá and Manizales were lower than New Delhi in India (44.0–106.0 mg/m^2) (Table 2).

RD_{10} loadings were higher and more variable in Bogotá than in Manizales (Figure 2, panel a). The three highest loadings in Bogotá (45.8, 23.1, and 21.1 mg/m^2 at ID points 8, 15, and 16, respectively, Figure 3) were sites located close to demolition/construction works in the southwest of the city, the same area where ambient PM_{10} is frequently exceeded. In Manizales, the three highest loadings (26.7, 11.7, and 8.5 mg/m^2 at ID points 1, 2, and 4, respectively, Figure 4) were found in sites with industrial activity and poor road pavement conditions in the eastern areas.

Table 2. Comparison of road dust loads from this study and others reported for different regions.

Source	City	Site Features	RD$_{10}$ (mg/m^2)	Season
[35]	Barcelona, Spain	City Center—Urban Zone	3.0–23.0	Summer
		Ring roads with heavy traffic	24.0–80.0	
		Urban tunnel	13.0	
		Demolition/construction area	2.5–471.0	
[8]	Barcelona, Spain	Urban Zone	3.7–23.1	Spring/ Summer
	Girona, Spain	Urban Zone	1.3–7.1	
		Demolition/construction area	48.7	
	Zürich, Switzerland	Urban Zone	0.2–1.3	
[42]	Andalucía, Spain	Urban Zone	2.0–22.0	Summer
[21]	Birmingham, UK	High traffic highway	3.8–21.8	Dry season
		High traffic tunnel	3.0–36.1	
	New Delhi, India	High traffic highway	44.0–106.0	
[17]	Paris, France	Urban Zone	0.7–2.2	Spring
		Cobblestone pavement	10.3	
[7]	Porto, Portugal	Paved road	0.1–0.9	Summer
		Cobblestone pavement	50.0	
[43]	Barcelona, Spain	Urban Zone	1.1–3.4	Summer
	Turin, Italy	Urban Zone	0.8–8.8	Summer and winter
		Roads in proximity to unpaved parks	12.3	
		Demolition/construction area	11.5–42.7	
Current study	Bogotá, Colombia	Urban Zone	1.8–45.5	Dry season
	Manizales, Colombia	Urban Zone	0.8–26.7	

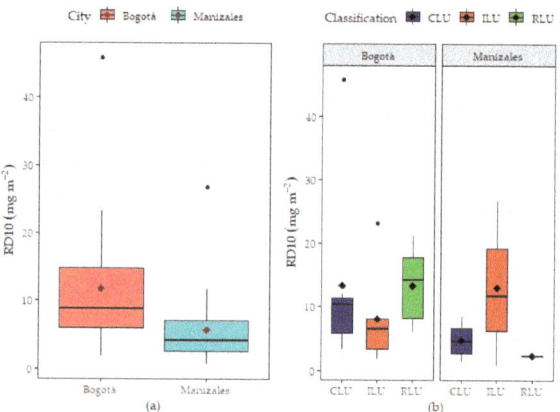

Figure 2. Road dust loads boxplots (**a**) for Bogotá and Manizales and (**b**) grouped by land use for Bogotá and Manizales—CLU: commercial land use; ILU—industrial land use; RLU—residential land use.

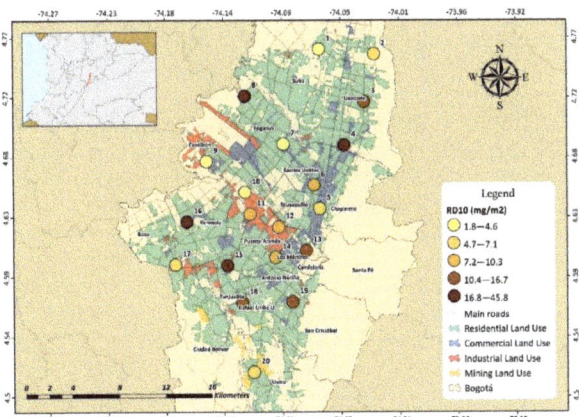

Figure 3. Spatial distribution of road dust loads in Bogotá.

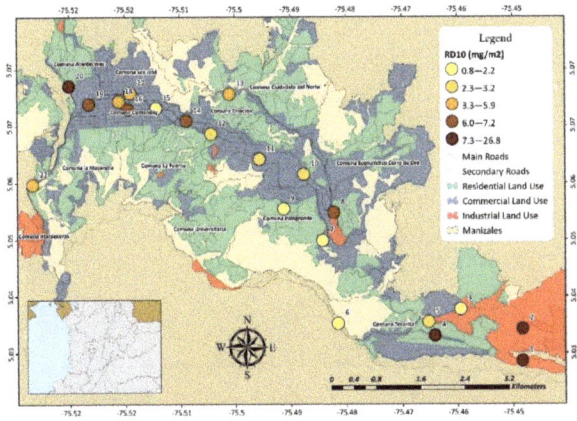

Figure 4. Spatial distribution of road dust loads in Manizales.

Differences in RD_{10} levels in Bogotá and Manizales can be partially explained by urban planning. As it can be identified from Figures 3 and 4, Manizales displays a central axis of commercial activity surrounded by residential areas. The industrial sector is located mainly towards the southeastern areas of the city. In contrast, industrial facilities in Bogotá are spread in the central and southwestern areas of the city, in conjunction with residential and commercial areas. These differences in land-use features determine, in part, levels of RD_{10}. The higher values in Bogotá were not only attributed to industrial zones but to areas with a mix of industries, heavy traffic, commercial facilities, and poor road condition, in addition to building and road construction.

Dust loadings in residential areas in Bogotá were larger than those observed in commercial or industrial zones. In contrast, RD_{10} levels were the highest under industrial land use in Manizales. Residential areas showed the lowest values (Figure 2, panel b). As it was described, urban development in Bogotá has resulted in zones where industrial and commercial sectors coexist with residential use. One of such zones is the southwest of the city (Figure 3). This area has heavy traffic, a higher fraction of unpaved roads and poor pavement conditions, quarrying/mining activity, and the presence of eroded soils. In Manizales, areas categorized under industrial land use also show heavy vehicular traffic and poor pavement quality, which explains the highest RD_{10} values. In residential areas with predominance of light vehicle circulation, dust loadings were the lowest (average

2.37 mg/m^2). Lastly, in areas with mixed land use (institutional, commercial, and services), the average RD$_{10}$ was 4.58 mg/m^2 (Figure 2, panel b and Figure 4).

3.2. Chemical Profile

Mineral elements such as Al, Ca, Fe, K, Mg, Mn, Na, and Ti represented 9.0% the total RD$_{10}$ mass in Bogotá, with an average load of 1020 µg/m^2; meanwhile, mineral contribution in Manizales comprised 37.8% of the RD$_{10}$ mass (1952 µg/m^2). Mineral compounds are abundant in the thoracic fraction of road dust [25] and can influence the mass percentage distribution. The mineral fraction was significantly larger in Manizales than Bogotá (Figure 5a). However, other studies have found greater contributions of the mineral component in RD$_{10}$ in Colombia, 62% ± 26% in Bogotá and 23% ± 18% in Barranquilla [24,25]. In cities such as Barcelona, New Delhi, and Fushun, the contribution was found to be in the range of 25–35% [21,35,44]. The contribution percentages of the main elements to total mass might be underestimated due to the fact that elements such as metalloids (Si), oxides (Al$_2$O$_3$, CO$_3$$^{-2}$, SiO$_2$), and organic matter were not analyzed.

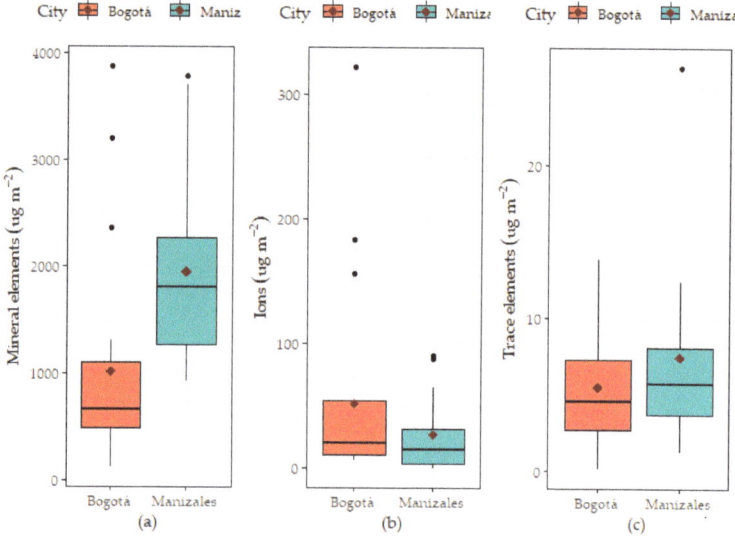

Figure 5. Total load of (**a**) mineral elements, (**b**) ions, and (**c**) trace elements determined for Bogotá and Manizales.

The fraction of water-soluble ions (SO$_4$$^{-2}$, NO$_3$$^-$ and Cl$^-$) represented less than 1.0% of the total mass in Bogotá (average load 51.52 µg/m^2) and Manizales (average load 26.64 µg/m^2) (Figure 5b). Previously, a larger ions contribution of 3.8% ± 1.1% was observed in Bogotá [24], similar to Barcelona, Spain (2.4%) [35], but higher than Fushun, China (0.5%) [44].

Trace metals (Ag, As, Be, Cd, Co, Cr, Cu, Hg, Mo, Ni, Pb, Sb, Se, and V), with an average load of 5.54 µg/m^2 and 7.48 µg/m^2, represented 0.05% and 0.13% of the total mass captured from RD$_{10}$ in Bogotá and Manizales, respectively (Figure 5c). In Bogotá, Barcelona, and Fushun, trace metals represented 0.5%, 0.36%, and 0.66%, respectively [24,35,44]. The Supplementary Materials Table S3 shows results of each of the chemical species analyzed.

In Bogotá, 89.4% of the mineral load was composed of four crustal metals: Al (33.6%), Ca (28.0%), Fe (19.5%), and Na (8.3%). The origin of these metals can be associated to: (i) poor road condition and unpaved roads; (ii) low or null vegetation cover [45]; (iii) road and building construction [17,35]; and (iv) quarries and mining areas [46] (Figure 6a). In Manizales, five crustal elements comprised 92.8% of the mineral components: Na (34.3%),

Al (20.5%), K (14.1%), Ca (14.0%), and Fe (9.9%). The sources of these elements are mainly related to the resuspension of fugitive dust (earth's crust material of volcanic geological formation, Figure 6b). In effect, previous studies in the Manizales area have highlighted the presence of high contents of Si, Al, and Fe, as well as compounds such as plagioclase feldspar (Ca-Na) and volcanic glass, among others, in the chemical composition of the soil derived from volcanic ash [47]. Likewise, Trejos et al. [36] found traces of volcanic ash, such as hydrated complexes of Al, Si, and K; heavy metals like As, Hg, Cd, and Pb; and specific compounds, such as ammonia salt and plagioclase feldspar (Ca-Na), in soil dust from Manizales. This volcanic influence may explain the higher loads of Al, K, and Na in Manizales in comparison to Bogotá (Figure 7).

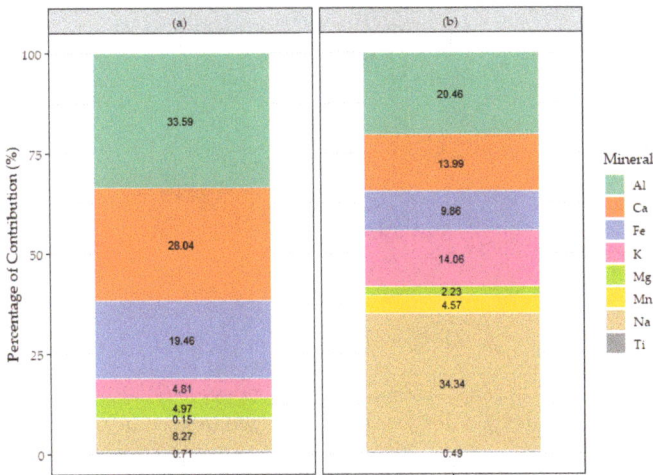

Figure 6. Average composition of main elements for: (**a**) Bogotá and (**b**) Manizales.

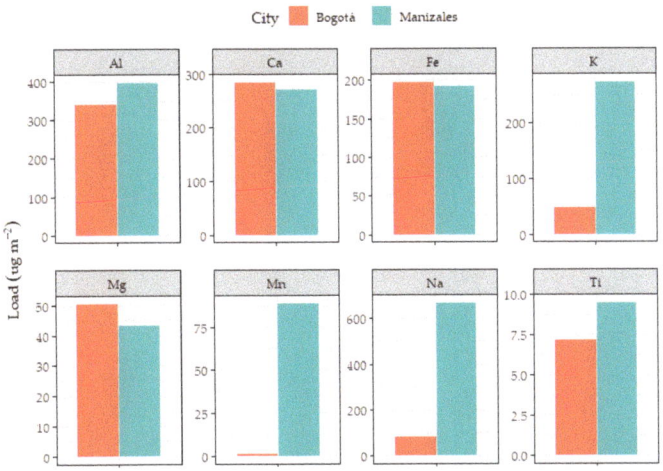

Figure 7. Individual load of main elements obtained in Bogotá and Manizales.

Despite their low fraction in mass, sulphate and nitrate were the most abundant ions in soil dust in Bogotá and Manizales (Figure 8). The precursors of these compounds are associated with pavement wear [46], vehicle exhaust emissions, and formation of secondary inorganic aerosols [48,49]. Cl⁻ showed a contribution of 7.4% in Bogotá and 20.9% in Manizales. The latter is mainly associated with the composition of soils derived from volcanic ash, where Cl^-, HCO_3^-, and SO_4^{-2} predominate among soluble anions [47] and the deposition of secondary particles formed from precursor gases, such as HCl [24], emitted from the Nevado del Ruiz volcano.

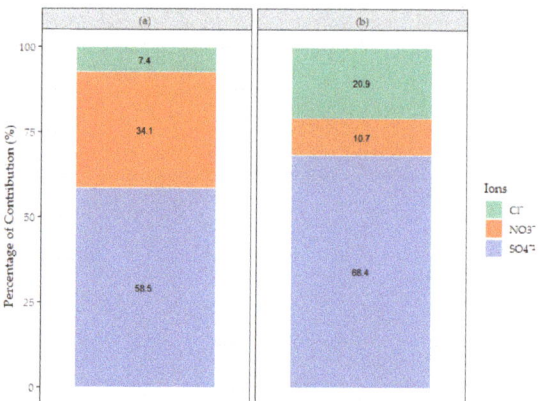

Figure 8. Water-soluble ion distribution for (**a**) Bogotá and (**b**) Manizales.

Trace elements, such as Cu, Pb, Cr, Ni, V, and Sb, comprised 96.0% of the mass attributed to this component in Bogotá (Figure 9). These metals are commonly associated with vehicle exhaust emissions, especially the use of antioxidants, additives, and lubricants (Cu and Pb), mechanical abrasion (Cu), and tire/brake wear (Cu, Pb, Ni, V, and Sb) [10,17,19]. In the case of Manizales, the contents of Cu and Pb were lower, but there was a significant mass of Mo (11%) in comparison to Bogotá (Figure 9). Molybdenum is mainly associated with emissions from the steel industry [50,51] and brake wear [42]. Both situations are relevant in Manizales, with a relatively large industrial sector and a complex topography that requires a strong use of brakes in steep streets with slopes that could be greater than 22% [52].

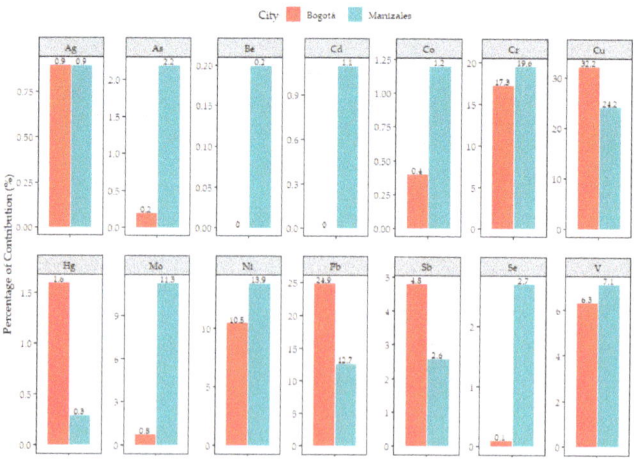

Figure 9. Average composition of traces for Bogotá and Manizales.

3.3. Source Exploration by EFs

Enrichment factors were estimated with the aim to explore the anthropogenic influence of some crustal elements (Ca, Fe, K, and Mn) and trace metals (As, Co, Cr, Cu, Mo, Ni, Pb, Sb, Se, and V). Aluminum was used as a reference element, given its abundance in the upper continental crust. In Bogotá, EFs showed extremely high values (EF > 40) for Mo and Sb; very high (20 < EF < 40) for Cu and Pb; high (5 < EF < 20) for Ni, Se, and Cr; and moderate (EF < 5) for Ca, Fe, V, and As. In Manizales, EFs were extremely high (EF > 40) for Mo, Se, Sb, and Mn; very high (20 < EF < 40) for Cu and As; high (5 < EF < 20) for Ni, Cr, and Pb; and moderate (1 < EF < 5) for K, Ca, V, Co, and Fe (Figure 10).

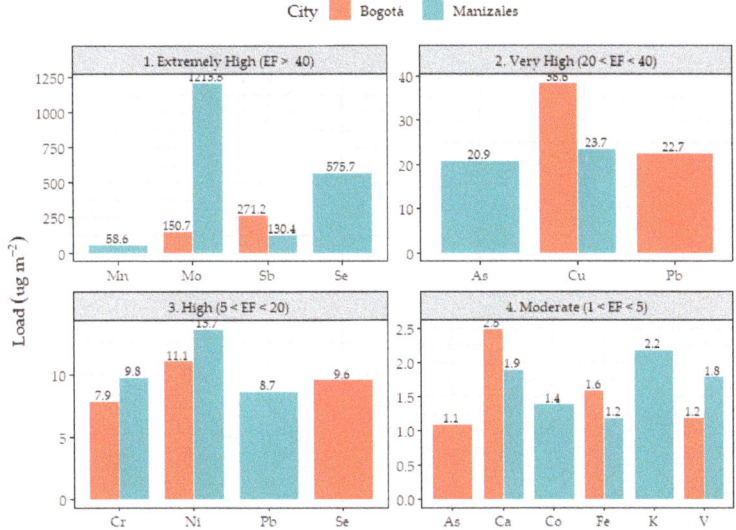

Figure 10. Enrichment factors in Bogotá and Manizales.

The presence of Sb, Ba, Cu, Fe, and Mn in road dust samples can be associated with brake wear [53]. Antimony was, in particular, the element that recorded the highest levels of enrichment in Bogotá (EF = 271), and it was among the highest in Manizales (EF = 130). Despite the relatively low number of vehicles (169,142), the complex topography and steep roads in Manizales imply the heavy use of brakes [36]. In Bogotá, the greater vehicular volume (approximately 2 million vehicles) and traffic congestion explain the frequent use of brakes.

The EF of Sb was higher than those reported in high-traffic cities such as Moscow, Russia (EF = 44) [19] and those registered in some roads in Barranquilla (EF close to 100) [25], but it was similar, and even lower, than those observed in high traffic roads in Viana do Castelo, Portugal (100 < EF <1000) [13]. Ramírez et al. [24] reported a Sb enrichment factor close to 140 for commercial-use areas in Bogotá, which was lower than those found in this study. In accordance with the chemical composition of the brake pads, a Cu/Sb ratio > 7 has been proposed for brake wear emissions in road dust [21,35]. An average Cu/Sb ratio of 7.6 for Bogotá and 9.2 for Manizales was observed, confirming the relevant contribution of brake wear to road dust.

Molybdenum registered an enrichment factor eight times higher in Manizales (EF = 1213) than Bogotá (EF = 151). The obtained EF values of Mb in cities such as Moscow (EF = 7) [19] and Toronto (EF = 0.9) [51] were much lower than the values observed in Colombia. Molybdenum has been associated with various industrial emissions, mainly those related to incinerators and with the mechanical/metallurgical industry [19]. Likewise, Mo is associated with brake pad abrasion [51]. A high correlation of Mo with Co (0.96), Hg

(0.73), Pb (0.74), Se (0.61), and V (0.94) in Manizales suggests a common source of origin, related with the industrial activity in the city (see Supplementary Materials Figure S1). In addition, the high correlation of Mo with elements found in volcanic ash, such as Cd (1.0), Pb (0.74), V (0.94), and Fe (0.84), suggests a potential contribution of volcanic emissions to the observed enrichment levels [36].

Selenium showed the second-highest EF value in Manizales (EF = 576), a level that was higher than those reported in Bogotá [24] and Viana do Castelo [13]. The enrichment of Se is commonly associated with anthropogenic emissions, including combustion (coal, oil, wood, and biomass), non-ferrous melting, manufacturing, and use of agricultural products. The correlations of Se with As (0.63), Cd (0.62), Mo (0.61), and V (0.63) (Figure S1) suggest a contribution from industrial activity and possible influence of the Nevado del Ruiz volcano [24,36,54].

Cu, Pb, Ni, and Cr presented high and very high EFs (5 < EF <40), widely associated with mechanical abrasion and tire/brake wear [19,24,51]. In Manizales, As also showed a high EF, possibly associated with coal combustion [55] and volcanic emissions (moderate correlation of As with SO_4^{-2} (0.62) and Se (0.63)).

3.4. Factors Associated to Sources in PCA Analysis

In the PCA analysis, 92.2% of the total variance could be explained by five factors in Bogotá and six factors in Manizales (Table 3). Factors that explain at least 10.0% of the data variability were considered. In Bogotá, PC1 explained 42.3% of the variance and showed high correlations with elements associated with dust resuspension, pavement wear, road traffic, and the use of antioxidants, additives, and vehicle lubricants (V, Al, Fe, Ti, As, K, Pb, Co, Mn, Ca, and Cr) [10,17]. PC2, explaining 25.9% of the variance, showed high correlations with Se, Na, NO_3, and Mg and a moderate relation with SO_4 and Ca. PC2 is associated with construction/demolition activities [35,46]. Lastly, PC3 (16.7% variance explained) is influenced by non-exhaust trace elements, such as Sb, Cu, Mo, and Ni [19].

In Manizales, the first component (PC1) explained 37.8% of the total variance and had high correlations with Co, V, Mo, Cd, Fe, Ca, Pb, Mg, and Ti, suggesting an influence of tire and brake wear, as well as combustion processes [42,50,51]. PC2, a component that explained 18.7% of the total variance, was mainly influenced by SO_4, As, and K with a lower influence of Sb, Mg, Ti, Al, and Cr. This factor may be associated with the road abrasion and volcanic ash emissions [24,36]. Lastly, PC3 (10.1% of the variance) was correlated with Na, K, and Al, suggesting a contribution related to the resuspension of fugitive dust and volcanic ash [36,47].

Table 3. Rotated component of PCA for road dust in Bogotá (n = 20) and Manizales (n = 14). Only significant values (>0.32) are presented. Highest values (>0.7) are shown in red.

Rotated Component Matrix [a]—RD_{10} Bogotá					Rotated Component Matrix [b]—RD_{10} Manizales						
Element	PC1	PC2	PC3	PC4	Element	PC1	PC2	PC3	PC4	PC5	PC6
V	0.97				Co	0.98					
Al	0.96				V	0.97					
Fe	0.96				Mo	0.96					
Ti	0.92				Cd	0.96					
As	0.85	0.35			Fe	0.91					
K	0.82	0.52			Ca	0.83					
Pb	0.78		0.4		Pb	0.79				0.49	
Co	0.78	0.47			Mg	0.75	0.54				
Mn	0.77	0.57			Ti	0.71	0.54				
Ca	0.75	0.61			SO_4		0.90				
Cr	0.71	0.38	0.52		As	0.35	0.79				
Se	0.34	0.90			K		0.77	0.55			
Na	0.33	0.88			Na	0.49		0.72		0.38	

Table 3. Cont.

Rotated Component Matrix [a]—RD$_{10}$ Bogotá					Rotated Component Matrix [b]—RD$_{10}$ Manizales						
Element	PC1	PC2	PC3	PC4	Element	PC1	PC2	PC3	PC4	PC5	PC6
NO$_3$		0.88			Ni				0.86		
Mg	0.54	0.77			Mn					0.97	
Sb			0.86		NO$_3$						0.90
Cu	0.35	0.36	0.83		Cu	0.43	0.39		0.53		0.52
Mo		0.45	0.80		Sb		0.61				0.46
Ni			0.72	0.42	Al	0.58	0.52	0.5			
Cl				0.92	Se	0.56	0.37		0.4	−0.38	
SO$_4$	0.49	0.63		0.55	Cr		0.52		−0.66		
Cd					Cl			−0.84			
Eigenvalues	8.9	5.4	3.5	1.5	Eigenvalues	8.3	4.1	2.2	2.1	1.9	1.7
Variance (%)	42.3	25.9	16.7	7.2	Variance (%)	37.8	18.7	10.1	9.3	8.5	7.7
Cum. (%)	42.3	68.3	85.0	92.2	Cum. (%)	37.8	56.5	66.6	76	84.5	92.2

Extraction method: principal component analysis. Rotation method: varimax with Kaiser normalization. [a] Rotation converged in 6 iterations. [b] Rotation converged in 14 iterations.

4. Conclusions

Road dust loadings and chemical composition were investigated in two Andean cities with different sizes, urban planning, and emission sources. RD$_{10}$ levels were larger in Bogotá (average of 11.8 mg/m^2) than in Manizales (average of 5.7 mg/m^2) due to a higher vehicular volume and a large mix of land use features. Residential areas in Manizales showed the lowest RD$_{10}$ values (average of 2.4 mg/m^2), whereas industrial zones contributed the largest dust loadings (average of 13.1 mg/m^2). Residential areas mixed with industrial and commercial activity showed significant levels of road dust in Bogotá (average of 13.4 mg/m^2). Construction and demolition activities were identified as relevant emitters of road dust (dust loadings between 45.8–21.1 mg/m^2).

Crustal elements (Al, Ca, Fe, K, and Na) were the most abundant elements in road dust in both cities. The complex topography in Manizales and the closeness to the Nevado del Ruiz volcano explain the high levels of crustal and trace metals in road dust, especially Mo, Se, Sb, and Mn. The volcanic activity was also associated with SO_4^{-2} and Cl^-. In Bogotá, Cu, Pb, Cr, Ni, V, Sb, and Mo were associated with combustion and non-exhaust (brake, tire, and road wear) emissions. Finally, the study of the influential factors and chemical composition of road dust, as well as its spatial variability, is crucial for public agencies and research centers to identify the origins of PM, formulate mitigation measures, and identify possible adverse effects on the population.

Supplementary Materials: The following are available online at https://www.mdpi.com/article/10.3390/atmos12091109/s1, Figure S1: Correlation matrix of chemically analyzed elements for road dust in the cities of (a) Bogota and (b) Manizales, Table S1: Calculation methodology for determining loads in RD$_{10}$, Table S2: Concentrations in upper continental crust, Table S3: Results of chemical species analyzed for each city.

Author Contributions: Conceptualization, B.H.A., O.R. and J.E.P.; data curation, S.V. and E.M.T.; formal analysis, S.V.; funding acquisition, B.H.A., O.R. and J.E.P.; investigation, S.V. and E.M.T.; methodology, S.V., E.M.T. and J.M.H.; project administration, B.H.A., O.R. and J.E.P.; resources, J.H.M., F.A. and L.F.O.S.; software, S.V. and E.M.T.; supervision, B.H.A., O.R., N.Y.R. and J.E.P.; validation, B.H.A., O.R., N.Y.R. and J.E.P.; visualization, S.V.; writing—original draft preparation, S.V. and E.M.T.; writing—review and editing, S.V., E.M.T., B.H.A., G.M.P., O.R., F.A., L.F.O.S., N.Y.R., C.Z. and J.E.P. All authors have read and agreed to the published version of the manuscript.

Funding: This research was funded by ECOPETROL under agreement 5224377; and CORPOCALDAS under agreement 107-2018.

Institutional Review Board Statement: Not applicable.

Informed Consent Statement: Not applicable.

Data Availability Statement: The data presented in this study are available in the Supplementary Materials file.

Acknowledgments: The authors are grateful for the financial support provided by ECOPETROL and CORPOCALDAS. The authors' viewpoint does not necessarily reflect the official opinion of their institutions. We thank our students from CLIMA Research Group and Hydraulic Engineering and Environmental Research Group who developed the field campaigns. In addition, we would like to thank Universidad Nacional de Costa Rica, who supported the chemical analysis of the road dust samples. The author Guilherme M. Pereira acknowledges the Brazilian foundation Fundação de Amparo à Pesquisa do Estado de São Paulo (FAPESP, São Paulo Research Foundation; Grants nos. 2019/01316-8 and 2018/07848-9).

Conflicts of Interest: The authors declare no conflict of interest. In addition, the funders had no role in the design of the study; in the collection, analyses, or interpretation of data; in the writing of the manuscript; or in the decision to publish the results.

References

1. Pant, P.; Harrison, R.M. Estimation of the contribution of road traffic emissions to particulate matter concentrations from field measurements: A review. *Atmos. Environ.* **2013**, *77*, 78–97. [CrossRef]
2. Grigoratos, T.; Martini, G. Brake wear particle emissions: A review. *Environ. Sci. Pollut. Res.* **2014**, *22*, 2491–2504. [CrossRef]
3. Charron, A.; Polo-Rehn, L.; Besombes, J.-L.; Golly, B.; Buisson, C.; Chanut, H.; Marchand, N.; Guillaud, G.; Jaffrezo, J.-L. Identification and quantification of particulate tracers of exhaust and non-exhaust vehicle emissions. *Atmos. Chem. Phys. Discuss.* **2019**, *19*, 5187–5207. [CrossRef]
4. Harrison, R.M.; Jones, A.M.; Gietl, J.; Yin, J.; Green, D. Estimation of the Contributions of Brake Dust, Tire Wear, and Resuspension to Nonexhaust Traffic Particles Derived from Atmospheric Measurements. *Environ. Sci. Technol.* **2012**, *46*, 6523–6529. [CrossRef]
5. Kumar, P.; Pirjola, L.; Ketzel, M.; Harrison, R.M. Nanoparticle emissions from 11 non-vehicle exhaust sources—A review. *Atmos. Environ.* **2013**, *67*, 252–277. [CrossRef]
6. Thorpe, A.; Harrison, R.M. Sources and properties of non-exhaust particulate matter from road traffic: A review. *Sci. Total Environ.* **2008**, *400*, 270–282. [CrossRef] [PubMed]
7. Alves, C.; Evtyugina, M.; Vicente, A.; Vicente, E.; Nunes, T.; Silva, P.; Duarte, M.; Pio, C.; Amato, F.; Querol, X. Chemical profiling of PM10 from urban road dust. *Sci. Total Environ.* **2018**, *634*, 41–51. [CrossRef]
8. Amato, F.; Pandolfi, M.; Moreno, T.; Furger, M.; Pey, J.; Alastuey, A.; Bukowiecki, N.; Prevot, A.; Baltensperger, U.; Querol, X. Sources and variability of inhalable road dust particles in three European cities. *Atmos. Environ.* **2011**, *45*, 6777–6787. [CrossRef]
9. Guttikunda, S. Estimating Health Impacts of Urban Air Pollution. *Public Health* **2008**, *16*. Available online: https://urbanemissions.info/wp-content/uploads/docs/SIM-06-2008.pdf (accessed on 20 August 2021).
10. Hetem, I.G.; de Fatima Andrade, M. Characterization of Fine Particulate Matter Emitted from the Resuspension of Road and Pavement Dust in the Metropolitan Area of São Paulo, Brazil. *Atmosphere* **2016**, *7*, 31. [CrossRef]
11. Kupiainen, K.J.; Tervahattu, H.; Räisänen, M.; Mäkelä, T.; Aurela, M.; Hillamo, R. Size and Composition of Airborne Particles from Pavement Wear, Tires, and Traction Sanding. *Environ. Sci. Technol.* **2004**, *39*, 699–706. [CrossRef] [PubMed]
12. Khan, R.K.; Strand, M.A. Road dust and its effect on human health: A literature review. *Epidemiol. Health* **2018**, *40*, e2018013. [CrossRef] [PubMed]
13. Alves, C.A.; Vicente, E.; Vicente, A.M.; Rienda, I.C.; Tomé, M.; Querol, X.; Amato, F. Loadings, chemical patterns and risks of inhalable road dust particles in an Atlantic city in the north of Portugal. *Sci. Total Environ.* **2020**, *737*, 139596. [CrossRef]
14. Gulia, S.; Goyal, P.; Goyal, S.K.; Kumar, R. Re-suspension of road dust: Contribution, assessment and control through dust suppressants—A review. *Int. J. Environ. Sci. Technol.* **2018**, *16*, 1717–1728. [CrossRef]
15. Ostro, B.; Tobias, A.; Querol, X.; Alastuey, A.; Amato, F.; Pey, J.; Pérez, N.; Sunyer, J. The Effects of Particulate Matter Sources on Daily Mortality: A Case-Crossover Study of Barcelona, Spain. *Environ. Health Perspect.* **2011**, *119*, 1781–1787. [CrossRef]
16. Meister, K.; Johansson, C.; Forsberg, B. Estimated Short-Term Effects of Coarse Particles on Daily Mortality in Stockholm, Sweden. *Environ. Health Perspect.* **2012**, *120*, 431–436. [CrossRef]
17. Amato, F.; Favez, O.; Pandolfi, M.; Alastuey, A.; Querol, X.; Moukhtar, S.; Bruge, B.; Verlhac, S.; Orza, J.; Bonnaire, N.; et al. Traffic induced particle resuspension in Paris: Emission factors and source contributions. *Atmos. Environ.* **2016**, *129*, 114–124. [CrossRef]
18. Basagaña, X.; Jacquemin, B.; Karanasiou, A.; Ostro, B.; Querol, X.; Agis, D.; Alessandrini, E.; Alguacil, J.; Artinano, B.; Catrambone, M.; et al. Short-term effects of particulate matter constituents on daily hospitalizations and mortality in five South-European cities: Results from the MED-PARTICLES project. *Environ. Int.* **2014**, *75*, 151–158. [CrossRef]
19. Vlasov, D.; Kosheleva, N.; Kasimov, N. Spatial distribution and sources of potentially toxic elements in road dust and its PM10 fraction of Moscow megacity. *Sci. Total Environ.* **2020**, *761*, 143267. [CrossRef]
20. Zhang, J.; Wu, L.; Zhang, Y.; Li, F.; Fang, X.; Mao, H. Elemental composition and risk assessment of heavy metals in the PM10 fractions of road dust and roadside soil. *Particuology* **2019**, *44*, 146–152. [CrossRef]
21. Pant, P.; Baker, S.J.; Shukla, A.; Maikawa, C.; Pollitt, K.G.; Harrison, R.M. The PM 10 fraction of road dust in the UK and India: Characterization, source profiles and oxidative potential. *Sci. Total Environ.* **2015**, *531*, 445–452. [CrossRef] [PubMed]

22. Pachón, J.E.; Galvis, B.; Lombana, O.; Carmona, L.G.; Fajardo, S.; Rincón, A.; Meneses, S.; Chaparro, R.; Nedbor-Gross, R.; Henderson, B. Development and Evaluation of a Comprehensive Atmospheric Emission Inventory for Air Quality Modeling in the Megacity of Bogotá. *Atmosphere* **2018**, *9*, 49. [CrossRef]
23. Pachon, J.E.; Vanegas, S.; Saavedra, C.; Amato, F.; Silva, L.F.O.; Blanco, K.; Chaparro, R.; Casas, O.M. Evaluation of factors influencing road dust loadings in a Latin American urban center. *J. Air Waste Manag. Assoc.* **2021**, *71*, 268–280. [CrossRef]
24. Ramírez, O.; de la Campa, A.M.S.; Amato, F.; Moreno, T.; Silva, L.; de la Rosa, J.D. Physicochemical characterization and sources of the thoracic fraction of road dust in a Latin American megacity. *Sci. Total Environ.* **2018**, *652*, 434–446. [CrossRef]
25. Ramírez, O.; da Boit, K.; Blanco, E.; Silva, L. Hazardous thoracic and ultrafine particles from road dust in a Caribbean industrial city. *Urban. Clim.* **2020**, *33*, 100655. [CrossRef]
26. Bogotá Cómo Vamos. *Informe de Calidad de Vida En Bogotá 2018*; Bogotá Cómo Vamos: Bogotá, Colombia, 2019.
27. Secretaría Distrital de Ambiente. *Inventario de Emisiones de Bogotá, Contaminantes Atmosféricos 2018*; Secretaría Distrital de Ambiente: Bogotá, Colombia, 2020.
28. Ramírez, O.; de la Campa, A.S.; Amato, F.; Catacolí, R.A.; Rojas, N.Y.; de la Rosa, J. Chemical composition and source apportionment of PM10 at an urban background site in a high–altitude Latin American megacity (Bogota, Colombia). *Environ. Pollut.* **2018**, *233*, 142–155. [CrossRef] [PubMed]
29. DANE. *Omisión Censal: Nivel Municipal y Departamental*; DANE: Bogotá, Colombia, 2019.
30. Cuesta-Mosquera, A.P.; Wahl, M.; Acosta-López, J.G.; García-Reynoso, J.A.; Aristizábal-Zuluaga, B.H. Mixing layer height and slope wind oscillation: Factors that control ambient air SO2 in a tropical mountain city. *Sustain. Cities Soc.* **2019**, *52*, 101852. [CrossRef]
31. González, C.; Gómez, C.; Rojas, N.; Acevedo, H.; Aristizábal, B. Relative impact of on-road vehicular and point-source industrial emissions of air pollutants in a medium-sized Andean city. *Atmos. Environ.* **2016**, *152*, 279–289. [CrossRef]
32. Universidad Nacional de Colombia. *Corpocaldas Aplicación de Herramientas de Simulación Atmosférica En El Estudio de La Calidad Del Aire En Manizales—Informe Final Convenio Interadministrativo No. 107-2018*; Universidad Nacional de Colombia: Bogotá, Colombia, 2019.
33. Carn, S.A.; Fioletov, V.E.; McLinden, C.; Li, C.; Krotkov, N. A decade of global volcanic SO2 emissions measured from space. *Sci. Rep.* **2017**, *7*, srep44095. [CrossRef]
34. Manizales Cómo Vamos. *Informe de Calidad de Vida Manizales 2019*; Manizales Cómo Vamos: Bogotá, Colombia, 2019.
35. Amato, F.; Pandolfi, M.; Viana, M.; Querol, X.; Alastuey, A.; Moreno, T. Spatial and chemical patterns of PM10 in road dust deposited in urban environment. *Atmos. Environ.* **2009**, *43*, 1650–1659. [CrossRef]
36. Trejos, E.M.; Silva, L.F.; Hower, J.C.; Flores, E.M.; González, C.M.; Pachón, J.E.; Aristizábal, B.H. Volcanic emissions and atmospheric pollution: A study of nanoparticles. *Geosci. Front.* **2021**, *12*, 746–755. [CrossRef]
37. Murillo, J.H.; Marín, J.F.R.; Álvarez, V.M.; Arias, D.S.; Guerrero, V.H.B. Chemical characterization of filterable PM 2.5 emissions generated from regulated stationary sources in the Metropolitan Area of Costa Rica. *Atmos. Pollut. Res.* **2017**, *8*, 709–717. [CrossRef]
38. Reimann, C.; de Caritat, P. Chemical Elements in the Environment. In *Factsheets for the Geochemist and Environmental Scientist*, 1st ed.; Springer: Berlin/Heidelberg, Germany, 1998; ISBN 978-3-642-72018-5.
39. Rudnick, R.; Gao, S. Composition of the Continental Crust. *Treatise Geochem.* **2003**, *3*, 1217–1232. [CrossRef]
40. Sutherland, R.A. Bed sediment-associated trace metals in an urban stream, Oahu, Hawaii. *Environ. Earth Sci.* **2000**, *39*, 611–627. [CrossRef]
41. Kaiser, H.F. The varimax criterion for analytic rotation in factor analysis. *Psychometrika* **1958**, *23*, 187–200. [CrossRef]
42. Amato, F.; Pandolfi, M.; Alastuey, A.; Lozano, A.; González, J.C.; Querol, X. Impact of traffic intensity and pavement aggregate size on road dust particles loading. *Atmos. Environ.* **2013**, *77*, 711–717. [CrossRef]
43. Padoan, E.; Ajmone-Marsan, F.; Querol, X.; Amato, F. An empirical model to predict road dust emissions based on pavement and traffic characteristics. *Environ. Pollut.* **2017**, *237*, 713–720. [CrossRef]
44. Kong, S.; Ji, Y.; Lu, B.; Chen, L.; Han, B.; Li, Z.; Bai, Z. Characterization of PM10 source profiles for fugitive dust in Fushun-a city famous for coal. *Atmos. Environ.* **2011**, *45*, 5351–5365. [CrossRef]
45. Ramírez, O.; de la Campa, A.M.S.; Sánchez-Rodas, D.; de la Rosa, J.D. Hazardous trace elements in thoracic fraction of airborne particulate matter: Assessment of temporal variations, sources, and health risks in a megacity. *Sci. Total Environ.* **2020**, *710*, 136344. [CrossRef]
46. Vega, E.; Mugica, V.; Reyes, E.; Sánchez, G.; Chow, J.; Watson, J. Chemical composition of fugitive dust emitters in Mexico City. *Atmos. Environ.* **2001**, *35*, 4033–4039. [CrossRef]
47. Herrera Ardila, M.C. Suelos Derivados de Cenizas Volcánicas En Colombia: Estudio Fundamental e Implicaciones En Ingeniería. *Rev. Int. Desastres Nat. Accid. Infraestruct. Civ.* **2006**, *6*, 167.
48. Cheng, Y.; Lee, S.-C.; Gu, Z.; Ho, K.F.; Zhang, Y.; Huang, Y.; Chow, J.C.; Watson, J.; Cao, J.; Zhang, R. PM2.5 and PM10-2.5 chemical composition and source apportionment near a Hong Kong roadway. *Particuology* **2013**, *18*, 96–104. [CrossRef]
49. Karanasiou, A.; Diapouli, E.; Cavalli, F.; Eleftheriadis, K.; Viana, M.; Alastuey, A.; Querol, X.; Reche, C. On the quantification of atmospheric carbonate carbon by thermal/optical analysis protocols. *Atmos. Meas. Tech.* **2011**, *4*, 2409–2419. [CrossRef]
50. Querol, X.; Viana, M.; Alastuey, A.; Amato, F.; Moreno, T.; Castillo, S.; Pey, J.; de la Rosa, J.D.; de la Campa, A.M.S.; Artinano, B.; et al. Source origin of trace elements in PM from regional background, urban and industrial sites of Spain. *Atmos. Environ.* **2007**, *41*, 7219–7231. [CrossRef]

51. Wiseman, C.L.; Levesque, C.; Rasmussen, P.E. Characterizing the sources, concentrations and resuspension potential of metals and metalloids in the thoracic fraction of urban road dust. *Sci. Total Environ.* **2021**, *786*, 147467. [CrossRef]
52. Findeter. *Plan Maestro de Movilidad de Manizales*; Findeter: Bogotá, Colombia, 2017.
53. Fujiwara, F.; Rebagliati, R.J.; Dawidowski, L.; Gómez, D.; Polla, G.; Pereyra, V.; Smichowski, P. Spatial and chemical patterns of size fractionated road dust collected in a megacitiy. *Atmos. Environ.* **2011**, *45*, 1497–1505. [CrossRef]
54. Manno, E.; Varrica, D.; Dongarrà, G. Metal distribution in road dust samples collected in an urban area close to a petrochemical plant at Gela, Sicily. *Atmos. Environ.* **2006**, *40*, 5929–5941. [CrossRef]
55. Liu, Y.; Xing, J.; Wang, S.; Fu, X.; Zheng, H. Source-specific speciation profiles of PM2.5 for heavy metals and their anthropogenic emissions in China. *Environ. Pollut.* **2018**, *239*, 544–553. [CrossRef]

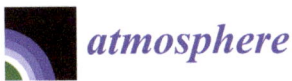

Article

The Content and Sources of Potentially Toxic Elements in the Road Dust of Surgut (Russia)

Dmitriy Moskovchenko [1,2,*], Roman Pozhitkov [1], Andrey Soromotin [2] and Valeriy Tyurin [3]

1. Tyumen Scientific Centre, Siberian Branch of Russian Academy of Sciences, 625026 Tyumen, Russia; pozhitkov-roma@yandex.ru
2. Institute of Earth Sciences, Tyumen State University, 625003 Tyumen, Russia; asoromotin@mail.ru
3. Institute of Natural and Technical Sciences, Surgut State University, 628412 Surgut, Russia; tyurin_vn@mail.ru
* Correspondence: moskovchenko1965@gmail.com; Tel.: +7-922-488-32-11

Abstract: The chemical and particle size composition of road dust in Surgut, which is a rapidly developing city in Western Siberia, was studied for the first time. Contents of major and trace elements were determined using ICP-MS and ICP-AES, respectively. It was found that the road dust had an alkaline pH (from 7.54 to 9.38) and that the particle size composition was dominated by the 100–250-µm fraction. The contamination assessment based on calculations of the enrichment factor (*EF*) showed that the road dust was significantly enriched in Sb and Cu and moderately enriched in Zn, Pb, Mo, Ni and W. The sources of these elements are probably associated with the abrasion of car tires and brake pads. Based on calculations of global pollution index (PIr) and total enrichment factor (*Ze*), the road dust of Surgut was characterized by a generally low level of potential ecological risk, except for stretches of road subject to regular traffic jams, where a moderate ecological risk level was identified. In comparison to the other Russian cities (Moscow, Chelyabinsk, Tyumen, etc.) where studies of road dust composition have been carried out, Surgut had similar contents of Cr and Cu and relatively lower contents of Sb, Cd, As and Pb.

Keywords: Western Siberia; urban pollution; road dust; potentially toxic elements; traffic-related contamination

1. Introduction

Road dust is currently one of the main materials used in assessments of the ecological state of urban and industrial environments. Studies on road dust composition help to assess the total accumulation of pollutants from the atmosphere, soils and technogenic sources and to forecast the effects of those pollutants on human health. The advantages of using road dust in such assessments include its ease of sampling, ubiquity and non-point source nature, as well as its strong relationship with car exhaust emissions [1].

The road dust deposited within transport zones is regarded as a multicomponent mixture of different fractions that are formed as a result of soil erosion, abrasion of road surfaces and vehicle parts, incomplete combustion of fuel, application of de-icing agents, etc. [2–5]. Particles of road dust can accumulate many potentially toxic metals, metalloids and organic compounds [6–9]. The deposition rates of road dust and its chemical composition depend on factors such as vehicle emissions; abrasion of road tarmac, road markings, car tires and brake pads; and the corrosion of metal parts of vehicles, as well as traffic densities, speed and frequencies of car maneuvers such as braking and stopping [10–12]. At the same time, resuspended particles can be one of the most important sources of microparticles in the atmosphere [13]. The high concentration of harmful substances in the dust makes it hazardous to human health. Microparticles can be lifted by air currents and inhaled by humans and, therefore, increase the risks of respiratory, cardiovascular and oncological diseases [14]. Globally, road dust is a major source of inhalable particulate matter in any urban environment [15].

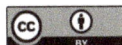

According to the Russian Federal Service for State Statistics, 75% of the country's population live in cities [16]. Numerous studies have reported that transport-related air pollution is one of the dominant sources of urban air pollution and is a continuously contributing emission [17–19]. In many cities of Russia, numerous dangerous environmental situations resulting from atmospheric air pollution have been repeatedly noted [20,21]. Therefore, ecological assessments of such cities are highly important for providing comfortable and safe conditions for their residents. However, the majority of such assessments are conducted in large cities, with a lack of attention given to medium-sized and smaller cities.

There have been few studies on road dust within the territory of the former Soviet Union. Determinations of road dust composition have been carried out in Moscow [13,22–26], cities of the Perm Region [27], Chelyabinsk [20] and Alushta [28]. In Tyumen (West Siberia), Konstantinova et al. [29] have analyzed 20 samples of road dust, which were found to have high concentrations of Cr, Ni and Co.

Surgut has one of the highest concentrations of motorized vehicles in Russia, with about 200,000 vehicles registered within this city. Busy highways running through Surgut connect different cities and numerous oil fields of Western Siberia. There is also a railway running across Surgut. The city streets and roads have a total length of 266.7 km, which corresponds to about 10% of the total area of urban constructions [30]. Such a high intensity of traffic has negative effects on the health of Surgut residents, in particular elevating the risks of cancer [31]. Traffic densities within the city drastically increase during certain peak hours of the mornings and evenings, when the traffic becomes very heavy and moves at an average speed of less than 10 km per hour. Nevertheless, the impacts of such traffic on the content of trace elements, including potentially toxic elements (PTEs), within the road dust of Surgut have not been studied until the present time. The objectives of this study were as follows: (i) to determine the total concentrations of major and trace elements, including PTEs, in the road dust of Surgut city, (ii) to assess the degree of contamination using contamination indices, (iii) to identify the potential sources of PTEs and (iv) to evaluate the human health risks of road dust.

2. Materials and Methods

2.1. Study Area

Surgut is located in the center of the West Siberian Plain, within the taiga zone. The climate is continental, with a mean annual temperature of $-1.8\ °C$ and a mean annual precipitation of 652 mm [32]. Southern and western winds prevail. The rapid development of Surgut began in the 1960s, following the discovery of numerous oil fields in the vicinities of the city. The population of Surgut grew from just over 6 thousand people in the early 1960s to 200 thousand in the mid-1980s and has reached nearly 400 thousand at the present time.

Surgut is one of the fastest growing cities in Russia. It is characterized by well-developed power engineering, food production, printing, building, publishing and sewing industries. Surgut's two largest gas-fired power stations, with a total output of 8.9 thousand MW, provide most of the regional power supply.

The ecological conditions of Surgut have been insufficiently studied, with only very few assessments within small areas. It has been found that the snowpack in Surgut is contaminated by heavy metals [33] and that Pb concentration in road-side soils exceeds its maximal permissible concentration [34]. Dumps of domestic and industrial waste also negatively affect the surrounding soils, where heavy metal concentrations exceed their maximal levels according to the ecological standards [35]. Moreover, there is a lack of data on the composition of the native soils of the Surgut region. It is only known that sandy soils with low contents of trace elements prevail within the Fedorovskoye Oil Field at distances of 20–50 km to the north of Surgut [36,37].

2.2. Sampling and Laboratory Analyses

Road dust sampling was undertaken in July 2021 during dry weather periods, i.e., no less than 36 h after any low-intensity rainfall. Samples of 200–300 g each were collected from road surfaces within 1 × 1 quadrats using a plastic brush and a scoop, placed into plastic bags and delivered to the laboratory. Sampling sites were located on roads with different traffic densities within different land use areas of the city. High, moderate and low traffic densities corresponded to >2, 1–2 and <1 thousand cars per hour. The traffic data were sourced from the municipal program for the development of transport infrastructure in Surgut [30]. The different types of land use were recorded at the sampling sites as follows:

(1) Industrial and warehouse area.
(2) High-rise residential area.
(3) Low-rise residential area.
(4) Power plant area.
(5) Public and business area.
(6) Transport hubs (railway station and airport).

A total of 25 samples were taken. It has been shown that a relatively low number of samples (16–31) is sufficient for evaluating the level of pollution of road dust in cities with a medium population, e.g., Thessaloniki, Greece [38], Ma'an City, Jordan [39] and Sakaka city, Saudi Arabia [40]. Locations of the sampling sites are shown in Figure 1. A detailed description of the sampling sites is presented in Supplementary Materials, Table S1.

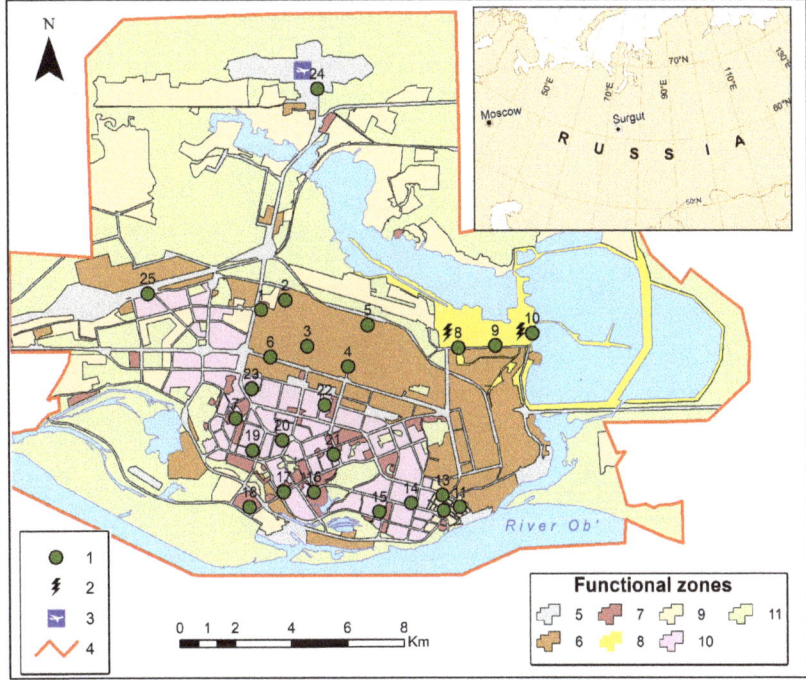

Figure 1. Sampling sites and land use areas within the city of Surgut: 1—sampling sites; 2—power plants; 3—airport; 4—city border; 5—transport area; 6—industrial and warehouse area; 7—public and business area; 8—power plant area; 9—low-rise area; 10—high-rise residential area; 11—recreation area, urban forests, green spaces.

In the laboratory, the samples were passed through a sieve with an aperture of 1 mm in order to remove coarse inclusions (fragments of plants, rubbish, etc.). Although the pollutant concentrations in fine fractions (PM1 and PM10) of road dust are known to be higher than those in coarse fractions [13], we analyzed bulk samples in order to be able to compare our results from Surgut with the data from other cities. Bulk samples have been used in the majority of studies on road dust composition, whereas fine fractions have been separately analyzed in only a few studies [7,13,26,41].

The pH values were measured potentiometrically in continuously mixed 1:2.5 dust:water suspensions using a Starter3100 conductivity meter (OHAUS, Baden-Wuerttemberg, Germany). The particle size distribution was determined using a Mastersizer 3000 laser diffraction particle size analyzer. Concentrations of 54 trace elements (Li, Be, Sc, V, Cr, Co, Ni, Cu, Zn, Ga, As, Se, Rb, Sr, Y, Zr, Nb, Mo, Rh, Pd, Ag, Cd, Sn, Sb, Te, Cs, Ba, La, Ce, Pr, Nd, Sm, Eu, Gd, Tb, Dy, Ho, Er, Tm, Yb, Lu, Hf, Ta, W, Re, Ir, Pt, Au, Hg, Tl, Pb, Bi, Th, U) and 8 major elements in weight percent oxide for the particulate fraction (Na_2O, MgO, Al_2O_3, P_2O_5, S, K_2O, CaO, Fe_2O_3) were measured by inductively coupled plasma mass spectrometry (ICP-MS) (Thermo Elemental—X7 spectrometer, Omaha, NE, USA) and inductively coupled plasma atom emission spectrometry (ICP-AES) (Thermo Scientific iCAP-6500 spectrometer, Thermo Fisher Scientific, Waltham, MA, USA), respectively. The analyzed samples, 100 mg each, were prepared by acid digestion in an open beaker system. The samples were placed in Teflon beakers (volume 50 mL); 0.1 mL of a solution containing 8 µg dm^{-3} 145Nd, 61Dy and 174Yb was added (control of the chemical yield during the sample decomposition procedure); and the mixture was moistened with several drops of deionized water. Then, 0.5 mL of $HClO_4$ (perchloric acid fuming 70% Supratur, Merck), 3 mL of HF (hydrofluoric acid 40% GR, ISO, Merck KGaA, Darmstadt, Germany) and 0.5 mL of HNO_3 (nitric acid 65%, max. 0.0000005%% GR, ISO, Merck) were added and evaporated until intense white vapors appeared. The beakers were cooled, their walls were washed with water and the solution was again evaporated to wet salts. Then, 2 mL of HCl (hydrochloric acid fuming 37% OR, ISO, Merck KGaA, Darmstadt, Germany) and 0.2 mL of 0.1 M H_3BO_3 solution (analytical grade) were added and evaporated to a volume of 0.5–0.7 mL. The resulting solutions were transferred into polyethylene bottles, 0.1 mL of a solution containing 10 mg L^{-1} In (internal standard) was added, diluted with deionized water to 20 mL and analysis was performed.

In addition to the studied samples, measurements were also taken for the blank and reference samples. We used the certified reference materials for soils—Gabbro Essexit STD-2A (GSO 8670-2005) and Andesite AGV-2 (United States Geological Survey)—in order to verify the accuracy of determinations. The comparison with the standard samples showed a sufficient repeatability (85–115%) for the majority of the analyzed elements, except for Sn (59%), Ba (70%), Ag (153%), Mo (78%) and W (63%), the measurements of which were excluded from the calculations. The analysis was performed in the Institute of Microelectronics Technology and High Purity Materials (Russian Academy of Sciences). The methods, recoveries, detection limits (DLs) and analytical results of the certified reference materials are given in the Supplementary Materials (Table S2).

2.3. Calculations and Data Processing

The processing of the statistical data was performed using Statistica 10.0 software (TIBCO, Palo Alto, CA, USA). Statistical parameters of the road dust composition (mean, standard deviation, maximum and minimum values) were determined. The significance of differences between the mean values for roads with different traffic intensities was assessed using the Mann–Whitney test.

Assessments carried out by two or more methods can improve the accuracy of the assessment result [42]. Therefore, to improve the accuracy of the result and make the assessment more comprehensive and systematic, additional methods were applied. Assessments of road dust contamination levels were based on calculations of generally accepted indices, including the global pollution index (*PIr*), enrichment factor (*EF*) and potential ecological risk index (E_r^i), as well as the total potential ecological risk index (*RI*) and total enrichment factor (*Ze*), the latter being commonly used in Russia.

The values of *PIr* were calculated using the following equation:

$$PIr = Cr/K, \qquad (1)$$

where Cr is the concentration of an element in road dust and K is the concentration of the same element in the upper continental crust [13].

The EF of an element, which is an important parameter for evaluating the contribution of human impact to its enrichment, is the normalization of a measured element against a reference element in a studied sample [43]. The EF was calculated according to the equation:

$$EF = \frac{Cx}{CAl}(sample) \bigg/ \frac{Cx}{CAl}(crust), \qquad (2)$$

where Cx (sample) is the measured concentration of the element of interest, Cx (crust) is the concentration of the same element in the Earth's crust and CAl is the concentration of the reference element (aluminum) in the same sample or the Earth's crust. Aluminum is most commonly used for calculations of EF [44–46]. The low mobility and crustal abundance of Al makes it a suitable reference element. The composition of the upper continental crust was used as a reference for normalization because of the lack of a background analogue for road dust, which is a specific anthropogenic object [13]. The same method of calculation was applied in the other Russian cities studied [13,20,24,26,28]. The use of world average values in the continental crust is acceptable only within regions where there are no geochemical anomalies associated with the features of the geological structure. In this case, the element contents of soils, which are the source of particles in the atmosphere, are close to continental crust values. According to the scientific research on the contents of some heavy metals and metalloids in Western Siberia soils [47,48], they are not very different from continental crust values. Indeed, the average contents of the elements in the soils of Western Siberia are as follows (mg kg^{-1}): Co—13, Cr—84, Cu—31, Ni—42, Pb—18, Zn—73 and Zr—295 [47]. These values are quite close to continental crust values according to Rudnick and Gao [49]. Therefore, comparisons with the distribution of elements in the Earth's crust are considered reasonable.

The potential ecological risk index E_r^i, which characterizes the degree of the ecological risk of a single element [50], was calculated by using the following equation:

$$E_r^i = PIr \cdot T_r^i \qquad (3)$$

where PIr is the global pollution index and T_r^i is the toxicity response coefficient. This index provides for the probability assessment of adverse ecological effects caused by exposure by to one or more pollutants [44]. In this study, we used the response T_r^i values according to [50] as follows: Zn, Mn, Fe, W, Sr = 1; Cr, Mo, Sn, Sb = 2; Pb, Cu, Co, Ni = 5; As = 10 and Cd = 30. For risk assessments, we adopted the following gradation: E_r^i < 40 describes low risk; 40 < E_r^i < 80 indicates moderate risk; 80 < E_r^i < 160 indicates considerable risk; 160 < E_r^i < 320 indicates high risk; and E_r^i > 320 indicates extreme risk [50,51].

The total rate of accumulation of PTEs and other chemical elements was estimated using two indices, the total potential ecological risk index (RI) and the total enrichment factor (Ze), because the use of different indices provides for the most accurate assessment of the ecological situation. The RI index, which characterizes the overall degree of the ecological risk of all metals under investigation [50], was calculated according to equation:

$$RI = \sum E_r^i \qquad (4)$$

where E_r^i is a potential ecological risk index of a single element. Risk levels were graded as follows: RI < 150, low; 150 < RI < 300, moderate; 300 < RI < 600, considerable and RI > 600, high ecological risk.

The values Ze were calculated using the following equation:

$$Ze = \sum EF - (n-1) \qquad (5)$$

where EF of n elements with EF > 1.5 were summed up [24].

Criteria for assessment of road dust contamination are presented in Table 1.

Table 1. Grades of enrichment factor (EF), potential ecological risk index (E_r^i), total potential ecological risk index (RI) and total enrichment factor (Ze).

Enrichment Factor		Potential Ecological Risk Index		Total Potential Ecological Risk Index		Total Enrichment Factor	
EF values	Enrichment level [1]	E_r^i grades [50]		RI values	RI levels [50]	Ze values	Environmental hazards [13,25,26]
$EF \leq 2$	Minimal	$E_r^i < 40$	Low	$RI < 150$	Low	<32	Non-hazardous
$2 < EF \leq 5$	Moderate	$40 < E_r^i < 80$	Moderate	$150 \leq RI < 300$	Moderate	32–64	Moderately dangerous
$5 < EF \leq 20$	Significant	$80 < E_r^i < 160$	Considerable	$200 \leq RI < 600$	High	64–128	Dangerous
$20 < EF \leq 40$	Very High	$160 < E_r^i < 320$	High	$RI \geq 600$	Very High	128–256	Very dangerous

Varimax-rotated principal component analysis (PCA) was applied to investigate the sources of PTEs. PCA is widely used to reduce data and to extract a small number of latent factors (principal components, PCs) for analyzing relationships among the observed variables [52].

The influence of road dust on the health of the Surgut population was evaluated using the U.S. Environmental Protection Agency (EPA) human health evaluation method [53]. This method implies that dust can induce negative effects when it is assimilated by the human body in three different pathways—ingestion, inhalation and dermal contact. Carcinogenic and non-carcinogenic risks can be calculated by summing up the risks from the three exposure pathways.

The calculations of such risks were based on the average daily dose (ADD) of the total assimilation of a certain element in three different ways. The equations and parameter values used for the calculations are presented in Table S3. Following the ADD calculations, we conducted determinations of non-carcinogenic hazard quotient (HQ) and carcinogenic risk assessment (CRA) using the following equation:

$$HQ = ADD/RfD,$$

where reference dose RfD (mg kg^{-1} day^{-1}) is an estimation of the maximum permissible risks to the human population through daily exposure with consideration of sensitive groups during their lifetime.

Hazard index (HI), the sum of HQ(Ing/Der/Inh), was used by us to estimate the health risk of different exposure pathways. HI values of ≤ 1 indicate no adverse health effects and HI values > 1 indicate possible adverse health effects [54].

For carcinogenic risk (CRA), the dose was multiplied by the corresponding slope factor (SF) to produce an estimate of cancer risk [55] as follows:

$$CRA = ADD\ ing, dermal, inh \times SF$$

Total cancer risk (CRAsum) was calculated as the sum of CRA for three exposure pathways (ingestion, inhalation and dermal contact).

3. Results

3.1. The pH and Particle Size Distribution

The analyzed dust had an alkaline reaction, with a pH ranging from 7.54 to 9.38. The roads with low, moderate and high traffic densities were characterized by mean pH values of 8.04, 7.80 and 7.82, respectively. The data on road dust pH in other cities of the world fall within generally the same range, between 7 and 9.5 [56–59]. The alkaline reaction of city road dust is explained by the presence of microparticles of building materials as well as different pollutants originating from vehicle exhaust emissions. Acidifying gaseous compounds (mainly nitrogen oxides) of car exhausts are removed by air currents, whereas alkaline particulate matter stays on the road surface. According to [34], the urban soils of

Surgut have neutral and alkaline pH values, as opposed to acid background soils around the city.

The particle size distribution of road dust was characterized by the predominance of the 100–250-μm size fraction (fine sand), which ranged from 19.5 to 50.1% with a mean of 39%. The content of the 100–250-μm size fraction (very fine sand) was significantly lower, with a mean of 14.4%. Sand-sized particles (>50 μm) composed between 45 and 95% of the total mass (with a mean of 82.5%). The 2–10-μm size fraction and the 10–50-μm size fraction had mean contents of 3.2 and 13.8%, respectively. The content of clay (<2 μm) ranged from 0.1 to 2.5%.

Sand (mainly fine sand) is known to be the predominant particle size fraction of road dust in many Russian cities. For example, in Chelyabinsk, which is not very far from Surgut, road dust is characterized by the predominance of particles from 30 to 300 μm [21]. In Moscow, road dust has the following mean contents of fractions: PM1—1.8%, PM10—12.8%, 10–50-μm size fraction—16.3% and >50 μm size fraction—69.1% [24]. The predominance of coarse particles in road dust has been reported from many cities of the world. For example, the urban sediments collected from Manchester were made up primarily of medium sand-sized particles ranging in size from 200 to 300 μm [60]. The 125–500-μm fraction was prevalent in the road dust of Thessaloniki, Greece [38].

It is generally believed that the predominance of particles of 180–240 μm in road dust is indicative of deposition of soil particles together with particles produced by the movement of vehicles, i.e., the abrasion of road surfaces, tires and metal parts of cars [61]. Smaller particles usually originate from industrial emissions [21]. It has been found that dust from metallurgical enterprises has a median particle size ranging from 1.0 to 200 mm and volumes of PM10 from 10 to 84% depending on the technological processes and the raw materials used [62]. Therefore, the composition of road dust from Surgut mainly resulted from the deposition of soil particles and particles produced by traffic, with only a low contribution of particles originating from industrial plants.

The distribution of fractions of road dust depending on traffic densities is shown in Table 2. The highest contents of PM10 particles, which are easily carried by winds and create the highest risks for human health, were observed on roads with moderate and high traffic densities. The lowest contents of fine particles combined with the predominance of sand were found on small roads with low traffic densities. However, such differences between the roads with different traffic intensities were only very small. The Mann–Whitney test showed that the differences between the mean values of contents of those particle size fractions were insignificant. The highest percentage (26.5%) of fine (<50 μm) particles was found within the public and business area, which is located in the southern part of Surgut (sampling sites 16–18, see Figure 1). Such a high content of fine particles can be explained by the predominance of fine-textured alluvial soils within that area.

3.2. The Chemical Composition of Road Dust

Summary statistics for the studied chemical element contents in the road dust of Surgut are presented in Table 3. The predominant major elements include Al_2O_3 (with a mean of 4.2%), CaO (3.9%), MgO (2.8%) and Fe_2O_3 (2.4%), with the other major elements having mean contents of <1%. The upper part of continental Earth's crust has a different descending order of major element concentrations: Al_2O_3 (15.4%), Fe_2O_3 (5.0%), CaO (3.6%), Na_2O (3.27%), K_2O (2.8%) and MgO (2.48%), according to [49]. In comparison with the latter, Surgut's road dust has relatively low contents of aluminum and iron but a relatively high content of magnesium.

The majority of trace elements in the road dust had lower contents as compared to those in the upper part of the continental Earth's crust, which was indicated by the PIr values (see Table 3). For example, the contents of Li, Be, Ga, As, Rb, Zr, Nb, all rare earth elements, Th and U were 3–10 times as low as their Clarke numbers. Most PTEs (Hg, As, Ni, Cr, Co, V) do not accumulate in the road dust of Surgut. Such low contents of trace elements can be explained by the predominance of sand fractions and low contents of fine fractions in the particle size composition of the studied samples. It has been repeatedly shown that fine particles are most enriched in trace elements [63,64].

Relative enrichment as compared to the world average values in the Earth's continental crust was observed in Sb, Cu, Zn, Cd and Pb (Table 3). The elements accumulated in Surgut's road dust can be defined as typical urban pollutants, including Cd, Pb, Sb, Ti, Ba, Zn and, to a lesser degree, Cu [65–68]. A similar assemblage of pollutants (Sb, Pb, Zn, Cd, Cu and Sn) has been found in the road dust of Moscow [13].

Table 2. The percentage of particle size fractions (mm) in road dust depending on (a) traffic densities and (b) land use within Surgut city.

Area	<0.002	0.002–0.01	0.01–0.05	0.05–0.1	0.1–0.25	0.25–0.5	0.5–1.0
			Traffic Densities:				
Low (n = 8)	0.5 ± 0.1 [1]	2.6 ± 0.7	14.9 ± 5.1	14.6 ± 6.7	36.7 ± 5.4	26.1 ± 7.4	4.4 ± 0.4
Moderate (n = 14)	0.7 ± 0.7	3.8 ± 3.2	14.0 ± 8.5	14.5 ± 4.0	40.0 ± 6.9	24.2 ± 7.8	2.7 ± 1.9
High (n = 3)	0.4 ± 0.1	2.1 ± 0.7	12.0 ± 5.1	15.0 ± 6.7	42.0 ± 5.4	26.2 ± 7.6	2.4 ± 0.4
			Land use Areas				
Industrial and warehouse area (n = 6)	0.25 ± 0.3	2.0 ± 1.1	8.9 ± 3.6	11.9 ± 2.8	44.4 ± 3.4	29.5 ± 4.6	3.1 ± 1.4
High-rise residential area (n = 6)	0.5 ± 0.32	2.6 ± 0.8	13.2 ± 5.7	16.0 ± 6.0	39.0 ± 5.0	25.1 ± 7.5	3.5 ± 1.9
Low-rise residential area (n = 5)	0.7 ± 1.0	4.4 ± 5.0	13.6 ± 13.8	12.2 ± 5.3	36.9 ± 9.4	27.1 ± 12.2	4.8 ± 3.9
Power plant area (n = 3)	0.9 ± 0.7	4.5 ± 2.6	14.5 ± 7.5	14.8 ± 2.4	39.3 ± 4,2	23.2 ± 7.3	3.1 ± 2.6
Public and business area (n = 3)	0.9 ± 0.6	3.0 ± 0.9	26.5 ± 13.4	21.0 ± 2.9	31.0 ± 9.4	15.8 ± 7.4	1.9 ± 0.9
Transport hubs (n = 2)	0.7 ± 0.2	3.6 ± 1.0	10.8 ± 5.8	11.9 ± 4.4	43.8 ± 3.4	27.3 ± 7.5	2.0 ± 0.6

[1] Mean ± SD.

Table 3. Summary statistics for the contents of PTEs and other chemical elements in Surgut's road dust, n = 25 (Na_2O- Fe_2O_3 in %, Li-U in mg kg^{-1}).

Element	DL	Mean	Sd	Min	Max	V, %	WA	PIr
Al_2O_3	0.009	4.2	0.97	2.6	6.68	23	15.4	0.3 (0.2–0.4)
CaO	0.005	3.9	1.42	2.0	7.81	36	3.59	1.1 (0.5–2.2)
Fe_2O_3	0.01	2.4	0.60	1.2	3.86	25	5.04	0.5 (0.2–0.8)
K_2O	0.002	0.80	0.16	0.55	1.26	20	2.8	0.3 (0.2–0.5)
MgO	0.005	2.8	1.06	1.4	5.48	37	2.48	1.1(0.5–2.2)
MnO	0.0004	0.043	0.013	0.024	0.071	29	0.1	0.4 (0.2–0.7)
Na_2O	0.001	0.91	0.22	0.65	1.48	24	3.27	0.3 (0.2–0.5)
P_2O_5	0.005	0.06	0.03	0.025	0.15	58	0.15	0.4 (0.2–1.0)
S	0.002	0.064	0.021	0.028	0.12	33	0.062	1.0 (0.4–2.0)
TiO_2	0.0005	0.27	0.09	0.12	0.55	35	0.64	0.4 (0.2–0.9)
As	0.1	1.29	0.65	0.4	3.3	51	4.8	0.3 (0.1–0.7)
Be	0.03	0.42	0.12	0.3	0.72	28	2.1	0.2(0.1–0.3)
Bi	0.01	0.067	0.046	0.02	0.22	69	0.16	0.4 (0.1–1.4)
Cd	0.04	0.11	0.15	0.04	0.66	136	0.09	1.2 (0.4–7.4)
Ce	0.008	15.5	8.1	8.4	45.4	52	63	0.2 (0.13–0.7)
Co	0.08	6.9	1.7	3.8	11.2	25	17.3	0.4 (0.2–0.7)
Cr	0.7	46.4	15.4	18.4	83.9	33	92	0.5 (0.2–0.9)
Cs	0.01	0.43	0.17	0.24	1.0	39	4.9	0.1 (0.05–0.2)
Cu	0.8	42.8	27.3	9.3	144.9	64	28	1.5 (0.3–5.2)
Dy	0.007	1.12	0.44	0.74	2.59	39	3.9	0.3 (0.2–0.7)
Er	0.003	0.60	0.24	0.40	1.34	39	2.3	0.3 (0.2–0.6)
Eu	0.006	0.40	0.19	0.26	1.17	47	1	0.4 (0.3–1.2)
Ga	0.1	3.74	0.84	2.6	6.1	23	17.5	0.2 (0.1–0.3)
Gd	0.007	1.20	0.53	0.77	3.13	44	4	0.3 (0.2–0.8)

Table 3. Cont.

Element	DL	Mean	Sd	Min	Max	V, %	WA	PIr
Hf	0.02	0.72	0.24	0.5	1.7	33	5.3	0.14 (0.1–0.3)
Ho	0.005	0.21	0.08	0.13	0.48	40	0.83	0.2 (0.2–0.6)
La	0.009	7.05	3.03	4.0	17.7	43	31	0.2 (0.13–0.6)
Li	0.03	5.16	1.04	3.7	7.57	20	24	0.2 (0.2–0.3)
Lu	0.005	0.091	0.035	0.06	0.20	39	0.31	0.3 (0.2–0.6)
Nb	0.02	2.85	1.55	1.5	8.9	55	12	0.2 (0.1–0.7)
Nd	0.009	6.78	3.83	3.86	22.5	56	27	0.3 (0.14–0.8)
Ni	0.7	41.1	17.0	12.1	90.1	41	47	0.9 (0.3–1.9)
Pb	0.06	19.0	25.5	5.6	126.1	134	17	1.1 (0.3–7.4)
Pr	0.005	1.77	0.96	0.95	5.50	54	7.1	0.2 (0.13–0.8)
Rb	0.1	19.8	4.21	13.0	33.3	21	84	0.2 (0.2–0.4)
Sb	0.06	0.89	0.57	0.38	3.13	64	0.4	2.2 (1.0–7.8)
Sc	0.09	5.62	1.30	3.7	8.5	23	14	0.4 (0.3–0.6)
Sm	0.004	1.42	0.73	0.85	4.26	51	4.7	0.3 (0.2–0.9)
Sr	0.07	119.6	27.8	91.0	210.6	23	320	0.4 (0.3–0.7)
Ta	0.01	0.19	0.13	0.1	0.7	69	0.88	0.2 (0.1–0.8)
Tb	0.004	0.18	0.08	0.12	0.48	44	0.7	0.3 (0.2–0.7)
Th	0.01	1.45	0.65	0.7	3.2	45	10.5	0.1 (0.07–0.3)
Tl	0.005	0.08	0.02	0.05	0.15	23	0.9	0.1 (0.06–0.16)
Tm	0.004	0.086	0.034	0.06	0.20	40	0.3	0.3 (0.2–0.7)
U	0.01	0.61	0.27	0.4	1.6	44	2.7	0.2 (0.1–0.6)
V	0.8	42.1	11.9	20.6	67.6	28	97	0.4 (0.2–0.7)
Y	0.02	6.03	2.29	4.1	13.2	38	21	0.3 (0.2–0.6)
Yb	0.003	0.66	0.27	0.45	1.54	41	2	0.3 (0.2–0.8)
Zn	0.5	89.9	50.6	35.6	262.7	56	67	1.3 (0.5–3.9)
Zr	0.04	28.6	10.1	18.2	68.8	35	193	0.1 (0.1–0.4)

Note: WA—world average [49]; Se, Rh, Pd, Te, Re, Ir, Pt, Hg and Au contents were below their detection limits in 50% samples, and hence, they were excluded from calculations.

The Pb, Cu and Zn contents in the soils of Western Siberia are similar to world average values and occasionally even lower [47]. It has also been shown that the Sb content in soils in the north of Western Siberia is below its world average value [69]. Therefore, enrichment in those trace elements in the road dust of Surgut is connected with the impact of anthropogenic sources, which is indirectly confirmed by significant variations in Cd (CV of 136%), Pb (134%) and Sb (64%). Elements originating predominantly from natural sources are expected to have a relatively lower variability, while those from anthropogenic sources should display a greater variability [70,71]. Significant variations in PTE concentrations indicate significant contributions from anthropogenic sources and a spatial heterogeneity of human impacts on the roads [13]. In addition, such variations reflect differences in the rates of pollution depending on road traffic, industrial emissions and street cleaning.

It should be mentioned that dust particles separated from the snowpack within Western Siberia, including remote background areas, are enriched in Sb, Zn, Cd and As [72]. Therefore, the assemblage of air pollutants within Surgut city is similar to the region-scale assemblage of air pollutants, which is indicative of their broad distribution. It is likely that the composition of atmospheric particulate matter within Western Siberia is generally predetermined by emissions from different cities and other point sources, the specific contributions of which can only be assessed when a larger database on such sources is available, but at the present time it is impossible to provide such an assessment with sufficient reliability.

The mean EF values of Sb (8.3) indicated significant enrichment. A very high level of enrichment (20 < EF < 40) in both Sb and Pb was observed in only one sample, which was collected from a stretch of road with a high traffic intensity within the industrial and warehouse area. Such a combined Sb and Pb contamination of road dust can be explained by emissions of those elements from worn car batteries that were made with the use of Sb–Pb alloys up until very recently [73].

Of the studied samples, 48% were significantly enriched in Cu, 32% in Zn, 20% in Ni, 12% in Pb and 4% in Cd. The mean EF values of Pb (4.3), Ni (3.3) and 36% EF of Cr were between 2 and 5, indicating moderate enrichment. Other trace elements were characterized by mean EF values of <2, i.e., belonging to the category of "deficiency to minimal enrichment" according to [1].

The data obtained on the distribution of EF, Ze and RI values over the city territory depending on the land use areas and road traffic intensities are shown in Table 4. The highest total contamination levels were observed in the industrial area and the roads with high traffic intensities (with the Ze values of 43 and 44, respectively). There was a clear relationship between the contamination level and the traffic density.

Table 4. The values of enrichment factor (EF), total potential ecological risk index (RI) and total enrichment factor (Ze) in the road dust of Surgut.

Area	Contamination Levels and EF Values		Ze	RI
	Significant (EF = 5–20)	Moderate (EF = 2–5)		
Land Use Areas				
Industrial and warehouse area (n = 6)	Sb 12 Pb 9 Cu 7	Ni 3	43	55
High-rise residential area (n = 6)	Cu 5 Zn 5	Ni 3 Pb 2	31	79
Low-rise residential area (n = 5)	Sb 6	Ni 4 Cu 4 Zn 4 Cr 2	27	47
Power plant area (n = 3)	Sb 9	Cu 5 Zn 5 Ni 4 Cr 2 Pb 2	32	39
Public and business area (n = 3)	Zn 7 Cu 6 Sb 6	Pb 2	29	87
Transport hubs (n = 2)	Sb 8	Cu 4 Ni 3 Zn 3 Fe 2	30	30
Traffic Density				
Low (n = 8)	Sb 5	Cu 4 Zn 3 Ni 3 Pb 2	28	39
Moderate (n = 14)	Sb 10 Cu 6 Pb 6	Zn 5 Ni 3	40	53
High (n = 3)	Zn 9 Sb 8 Cu 8	Ni 4 Pb 3 Cd 2	44	144
Total for Surgut	Sb 8.1 Cu 5.5	Zn 4.9 Pb 4 Ni 4	37	59

Note: the numbers after the elements correspond to their mean EF values. Elements with EF < 2 are not shown.

The dust samples from roads with low traffic densities only had a significant enrichment in Sb. Roads with heavier traffic were characterized by dust enrichment in practically all pollutants, including Sb, Zn, Cu and Pb. In particular, the roads with moderate and high traffic intensities as compared to the roads with low traffic intensities were characterized by the following increases in pollutant concentrations: Zn by multiples of 1.4–2.8, Cu—1.3–1.7, Pb—1.1–2.5, Cd—1.3–2.8, Sb—1.5–1.9 and Bi by multiples of 1.7–2.0. Verification using the Mann–Whitney test showed that small roads significantly differ from medium and large ones in the enrichment of road dust with Zn, Sb and Pb (p = 0.01). The dust samples from roads with low, moderate and high traffic densities were characterized the total enrichment factor Ze values of 28, 40 and 44, respectively, with an overall mean of 37. As compared to Moscow, where the mean for Ze is 54 [13], Surgut has a lower level of road dust contamination, which can be easily explained by Moscow's much higher intensities of traffic and industrial emissions, both being sources of PTEs. However, it should be taken into account that concentrations of some elements (Mo, W and Sn) were excluded from the calculations, and therefore, the index values could be slightly underestimated.

The spatial distribution of Ze values is shown in Figure 2. The highest values are found within the road stretches where traffic jams regularly occur, which causes the increase in emissions of fine particles and soot.

The total potential ecological risk index (RI) had values between 150 and 300 in only two samples, which corresponded to the category of "moderate risk" according to [50]. Those abnormal values resulted from a sporadic occurrence of high Cd concentrations in the road dust. The samples from business areas had high Cd concentrations (0.33 and 0.66 mg kg^{-1}) as well as a high concentration of Zn. Solid waste incinerators are known to be an important source of both Cd and Zn [74]. It is likely that solid waste incineration was practiced near our sampling sites. In addition, car tire wear is also a source of Cd [75]. All other studied samples belonged to the category of low risk, with the maximal values of total potential ecological risk index *RI* found on roads with high traffic densities.

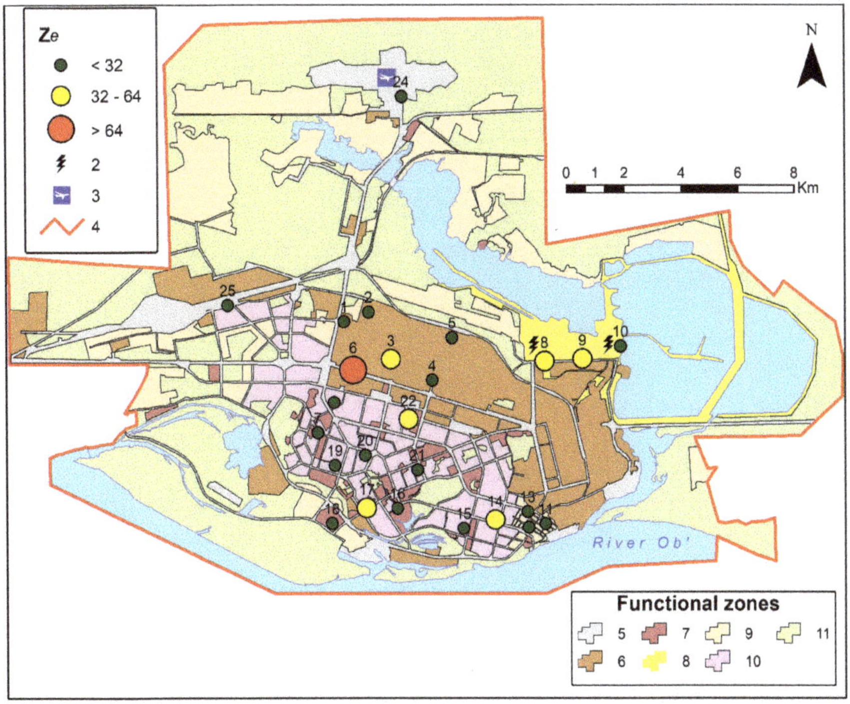

Figure 2. Spatial distribution of *Ze* values: 1—sampling sites; 2—power plants; 3—airport; 4—city border; 5—industrial and warehouse area; 6—high-rise residential area; 7—low-rise residential area; 8—power plant area; 9—public and business area; 10—modern business zones; 11—recreational area, urban forests, green spaces.

3.3. Source Identification

The most significant contributors to PTE pollution from vehicles are considered to be brake wear, tire erosion, exhaust emissions and oil losses [76]. The other source of PTEs, which include V, Cr, Co, Ni, Cu, Zn and Pb, is the abrasion of road tarmac [77,78]. Calculations of *EF* values showed that Sb, Zn, Mo, Cu and Pb were the main pollutants of Surgut's road dust (See Table 3). The main source of Sb in road dust is brake wear [79]. Antimony pentasulfide is used as a pigment in the production of car tires [80]. On the road stretches where traffic regularly slows and stops (traffic lights, cross-roads, etc.), Sb concentrations are generally eight times as high as those in the background [81]. Antimony is also used for the production of car batteries.

Tire erosion is also a source of Zn, because zinc oxide is used as a vulcanization agent in tire production [78,82]. The concentration of Zn in car tires is about 1% [77]. Research on the variability in the chemical composition of road dust in Spain by Amato et al. [7] has shown that contents of Sb, Zn and Mo are increased within stretches of roads where traffic slows and stops, which confirms their relationship with tire wear.

Principal sources of Cu in the atmosphere include fossil fuel burning, traffic emissions, fuel combustion and industrial combustion [83]. The erosion of brake pads is an important source of Cu in road dust. It is known that up to 47% of Cu in urban sewage is also sourced from brake pad wear [84]. The degradation of brake pads over time contributes Fe, Cu, Pb, Cr, Zn and Sb to road dust [85].

It should be noted that Cu and Zn are the main PTE components within high-rise residential areas that have the highest number of traffic lights (see Figure 2). Traffic jams where vehicles move at a speed of 20 km/h result in a 30% increase in car exhaust emissions [86]. Therefore, we believe that the high content of Cu in the road dust of Surgut mainly resulted from brake pad erosion.

To verify the sources of pollution, we conducted a PCA analysis of the obtained data set on the contents of PTEs, pH values and the content of fine particles (<2 and 2–10 μm). Elements of geogenic origin with concentrations similar to their world crust average were excluded from the analysis, which therefore included only the ecologically hazardous elements (Cr, Co, V, etc.). Our choice of the fine fraction was based on the fact that fine fractions have the highest PTE contents, e.g., the PM10 fraction of Moscow's road dust is 1.2–6.4 times more polluted by PTEs than bulk samples of the dust [13].

The essence of PCA analysis is to restrict a multicomponent data set to a limited, user-selected number of factors that determine the sample variance. The results obtained made it possible to identify four main factors which predetermine the chemical composition of road dust (Table 5).

Table 5. Varimax principal component loadings for PTE concentrations, pH and PM10 in the studied samples of road dust.

Elements and Parameters	PC1	PC2	PC3	PC4
V	0.61	0.04	−0.04	0.52
Cr	0.78	0.06	0.23	0.15
Co	0.86	0.14	−0.01	0.16
Ni	0.85	−0.03	−0.02	−0.28
Cu	0.16	0.57	0.28	0.41
Zn	0.16	0.92	0.10	0.17
As	0.55	0.01	−0.18	0.17
Cd	0.09	0.87	−0.06	0.05
Sb	0.18	0.16	0.90	−0.01
Pb	−0.10	0.05	0.94	−0.01
pH	−0.10	−0.0	0.01	−0.69
PM10	0.70	0.073	0.13	0.12
Expl. Var	3.39	2.62	1.97	1.33
Prp. Totl	0.26	0.20	0.15	0.10

The four PCs together account for 71% of the variance. The first PC explains 26% of the total variance and has a strong loading of Cr, Co, Ni and PM10. The concentrations of Cr, Co and Ni in Surgut's road dust were generally low as compared to their world crust average values (PIr = 0.4–0.5). However, some sampling sites, in particular within the low-rise residential area and the power plant area, were characterized by Ni enrichment. Relatively higher concentrations of metals such as Ni and Co are caused by the adsorption of these metals by Fe–Mn colloids [87]. Both Ni and Co originate from geogenic sources. The abrasion of road surfaces is an additional source of Ni, which is a component of asphalt bitumen and gabbro rock material [88]. High Ni contents have also been noted in gabbro rocks of the Ural Mountains [89], which are not far from Surgut.

The PC2 is dominated by Zn and Cd. Our observations showed that Zn and Cd probably originated from the same anthropogenic source. Previous studies [90–92] have reported that vehicle emissions and diesel and fossil fuel combustion are known as the primary anthropogenic sources of Cd and Zn atmospheric pollution. PC 3 is dominated by Sb and Pb, accounting for 15% of the total variance. This group of elements, as shown above, is associated with traffic. PC4, dominated by pH, explains 10% of the total variance. The soil acidity to a large extent predetermines the mobility of metals [65] and, therefore, their concentrations in soils.

3.4. Comparisons with Other Cities

Table 6 compares the concentrations of PTEs in this study with some other world cities. Our selection of cities for such a comparison was based on the presence of comparable assemblages of the analyzed elements. A comparison allowed us to determine the geochemical properties of the road dust of Surgut as follows: low contents of As, Cd, Sb and Zn but a 1.6–2 times higher content of Ni in comparison with those in Moscow and Chelyabinsk. The high content of Ni has been previously identified in the road dust of Tyumen, which is a large city in Western Siberia [29]. The latter is explained by the fact that the road construction there involved the use of fine gravel of ultramafic and mafic rocks imported from the Urals. High concentrations of Ni and Cr are often mentioned in descriptions of Uralian ultramafic rocks such as gabbro [89]. Regarding the levels of Cu, Co and Cr in road dust, Surgut occupies an intermediate position among other cities.

Table 6. Literature data on published metal median concentrations (mg kg^{-1}) in street dust from cities around the world.

City	Cr	Co	Ni	Cu	Zn	As	Cd	Pb	Sb	Reference
Surgut, this study	46	6.9	41.1	42.8	89.9	1.3	0.11	19.0	0.89	This study
Chelyabinsk	48.5	6.3	21.9	55.9	154	3.8	0.4	14.4	1.3	[20]
Moscow	50	8.0	26	93	252	2.8	0.61	53	4.6	[23]
Alushta	31	7.4	33	44	127	8.0	0.3	37	1.5	[28]
Tyumen	415	25.6	324	51.3	105	8.8	0.19	20.1	1.83	[29]
Ahvaz, Iran	51.5	9.2	59.7	74.4	309	-	0.5	85.4	2.1	[93]
Hangzhou, China	51	20	26	116	321	-	1.59	202	-	[94]
Houston, TX, USA	67	4.8	119	183	557	-	-	40	-	[95]
Kabul, Afganistan	38.4	8.52	66.4	43.6	122.5	-	1.16	28.7	-	[96]
Kuala Lumpur, Malaysia	74.1	3.36	11.3	87.0	314	68.8	0.71	98.8	-	[19]
Katowice, Poland	211	-	43.7	239	**2030**	-	0.35	430	-	[97]
Luanda, Angola	26	2.9	10	42	317	5.0	1.1	351	3.4	[98]
Nicosia, North Cyprus	321	-	65	52	136	17.5	-	35.6	-	[99]
Ottawa, Canada	43.3	8.3	15.2	65.8	112	1.3	0.6	39	0.89	[100]
Seul, Korea	151	-	-	396	795	-	-	144	-	[101]
Shanghai, China	159	-	84	197	734	-	1.23	295	-	[102]
Thessaloniki, Greece	105	-	89	**662**	452	-	**1.76**	209	-	[17]
Tongchuan, China	106.5	31.7	25.3	32.4	142	6.7	-	75.2	-	[103]
Toronto, Canada	198	-	58.8	162	233	-	0.51	183	-	[12]
Xi'an, China	145	30.9	30.8	54.7	268.6	-	-	125	-	[104]

Note: the values in bold font correspond to the highest concentration in the areas compared.

4. Exposure and Risk Assessment

The results of calculations of non-carcinogenic and carcinogenic risk indices through all exposure pathways (ingestion, inhalation and dermal contact) are presented in Tables 7 and 8.

Table 7. Non-carcinogenic hazard quotient (HQ) and hazard index (HI) values of trace elements through all exposure pathways in Surgut city.

Element	HQ Ing		HQ Derm		HQ Inh		HI	
	Childr	Adults	Childr	Adults	Childr	Adults	Childr	Adults
Pb	3.4×10^{-2}	3.8×10^{-3}	2.5×10^{-4}	2.8×10^{-5}	1.6×10^{-4}	2.7×10^{-4}	3.4×10^{-2}	3.8×10^{-3}
Ni	2.4×10^{-2}	2.7×10^{-3}	4.4×10^{-4}	4.9×10^{-5}	4.9×10^{-2}	8.1×10^{-2}	7.3×10^{-2}	8.4×10^{-2}
Cu	2.7×10^{-2}	3.1×10^{-3}	3.5×10^{-5}	4.0×10^{-6}	3.2×10^{-5}	5.4×10^{-5}	2.7×10^{-2}	3.1×10^{-3}
Zn	1.9×10^{-3}	2.2×10^{-4}	1.4×10^{-5}	1.6×10^{-6}	4.5×10^{-5}	7.6×10^{-5}	1.9×10^{-3}	2.2×10^{-4}
As	2.7×10^{-2}	3.1×10^{-3}	2.1×10^{-5}	2.4×10^{-6}	9.1×10^{-5}	1.5×10^{-4}	2.8×10^{-2}	3.2×10^{-3}
Cd	6.9×10^{-4}	7.7×10^{-5}	2.0×10^{-5}	2.3×10^{-6}	1.1×10^{-3}	1.9×10^{-3}	1.8×10^{-3}	2.0×10^{-3}
Sb	1.4×10^{-2}	1.6×10^{-3}	7.0×10^{-5}	7.9×10^{-6}	3.2×10^{-4}	5.3×10^{-4}	1.5×10^{-2}	2.1×10^{-3}

Table 8. Carcinogenic risk (CRA) values of Pb and As through all exposure pathways in Surgut city.

Element	CRA Ing		CRA Derm		CRA Inh		CRA Sum	
	Childr	Adults	Childr	Adults	Childr	Adults	Childr	Adults
Pb	1.0×10^{-6}	1.2×10^{-6}	7.6×10^{-9}	8.5×10^{-10}	2.4×10^{-8}	4.0×10^{-8}	1.1×10^{-6}	1.6×10^{-7}
As	1.2×10^{-5}	1.4×10^{-6}	9.5×10^{-9}	1.1×10^{-9}	5.9×10^{-7}	9.8×10^{-7}	1.3×10^{-5}	2.4×10^{-6}

The non-carcinogenic risk assessment was based on metal concentrations, which were above their Clarke (world crust average) values ($PIr > 1$). The results showed that non-carcinogenic risk in Surgut was mainly associated with the ingestion of dust particles. Data from other cities confirm that ingestion is the most hazardous pathway [21,40,96,98,105]. Children tend to be at higher risk than adults, because their relatively lower body weight implies that the impact of road dust contaminated with heavy metals can be relatively higher. The obtained HI values show that Sb, Ni, Cu and As are generally the most harmful elements within Surgut, with additional health risks associated with Cd and Pb within some areas of the city. It should be noted that despite the low Ni enrichment of road dust, its health risk is high due to the high toxicity of this element.

The carcinogenic risks of As and Pb were also mainly associated with the ingestion pathway, whereas the risks from dermal contact are very low. The total carcinogenic risk values (CRA sum, see Table 8) ranged from 10^{-5} to 10^{-7}. According to the U.S. EPA, any value of cancer risk within the range of 10^{-6} to 10^{-4} is an acceptable or tolerable risk, and any value below 10^{-6} can be ignored. Therefore, the present study showed that carcinogenic risks from the PTEs in the road dust of Surgut were insignificant due to their low concentrations.

5. Conclusions

The road dust of Surgut, as in the majority of cities of the world, has an alkaline reaction due to the presence of carbonate microparticles. The 100–250 μm fraction, which was predominant in the particle size distribution of the studied dust samples, originates from geogenic sources and abrasion processes caused by road traffic. Fine particles (<50 μm), which mainly originate from industrial emissions, had a mean content of 17.5% in the studied samples. Therefore, the composition of road dust was mainly predetermined by contributions from sources associated with road traffic and soil erosion. The texture of Surgut's road dust is relatively homogeneous. Fluctuations in the particle size distribution for roads of different categories and different land use areas are small.

It was found that Surgut's road dust was rich in Sb, Cu, Zn, Cd and Pb as compared to their mean contents in the upper part of the Earth's crust. These elements are regarded as typical urban pollutants that accumulate in the road dust of many cities. Those element concentrations in the road dust of Surgut increased by multiples of 1.4–2.8 on average with increasing traffic densities. The highest concentrations were found within stretches of roads, where traffic jams regularly occur. The main source of these elements is from the abrasion of car tires and brake pads. In addition to traffic densities, the road dust composition was influenced by solid waste incineration, which led to the Cd and Zn contamination of the studied samples.

Based on the values of the total potential eco-logical risk index (PI) and the total enrichment factor (Ze), levels of the total contamination of Surgut's road dust were mostly low. The moderate contamination levels were only detected in samples from high-traffic roads. The generally low contamination can be explained by the predominance of coarse particles in the road dust. Taking into account that the PTE concentrations in fine fractions (PM10) is significantly higher than in the coarse fraction, further research should focus on the analysis of the fine fraction.

The present study on PTEs showed that their greatest potential risks to human health were associated with the ingestion pathway; however, both carcinogenic and non-carcinogenic risks of such PTEs were generally acceptable or tolerable due to their low concentrations in the road dust of Surgut.

The results obtained in this study can be used in the planning and further development of the transport network of Surgut city and also help improve the efficiency of the street cleaning practices by the municipal services.

Supplementary Materials: The following are available online at https://www.mdpi.com/article/10.3390/atmos13010030/s1, Table S1: Description of sampling sites, Table S2: Methods of analysis, analytical results and recovery of certified reference material, Table S3: Exposure parameters used for the health risk assessment.

Author Contributions: D.M.: conceptualization, original draft writing; R.P.: sample collection, data processing; A.S.: conceptualization, visualization, reviewing the manuscript; V.T. sample collection, reviewing the manuscript. All authors have read and agreed to the published version of the manuscript.

Funding: This research was funded by the Russian Foundation for Basic Research (project no. 19-05-50062) and project no. 121041600045-8 of RAS Siberian Branch.

Institutional Review Board Statement: Not applicable.

Informed Consent Statement: Not applicable.

Data Availability Statement: The datasets generated during and/or analyzed during the current study are available from the corresponding author on reasonable request.

Acknowledgments: We would like to thank the Russian Foundation for Basic Research for the financial support (19-05-50062). The authors are especially grateful to Vasiliy Karandashev for the element determination.

Conflicts of Interest: The authors declare no conflict of interest.

References

1. Sutherland, R. Bed sediment-associated trace metals in an urban stream, Oahu, Hawaii. *Environ. Geol.* **2000**, *39*, 611–627. [CrossRef]
2. Chow, J.; Watson, J.; Lu, Z. Descriptive analysis of PM(2.5) and PM(10) at regionally representative locations during SJ-VAQS/AUSPEX 1996. *Atmos. Environ.* **1996**, *30*, 2079–2112. [CrossRef]
3. Kupiainen, K. Monograph of Boreal Environment Research. In *Road Dust from Pavement Wear and Traction Sanding*; Finnish Environment Institute: Helsinki, Finland, 2007; 50p, Available online: http://hdl.handle.net/10138/39334 (accessed on 18 November 2021).
4. Mazzei, F.; D'alessandro, A.; Lucarelli, F.; Nava, S.; Prati, P.; Valli, G.; Vecchi, R. Characterization of particulate matter sources in an urban environment. *Sci. Total Environ.* **2008**, *401*, 81–89. [CrossRef]
5. Kosheleva, N.E.; Vlasov, D.V.; Korlyakov, I.D.; Kasimov, N.S. Contamination of urban soils with heavy metals in Moscow as affected by building development. *Sci. Total Environ.* **2018**, *636*, 854–863. [CrossRef] [PubMed]
6. Varrica, D.; Dongarra, G.; Sabatino, G.; Monna, F. Inorganic geochemistry of roadway dust from the metropolitan area of Palermo, Italy. *Environ. Geol.* **2003**, *44*, 222–230. [CrossRef]
7. Amato, F.; Pandolfi, M.; Viana, M.; Querol, X.; Alastuey, A.; Moreno, T. Spatial and chemical patterns of PM10 in road dust deposited in urban environment. *Atmos. Environ.* **2009**, *43*, 1650–1659. [CrossRef]
8. Amato, F.; Cassee, F.R.; Denier van der Gon, H.A.C.; Gehrig, R.; Gustafsson, M.; Hafner, W.; Harrison, R.M.; Jozwicka, M.; Kelly, F.J.; Moreno, T.; et al. Urban air quality: The challenge of traffic non-exhaust emissions. *J. Hazard. Mater.* **2014**, *275*, 31–36. [CrossRef]
9. Denier van der Gon, H.A.C.; Gerlofs-Nijland, M.E.; Gehrig, R.; Gustafsson, M.; Janssen, N.; Harrison, R.M.; Hulskotte, J.; Johansson, C.; Jozwicka, M.; Keuken, M.; et al. The policy relevance of wear emissions from road transport, now and in the future—An international workshop report and consensus statement. *J. Air Waste Manag.* **2013**, *63*, 136–149. [CrossRef]
10. Murakami, M.; Nakajima, F.; Furumai, H.; Tomiyasu, B.; Owari, M. Identification of particles containing chromium and lead in road dust and soakaway sediment by electron probe microanalyser. *Chemosphere* **2007**, *67*, 2000–2010. [CrossRef] [PubMed]
11. Irvine, K.N.; Perrelli, M.F.; Ngoen-klan, R.; Droppo, I.G. Metal levels in street sediment from an industrial city: Spatial trends, chemical fractionation, and management implications. *J. Soils Sedim.* **2009**, *9*, 328–341. [CrossRef]
12. Nazzal, Y.; Rosen, M.A.; Al-Rawabden, A.M. Assessment of metal pollution in urban road dusts from selected highways of the Greater Toronto Area in Canada. *Environ. Monit. Assess.* **2013**, *185*, 1847–1858. [CrossRef] [PubMed]

13. Vlasov, D.V.; Kosheleva, N.E.; Kasimov, N.S. Spatial distribution and sources of potentially toxic elements in road dust and its PM10 fraction of Moscow megacity. *Sci. Total Environ.* **2021**, *761*, 143267. [CrossRef] [PubMed]
14. Tager, I.B. Health effects of aerosols: Mechanisms and epidemiology. In *Aerosols Handbook: Measurement, Dosimetry, and Health Effects*; Ruzer, L.S., Harley, N.H., Eds.; CRC Press: Boca Raton, FA, USA, 2005; pp. 619–696.
15. Jose, J.; Srimuruganandam, B. Investigation of road dust characteristics and its associated health risks from an urban environment. *Environ. Geochem. Health* **2020**, *42*, 2819–2840. [CrossRef]
16. Demographics. Federal State Statistics Service. 2021. Available online: https://rosstat.gov.ru/folder/12781 (accessed on 18 November 2021).
17. Li, F.; Zhang, J.; Huang, J.; Huang, D.; Yang, J.; Song, Y.; Zeng, G. Heavy metals in road dust from Xiandao District, Changsha City, China: Characteristics, health risk assessment, and integrated source identification. *Environ. Sci. Pollut. Res.* **2016**, *23*, 13100–13113. [CrossRef] [PubMed]
18. Gulia, S.; Goyal, P.; Goyal, S.K.; Kumar, R. Re-suspension of road dust: Contribution, assessment and control through dust suppressants—A review. *Int. J. Environ. Sci. Technol.* **2019**, *16*, 1717–1728. [CrossRef]
19. Othman, M.; Latif, M.T. Pollution characteristics, sources, and health risk assessments of urban road dust in Kuala Lumpur City. *Environ. Sci. Pollut. Res.* **2020**, *27*, 11227–11245. [CrossRef]
20. Kasimov, N.S.; Bityukova, V.R.; Malkhazova, S.M.; Kosheleva, N.E.; Nikiforova, E.M.; Shartova, N.V.; Vlasov, D.V.; Timonin, S.A.; Krainov, V.N. *Regions and Cities of RUSSIA: The Integrated Assessment of the Environment*; Filimonov MV Publishing: Moscow, Russia, 2014; 560p. (In Russian)
21. Krupnova, T.G.; Rakova, O.V.; Gavrilkina, S.V.; Antoshkina, E.G.; Baranov, E.O.; Yakimova, O.N. Road dust trace elements contamination, sources, dispersed composition, and human health risk in Chelyabinsk, Russia. *Chemosphere* **2020**, *261*, 127799. [CrossRef]
22. Ladonin, D.V.; Plyaskina, O.V. Isotopic composition of lead in soils and street dust in the Southeastern administrative district of Moscow. *Eurasian Soil Sci.* **2009**, *42*, 93–104. [CrossRef]
23. Ladonin, D.V.; Mikhaylova, A.P. Heavy Metals and Arsenic in Soils and Street Dust of the Southeastern Administrative District of Moscow: Long-Term Data. *Eurasian Soil Sci.* **2020**, *53*, 1635–1644. [CrossRef]
24. Vlasov, D.V.; Kasimov, N.S.; Kosheleva, N.E. Geochemistry of the road dust in the Eastern district of Moscow. *Vestn. Mosk. Univ. Geogr.* **2015**, *1*, 23–33. (In Russian)
25. Kasimov, N.S.; Vlasov, D.V.; Kosheleva, N.E.; Nikiforova, E.M. *Geochemistry of Landscapes of Eastern Moscow*; APR Publishing: Moscow, Russia, 2016; 276p. (In Russian)
26. Kasimov, N.S.; Vlasov, D.V.; Kosheleva, N.E. Enrichment of road dust particles and adjacent environments with metals and metalloids in eastern Moscow. *Urban Clim.* **2020**, *32*, 100638. [CrossRef]
27. Kaygorodov, R.V.; Tiunova, M.I.; Druzshinina, A.A. Polluting substances in a dust of travellers of parts and in wood vegetation of roadside strips of a city zone. *Vestn. Permsk. Univ. Seriya Biol.* **2009**, *10*, 141–146. (In Russian)
28. Kasimov, N.S.; Bezberdaya, L.A.; Vlasov, D.V.; Lychagin, M.Y. Metals, Metalloids, and benzo[a]pyrene in PM10 particles of soils and road dust of Alushta City. *Eurasian Soil Sci.* **2019**, *52*, 1608–1621. [CrossRef]
29. Konstantinova, E.; Minkina, T.; Konstantinov, A.; Sushkova, S.; Antonenko, E.; Kurasova, A.; Loiko, S. Pollution status and human health risk assessment of potentially toxic elements and polycyclic aromatic hydrocarbons in urban street dust of Tyumen city, Russia. *Environ. Geochem. Health* **2020**. [CrossRef] [PubMed]
30. Program for the Integrated Development of the Transport Infrastructure of the Municipal Formation "Urban District of the City of Surgut" for the Period up to 2035. 2017. Available online: https://www.dumasurgut.ru/getattachment/2be92a61-ce22-4fec-970b-ac2456e2a195/221-VI%20%D0%94%D0%93.aspx (accessed on 18 November 2021).
31. Vinokurova, M.V.; Vinokurov, M.V.; Voronin, S.A. Effect of auto-road complex in the city of Surgut on air pollution and population health. *Gig. Sanit.* **2015**, *94*, 57–61. (In Russian)
32. *Reference Book on the USSR Climate. Series 2. Issue 17. Tyumen and Omsk Regions*; Gidrometeoizdat: S.-Petersburg, Russia, 1998; 702p. (In Russian)
33. Nasratinova, R.M.; Shantarin, V.D. Ecological monitoring of snow cover in the Town of Surgut. *Oil Gas* **2014**, *6*, 120–123. (In Russian)
34. Gorban, M.V.; Nakonechniy, N.V.; Vdovkin, R.S.; Bashkatova, Y.V. The condition assessment of Surgut City soils experiencing the influence of motor transport. *Vestn. KrasGAU* **2014**, *9*, 53–58. (In Russian)
35. Samoylenko, Z.A.; Bezuglaya, V.V.; Guselnikova, M.V.; Pyatova, P.N. Content of heavy metals in soils under the influence of unauthorized dumps in Surgut. *J. Agric. Environ.* **2021**, *3*, 1–6. (In Russian)
36. Slashcheva, A.V. Ecological and geochemical assessment of the Surgut lowland territory. *Reg. Environ. Issues* **2011**, *3*, 35–44. (In Russian)
37. Moskovchenko, D.V. *Ecogeochemistry of Oil and Gas Producing Regions of Western Siberia*; Academic Publishing House "Geo": Novosibirsk, Russia, 2013; 259p. (In Russian)
38. Bourliva, A.; Christophoridis, C.; Papadopoulou, L.; Giouri, K.; Papadopoulos, A.; Mitsika, E.; Fytianos, K. Characterization, Heavy metal content and health risk assessment of urban road dusts from the historic center of the city of Thessaloniki, Greece. *Environ. Geochem. Health* **2017**, *39*, 611–634. [CrossRef] [PubMed]

39. Alsbou, E.; Zaitoun, M.A.; Alasoufi, A.M.; Al Shra'Ah, A. Concentration and Source Assessment of Polycyclic Aromatic Hydrocarbons in the Street Soil of Ma'an City, Jordan. *Arch. Environ. Contam. Toxicol.* **2019**, *77*, 619–630. [CrossRef] [PubMed]
40. Alsohaimi, I.H.; El-Hashemy, M.A.; Al-Ruwaili, A.G.; El-Nasr, T.A.S.; Almuaikel, N.S. Assessment of Trace Elements in Urban Road Dust of a City in a Border Province Concerning Their Levels, Sources, and Related Health Risks. *Arch. Environ. Contam. Toxicol.* **2020**, *79*, 23–38. [CrossRef]
41. Padoan, E.; Romè, C.; Ajmone-Marsan, F. Bioaccessibility and size distribution of metals in road dust and roadside soils along a peri-urban transect. *Sci. Total Environ.* **2017**, *601*, 89–98. [CrossRef]
42. Trujillo-Gonzalez, J.M.; Torres-Mora, M.A.; Keesstra, S.; Brevik, E.C.; Jimenez-Ballesta, R. Heavy metal accumulation related to population density in road dust samples taken from urban sites under different land uses. *Sci. Total Environ.* **2016**, *553*, 636–642. [CrossRef] [PubMed]
43. Al-Awadhi, J.M.; AlShuaibi, A.A. Dust fallout in Kuwait City: Deposition and characterization. *Sci. Total Environ.* **2013**, *461*, 139–148. [CrossRef]
44. Li, F.; Huang, J.; Zeng, G.; Huang, X.; Liu, W.; Wu, H.; Yuan, Y.; He, X.; Lai, M. Spatial distribution and health risk assessment of toxic metals associated with receptor population density in street dust: A case study of Xiandao District, Changsha, Middle China. *Environ. Sci. Pollut. Res.* **2015**, *22*, 6732–6742. [CrossRef]
45. Kara, M.; Dumanoglu, Y.; Altiok, H.; Elbir, T.; Odabasi, M.; Bayram, A. Seasonal and spatial variations of atmospheric trace elemental deposition in the Aliaga industrial region, Turkey. *Atmos. Res.* **2014**, *149*, 204–216. [CrossRef]
46. Bourennane, H.; Douay, F.; Sterckeman, T.; Villanneau, E.; Ciesielski, H.; King, D.; Baize, D. Mapping of anthropogenic trace elements inputs in agricultural topsoil from Northern France using enrichment factors. *Geoderma* **2010**, *157*, 165–174. [CrossRef]
47. Syso, A.I. *Patterns of Distribution of Chemical Elements in Soil-Forming Rocks and Soils of Western Siberia*; Publishing House of SB RAS: Novosibirsk, Russia, 2007; 227p. (In Russian)
48. Moskovchenko, D.V. *Oil and Gas Production and the Environment: Ecological and Geochemical Analysis of the Tyumen Region*; Nauka, Sib.predpriyatie RAS: Novosibirsk, Russia, 1998; 112p. (In Russian)
49. Rudnick, R.L.; Gao, S. Composition of the continental crust. In *Treatise on Geochemistry*, 3rd ed.; Elsevier Science: New York, NY, USA, 2003; pp. 1–64.
50. Hakanson, L. An ecological risk index for aquatic pollution control. A sedimentological approach. *Water Res.* **1980**, *14*, 975–1001. [CrossRef]
51. Zhang, X.; Wang, Y.; Guo, S.; Li, H.; Liu, J.; Zhang, Z.; Yan, L.; Tan, C.; Yang, Z.; Guo, X. Concentration and speciation of trace metals and metalloids from road-deposited sediments in urban and rural areas of Beijing, China. *J. Soils Sediments* **2020**, *20*, 3487–3501. [CrossRef]
52. Yongming, H.; Peixuan, D.; Junji, C.; Posmentier, E.S. Multivariate analysis of heavy metal contamination in urban dusts of Xi'an, Central China. *Sci. Total Environ.* **2006**, *355*, 176–186. [CrossRef]
53. US EPA (US Environmental Protection Agency). *Risk Assessment Guidance for Superfund. Volume I: Human Health Evaluation Manual (Part A). Interim Final (EPA/ 540/1-89/002)*; Office of Emergency and Remedial Response: Washington, DC, USA, 1989.
54. Kong, S.; Lu, B.; Bai, Z.; Zhao, X.; Chen, L.; Han, B.; Li, Z.; Ji, Y.; Xu, Y.; Liu, Y.; et al. Potential threat of heavy metals in re-suspended dusts on building surfaces in oilfeld city. *Atmos. Environ.* **2011**, *25*, 4192–4204. [CrossRef]
55. Zheng, N.; Liu, J.; Wang, Q.; Liang, Z. Health risk assessment of heavy metal exposure to street dust in the zinc smelting district, Northeast of China. *Sci. Total Environ.* **2010**, *408*, 726–733. [CrossRef]
56. Li, R.P.; Cai, G.Q.; Wang, J.; Wei, O.Y.; Cheng, H.G.; Lin, C.Y. Contents and chemical forms of heavy metals in school and roadside topsoils and road-surface dust of Beijing. *J. Soils Sediments* **2014**, *14*, 1806–1817. [CrossRef]
57. Al-Khashman, O.A. The investigation of metal concentrations in street dust samples in Aqaba city, Jordan. *Environ. Geochem. Health* **2007**, *29*, 197–207. [CrossRef] [PubMed]
58. Acosta, J.A.; Faz, A.; Kalbitz, K.; Jansen, B.; Martínez-Martínez, S. Heavy metal concentrations in particle size fractions from street dust of Murcia (Spain) as the basis for risk assessment. *J. Environ. Monit.* **2011**, *13*, 3087–3096. [CrossRef] [PubMed]
59. Li, X.; Zhang, Y.; Luo, J.; Wang, T.; Lian, H.; Ding, Z. Bioaccessibility and health risk of arsenic, mercury and other metals in urban street dusts from a mega-city, Nanjing, China. *Environ. Pollut.* **2011**, *159*, 1215–1221. [CrossRef]
60. Robertson, D.J.; Taylor, K.G.; Hoon, S.R. Geochemical and mineral magnetic characterisation of urban sediment particulates, Manchester, UK. *Appl. Geochem.* **2003**, *18*, 269–282. [CrossRef]
61. Christoforidis, A.; Stamatis, N. Heavy metal contamination in street dust and roadside soil along the major national road in Kavala's region, Greece. *Geoderma* **2009**, *15*, 257–263. [CrossRef]
62. Zaytseva, N.V.; May, I.V.; Maks, A.A.; Zagorodnov, S.Y. Analysis of the dispersion and component composition of the dust for the assessment of the exposure to the population in the areas of influence of industrial emissions of stationary source. *Hyg. Sanit.* **2013**, *5*, 19–23. (In Russian)
63. Lanzerstorfer, C. Heavy metals in the finest size fractions of road-deposited sediments. *Environ. Pollut.* **2018**, *239*, 522–531. [CrossRef] [PubMed]
64. Cowan, N.; Blair, D.; Malcolm, H.; Graham, M. A survey of heavy metal contents of rural and urban roadside dusts: Comparisons at low, medium and high traffic sites in Central Scotland. *Environ. Sci. Pollut. Res.* **2021**, *28*, 7365–7378. [CrossRef]
65. Kabata-Pendias, A. *Trace Elements in Soils and Plants*, 3rd ed.; CRC press: Boca Raton, FL, USA, 2000; 432p. [CrossRef]

66. De Miguel, E.; Llamas, J.F.; Chacón, E.; Berg, T.; Larssen, S.; Røyset, O.; Vadset, M. Origin and patterns of distribution of trace elements in street dust: Unleaded petrol and urban lead. *Atmos. Environ.* **1997**, *31*, 2733–2740. [CrossRef]
67. Shi, G.; Chen, Z.; Bi, C.; Wang, L.; Teng, J.; Li, Y.; Xu, S. A comparative study of health risk of potentially toxic metals in urban and suburban road dust in the most populated city of China. *Atmos. Environ.* **2011**, *45*, 764–771. [CrossRef]
68. Siddiqui, Z.; Khillare, P.S.; Jyethi, D.S.; Aithani, D.; Yadav, A.K. Pollution characteristics and human health risk from trace metals in roadside soil and road dust around major urban parks in Delhi city. *Air Qual. Atmos. Health* **2020**, *13*, 1271–1286. [CrossRef]
69. Opekunova, M.G.; Opekunov, A.Y.; Kukushkin, S.Y.; Ganul, A.G. Background contents of heavy metals in soils and bottom sediments in the north of Western Siberia. *Eurasian Soil Sci.* **2019**, *52*, 380–395. [CrossRef]
70. Yuan, G.L.; Sun, T.H.; Han, P.; Li, J.; Lang, X.X. Source identification and ecological risk assessment of heavy metals in topsoil using environmental geochemical mapping: Typical urban renewal area in Beijing, China. *J. Geochem. Explor.* **2014**, *136*, 40–47. [CrossRef]
71. Cao, Z.; Chen, Q.; Wang, X.; Zhang, Y.; Wang, S.; Wang, M.; Zhao, L.; Yan, G.; Zhang, X.; Zhang, Z.; et al. Contamination characteristics of trace metals in dust from different levels of roads of a heavily air-polluted city in north China. *Environ. Geochem. Health* **2018**, *40*, 2441–2452. [CrossRef] [PubMed]
72. Shevchenko, V.P.; Pokrovsky, O.S.; Vorobyev, S.; Krickov, I.V.; Manasypov, R.M.; Politova, N.V.; Kopysov, S.G.; Dara, O.M.; Auda, Y.; Shirokova, L.S.; et al. Impact of snow deposition on major and trace element concentrations and elementary fluxes in surface waters of the Western Siberian Lowland across a 1700 km latitudinal gradient. *Hydrol. Earth Syst. Sci.* **2017**, *21*, 5725–5746. [CrossRef]
73. Pavlov, D.; Dakhouche, A.; Rogachev, T. Influence of arsenic, antimony and bismuth on the properties of lead/acid battery positive plates. *J. Power Sources* **1990**, *1*, 117–129. [CrossRef]
74. Nriagu, J.O.; Pacyna, J.M. Quantitative assessment of worldwide contamination of air, water and soils by trace metals. *Nat. Cell Biol.* **1988**, *333*, 134–139. [CrossRef]
75. Mugica-Alvarez, V.; Maubert, M.; Torres-Rodríguez, M.; Muñoz, J.; Rico, E. Temporal and spatial variations of metal content in TSP and PM10 in Mexico City during 1996. *J. Aerosol Sci.* **2002**, *33*, 91–102. [CrossRef]
76. Napier, F.; D'Arcy, B.; Jefferies, C. A review of vehicle related metals and polycyclic aromatic hydrocarbons in the UK environment. *Desalination* **2008**, *226*, 143–150. [CrossRef]
77. Adachi, K.; Tainosho, Y. Characterization of heavy metal particles embedded in tire dust. *Environ. Int.* **2004**, *30*, 1009–1017. [CrossRef] [PubMed]
78. Mummullage, S.; Egodawatta, P.; Ayoko, G.A.; Goonetilleke, A. Use of physicochemical signatures to assess the sources of metals in urban road dust. *Sci. Total Environ.* **2015**, *541*, 1303–1309. [CrossRef] [PubMed]
79. Miazgowicz, A.; Krennhuber, K.; Lanzerstorfer, C. Metals concentrations in road dust from high traffic and low traffic area: A size dependent comparison. *Int. J. Environ. Sci. Technol.* **2020**, *17*, 3365–3372. [CrossRef]
80. Councell, T.B.; Duckenfield, K.U.; Landa, E.R.; Callender, E. Tire wear particles as a source of zinc to the environment. *Environ. Sc. Technol.* **2004**, *38*, 4206–4214. [CrossRef] [PubMed]
81. Hjortenkrans, D.; Bergbäck, B.; Häggerud, A. New metal emission patterns in road traffic environments. *Environ. Monit. Assess.* **2006**, *117*, 85–98. [CrossRef] [PubMed]
82. Dall'Osto, M.; Beddows, D.C.; Gietl, J.K.; Olatunbosun, O.A.; Yang, X.; Harrison, R.M. Characteristics of tyre dust in polluted air: Studies by single particle mass spectrometry (ATOFMS). *Atmos. Environ.* **2014**, *94*, 224–230. [CrossRef]
83. Nriagu, J.O. A History of Global Metal Pollution. *Science* **1996**, *272*, 223. [CrossRef]
84. Davis, A.P.; Shokouhian, M.; Ni, S. Loading estimates of lead, copper, cadmium, and zinc in urban runoff from specific sources. *Chemosphere* **2001**, *44*, 997–1009. [CrossRef]
85. Thorpe, A.; Harrison, R.M. Sources and properties of non-exhaust particulate matter from road traffic: A review. *Sci. Total Environ* **2008**, *400*, 270–282. [CrossRef]
86. Bityukova, V.R.; Mozgunov, N.A. Spatial Features transformation of emission from motor vehicles in Moscow. *Geogr. Environ. Sustain.* **2019**, *12*, 57–73. [CrossRef]
87. Al-Khashman, O.A. Assessment of heavy metals contamination in deposited street dusts in different urbanized areas in the city of Ma'an, Jordan. *Environ. Earth Sci.* **2013**, *70*, 2603–2612. [CrossRef]
88. Lindgren, A. Asphalt Wear and Pollution Transport. *Sci. Total Environ.* **1996**, *189*, 281–286. [CrossRef]
89. Lesovaya, S.N.; Goryachkin, S.V.; Polekhovskii, Y.S. Soil formation and weathering on ultramafic rocks in the mountainous tundra of the Rai-Iz massif, Polar Urals. *Eurasian Soil Sci.* **2012**, *45*, 33–44. [CrossRef]
90. Aminiyan, M.M.; Baalousha, M.; Mousavi, R.; Aminiyan, F.M.; Hosseini, H.; Heydariyan, A. The ecological risk, Source identification, and pollution assessment of heavy metals in road dust: A case study in Rafsanjan, SE Iran. *Environ. Sci. Pollut. Res.* **2018**, *25*, 13382–13395. [CrossRef] [PubMed]
91. Kabata-Pendias, A.; Mukherjee, A.B. *Trace Elements from Soil to Human*; Springer: Berlin/Heidelberg, Germany, 2007; 550p.
92. Wei, B.; Jiang, F.; Li, X.; Mu, S. Spatial distribution and contamination assessment of heavy metals in urban road dusts from Urumqi, NW China. *Microchem. J.* **2009**, *93*, 147–152. [CrossRef]
93. Najmeddin, A.; Keshavarzi, B.; Moore, F.; Lahijanzadeh, A. Source apportionment and health risk assessment of potentially toxic elements in road dust from urban industrial areas of Ahvaz megacity, Iran. *Environ. Geochem. Health* **2018**, *40*, 1187–1208. [CrossRef] [PubMed]

94. Zhang, M.K.; Wang, H. Concentrations and chemical forms of potentially toxic metals in road-deposited sediments from different zones of Hangzhou, China. *J. Environ. Sci.* **2009**, *21*, 625–631. [CrossRef]
95. Fiala, M.; Hwang, H.M. Influence of Highway Pavement on Metals in Road Dust: A Case Study in Houston, Texas. *Water Air Soil Pollut.* **2021**, *232*, 185. [CrossRef]
96. Jadoon, W.; Khpalwak, W.; Chidya, R.C.G.; Abdel-Dayem, S.M.M.A.; Takeda, K.; Makhdoom, M.A.; Sakugawa, H. Evaluation of Levels, Sources and Health Hazards of Road-Dust Associated Toxic Metals in Jalalabad and Kabul Cities, Afghanistan. *Arch. Environ. Contam. Toxicol.* **2018**, *74*, 32–45. [CrossRef] [PubMed]
97. Adamiec, E.; Jarosz-Krzemińska, E.; Wieszała, R. Heavy metals from non-exhaust vehicle emissions in urban and motorway road dusts. *Environ. Monit. Assess.* **2016**, *188*, 369. [CrossRef]
98. Ferreira-Baptista, L.; De Miguel, E. Geochemistry and risk assessment of street dust in Luanda, Angola: A tropical urban environment. *Atmos. Environ.* **2005**, *39*, 4501–4512. [CrossRef]
99. Musa, A.A.; Hamza, S.M.; Kidak, R. Street dust heavy metal pollution implication on human health in Nicosia, North Cyprus. *Environ. Sci. Pollut. Res.* **2019**, *26*, 28993–29002. [CrossRef]
100. Rasmussen, P.; Subramanian, K.; Jessiman, B. A multi-element profile of house dust in relation to exterior dust and soils in the city of Ottawa, Canada. *Sci. Total Environ.* **2001**, *267*, 125–140. [CrossRef]
101. Kim, W.; Doh, S.J.; Park, Y.H.; Yun, S.T. Two-year magnetic monitoring in conjunction with geochemical and electron microscopic data of roadside dust in Seoul, Korea. *Atmos. Environ.* **2007**, *41*, 7627–7641. [CrossRef]
102. Shi, G.; Chen, Z.; Xu, S.; Zhang, J.; Wang, L.; Bi, C.; Teng, J. Potentially toxic metal contamination of urban soils and roadside dust in Shanghai, China. *Environ. Pollut.* **2008**, *156*, 251–260. [CrossRef]
103. Zhang, M.; Lu, X.; Chen, H.; Gao, P.; Fu, Y. Multi-element characterization and source identification of trace metal in road dust from an industrial city in semi-humid area of Northwest China. *J. Radioanal. Nucl. Chem.* **2015**, *303*, 637–646. [CrossRef]
104. Pan, H.; Lu, X.; Lei, K. A comprehensive analysis of heavy metals in urban road dust of Xi'an, China: Contamination, source apportionment and spatial distribution. *Sci. Total Environ.* **2017**, *609*, 1361–1369. [CrossRef]
105. Li, H.; Qian, X.; Hu, W.; Wang, Y.; Gao, H. Chemical speciation and human health risk of trace metals in urban street dusts from a metropolitan city, Nanjing, SE China. *Sci. Total Environ.* **2013**, *456*, 212–221. [CrossRef] [PubMed]

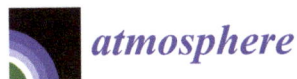

Article

Pollution Caused by Potentially Toxic Elements Present in Road Dust from Industrial Areas in Korea

Hyeryeong Jeong [1,2], Jin Young Choi [1], Jaesoo Lim [3] and Kongtae Ra [1,2,*]

1   Marine Environmental Research Center, Korea Institute of Ocean Science and Technology (KIOST), Busan 49111, Korea; hrjeong@kiost.ac.kr (H.J.); jychoi@kiost.ac.kr (J.Y.C.)
2   Department of Ocean Science (Oceanography), KIOST School, University of Science and Technology (UST), Daejeon 34113, Korea
3   Geological Research Division, Korea Institute of Geosciences and Mineral Resources (KIGAM), Daejeon 34132, Korea; limjs@kigam.re.kr
*   Correspondence: ktra@kiost.ac.kr

Received: 2 November 2020; Accepted: 14 December 2020; Published: 17 December 2020

Abstract: We examined the pollution characteristics of potentially toxic elements (PTEs) in road dust (RD) from nine industrial areas in South Korea to assess PTE pollution levels and their environmental risks for devising better strategies for managing RD. The median concentrations (mg/kg) were in the order Zn (1407) > Cr (380) > Cu (276) > Pb (260) > Ni (112) > As (15) > Cd (2) > Hg (0.1). The concentration of PTEs was the highest at the Onsan Industrial Complex, where many smelting facilities are located. Our results show that Onsan, Noksan, Changwon, Ulsan, Pohang, and Shihwa industrial areas are heavily polluted with Cu, Zn, Cd, and Pb. The presence of these toxic elements in RD from the impervious layer in industrial areas may have a moderate to severe effect on the health of the biota present in these areas. The potential ecological risk index (E_r^i) for PTEs was in the decreasing order of Cd > Pb > Hg > Cu > As > Zn > Ni > Cr, indicating that the dominant PTE causing ecological hazards is Cd owing to its high toxicity. Our research suggests the necessity for the urgent introduction of an efficient management strategy to reduce RD, which adds to coastal pollution and affects human health.

Keywords: potentially toxic metal; road dust; industrial area; pollution assessment; ecological risk

1. Introduction

In view of rapid and intense industrialization, several studies have been conducted on soils [1,2], stream sediments [3,4], river sediments [5] and road dust (RD) or road-deposited sediments [6,7] around industrial areas that are significantly contaminated with potentially toxic elements (PTEs). The levels of PTEs in soils and RD are comparatively higher in industrial areas than in urban areas [8,9]. Trace metals present in soils are difficult to migrate owing to their long residual time and strong concealment [4]. Pollution caused by PTEs present in RD has become an interesting topic of research because RD is an important carrier of PTEs and can contribute as a non-point source to runoff pollution in urban areas [6,10].

Industrial activities, such as metal processing and smelting, and industrial emissions are major sources of PTE pollution in industrial areas [11,12]. Hg pollution in agricultural soils is attributed to the atmospheric deposition of Hg through industrial emission [13]. Ma et al. [14] reported that nonferrous metal industries released approximately 88 tons of Cd into the environment. Particles emitted into the atmosphere from industrial sources and waste incineration can be deposited directly on the top surface of roads and soil, as well as on the leaves of crop plants [15,16]. Therefore, in the past decade, there has been an interest in the quality of ambient air subjected to dry deposition [17–19] and in the pollution status of soil and other nature in industrial areas [20,21]. The main sources of ambient pollution in industrial areas are not only coal-based power generation and industrial activities but also traffic activity and resuspension on the road [22]. However, unlike in metropolitan and urban areas, pollution caused by RD in industrial areas has not been studied, and there are no strategies in place to manage it.

A large proportion of industrial areas are covered with impervious areas, such as roads, and are being zoned for industrial use. RD from impervious areas contains large amounts of PTEs. During rainfall, RD can be transported through stormwater runoff to the surrounding aquatic environments without any treatment; thus, streams, rivers, and marine sediments can be contaminated with toxic elements [7,23–25]. We reported the contamination of coastal sediments near industrial complexes with PTEs compared with urban areas in Korea [26].

RD can easily be resuspended in the atmosphere by wind and vehicular movement and can spread PTEs over large areas [27,28]. Bi et al. [29] reported that industrial and combustion emissions were the major sources of Pb in dust and vegetables. PTEs present in RD continues to contaminate crops, water, sediments, and the atmosphere, posing a threat to human health. Therefore, RD pollution in industrial complexes should be considered an important factor in the maintenance of the surrounding areas; human health, pollution level, environmental risk, and mobility of RD should be investigated to establish an effective management strategy.

The objectives of this study were (1) to investigate the extent of pollution caused by PTEs present in RD collected from nine industrial areas in Korea; (2) to quantify the potential ecological risk of PTEs present in RD; and (3) to discuss environmental concerns that may be posed by runoff and resuspension of RD. The results presented here provide valuable information for managing RD in industrial areas.

2. Materials and Methods

2.1. Sampling Area

After the 1960s, Korea implemented an export-driven industrialization policy to promote industrialization. In the 1970s, the development strategy focused on the heavy and chemical industries such as steel, nonferrous metal, refinery, machinery, shipbuilding, electronic and chemicals and large-scale industrial area were created in cities of coastal areas in Korea [30]. There are 27 national industrial complexes and 133 local industrial complexes located along the coast of Korea, but the total area is 3.7 times higher than that of national industrial complexes. Most of the industrial complexes in Korea were developed during the 1960s–1970s when there was little environmental interest; therefore, environmental problems continuously arise from the planning stage [31]. Coastal sediments and airborne particles in industrial areas are reported to be contaminated with metals and metalloids [32,33], but there are little data on PTEs in RD. Therefore, this study was conducted in 9 industrial complexes (Shihwa; SH, Gunsan; GS, Daebul; DB, Gwangyang; GW, Changwon; CW, Noksan; NS, Onsan; OS, Ulsan; US, Pohang; PH) selected in consideration of representative industries of Korea's major industries.

The average temperature in December 2013 in Korea was 1.5 °C, like the average level (1.5 °C), and the average precipitation was 84% higher than that of the 10-year average level. Sampling was conducted from 1st to 6th December 2013. During the sampling duration, the average temperature and relative humidities were 0–5.4 °C and 47–80 (%), respectively, in the regions of sampling. The climate of the regions in the north was low and humid, and those in the south were high and dry. Detailed climate information of the sampling regions is shown in the Supplementary Table S1.

2.2. Road Dust Sampling

RD samples were collected from 165 sampling sites in eight national industrial complexes and one steel industrial complex of South Korea (Figure 1 and Table 1) following antecedent dry-weather periods of approximately 10 days. RD samples were collected using a cordless vacuum cleaner (DC-35, Dyson Co., Malmesbury, UK) from a 0.5 m × 0.5 m area along the curb. The dry vacuum cleaning method is a method adopted in several RD studies and is designed to collect even fine particles on the road surface [34]. Because of road design, it is reported that 95% of the RD on the total road areas is accumulated in the curb and 1 m inside the road by Novotny and Chesters [35]. In one industrial region, 14–25 sampling points were selected at equal intervals within the complex to evenly reflect road pollution in every sampling region. Four or more subsamples were taken per site and then composited to ensure representativeness for each sampling site. The vacuum cleaner was replaced or cleaned to prevent cross-contamination between a sampling of a single point. The collected RD was dried in an oven at 40 °C, weighed, sealed and stored in a zipper bag until analysis.

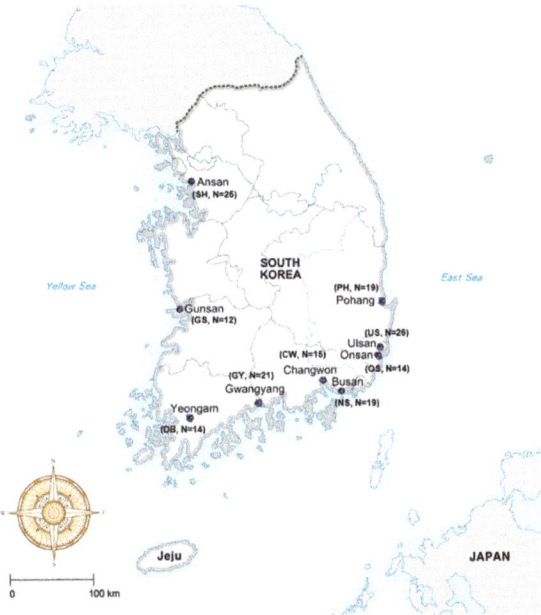

Figure 1. Map of the study area showing road dust sampling locations from 9 different industrial areas of Korea.

2.3. Particle Size and Magnetic Susceptibility Analysis

Before analysis, large contaminants such as leaves, petals, metal lumps, and garbage were removed by hand, and particles larger than 1000 µm were removed using a standard test sieve (1000 µm) from every raw RD sample. The particle size of RDS samples was measured using a laser particle size analyzer (Mastersizer 2000, Malvern Instruments, Malvern, UK) after removing organic matter with 30% hydrogen peroxide and carbonate with 1 N HCl, respectively. The determination of magnetic susceptibility was conducted with a magnetic susceptibility meter (MS2, Bartington Instruments Ltd., Oxford, UK) and was performed three times.

Table 1. Information on the number of operating facilities, designated area (km^2), the number of employees, residents and major industrial types in different industrial regions collected from the road dust (RD) of this study.

Region	No. of Facilities (N)	Designated Area (km^2)	No. of Employees (N)	No. of Residents (N)	No. of Sampling (N)	Major Industrial Types
Ansan (Shihwa; SH)	18,809	30.8	292,070	650,918	25	Assembled metal, metal processing, electronics components
Gunsan (Gunsan; GS)	519	19.2	9.573	270,131	12	Manufacture of assembly metals related to automobiles
Yeongam (Daebul; DB)	245	10.7	6.172	54,593	14	Transportation equipment, steel, machinery manufacturing
Gwangyang (Gwangyang; GY)	92	16.6	4.643	156,750	21	Steel and steel-related works, container terminal
Changwon (Changwon; CW)	2469	24.4	116.436	1,044,740	15	Industrial machinery industry, electrical equipment, transportation machinery
Busan (Noksan; NS)	1459	6.0	35.208	3,413,841	19	Precision machinery manufacturing, assembled metal, automobile
Onsan (Onsan; OS)	296	16.6	17.220	223,167	14	Nonferrous metals processing, shipbuilding equipment, oil refining
Ulsan (Ulsan; US)	757	37.1	106.075	1,148,019	26	Petrochemicals, automobile and transportation equipment
Pohang (Pohang; PH)	78	3.9	7.134	507,025	19	Steel-related primary metal manufacturing industry

2.4. Potentially Toxic Metal Analysis

For the determination of PTEs (Cr, Ni, Cu, Zn, As, Cd, Pb, and Hg), RD samples were pulverized and homogenized using a mechanical mortar (Pulverisette 6, Fritsch Co., Markt Einersheim, Germany). Total digestion of samples with mixed acids was performed. Briefly, 0.1 g of ground samples were placed in Teflon digestion vessels and digested with nitric acid, hydrofluoric acid and perchloric acid (Ultra-100 grade, Kanto Chemical, Tokyo, Japan) on a hot plate at 180 °C for 24 h. After dryness, the digested samples were dissolved with 1% nitric acid (v/v) to a final volume of 10 mL. Al, Li, Cr, Co, Ni, Cu, Zn, As, Cd and Pb concentrations were measured by inductively coupled plasma mass spectrometry (ICP-MS; iCAP-Q, Thermo Scientific Co., Bremen, Germany). Hg was analyzed using an automated direct Hg analyzer (Hydra-C, Leeman Labs, Hudson, NH, USA) according to the USEPA 7473 method.

The blanks and triplicate determinations were performed. Data accuracies were checked using two types of certified reference materials, MESS-4 and PACS-3 (National Research Council, Ottawa, ON, Canada). Metals and metalloid recoveries ranged from 94.7% to 104.3%.

2.5. Pollution and Ecological Risk Assessment

The geo-accumulation index (I_{geo}), potential ecological risk factor (E_r^i) and potential ecological risk index (PER) for eight PTEs (Cr, Ni, Cu, Zn, As, Cd, Pb, and Hg) were used to assess the PTEs pollution in RD of this study.

The geo-accumulation index (I_{geo}) was calculated using the following equation proposed by Müller [36]:

$$I_{geo} = \log_2(C_n/(1.5 \times B_n)) \quad (1)$$

where C_n represents the metals and metalloids concentrations in RD of this study. B_n represents the natural background values of the soils in Korea, and its values (mg/kg) of Cr, Ni, Cu, Zn, As, Cd, and Pb are 25.4, 17.6, 15.3, 54.3, 6.8, 0.05, and 18.4, respectively [37]. The background value of Hg was not presented in Korea, so the value of the upper continental crust was used [38]. Müller [36] defined seven classes of I_{geo} index ranging from Class 0 ($I_{geo} < 0$, unpolluted) to Class 6 ($I_{geo} > 5$, extremely polluted).

The potential ecological risk factor (E_r^i) was also calculated using the following equation by Håkanson [39].

$$E_r^i = T_r^i \times (C_n/B_n) \quad (2)$$

where, T_r^i is the metals and metalloid toxicity response factors (Hg = 40, Cd = 30, As = 10, Cu = Ni = Pb = 5, Cr = 2, Zn = 1). C_n and B_n represent the same in I_{geo} calculation. The E_r^i values were classified into five classes: low risk ($E_r^i < 40$), moderate risk ($40 < E_r^i < 80$), considerable risk ($80 < E_r^i < 160$), high risk ($160 < E_r^i < 320$), serious risk ($E_r^i > 320$).

The comprehensive ecological risk (PER) is the sum of E_r^i of eight PTEs in RD. PER value illustrates the potential ecological risks caused by the overall contamination for eight PTEs. The PER values were classified into four classes of potential ecological risk: low-grade (PER < 150), moderate (150 < PER < 300), severe (300 < PER < 600) and serious (PER > 600) [39].

3. Results and Discussion

3.1. Characteristics of PTEs Concentrations

A comparison of particle size, magnetic susceptibility, and concentration of PTEs in RD from the sampling sites is presented in Figure 2 and Table S2. The median RD surface load and the median size of particles were 1652 g/m^2 and 355 μm, respectively, with the highest concentrations observed at the Daebul Industrial Complex. The median magnetic susceptibility of RD ranged from 76 × 10^{-6} to 346 × 10^{-6} SI units, with the highest value observed at the Pohang Steel Industrial Complex (PH) and the lowest value observed at the Gunsan Industrial Complex (GS) (Figure 2). Al and Li were present at high concentrations at the Ulsan Industrial Complex (US); however, differences in median concentrations of these elements between industrial areas were very small compared with those of the other toxic elements.

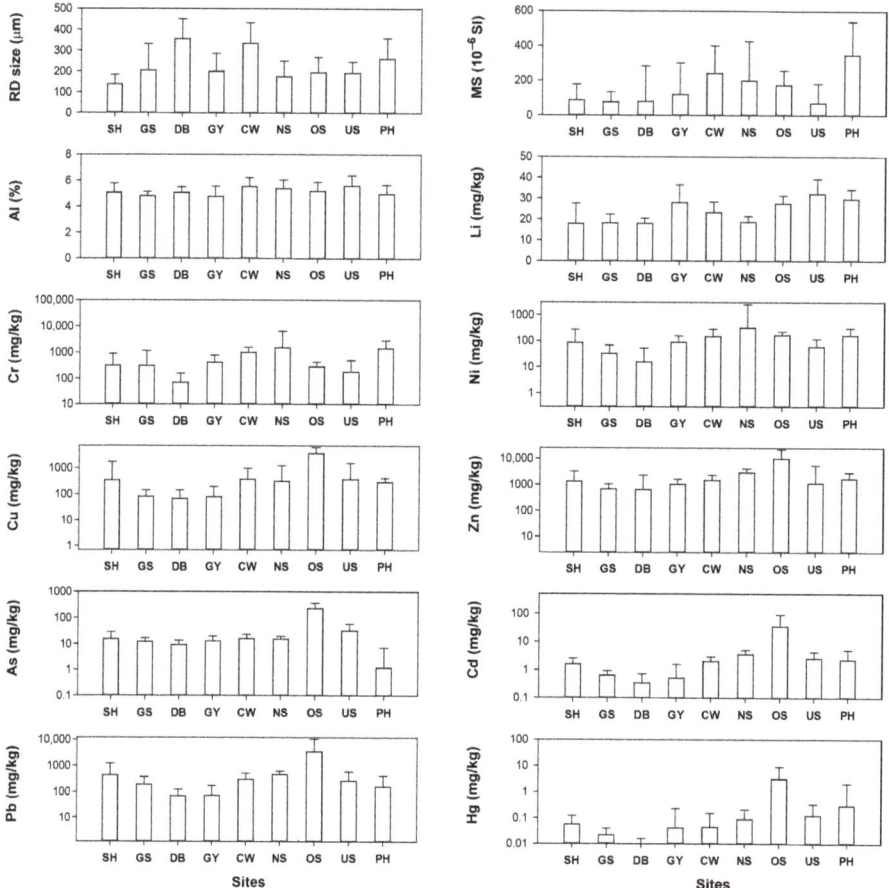

Figure 2. Comparison of PTEs concentrations in RD from different Industrial areas of Korea. The bar height and error bar represents the median values and standard deviation (SD) of the data (note the log scale on the y–axis).

The median concentrations of PTEs were in the following order: Zn (1407 mg/kg) > Cr (380 mg/kg) > Cu (276 mg/kg) > Pb (260 mg/kg) > Ni (112 mg/kg) > As (15 mg/kg) > Cd (2 mg/kg) > Hg (0.1 mg/kg). The median concentrations of Cr and Ni in RD samples were 1486 and 315 mg/kg, respectively, with the highest values observed at the Noksan Industrial Complex. Relatively higher values for Cr and Ni were also observed at the Pohang Steel Industrial Complex than in other areas because of the presence of many industrial facilities, such as steel-related metal manufacturing, precision machinery manufacturing using stainless steel, and automobile manufacturing. Cr and Ni are major conventional pollutants emitted from blast furnaces during the manufacture of iron and steel [40].

The coefficient of variation (CV) describes the degree of variation in the concentrations of PTEs present in RD samples investigated in this study. CVs over 100% are considered exceptionally highly variable among the sampling sites. The mean CVs for the concentrations of PTEs in RD samples decreased in the following order: Hg (360%) > Ni (342%) > Cd (334%) > Pb (302%) > Cr (215%) > As (210%) > Cu (196%) > Zn (189%). The large CV values indicate that the pollution sources of these metals greatly differed among the sampling sites. There is no specific major source of pollution in a particular industrial complex. Although the dominant industrial type differs among the nine industrial regions, there are many different types of factories around the sampling sites from where RD samples were collected. Considering the spatial distribution and large variability in the concentration of PTEs, the contamination of RD samples with PTEs seems to reflect the various types of industries rather than the difference in the degree of pollution according to the distance from individual metal pollution sources.

The median concentrations of Cu, Zn, As, Cd, Pb, and Hg were the highest in the Onsan Industrial Complex, where the largest nonferrous metal processing facilities in Korea are located. Significant differences ($p < 0.05$) in the concentrations of these PTEs between Onsan Industrial Complex and those of other industrial areas were observed (Table S2). The pollution of RD with PTE caused by the smelting activity was found to be severe. The lowest concentrations of Cr, Ni, Cu, Cd, Pb, and Hg were observed at the Daebul Industrial Complex, and those of Zn and As were observed at the Gunsan and Pohang Industrial complexes, respectively. Based on the sum of the concentrations of the eight PTEs, the descending order of predominance in RD from different areas was as follows: OS > NS > PH > SH > CW > US > GY > GS > DB. According to a previous study, PTEs concentrations in RD samples from industrial areas were 3.5–24.3 times higher than those of urban areas in Korea [41].

PTEs are bound to RD, which is a mixture of various particles, are derived from diverse sources, such as traffic activities (e.g., wear of brake pads, tires, and vehicles; engine exhaust; wear of roads) and industrial activities (e.g., transportation and processing of industrial raw materials) [7,42–45].

A principal component analysis (PCA) was performed to identify the differences in the parameters measured in this study (Table 2). Three significant principal components (PC1–PC3) were determined. PC1 was dominant for Cu, Zn, As, Cd, Pb, and Hg, explaining 35.5% of the total variance. There was a strong positive correlation between these elements (Table S3). These PTEs did not show significant relationships with the other measured parameters. The major source of Cu and Zn in urban RD is the brake pads and tires wearing [44]. The Zn/Cu ratio in RD from urban areas is widely used as a potential tool to assess the contribution of traffic activities related to the abrasion of brake pads and tires [25,46]. The Zn/Cu ratio in RD samples from urban areas was reported to be 2.6–5.1 in the USA and 4.5 in Korea. In this study, the average Zn/Cu ratio was found to be 7.8 and ranged from 0.4 to 62.0. The mean CV of the Zn/Cu ratio was 93%, indicating a high variability, depending on the sampling site. In industrial regions, the traffic of large vehicles is higher than that in urban regions. Therefore, traffic activity would have caused RD pollution with PTEs in industrial regions. Considering the higher concentration of PTEs, the Zn/Cu ratio, and the large difference in concentrations between industrial regions, the effect of industrial activities, such as the transport of raw materials and industrial emissions, on ambient pollution would be greater than that of traffic activity. Hwang et al. [46] reported that the proportion of Zn in RD samples from urban areas is also affected by climatic factors. Our results show a relatively higher Zn/Cu ratio and Zn concentration from industrial areas than those in RD samples from urban areas.

High-strength galvanized steel sheet is widely used in the form of Zn alloy and for Zn plating of metals containing iron because of its excellent resistance to corrosion [47,48]. It is also used worldwide in the construction industry owing to its low cost and easy maintenance [49,50]. Indeed, most factories in industrial areas are assembled using galvanized steel panels. In addition, all industrial complexes included in this study were located along the coast. The average humidity in the study areas was 61%, ranging from 47% to 80%. Corrosion of galvanized steel sheets is accelerated by the influence of sea salt and high humidity. A large amount of Zn accumulates on the road surface. Therefore, in this study, Cu, Zn, As, Cd, Pb, and Hg contamination in RD samples may have been affected by a combination of traffic and industrial activities.

Table 2. Principal component factor scores and eigenvalues of the measured parameter of this study. The results of the principal component analysis (PCA) (PCA loadings > 0.5) are shown in Bold.

Parameter	Component		
	PC1	PC2	PC3
Eigenvalue	4.25	2.22	1.3
Variance (%)	35.5%	18.5%	10.9%
Particle size	−0.093	−0.024	−0.523
Magnetic susceptibility	0.063	**0.504**	−0.383
Al	−0.122	−0.095	**0.803**
Li	0.057	−0.070	**0.538**
Cr	−0.051	**0.962**	−0.022
Ni	−0.001	**0.947**	−0.006
Cu	**0.797**	−0.002	−0.079
Zn	**0.890**	0.036	−0.111
As	**0.774**	−0.044	0.238
Cd	**0.929**	−0.015	−0.014
Pb	**0.938**	−0.013	0.010
Hg	**0.671**	0.032	0.106

PC2 was dominated by magnetic susceptibility, Cr, and Ni, explaining 18.5% of the total variance (Table 2). According to Pearson's correlation, magnetic susceptibility shows a strong positive relationship with the concentration of Cr and Ni (Table S3). In several studies, a good relationship of magnetic susceptibility with Cr, Ni, Pb, Cu, and Zn present in soils from industrial areas has been reported [51–53]. The presence of hematite and magnetite as primary and secondary minerals in soil and solid waste, and the content of Fe, Mn, Cr, Co, and Ni affect the magnetic susceptibility of soil [54]. The pollution levels of Cr and Ni in this study were lower than those of Cu, Zn, Cd, Pb, and Hg comprising the PC1 component. PC3 was dominated by Al and Li, explaining 10.9% of the total variance. Al and Li were not correlated with the other measured parameters (Table S3), indicating that these elements were mainly derived from natural sources.

3.2. PTEs Pollution and Ecological Risk Assessments

The New York State Department of Environmental Conservation (NYSDEC) [55] has proposed three types of freshwater sediment guidance values. Class A considered low risk to aquatic life. Class B is slight to moderately contaminated, and Class C is considered to be highly contaminated. If the PTE concentration lies between that in Class A and Class C, the sediments pose potential risks to aquatic life. If the PTE concentration exceeds the Class C threshold value, the sediment could potentially present a high risk to the aquatic life. Among the 165 RD samples, the concentrations of Cr, Ni, Cu, Zn, and Pb exceeded the Class C threshold values in 88%, 76%, 68%, 90%, and 75% of the samples, respectively (Table 3). The concentrations of As, Cd, and Hg exceeded the Class C threshold values in 10–18% of the RD samples, most of which were samples at the Onsan Industrial Complex. In the RD samples from Onsan Industrial Complex, the concentrations of Cr, Ni, Cu, Zn, As, Cd, Pb, and Hg significantly exceeded the Class C threshold values, implying that the PTEs present in RD samples would pose a very high risk to the aquatic life. In Shihwa, Changwon, Noksan, and Pohang Industrial complexes, the concentrations of only five PTEs, namely Cr, Ni, Cu, Zn, and Pb, exceeded the Class C threshold values.

Table 3. Comparison of sediment criteria and percent exceedance samples (in parentheses) using freshwater sediment guidance values (class A, B, and C) in all RD samples (N = 165) of this study.

	Cr	Ni	Cu	Zn	As	Cd	Pb	Hg
<Class A	6	16	6	0	43	61	4	117
(% samples)	(4%)	(10%)	(4%)	(0%)	(26%)	(37%)	(2%)	(71%)
Class B	13	24	46	16	93	81	37	32
(% samples)	(8%)	(15%)	(28%)	(10%)	(56%)	(49%)	(22%)	(19%)
>Class C	146	125	113	149	29	23	124	16
(% samples)	(88%)	(76%)	(68%)	(90%)	(18%)	(14%)	(75%)	(10%)
Class A	<43	<23	<32	<120	<10	<1	<36	<0.2
Class B	43–110	23–49	32–150	120–460	10–33	1–5	36–130	0.2–1
Class C	>110	>49	>150	>460	>33	>5	>130	>1

The geoaccumulation index (I_{geo}) was applied to compare RD pollution with PTEs in different industrial areas (Table 4). Cd has the highest median I_{geo} value among toxic metals. The median I_{geo} values were in the following order: Cd (4.5) > Zn (4.1) > Cu (3.6) > Pb (3.2) > Cr (3.3) > Ni (2.1) > As (0.6) > Hg (–0.02). The Shihwa Industrial Complex is heavily contaminated with Cr, Cu, and Pb and is heavily to extremely contaminated with Cd and Zn. The median I_{geo} values revealed that RD from the Daebul Industrial Complex is not heavily contaminated with Cr, Ni, Cu, As, Cd, Pb, and Hg. The Gwangyang Industrial Complex is heavily contaminated with Cr and Zn. The Changwon Industrial Complex is heavily to extremely contaminated with Cr, Cu, Zn, and Cd. The Noksan Industrial Complex is heavily to extremely contaminated with Ni, Cu, and Pb, whereas it is extremely contaminated with Cr, Zn, and Cd. Our results show that RD at the Onsan Industrial Complex is extremely contaminated with Cu, Zn, Cd, Pb, and Hg, heavily to extremely contaminated with As, and moderately contaminated with Cr and Ni. The Ulsan Industrial Complex is extremely contaminated with Cd. The Pohang Industrial Complex is extremely contaminated with Cr and heavily to extremely contaminated with Zn and Cd.

Table 4. Comparison of median I_{geo} values in RD from 9 different industrial areas of Korea.

	SH	GS	DB	GY	CW	NS	OS	US	PH
Cr	3.0	3.0	0.9	3.4	4.7	5.3	2.9	2.2	5.2
Ni	1.7	0.3	–0.8	1.7	2.5	3.6	2.7	1.2	2.6
Cu	3.9	1.8	1.5	1.8	4.0	3.7	7.3	4.0	3.7
Zn	4.0	3.0	3.0	3.7	4.2	5.2	6.9	3.8	4.3
As	0.6	0.2	–0.2	0.3	0.6	0.6	4.5	1.6	–3.1
Cd	4.3	3.0	2.1	2.7	4.6	5.5	8.8	5.0	4.8
Pb	3.9	2.8	1.3	1.3	3.4	4.0	6.9	3.2	2.5
Hg	–0.4	–1.8	–2.9	–0.9	–0.8	0.2	5.3	0.7	1.9

Extremely contaminated | Heavily to extremely contaminated
Heavily contaminated | Moderately to heavily contaminated
Moderately contaminated | Uncontaminated to moderately contaminated.

Pollution assessments using I_{geo} values and comparisons with sediment guidance values have the advantage of classifying the pollution status for each metal; however, these assessment tools are limited as they cannot comprehensively assess metallic pollution in environmental samples. Therefore, the ecological risk assessment was used to evaluate the potential ecological risk of each metal and the comprehensive toxicity of metals in this study.

The ecological risk factor, E_r^i, and potential ecological risk (PER) for RD from the nine industrial areas of Korea are presented in Figure 3. The decreasing order of potential E_r^i for PTEs was as follows: Cd (2573) > Hg (584) > Pb (305) > Cu (139) > As (85) > Zn (45) > Ni (24) > Cr (19). Cd poses a serious potential ecological risk to the environment. A value of 88% of Cr and 92% of Ni in RD samples was categorized as below low ecological risk. Values of 57% of Cu, 22% of Zn, 38% of As, 100% of Cd, 75% of Pb, and 60% of Hg exceeded the moderate ecological risk level ($E_r^i > 40$) (Figure 3). For Cd,

72% of the RD samples were classified to pose a serious ecological risk ($E_r^i > 320$). The industrial areas where Cd posed a serious ecological risk were SH, CW, NS, OS, and US. Among them, in the Onsan Industrial Complex, most E_r^i values indicated serious ecological risk posed by Cu, Pb, As, and Hg ($E_r^i > 320$). The highest median PER value of 25,489 was recorded at the Onsan Industrial Complex (OS), whereas the lowest median PER value of 250 was observed at the Daebul Industrial Complex (DB). Based on the PER classification, 4.8% of the total RD-sampling sites were placed in the low ecological risk category (PER < 150); 7.9% in the moderate risk category (150 < PER < 300); 20.0% in the severe risk category (300 < PER < 600); and 67.3% in the serious risk category (PER > 600).

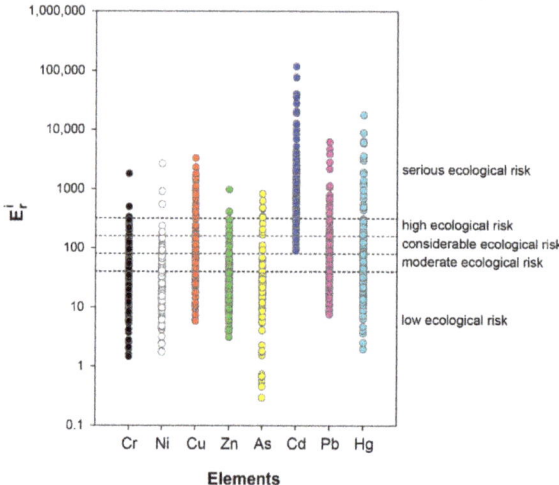

Figure 3. Ecological risk factors (E_r^i) of individual toxic elements in RD samples in this study.

3.3. RD as a Potential Pollution Source for Coastal Environments and Atmosphere

The median total load of RD at the nine industrial complexes considered in this study was 822 g/m², ranging from 334 to 1669 g/m². The total load of RD in the industrial areas was 2.1–6.5 and 15–16.4 times higher than that in the heavy traffic (126–393 g/m²) and urban (50 g/m² in commercial areas; 54 g/m² in residential areas) areas of Korea, respectively [10,41].

The decreasing order of median PTE load (mg/m²) in RD samples from the study areas was as follows: Zn (2667.6) > Cu (839.4) > Pb (824.9) > Cr (722.5) > Ni (198.6) > As (42.2) > Cd (6.5) > Hg (0.6). The highest PTE loads in RD were found at the Noksan Industrial Complex for Cr and Ni and at the Onsan Industrial Complex for Cu, Zn, As, Cd, Pb, and Hg (Figure 4).

The median total PTE load (for Cr, Ni, Cu, Zn, As, Cd, Pb, and Hg) in RD samples was 5302 mg/m², ranging from 574 mg/m² in Gunsan to 26,011 mg/m² in Onsan. The median PTE load in RD was 120-times higher than that in the urban areas of Korea [41]. Zn occupied a large proportion of the total load (50.3%), and Cr, Cu, Zn, and Pb accounted for 95.3% of the total load. The total metal load of eight metals was highest in the Onsan Industrial Complex (Figure 4).

The particle size distribution in RD samples from different industrial areas investigated in this study is shown in Figure 5. The median relative proportions of particles less than 10 and 125 μm in size in the RD samples were 6.7% (5.0–8.3%) and 36.2% (23.4–46.2%), respectively. Generally, the highest PTE concentrations are found in finer size fractions [56,57]. Considering the total area and the total length of roadways in industrial areas, enormous amounts of RD and PTEs would have accumulated on the road surface.

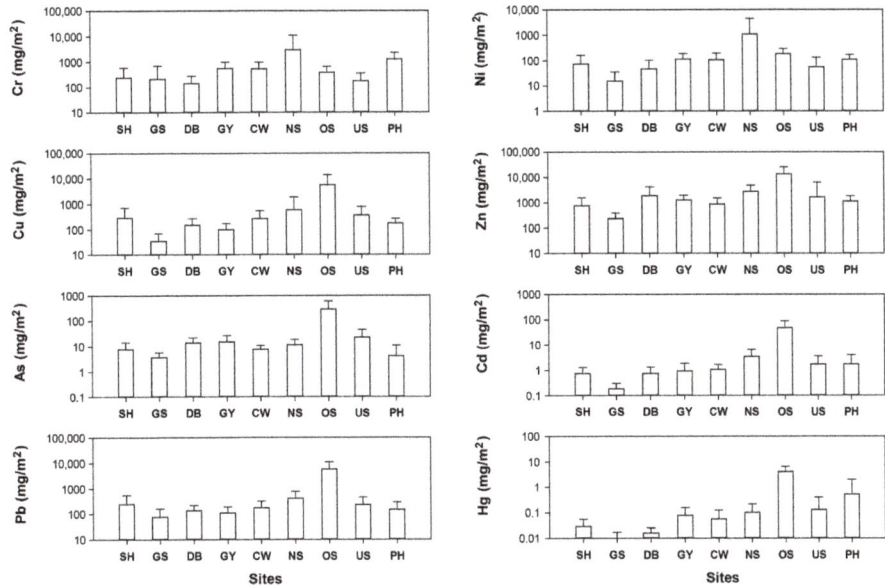

Figure 4. Comparison of median potentially toxic elements (PTEs) load (mg/m^2) in RD samples from different industrial areas in this study. Log-scale was used for arithmetic scaling of the y-axis. Values are expressed as median ± standard deviation (SD) of the measured metal data.

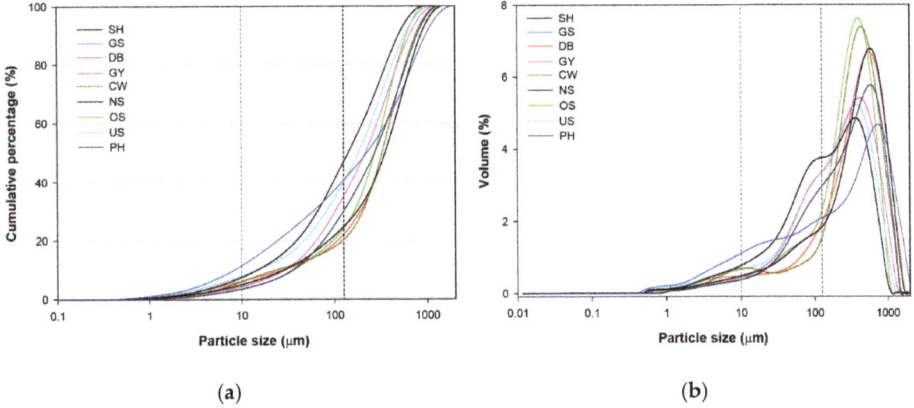

Figure 5. Cumulative curves (a) and particle size distributions (b) in the RD samples from different national industrial areas of this study.

Runoff and resuspension of RD are important contributors to aquatic environments and ambient particulate matter (PM) in the urban area [7,58–61]. Therefore, RD has increased environmental problems, such as water, sediment, and air pollution, and there are concerns regarding human health associated with RD [25,62–64].

Stormwater runoff derives from the wash-off of RD, which is contaminated with PTEs and thus imposes an increasing threat to aquatic and coastal environments [65,66]. Aryal et al. [24] reported that the particle size < 75 µm made up between 6% and 10% of the entire particle size distribution in runoff from motorways, and such particles contributed to more than 90% of the trace metal content.

In a previous study [7], we reported that road-deposited sediment (<125 μm) contributed to 41% of a total load of suspended solids in stormwater runoff at intensive industrial areas of Korea. The relative contribution of road-deposited sediment to the total PTE load of suspended solids in runoff was 10–25% in urban areas [67] and 22.1% in industrial areas [7]. RD and associated PTEs are ultimately discharged into coastal environments during wet seasons without any treatment. It has been reported that the concentration of trace metals around the Onsan Industrial complex is the highest among that in marine sediments along the coast of Korea [26,32] as well as in stream sediments [68]. One of the important sources of PTE pollution in coastal sediments around industrial areas is possibly RD, which is accumulated on impervious surfaces such as roads.

RD resuspension is also a major source of urban air pollution and contributes to non-exhaust emission (for example, from the wear of brake pads and tires and abrasion of the road surface) emanating from road transport [63,69,70]. Rexeis and Hausberger [71] reported that 80–90% of the total particulate matter emission due to traffic came from non-exhaust emission until 2020.

In Korea, it has been reported that resuspension dust or fugitive dust from paved roads contributes more than 60% of fine dust [72,73]. The mean traffic in the National Industrial Complex was 52,012 vehicles/day in 2017, comprising 77.4%, 1.9%, and 20.7% of cars, buses, and trucks, respectively [74]. Therefore, resuspended dust in industrial areas is higher than that in urban areas owing to the accumulation of large amounts of RD and the increase in traffic-induced turbulence by large trucks. The fine particles present in RD are inhaled by humans and may have harmful effects on the respiratory system [75,76].

In Korea, the importance of resuspended dust (fugitive dust) has been emphasized recently, and roads in urban areas are periodically cleaned using road-cleaning vehicles with vacuum-assisted rotary sweepers. However, in industrial areas, although the amount of RD accumulated on the road surface and the concentration of PTEs are very high compared to that in urban areas, there is a lack of awareness regarding the importance of road cleaning. In addition, industrial complexes in Korea were created several decades ago; many vehicles are parked on roads around the facility because of the lack of parking spaces. Large cities are established around the industrial areas where a large population resides (Table 1). Therefore, it is important to establish a strategy to efficiently remove RD in industrial areas to protect the health of employees and residents around industrial complexes as well as to reduce coastal pollution induced by RD wash-off during rainfall events.

4. Conclusions

This study examined the pollution characteristics of PTEs in road dust from nine different industrial areas in Korea. The PTEs contamination in RD samples was affected by a combination of traffic and industrial activities, such as corrosion of galvanized steel sheets in factories, transportation of raw industrial materials, and the presence of smelters. The concentration of Zn in RD was the highest, but Cd was more severe than that of other elements in terms of pollution and ecological risk assessment. Considering the total length of the roads, enormous amounts of Cu, Zn, Cr, and Pb would have accumulated on road surfaces in industrial areas of Korea. Additionally, the mean proportions of particles < 10 and < 125 μm in size were 6.7% and 36.2% of the total particles in RD, respectively. PTEs accumulated on the impervious layers, especially road surfaces, may be diffused by the wind, affecting the surrounding cities and transported to coastal environments without any treatment as a non-point source, causing coastal pollution. This study provides a scientific basis for solving public and environmental concerns caused by RD highly contaminated with PTEs and proposes the necessity of introducing an efficient management strategy to reduce RD, which affects coastal pollution and human health. Furthermore, it would be important to conduct additional surveys on the impact of small-sized RD on the health of industrial employees and residents living around industrial areas.

Supplementary Materials: The following are available online at http://www.mdpi.com/2073-4433/11/12/1366/s1, Table S1: Detailed climate information of the sampling regions in this study, Table S2: Median, minimum, and maximum values (in parentheses) for amount of road dust surface loading (g/m2), median particle size (µm), magnetic susceptibility (10–6 SI), PTEs concentrations and pollution assessment indices in road dust from 9 different Industrial regions of this study, Table S3: Pearson's correlation coefficient between the measured parameters in the RD of this study. Marked correlations (bold) are significant at the 0.01 level (2–tailed).

Author Contributions: Conceptualization, field sampling, methodology, writing—original draft, H.J. and K.R.; methodology, writing—review and editing, J.Y.C. and J.L. All authors have read and agreed to the published version of the manuscript.

Funding: This research was funded by the Korea Institute of Ocean Science and Technology (PE99812).

Acknowledgments: We thank Seung-yong Lee for helping us with road dust sampling.

Conflicts of Interest: The authors declare no conflict of interest.

References

1. Gabarrón, M.; Faz, A.; Martínez-Martínez, S.; Zornoza, R.; Acosta, J.A. Assessment of metals behaviour in industrial soil using sequential extraction, multivariable analysis and a geostatistical approach. *J. Geochem. Explor.* **2017**, *172*, 174–183. [CrossRef]
2. Radziemska, M.; Bęś, A.; Gusiatin, Z.M.; Majewski, G.; Mazur, Z.; Bilgin, A.; Jaskulska, I.; Brtnický, M. Immobilization of potentially toxic elements (PTE) by mineral-based amendments: Remediation of contaminated soils in post-industrial sites. *Minerals* **2020**, *10*, 87. [CrossRef]
3. Srarfi, F.; Rachdi, R.; Bol, R.; Gocke, M.I.; Brahim, N.; SlimShimi, N. Stream sediments geochemistry and the influence of flood phosphate mud in mining area, Metlaoui, Western south of Tunisia. *Environ. Earth Sci.* **2019**, *78*, 211. [CrossRef]
4. Wei, J.; Duan, M.; Li, Y.; Nwankwegu, A.S.; Ji, Y.; Zhang, J. Concentration and pollution assessment of heavy metals within surface sediments of the Raohe Basin, China. *Sci. Rep.* **2019**, *9*, 1–7. [CrossRef] [PubMed]
5. Gabrielyan, A.V.; Shahnazaryan, G.; Minasyan, S. Distribution and identification of sources of heavy metals in the Voghji River Basin impacted by mining activities (Armenia). *J. Chem.* **2018**, *2018*, 7172426. [CrossRef]
6. Zhao, H.; Li, X.; Wang, X. Heavy metal contents of road-deposited sediment along the urban-rural gradient around Beijing and its potential contribution to runoff pollution. *Environ. Sci. Technol.* **2011**, *45*, 7120–7127. [CrossRef] [PubMed]
7. Jeong, H.; Choi, J.Y.; Lee, J.; Lim, J.; Ra, K. Heavy metal pollution by road-deposited sediments and its contribution to total suspended solids in rainfall runoff from intensive industrial areas. *Environ. Pollut.* **2020**, *265*, 115028. [CrossRef] [PubMed]
8. Jeong, H.; Kim, K.T.; Kim, E.S.; Ra, K.; Lee, S.Y. Sediment quality assessment for heavy metals in streams around the Shihwa Lake. *J. Korean Soc. Mar. Environ. Energy* **2016**, *19*, 25–36, (in Korean with English abstract). [CrossRef]
9. Kelepertzis, E.; Argyraki, A.; Chrastny, V.; Botsou, F.; Skordas, K.; Komarek, M.; Fouskas, A. Metal(loid) and isotopic tracing of Pb in soils, road and house dusts from the industrial area of Volos (central Greece). *Sci. Total Environ.* **2020**, *725*, 138300. [CrossRef]
10. Kim, D.G.; Kang, H.M.; Ko, S.O. Reduction of non-point source contaminants associated with road-deposited sediments by sweeping. *Environ. Sci. Pollut. Res.* **2019**, *26*, 1192–1207. [CrossRef]
11. Zhang, X.; Yang, L.; Li, Y.; Li, H.; Wang, W.; Ye, B. Impacts of lead/zinc mining and smelting on the environment and human health in China. *Environ. Monit. Assess.* **2012**, *184*, 2261–2273. [CrossRef] [PubMed]
12. Xia, Q.; Zhang, J.; Chen, Y.; Ma, Q.; Peng, J.; Rong, G.; Tong, Z.; Liu, X. Pollution, sources and human health risk assessment of potentially toxic elements in different land use types under the background of industrial cities. *Sustainability* **2020**, *12*, 2121. [CrossRef]
13. Xu, X.; Zhao, Y.; Zhao, X.; Wang, Y.; Deng, W. Sources of heavy metal pollution in agricultural soils of a rapidly industrializing area in the Yangtze Delta of China. *Ecotoxicol. Environ. Saf.* **2014**, *108*, 161–167. [CrossRef] [PubMed]
14. Ma, C.Y.; Cai, D.J.; Yan, H. Soil Cd pollution and research progress of treatment techniques. *Henan Chem. Ind.* **2013**, *30*, 17–22. (In Korean)
15. Shi, J.; Liang, L.; Yuan, C.; He, B.; Jiang, G. Methylmercury and total mercury in sediments collected from the East China Sea. *Bull. Environ. Contam. Toxicol.* **2005**, *74*, 980–987. [CrossRef]
16. Luo, L.; Ma, Y.; Zhang, S.; Wei, D.; Zhu, Y.G. An inventory of trace element inputs to agricultural soils in China. *J. Environ. Manag.* **2009**, *90*, 2524–2530. [CrossRef]

17. Fang, W.; Yang, Y.; Xu, Z. PM10 and PM2.5 and health risk assessment for heavy metals in a typical factory for Cathode Ray tube television recycling. *Environ. Sci. Technol.* **2013**, *47*, 12469–12476. [CrossRef]
18. Hsu, C.Y.; Chiang, H.C.; Chen, M.J.; Chuang, C.Y.; Tsen, C.M.; Fang, G.C.; Tsai, Y.I.; Chen, N.T.; Lin, T.Y.; Lin, S.L.; et al. Ambient PM2.5 in the residential area near industrial complexes: Spatiotemporal variation, source apportionment, and health impact. *Sci. Total Environ.* **2017**, *590–591*, 204–214. [CrossRef]
19. Jia, J.; Cheng, S.; Yao, S.; Xu, T.; Zhang, T.; Ma, Y.; Wang, H.; Duan, W. Emission characteristics and chemical components of size-segregated particulate matter in iron and steel industry. *Atmos. Environ.* **2018**, *182*, 115–127. [CrossRef]
20. Song, X.; Shao, L.; Zheng, Q.; Yang, S. Mineralogical and geochemical composition of particulate matter (PM10) in coal and non-coal industrial cities of Henan Province, North China. *Atmos. Res.* **2014**, *143*, 462–472. [CrossRef]
21. Li, Y.; Zhang, B.; Liu, Z.; Wang, S.; Yao, J.; Borthwick, A.G.L. Vanadium contamination and associated health risk of farmland soil near smelters throughout China. *Atmos. Environ.* **2018**, *182*, 115–127. [CrossRef] [PubMed]
22. Konieczynski, J.; Zajusz-Zubek, E.; Jablonska, M. The release of trace elements in the process of coal coking. *Sci. World J.* **2012**, *2012*, 1–8. [CrossRef] [PubMed]
23. Liu, A.; Liu, L.; Ii, D.; Guan, Y. Characterizing heavy metal build-up on urban road surfaces: Implication for stormwater reuse. *Sci. Total Environ.* **2015**, *515–516*, 20–29. [CrossRef] [PubMed]
24. Aryal, R.; Beecham, S.; Sarkar, B.; Chong, M.N.; Kinsela, A.; Kandasamy, J.; Vigneswaran, S. Readily wash-off road dust and associated heavy metals on motorways. *Water Air Soil Pollut.* **2018**, *228*, 1. [CrossRef]
25. Jeong, H.; Choi, J.Y.; Lim, J.; Shim, W.J.; Kim, Y.O.; Ra, K. Characterization of the contribution of road deposited sediments to the contamination of the close marine environment with trace metals: Case of the port city of Busan (South Korea). *Mar. Pollut. Bull.* **2020**, *161*, 111717. [CrossRef]
26. Ra, K.; Kim, E.S.; Kim, K.T.; Kim, J.G.; Lee, J.M.; Choi, J.Y. Assessment of heavy metal contamination and its ecological risk in the surface sediments along the coast of Korea. *J. Coast. Res.* **2013**, *65*, 105–110. [CrossRef]
27. Hussein, T.; Johansson, C.; Karlsson, H.; Hansson, H.C. Factors affecting non-tailpipe aerosol particle emissions from paved roads: On-road measurements in Stockholm, Sweden. *Atmos. Environ.* **2008**, *42*, 688–702. [CrossRef]
28. Chen, J.; Wang, W.; Liu, H.; Ren, L. Determination of road dust loading and chemical characteristics using resuspension. *Environ. Monit. Assess.* **2011**, *184*, 1693–1709. [CrossRef]
29. Bi, C.; Zhou, Y.; Chen, Z.; Jia, J.; Bao, X. Heavy metals and lead isotopes in soils, road dust and leafy vegetables and health risks via vegetable consumption in the industrial areas of Shanghai, China. *Sci. Total Environ.* **2018**, *619–620*, 1349–1357. [CrossRef]
30. Kim, K.S.; Gallent, N. Industrial park development and planning in South Korea. *Reg. Stud.* **1997**, *31*, 424–430.
31. Choi, J.S. A study on problems of environmental facilities in industrial complexes and some policy recommendations. *J. Korean Urban Manag. Assoc.* **2009**, *22*, 117–144. (In Korean)
32. Ra, K.; Kim, J.K.; Hong, S.H.; Yim, U.H.; Shim, W.J.; Lee, S.Y.; Kim, Y.O.; Lim, J.; Kim, E.S.; Kim, K.T. Assessment of pollution and ecological risk of heavy metals in the surface sediments of Ulsan Bay, Korea. *Ocean Sci. J.* **2014**, *49*, 279–289. [CrossRef]
33. Kang, B.W.; Kim, M.J.; Baek, K.M.; Seo, Y.K.; Lee, H.S.; Kim, J.H.; Han, J.S.; Baek, S.O. A study on the concentration distribution of airborne heavy metals in major industrial complexes in Korea. *J. Korean Soc. Atmos. Environ.* **2018**, *34*, 269–280, (In Korean with English abstract). [CrossRef]
34. Gundawardena, J.; Ziyath, A.M.; Egodawatta, P.; Ayoko, G.A.; Goonetilleke, A. Mathematical relationships for metal build-up on urban road surfaces based on traffic and land use characteristics. *Chemosphere* **2014**, *99*, 267–271. [CrossRef]
35. Novotny, V.; Chesters, G. *Handbook of Nonpoint Pollution Sources and Management*; Van Nostrand Reinhold Company: New York, NY, USA, 1981; p. 255.
36. Müller, G. Index of geoaccumulation in sediments of the Rhine River. *Geojournal* **1969**, *2*, 108–118.
37. Yoon, J.K.; Kim, D.H.; Kim, T.S.; Park, J.G.; Chung, I.R.; Kim, J.H.; Kim, H. Evaluation on natural background of the soil heavy metals in Korea. *J. Soil Groundw. Environ.* **2009**, *14*, 32–39. (In Korean)
38. Rudnick, R.L.; Gao, S. Composition of the continental crust. *Treatise Geochem.* **2003**, *3*, 1–64. [CrossRef]
39. Håkanson, L. An ecological risk index for aquatic pollution control. A sedimentological approach. *Water. Res.* **1980**, *14*, 975–1001. [CrossRef]

40. Wang, K.; Tian, H.; Hua, S.; Zhu, C.; Gao, J.; Xue, Y.; Hao, J.; Wang, Y.; Zhou, J. A comprehensive emission inventory of multiple air pollutants from iron and steel industry in China: Temporal trends and spatial variation characteristics. *Sci. Total Environ.* **2016**, *559*, 7–14. [CrossRef]
41. Jeong, H.; Choi, J.Y.; Ra, K. Characteristics of heavy metal pollution in road dust from urban areas: Comparison by land use types. *J. Environ. Anal. Health Toxicol.* **2020**, *23*, 101–111. [CrossRef]
42. Gunawardena, J.; Ziyath, A.M.; Egodawatta, P.; Ayoko, G.A.; Goonetilleke, A. Sources and transport pathways of common heavy metals to urban road surfaces. *Ecol. Engin.* **2015**, *77*, 98–102. [CrossRef]
43. Mummullage, S.; Egodawatta, P.; Ayoko, G.A.; Goonetilleke, A. Use of physiochemical signatures to assess the sources of metals in urban road dust. *Sci. Total Environ.* **2015**, *541*, 1303–1309. [CrossRef] [PubMed]
44. Hong, N.; Zhu, P.; Liu, A.; Zhao, X.; Guan, Y. Using an innovative flag element ratio approach to tracking potential source of heavy metals on urban road surfaces. *Environ. Pollut.* **2018**, *243*, 410–417. [CrossRef] [PubMed]
45. Jeong, H.; Choi, J.; Ra, K. Assessment of metal pollution of road-deposited sediments and marine sediments around Gwangyang Bay, Korea. *J. Korean Soc. Oceanogr.* **2020**, *25*, 42–53. (in Korean) [CrossRef]
46. Hwang, H.M.; Fiala, M.J.; Park, D.; Wade, T.L. Review of pollutants in urban road dust and stormwater runoff: Part 1. Heavy metals released from vehicles. *Int. J. Urban Sci.* **2016**, *20*, 334–360. [CrossRef]
47. Helmreich, B.; Hilliges, R.; Schriewer, A.; Horn, H. Runoff pollutants of a highly trafficked urban road-Correlation analysis and seasonal influences. *Chemosphere* **2010**, *80*, 991–997. [CrossRef]
48. Huber, M.; Welker, A.; Helmreich, B. Critical review of heavy metal pollution of traffic area runoff: Occurrence influencing factors and partitioning. *Sci. Total Environ.* **2016**, *541*, 895–919. [CrossRef]
49. Sere, P.R.; Deya, C.; Elsner, C.I.; Di Sarli, A.R. Corrosion of painted galvanneal steel. *Procedia Mater. Sci.* **2015**, *8*, 1–10. [CrossRef]
50. Ji, C.; Ma, X.; Zhai, Y.; Zhang, R.; Shen, X.; Zhang, T.; Hong, J. Environmental impact assessment of galvanized sheet production: A case study in Shandong Province, China. *Int. J. Life Cycle Assess.* **2020**, *25*, 760–770. [CrossRef]
51. Lu, S.G.; Bai, S.Q.; Xue, Q.F. Magnetic properties as indicators of heavy metals pollution in urban topsoils: A case study from the city of Luoyang, China. *Geophys. J. Int.* **2007**, *171*, 568–580. [CrossRef]
52. Cao, L.; Appel, E.; Hu, S.; Yin, G.; Lin, H.; Rosler, W. Magnetic response to air pollution recorded by soil and dust-loaded leaves in a changing industrial environment. *Atmos. Environ.* **2015**, *119*, 304–313. [CrossRef]
53. Jaffar, S.T.A.; Chen, L.Z.; Younas, H.; Ahmad, N. Heavy metals pollution assessment in correlation with magnetic susceptibility in topsoils of Shanghai. *Environ. Earth Sci.* **2017**, *76*, 277. [CrossRef]
54. Brempong, F.; Mariam, Q.; Preko, K. The use of magnetic susceptibility measurements to determine pollution of agricultural soils in road proximity. *Afr. J. Environ. Sci. Technol.* **2016**, *10*, 263–271. [CrossRef]
55. NYSDEC (New York State Department of Environmental Conservation). *Screening and Assessment of Contaminated Sediment*; Division of Fish, Wildlife and Marine Resources: Albany, NY, USA, 2014; p. 66.
56. Zhao, H.; Li, X.; Wang, X.; Tian, D. Grain size distribution of road-deposited sediment and its contribution to heavy metal pollution in urban runoff in Beijing, China. *J. Hazard. Mater.* **2010**, *183*, 203–210. [CrossRef] [PubMed]
57. Lanzerstorfer, C. Heavy metals in the finest size fractions of road-deposited sediments. *Environ. Pollut.* **2018**, *239*, 522–531. [CrossRef]
58. Han, S.; Youn, J.S.; Jung, Y.W. Characterization of PM10 and PM2.5 source profiles for resuspended road dust collected using mobile sampling methodology. *Atmos. Environ.* **2011**, *45*, 3343–3351. [CrossRef]
59. Ram, S.S.; Kumar, R.V.; Chaudhuri, P.; Chanda, S.; Santra, S.C.; Sudarshan, M.; Chakraborty, A. Physico-chemical characterization of street dust and re-suspended dust on plant canopies: An approach for fingerprinting the urban environment. *Ecol. Indic.* **2014**, *36*, 334–338. [CrossRef]
60. Alves, C.A.; Evtyugina, M.G.; Vicente, A.M.P.; Vicente, E.; Nunes, T.; Silva, P.M.A.; Duarte, M.A.C.; Pio, C.A.; Amato, F.; Querol, X. Chemical profiling of PM10 from urban road dust. *Sci. Total Environ.* **2018**, *434*, 41–51. [CrossRef]
61. Lanzerstorfer, C. Toward more intercomparable road dust studies. *Crit. Rev. Environ. Sci. Technol.* **2020**, 1737472. [CrossRef]
62. Yang, Q.; Li, Z.; Lu, X.; Duan, Q.; Huang, L.; Bi, J. A review of soil heavy metal pollution from industrial and agricultural regions in China: Pollution and risk assessment. *Sci. Total Environ.* **2018**, *642*, 690–700. [CrossRef]

63. Pun, V.C.; Tian, L.; Ho, K.F. Particulate matter from re-suspended mineral dust and emergency cause-specific respiratory hospitalizations in Hong Kong. *Atmos. Environ.* **2017**, *165*, 191–197. [CrossRef]
64. Askariyeh, M.H.; Venugopal, M.; Khreis, H.; Birt, A.; Zietsman, J. Near-road traffic-related air pollution: Resuspended PM2.5 from highways and arterials. *Int. J. Environ. Res. Public Health* **2020**, *17*, 2851. [CrossRef] [PubMed]
65. Huang, J.; Li, F.; Zeng, G.; Liu, W.; Huang, X.; Xiao, Z.; Wu, H.; Gu, Y.; Li, X.; He, X.; et al. Integrating hierarchical bioavailability and population distribution into potential eco-risk assessment of heavy metals in road dust: A case study in Xiandao District, Changsha City, China. *Sci. Total Environ.* **2016**, *541*, 969–976. [CrossRef] [PubMed]
66. Wang, Q.; Zhang, Q.; Dzakpasu, M.; Chang, N.; Wang, X. Transferral of HMs pollution from road-deposited sediments to stormwater runoff during transport processes. *Front. Environ. Sci. Eng.* **2019**, *13*, 13. [CrossRef]
67. Zhao, H.; Li, X. Risk assessment of metals in road-deposited sediment along an urban-rural gradient. *Environ. Pollut.* **2013**, *174*, 297–304. [CrossRef]
68. Jeong, H.; Choi, J.Y.; Ra, K. Heavy metal pollution assessment in stream sediments from urban and different types of industrial areas in South Korea. *Soil Sediment Contam.* **2021**. under review.
69. Pant, P.; Harrison, R.M. Estimation of the contribution of road traffic emissions to particulate matter concentrations from field measurements: A review. *Atmos. Environ.* **2013**, *77*, 78–97. [CrossRef]
70. Valotto, G.; Rampazzo, G.; Visin, F.; Bonella, F.; Cattaruzza, E.; Slisenti, A.; Formenton, G.; Tieppo, P. Environmental and traffic related parameters affecting road dust composition: A multi-technique approach applied to Venice area (Italy). *Atmos. Environ.* **2015**, *122*, 596–608. [CrossRef]
71. Rexeis, M.; Hausberger, S. Trend of vehicle emission levels until 2020—Prognosis based on current vehicle measurements and future emission legislation. *Atmos. Environ.* **2009**, *43*, 4689–4698. [CrossRef]
72. Jung, Y.W.; Han, S.; Won, K.H.; Jang, K.W.; Hong, J.H. Present status of emission estimation methods of resuspended dusts from paved roads. *J. Korean Soc. Environ. Eng.* **2006**, *28*, 1126–1132, (in Korean with English abstract).
73. Yoo, E.C.; Dou, W.G.; Cho, J.G. Study for the control of re-suspend dust from paved road. *Annu. Rep. Busan Metropolitan City Inst. Health. Environ.* **2009**, *19*, 177–186, (In Korean with English abstract).
74. MOLIT (Ministry of Land, Infrastructure and Transport). *National Traffic Survey in 2017 (Freight Transport Surveys)*; MOLIT: Sejong City, Korea, 2017; p. 328.
75. Bian, B.; Lin, C.; Wu, H.S. Contamination and risk assessment of metals in road-deposited sediments in a medium-sized city of China. *Ecotox. Environ. Safe* **2015**, *112*, 87–95. [CrossRef] [PubMed]
76. Adamiec, E.; Jarosz-Krzeminska, E. Human Health risk assessment associated with contaminants in the finest fraction of sidewalk dust collected in proximity to trafficked roads. *Sci. Rep.* **2019**, *9*, 16364. [CrossRef] [PubMed]

Publisher's Note: MDPI stays neutral with regard to jurisdictional claims in published maps and institutional affiliations.

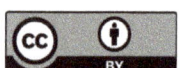

© 2020 by the authors. Licensee MDPI, Basel, Switzerland. This article is an open access article distributed under the terms and conditions of the Creative Commons Attribution (CC BY) license (http://creativecommons.org/licenses/by/4.0/).

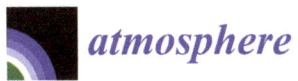

Article

Assessment of Pollution Sources and Contribution in Urban Dust Using Metal Concentrations and Multi-Isotope Ratios (^{13}C, $^{207/206}Pb$) in a Complex Industrial Port Area, Korea

Min-Seob Kim [1,*], Jee-Young Kim [1], Jaeseon Park [1], Suk-Hee Yeon [1], Sunkyoung Shin [2] and Jongwoo Choi [1,*]

[1] Environmental Measurement & Analysis Center, Fundamental Environmental Research Department, National Institute of Environmental Research (NIER), Incheon 22689, Korea; jykim1984@korea.kr (J.-Y.K.); jspark0515@korea.kr (J.P.); yoonsh1120@korea.kr (S.-H.Y.)

[2] Fundamental Environmental Research Department, National Institute of Environmental Research (NIER), Incheon 22689, Korea; shinsun1004@korea.kr

* Correspondence: candyfrog77@gmail.com (M.-S.K.); cjw111@korea.kr (J.C.)

Abstract: The metal concentrations and isotopic compositions (^{13}C, $^{207/206}Pb$) of urban dust, topsoil, and PM_{10} samples were analyzed in a residential area near Donghae port, Korea, which is surrounded by various types of industrial factories and raw material stockpiled on empty land, to determine the contributions of the main pollution sources (i.e., Mn ore, Zn ore, cement, coal, coke, and topsoil). The metal concentrations of urban dust in the port and residential area were approximately 85~112 times higher (EF > 100) in comparison with the control area (EF < 2), especially the Mn and Zn ions, indicating they were mainly derived from anthropogenic source. These ions have been accumulating in urban dust for decades; furthermore, the concentration of PM_{10} is seven times higher than that of the control area, which means that contamination is even present. The isotopic (^{13}C, $^{207/206}Pb$) values of the pollution sources were highly different, depending on the characteristics of each source: cement (−19.6‰, 0.8594‰), Zn ore (−24.3‰, 0.9175‰), coal (−23.6‰, 0.8369‰), coke (−27.0‰, 0.8739‰), Mn ore (−24.9‰, 0.9117‰), soil (−25.2‰, 0.7743‰). As a result of the evaluated contributions of pollution source on urban dust through the Iso-source and SIAR models using stable isotope ratios (^{13}C, $^{207/206}Pb$), we found that the largest contribution of Mn (20.4%) and Zn (20.3%) ions are derived from industrial factories and ore stockpiles on empty land (Mn and Zn). It is suggested that there is a significant influence of dust scattered by wind from raw material stockpiles, which are stacked near ports or factories. Therefore, there is evidence to support the idea that port activities affect the air quality of residence areas in a city. Our results may indicate that metal concentrations and their stable isotope compositions can predict environmental changes and act as a powerful tool to trace the past and present pollution history in complex contexts associated with peri-urban regions.

Keywords: urban dust; metal concentration; multi-stable isotopes (^{13}C, $^{207/206}Pb$); contamination assessment; source identification

1. Introduction

Rapid urban development, explosive population growth, industrial activities, and increases in automobile exhaust have caused widespread pollution in the surrounding environment [1–4]. Pollutants steadily accumulate in urban areas, and toxic substances, especially heavy metals, are excessively concentrated [4]. Urban dust (house and road) and topsoil are environmental key indicators due to the fact that they contain complex particle mixtures and heavy metal ions from atmospheric deposition [5–7]. Therefore, studies on metal enrichment in urban dust and surface topsoil has been reported in the numerous scientific literature [8–16]. It is generally derived from several sources, such as crustal material, atmospheric sediment, industrial activity, coal combustion, biomass burning, and traffic activity (emissions, tire wear, brake wear, and road wear) [13], and

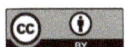

can be easily transported by runoff or resuspended by wind [14]. These pollutants in industrial complexes and ports, and frequent exposure to residents in adjacent living areas, can cause various health problems, such as respiratory disease, lung disease, heart disease, and rhinitis [17–25]. Thus, tracking the source of heavy metal ions and investigating the quantitative contribution of pollutants as an environmental forensic science is critical to understanding their environmental behavior and controlling exposure risk [26,27].

Previous studies have developed numerous methods to trace various types of environmental pollutions that are often difficult to identify. Metal concentrations and statistical analyses, such as clustering analysis, principal component analysis (PCA), and multivariate and geostatistical analysis, are frequently used to identify environmental pollution sources and the routes of metal contamination [3,28–37]. These methods are easy to use, but typically only offer general information on the sources. Another approach is the use of metal ratios of some crustal elements, such as Al and Fe (Enrichment Factor, [3]). These methods may provide useful information on potential enrichments, but the determination of sources based on these measurements is often uncertain. Isotopic fingerprinting, which is based on stable isotopic ratios, is a superior and in-depth method used to identify the origins of various contaminants because isotopic ratios are highly sensitive tracers, as different pollutant sources have difference isotopic values [38–43]. The stable C isotope ratio ($\delta^{13}C$) of various types of environmental samples reflects the isotope ratio of their source material and isotopic fractionations related to their generation processes. Samples (e.g., urban dust, topsoil, and atmospheric PM) with C derived from different plant materials (C_3 and C_4 plants), different fossil fuels (coal, diesel, gasoline, natural gas, and crude oil), different combustion conditions, and different degrees of post-emission transformation can be differentiated using their $\delta^{13}C$ compositions. Therefore, the $\delta^{13}C$ values of samples have been determined in various studies and used for source apportionment [25,42,44–46]. A number of studies have used Pb isotope ratios to identify the sources and transport pathways of Pb in atmospheric PM because the Pb isotope ratio does not change during industrial or environmental processing, retaining its characteristic ratio inherited at its source [47,48]. Kelepertzis (2016) analyzed the origin of natural Pb originating from soil and Pb from concrete, asphalt, automobile exhaust gas, and various types of plants [49]. Han (2016) examined the contribution from external sources using the $^{206}Pb/^{207}Pb$ isotope ratios of road dust (anthropogenic source) and crust (natural source) [50]. Li (2018) used Pb isotope consumption to reveal that residential dust originates from coal combustion, while road dust is an automobile exhaust gas emission [3]; Kumar (2013) found that road dust in residential areas and adjacent highway dust have different origins [51]. Identifying a definite source with this information, however, is sometimes difficult due to the uncertainty associated with the isotope composition of the source (distributed over a wide range) or occasionally overlapping sources. Because the use of the single isotope ratio has some limitations in pollution research, better results can be obtained by multiple isotope systems [3,12,52,53]. Therefore, presents studies have now proposed a new paradigm based on the understanding of pollution sources of urban dust and topsoil, which indicate that the combination of multiple approaches should provide more detailed information rather than the application of only one method. In this study, C and Pb isotopic fingerprints were determined in main urban pollutant sources such as stockpiles of Mn and Zn ore, cement, coal, cokes, and topsoil collected from the industrial and residential areas of Donghae port. This port is one of five major trading ports in Korea, is characterized by international trade exchanges, and has serious problems with air quality.

Here, the objectives of this study are to (1) determine the metal concentrations in urban dust (house and road) topsoil, and PM_{10} samples in industrial, residential, and port areas; (2) evaluate the spatial distribution of metal concentrations; (3) asses the metal pollution level; and (4) reveal the potential sources and their contribution through multi isotopic (C, Pb) compositions. To the best of our knowledge, this is the first study that combines metal concentrations and multi stable isotope (C and Pb) approaches to address the behavior of urban dust and the contributions of anthropogenic pollution sources in a complex industrial area near an international shipping port. Our results should provide an improved understanding of the metal behavior in urban dusts and the ability to effectively manage human and environmental exposure risks.

2. Materials and Methods

2.1. Site Information

Donghae port (37.4° S, 129.12° N) is an artificial port that was built in 1974, with an area of 13,542 thousand m^2. The port is characterized by a small difference in tides, and is the largest trading port of the East Sea, which allows entry and departure at all times. The world's largest cement plant, Korea's largest ferroalloy production plant, a steel plant, a small-scale industrial complex, and a thermal power plant are located adjacent to Donghae port. Logistics warehousing and stevedoring businesses are prospering at the port, with a total annual cargo volume of 30,000 tons and a maximum simultaneous berthing capacity of 16 thousand tons (50,000 tons, class 8 ships) for a total of 3000 ships. By cargo type, the port stores ore products (12,400 thousand tons) and cement and coal (11,645 thousand tons and 4290 thousand tons, respectively) [54]. However, due to a lack of warehouses and logistical planning, raw materials (Mn and Zn ore, cement, zinc, coke, and briquettes, among others) shipped to the port have been stacked as a stockpile in surrounding empty land and have been left unattended for decades. There is no minimum cover facility at the port. Ore materials, transported by means of trucks, are also stacked uncovered in the ore processing area and are scattered to adjacent areas via wind, such that the constant exposure of residential areas or adjacent soil is a substantial problem that has been causing numerous diseases for decades. In addition because the residential area is located between the port and an industrial complex, residents have been exposed to various pollutants for an extended period (more than 30 years), resulting in lung diseases (pneumonia, lung nodules, atelectasis, and calcification), respiratory disorders, and other chronic health damage. Currently, 16,000 people live in adjacent residential areas; however, this population decreases every year.

2.2. Sampling

Urban dust (road and house), topsoil, PM_{10}, and pollution source (Mn and Zn ore, coal, cokes, and cement) samples were collected in June 2016. All samples were taken in duplicate. The sampling sites were located in different functional areas, including port, industrial, and residential areas, as shown in Figure 1. In order to compare with the study area, rural topsoil from 30 km away, in an area that is not affected by industrial complexes, was selected as a control. Pollution source samples were collected directly at the stockpiles using a plastic seedling shovel and transferred to 200 mL glass vials for storage. Urban dust samples were collected from the rooftops and windows of houses in residential areas, and road dust samples were collected from roads adjacent to the port, using a brush and plastic dustpan at least three times within 0.5 m. Repeatedly, the total weight was carefully swept over 300 g. Collected samples were stored in sealed plastic bags and immediately transferred to the laboratory. Sample were air-dried in the laboratory for 15 days, then sieved through a 500 μm nylon sieve to remove small stones and bricks, leaves, cigarette butts, and other debris, and were finally stored in a refrigerator at 4 °C. Topsoil samples were taken three times from the surface to a depth of 1 cm within the upper 1 m^2 range using a stainless steel shovel at the site. The samples were then sealed in a clean polyethylene plastic bag and transferred to the laboratory. After drying the sample for weeks, foreign substances, such as leaves and large stones, were removed with a 500 μm nylon sieve, and the samples were pulverized into particles using a mortar and pestle. The pulverized sample was stored in a refrigerator at 4 °C. PM_{10} sample collectors were installed on the rooftops of schools, buildings, and houses in residential, urban, and control areas. PM_{10} samples were collected for 72 h once a week from Monday to Wednesday using a high-volume air sampler (HV-1000R, Sibata, Japan), adapted with a PM_{10} impactor (Sibata, Japan). PM_{10} were sampled in quartz microfiber filters (254 mm × 203 mm × 2.2 mm) that were pre-combusted to 700 °C for 2 h to remove any volatile organic compound before sampling.

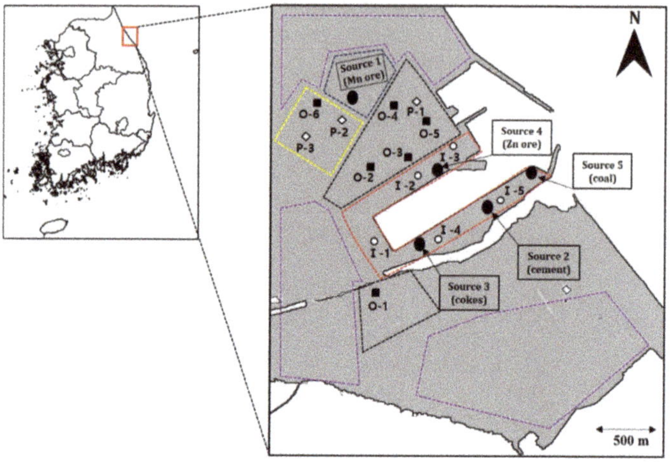

Figure 1. Map showing the location of the sampling sites in Donghae port, Korea.

2.3. Trace Elemental Analysis

All samples were processed and analyzed in a trace metal clean HEPA filtered laboratory, using high purity acids and milliQ water. The ground samples (10 g, minimum) and quartz filters were digested in a Teflon tube with 50 mL of high-purity mixture acids (HF/HCl/HNO$_3$, 1:6:2), sonicated for 2 h, and heated on a hot-block at 100 °C for 4 h. The obtained solutions were cooled, filtered through Whatman No. 40 filter paper, and diluted in 10 mL of 2% HNO$_3$ for subsequent analysis [55]. This digestion procedure was repeated twice. The solution samples were analyzed by inductively coupled plasma optical emission spectrometry (ICP-OES, Optima 5300 DV, Perkin Elmer, Wellesley, MA, USA) for Cr, Mn, Co, Ni, Cu, Zn, As, Cd, Pb, Sr, Ba, and Ni.

2.4. Stable Isotope Analysis

For Pb isotope ratio determination, the extracted solutions were purified with exchange resin (AG1x8, anionic resin), and were adjusted to a Pb concentration of 20 μg L^{-1} using 2% HNO$_3$ to monitor the performance of the instrument. The ^{206}Pb/^{204}Pb, ^{207}Pb/^{204}Pb, ^{208}Pb/^{204}Pb, ^{208}Pb/^{206}Pb, and ^{207}Pb/^{206}Pb ratio analyses were carried out on an MC-ICP-MS (Nu plasma II, Nu). To inject the samples into the MC-ICP-MS, a DSN-100 desolvating system equipped with a micromist nebulizer was employed.

Thallium (Tl, NIST 997), as an internal standard material, was added to all samples to correct for instrumental drift and Pb mass fractionation, which improved the reproducibility of the isotope value. In addition, Pb isotope ratios were corrected using a standard reference material (NIST 981, National Institute of Standards and Technology, USA) through the standard bracketing method. The NIST SRM 981 standard was separately run after every five samples to compensate for any mass bias and to assess precision. The combination of Tl normalization and the classic bracketing method provided an analytical precision of 0.0021, 0.0005, and 0.0002 for ^{208}Pb/^{206}Pb, ^{207}Pb/^{206}Pb, and ^{206}Pb/^{204}Pb, respectively.

To analyze the C isotope ratios of the dust, pollution source, and soil samples, carbonate was removed using concentrated 1 N HCl for 6 h [56]. Triplicate samples placed in acid with an HCl fume were compared with samples that were not placed in acid with an HCl fume. This test showed no differences in the δ^{13}C isotope values at less than 0.2‰. Therefore, no pre-treatment was necessary for the isotope analysis. The stable C isotopic ratios

(δ^{13}C) in all samples were measured by an isotope ratio mass spectrometer (IRMS) with an elemental analyzer (Vario MicroCube-Isoprime 100; Elementar-GV Instruments, UK).

The δ values (‰) were calculated using the following equation:

$$\delta\ (‰) = [(R_{sample})/(R_{standard}) - 1] \times 1000 \quad (1)$$

where R = (^{13}C/^{12}C). The international reference standard materials for the stable isotope analysis of δ^{13}C, i.e., Vienna Pee Dee Belemnite (VPDB), were used. The reference materials were procured from the International Atomic Energy Agency, Vienna, Austria. The δ^{13}C value was standardized using IAEA-CH-6 (Sucrose) and USGS24 (Graphite). The analytical precision for the standardization of the reference materials was 0.1‰.

2.5. Assessment of Heavy Metal Pollution

To assess the heavy metal contamination of urban dust, the enrichment factor (EF) was used:

$$EF = (Metal/Li)sample/(Metal/Li)background \quad (2)$$

where (Metal/Li)$_{sample}$ is the concentration of the heavy metal and Li in the sample and (Metal/Li)$_{background}$ is the concentration of the heavy metal and Li in the control area. For the background concentration, the average perceptual concentration reported in Rudnick and Gao (2003) was used [57]. Al, Fe, and Li are generally used as normalizing elements [58,59]. Because Al and Fe hydroxides can precipitate when the salinity is changed in the estuary environment, Li can be more suitable for normalizing than Al and Fe. Additionally, for road dust, Li has been used frequently as a normalizing element [4,12,15,17]. The EF is divided into five classes according to each heavy metal type as follows: EF < 2, minimal enrichment; 5 < EF > 2, moderate enrichment; 20 < EF > 5, significant enrichment; 40 < EF > 20, very high enrichment; and EF > 40, extremely high enrichment [60,61].

2.6. Mixing Model

Statistical analyses were performed using the SIAR (Stable Isotope Analysis) Bayesian mixing model in R (version 3.1.10, [62]). Before the analysis, all data were verified for normality and homogeneity of variances. Correlations between variables were valuated using Pearson correlation coefficients.

3. Results and Discussion

3.1. Heavy Metals in Urban Dust, Topsoil and PM$_{10}$

The concentrations of Co, Sr, and Ba in urban dust (house and road) and topsoil are similar to the concentration of topsoil in the control area, whereas the concentrations of Mn, Ni, Cu, Cr, Zn, As, Cd, and Pb are significantly higher than those in the control topsoil (Table 1). This suggests that Co, Sr, and Ba in urban dust and topsoil are likely predominantly derived from natural sources; however, Mn, Ni, Cu, Cr, Zn, As, Cd, and Pb may be influenced by anthropogenic sources. The average concentrations of Mn, Zn, Pb, and Cd in urban dust are 84-, 111-, 25-, and 56-fold higher and are 241-, 43-, 17-, and 18-fold higher in topsoil compared with those of topsoil in the control area, respectively. In addition, the average concentrations for those of PM$_{10}$ in urban area are also approximately 1.3–7.0 times higher compared with the control area, which means that contamination is even present (Table 2). When compared with the metal concentrations and enrichment factors of urban dust in other environments worldwide, the levels of Mn, Zn, and Cd were dozens of time higher; Pb also shows high concentrations, except for in a few studies (Tables 1 and 3). It is indicated that the study area exhibited severe Mn, Zn, Cd, and Pb pollution. Therefore, we focused on metals of environmental concern: Mn, Zn, Cd, and Pb.

Table 1. Results of metal concentration in pollution source, control soil, and urban dust samples of this study and other literature values.

Location	Type		Metal Ion (mg/kg)											Reference
			Cr	Mn	Co	Ni	Cu	Zn	As	Cd	Pb	Sr	Ba	
Donghae, Korea	urban dust (Port area, n = 5)	Minimum	24.6	2537	7.2	14.8	50.8	364	11.5	2.5	15.9	120	17.5	This study
		Maximum	56.0	38,583	35.9	29.2	866	57,584	127	192	680	286	213	
		Mean	35.5	13,736	15.1	19.6	244	13,860	36.7	47.7	209	164	95.7	
		Median	33.1	10,988	10.8	18.3	110	1469	12.9	9.0	37.7	127	77.6	
		SD	11.9	14,794	11.7	5.6	350	24,677	50.8	81.6	286	70.3	71.7	
	urban dust (Residence area, n = 6)	Minimum	59.9	19,139	18.5	29.9	103	5255	11.4	5.5	19.2	101	29.0	
		Maximum	496	157,119	46.0	136	439	35,570	85.9	119	3389	250	181	
		Mean	232	68,793	28.4	84.0	276	12,114	42.5	41.2	794	154	86.3	
		Median	221	52,293	23.4	81.9	257	6400	27.0	14.9	242	149	69.6	
		SD	164	52,374	11.7	42.4	125	12,799	31.2	48.2	1295	54.8	64.2	
	topsoil (Residence area, n = 3)	Minimum	105	86,525	30.5	49.3	131	2620	12.2	9.8	33.6	190	92	
		Maximum	583	144,214	37.7	97.3	241	7366	29.3	24.2	751.1	384	1444	
		Mean	329	117,798	34.7	74.0	177	5080	22.4	14.9	338	277	557	
		Median	198	122,753	35.8	75.4	158	5256	25.7	10.5	227	256	135	
		SD	241	29,211	3.7	24.0	57.1	2378	9.0	8.1	371.1	98.5	768.4	
	Pollution source	Mn Ore Mean	1.4	411,439	54	14	5	101	5.4	0.6	1.2	56	124	
		Coal Mean	25	75	3.8	5.1	26	37	7.3	0.7	5.3	136	64	
		Cokes Mean	10	17	2.5	360	3	37	1.8	0.7	0.7	3.6	5.8	
		Cement Mean	6.8	895	17	68	140	337	30	0.9	34	242	144	
		Zn ore Mean	21	15,419	658	35	9398	450,428	22	925	210	3.2	3.8	
	topsoil (Control, rural area)		51	488	9.6	11	39	116	5.8	0.8	20	71	309	

120

Table 1. *Cont.*

Location	Type	Cr	Mn	Co	Ni	Cu	Zn	As	Cd	Pb	Sr	Ba	Reference
Seoul, Korea	dust (urban)	58			20	70	179		1.0	35			[63]
Ulsan, Korea	dust (industry)				18	119	136		1.4	82			[64]
Shihwa, Korea	dust (industry)	468	660	17	181	1034	1261	21	16	1.9	1418		[4]
Gary, USA	dust (industry)	153	2668			30	202				207	302	[65]
Stratoni, Greece	dust (mining)		1250			446	2720		10	1660			[66]
Volos, Greece	dust (industry)	745	3021		93.5	154	2169	57.3	6.2	300			[11]
Beijing, China	dust (urban)	114.3	685	12.3	30.4	62.3	318	5.6	0.9	85.3	349	754	[67]
Hangzhou, China	dust (urban)		616						0.6	1165			[3]
Huludao, China	dust (industry)					264	5271		72.8	533			[68]
Sonora, Mexico	dust (urban)	11.1		2.2	4.7	26.3	387.9		4.2	36.1			[69]
Hong Kong	dust (industry)	124			29	110	3840	67		120			[70]
Hamilton, USA	dust (urban)	34	793		38	245	611	4		468	128		[71]
Newcastle, UK	dust (urban)				26	132	421	6.4	1.0	992			[72]
Baghdad, Iraq	dust (urban)	32	322		80	24	94		0.9	156			[73]

Table 2. The concentration of metal ion of PM$_{10}$ samples in the study area.

Location	Type		Metal Ion (ng/m^3)										
			Cr	Mn	Co	Ni	Cu	Zn	As	Cd	Pb	Sr	Ba
Donghae, Korea	PM$_{10}$ (Urban area, n = 15)	Minimum	48.3	136.3	1.9	9.7	11.7	97.6	11.9	0.8	15.1	43.5	386.5
		Maximum	54.3	781.4	2.4	12.9	902.5	360.0	14.3	2.0	38.0	57.0	539.1
		Mean	50.6	452.6	2.1	11.1	222.7	161.6	13.3	1.0	21.3	50.7	456.3
		Median	2.7	253.1	0.2	1.2	381.8	111.5	1.0	0.5	9.5	4.9	57.5
		SD	49.4	379.2	2.2	11.2	51.9	120.6	13.5	0.8	16.9	51.0	461.8
	PM$_{10}$ (Control area, n = 3)	Minimum	20.0	53.8	1.4	7.9	6.6	75.6	9.8	0.6	11.7	0.6	284.8
		Maximum	58.8	72.3	2.7	11.5	13.3	167.6	21.5	0.7	20.7	0.7	502.4
		Mean	43.8	64.3	1.9	9.4	9.8	112.7	13.9	0.7	15.7	0.7	358.3
		Median	20.9	9.5	0.8	1.8	3.3	48.5	6.6	0.1	4.6	0.1	124.9
		SD	52.7	66.8	1.4	8.8	9.4	95.0	10.4	0.7	14.8	0.7	287.6

Specifically, the concentrations of Zn in urban dust (max = 57,584 mg/kg, mean = 12,987 mg/kg) and topsoil (max = 7366 mg/kg, mean = 5080 mg/kg) around residence and port areas are significantly higher than those of topsoil in the control area (116 mg/kg). Zinc can provide parts made of ferrous metal with very efficient anti-corrosion protection in the long run. It is used as a protective coating for steel products and can be galvanized, sheradized, or electroplated; it is also a component of zinc rich paint and printing ink for corrosion protection [4,74,75]. Because there is a Zn smelting plant and steel-related and auto-parts manufactures located in the study area, it is estimated that the particles generated from them contributed to the dust in urban area. In addition, frequent transportation by automobile from the port to the ferroalloy and steel production plants would have affected urban dust, because Zn is closely related to traffic activities such as tire and brake pad wear [76]. A comparison of the metal concentration in urban dust with scientific reports are shown in Table 1. Our results were dozens of times higher compared to those in domestic industrial complexes [4,12] and other regions of worldwide: Yeung et al. (2003) in Hong Kong [70], Argyraki (2014) in Greece [66], Yu et al. (2016) in China [8], and Dietrich et al. (2019) in the USA [65]. The reasons for this trend could be due to the possibility that there are other major pollutants except for the known Zn sources previously described. It may result that the particles scattered by the wind from the Zn ore stockpile containing a high Zn concentration have accumulated in urban dust. Therefore, stockpiles of raw materials could have a greater impact in urban dust than traffic activities or steel-related factory operation.

The concentration of Mn in urban dust (max = 157,119 mg/kg, mean = 41,265 mg/kg) and topsoil (max = 144,214 mg/kg, mean = 117,797 mg/kg) around residence and port areas are significantly higher than those of topsoil in the control area (488 mg/kg). Manganese has a very important position in the steel industry. The majority of Mn used in the steel industry is for strengthening and desulfurization of steel, while the remaining 5% is used in chemical and battery industries. This is because Mn improves toughness, hardness, and strength and is used in steel alloy applications [77]. It is also widely used in batteries, metallurgy, glass materials, ceramic objects, pigments, dyes, glass, fireworks, food, and medicine [78,79]. Many Mn-related factories are located in the study area, and higher Mn concentration in the urban dust may result from industrial processes from steel, battery, and chemical plants. It is indicated that particles derived from Mn-related industries may be deposited in the urban dust. However, Mn concentrations were 15- to 60-fold higher than in domestic industries with the most Mn-related factories [4,12] as well as industries of the world (Table 1). These results suggest that there is another major Mn source apart from the known sources previously described; the particles scattered by the wind from the uncovered Mn ore stockpile in the factory and port area might be deposited in the surrounding urban and road dust.

The concentrations of Cd in urban dust (max = 192 mg/kg, mean = 44.5 mg/kg) and topsoil (max = 119 mg/kg, mean = 18.5 mg/kg) around residence and port areas are significantly higher than those of topsoil in the control area (0.8 mg/kg). It is indicated that the Cd from various industries might be deposited in the surrounding environment. Cd and Cd compounds are used in a variety of industries, including in the manufacture of Ni-Cd batteries and pigment manufacturing [80]. In addition, car tires, body corrosion, and the lubrication and wear of galvanized parts of vehicles have been reported as a major source of Cd contamination [81]. Cd is 3-fold higher than in the Shihwa industrial complex in Korea [4,12] and 4- to 10-fold higher than in most of the literature data in the world (Table 1). Therefore, industrial activities, transportation by means of automobile, and the manufacturing and processing of raw materials could have a greater impact on Cd concentration in urban dust. In addition, because the Zn ore stockpile itself contains a very high Cd concentration, it is very likely that the particles from the Zn ore stockpile have affected the Cd concentration in urban dust.

The concentrations of Pb in urban dust (max = 3389 mg/kg, mean = 501 mg/kg) and topsoil (max = 751 mg/kg, mean = 337 mg/kg) around residence and port areas are significantly higher than those of topsoil in control area (19.8 mg/kg). Lead is mainly derived from coal power plants, burning fossil fuels, metal coatings, paint factories, lead batteries, leather whipping, and waste pyromania, and it is also used as a component in plastics and rubber [82–84]. In Korea, high Pb concentrations (82 mg/kg) occur in urban dust from the Ulsan industrial complex, where large factories are located [64]. Argyraki (2014) reported Pb concentrations of 1660 mg/kg [66], Li et al. (2018) reported 1165 mg/kg in China [3], and Kelepertizis et al. (2020) reported 85.3 mg/kg in Greece [11] (Table 1). However, unlike Mn, Zn, and Cd, Pb-ion concentrations are higher than those in domestic industrial complexes, but lower than those in other urban area in the world. This is because lead smelting facilities and PCB manufactures are few in Donghae port.

The study area is a port where raw materials are loaded and moved more frequently than in urban are, and the number of industrial facilities (metal manufacturing, ore processing) and power plant operated per unit area is the highest in Korea. The main sources of urban dust may be pollutants emitted from industrial complexes (steel, cement, coal, alloy factories), construction and repair activities largely operating in the city and asphalt pavement weathering, pollutants generated during cargo entry and unloading operations, pollutants generated from vehicles passing through the port and surrounding roads for transportation, and spills from adjacent industrial areas. However, this study area has unique characteristics compared to other area. Due to a lack of storage warehouses, raw materials (Mn and Zn ore, coal, coke, cement) are stockpiled in the surrounding area of the port and steel related plants, all within 3 km of the residence, and they are often left for decades. Therefore, particles scattered by wind from stockpiles (Mn and Zn ore, coal, coke, cement), which are stacked near ports or factories, is considered to be the main pollutant source. Among the stockpiles of raw material in the port area, the Mn ore stockpile has a very high Mn concentration, and the Zn ore stockpile has a high Zn, Cd, and Pb concentration in comparison with other ions, which supports the preceding hypothesis.

3.2. Spatial Distribution of Metals in Urban Dust

The concentration of heavy metals in the urban dust samples was examined as a spatial distribution (Figure 2). The Zn concentration was the highest, with an average of 13,860 mg/kg for urban dust in port area, followed by Mn > Cu > Pb > Sr > Ba > Cd > As > Cr > Ni > Co. In particular, the maximum concentration (57,584 mg/kg) occurs at the I-3 site closest to the port, where the Zn ore stockpile is located, with the concentration being 4-fold higher than the average value and 494-fold higher than the control area, indicating severe Zn contamination. The Mn concentration was the highest, with an average of 68,793 mg/kg for urban dust in residence area, followed by Zn > Pb > Cu > Sr > Cr > Ba > Ni > Cd > As > Co. The maximum concentration (157,119 mg/kg) occurred at the O-4 site adjacent to the ferroalloy and Mn-related plant where the Mn ore stockpile is located, with severe Mn contamination being twice the average value and 321-fold higher than that in the control area (Figure 2). The Cd and Pb concentrations are, respectively, dozens of orders of magnitude higher at I-3 and O-1 than those in the control area. The I-3 site, closest to the port where the Zn ore stockpile is located, is thought to have an effect on the Cd concentration. Mn, Zn, Cd, and Pb in urban dust showed a smooth decrease with distance from the pollution source (Mn: $R^2 = 0.67$, Zn: $R^2 = 0.67$, Cd: $R^2 = 0.69$, Pb: $R^2 = 0.69$) (Figure 2), which indicates that atmospheric deposition from pollutants (Mn and Zn ore stockpiles) is the main source of heavy metals in urban dust.

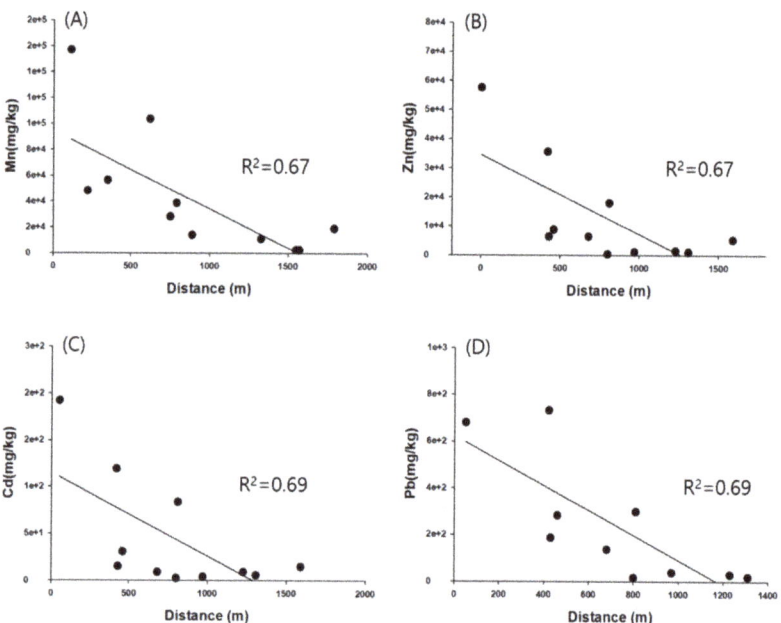

Figure 2. Spatial distribution of (**A**) Mn, (**B**) Zn, (**C**) Cd, and (**D**) Pb in topsoil and urban dust in Donghae port.

As the distance increases, it is less susceptible to being transported or scattered by the wind. Nevertheless, the Mn concentration was 39-fold higher than in the control area, while the Zn concentration was 3-fold higher than in the control area at site O-1, which is farthest from the ferroalloy plant. In this study, the general spatial distribution indicates that the Mn ore stockpile in the ferroalloy production plant and the Zn ore stockpile on empty space in the port area are the main sources of Mn and Zn in urban dust. However, several factors may affect the concentration of Mn and Zn ion observed within a specific spatial region. There are relevant contributions from vehicular and pedestrian traffic, agricultural activities, street sweeping, specific industrial processes, and incineration and construction operations [85–87]. Street dust and the fine soil resuspension fractions are enriched in anthropogenic trace elements, which, if resuspended, can make a notable contribution to the inhalable trace element load of an urban aerosol [4]. Furthermore, the emissions profile of refuse incineration depends on a number of process factors; Pacyna (1983) and Kowalczyk et al. (1982) reported that incineration is a major source of Zn, Cd, and Sb [88,89]. Wadge et al. (1986) found high levels of Pb and Cd in the finest fraction of refuse incineration fly ash [90]. However, the concentrations of Mn, Zn, Cd, and Pb in our studies are dozens to hundreds of times higher than those reported in the literature; the previously described processes cannot be regarded as the origin of urban dust. Therefore, it indicates that the origin of the main pollutants in urban dust in this study area is the Mn and Zn ore stockpiles.

3.3. Metal Enrichment in Urban Dust: Heavy Metal Pollution Assessment

To assess the anthropogenic contamination level, we calculated the EF against the local baseline (Table 3). Co, Ba, and Sr showed a range from $2 \leq EF \leq 5$ in all samples, indicating that they are mainly of crustal origin. Cr, Ni, Cu, and As were characterized by moderate enrichment on average ($2 \leq EF \leq 5$), but some samples showed $5 \leq EF \leq 10$, suggesting that they were affected by anthropogenic pollutants. These results may reflect the impact of intensive industrial activities, especially metal processing industries, in this region. Cd and Pb were characterized by moderate enrichment or higher, and Mn and Zn especially had extremely high enrichment values of EF exceeding 200, often reaching 400; as the distance decreases from the ore stockpile, the EF tends to increase. These results also exhibit a similar trend as in recent studies [4,12]. In the case of Mn, EF is the highest in the topsoil in residential areas, and this is the closest place to the Mn ore stockpile in the factory.

Table 3. Comparison of EF value in pollution source, control soil and urban dust sample of this study and other literature values. (EF < 2, minimal enrichment; 5 < EF > 2, moderate enrichment; 20 < EF > 5, significant enrichment; 40 < EF > 20, very high enrichment; and EF > 40, extremely high enrichment).

Location	Type	Metal Ion (mg/kg)											Reference
		Cr	Mn	Co	Ni	Cu	Zn	As	Cd	Pb	Sr	Ba	
	Urban dust (Port area)	0.7	28.1	1.6	1.7	6.2	119.0	6.4	60.2	10.6	2.3	0.3	This study.
Donghae, Korea	Urban dust (Residence area)	4.6	140.9	3.0	7.4	7.0	104.0	7.4	51.9	40.1	2.2	0.3	
	topsoil (Residence area)	6.5	241.2	3.6	6.5	4.5	43.6	3.9	18.7	17.1	3.9	1.8	
Shihwa, Korea	dust (industry)	6.3	1.0	1.2	4.7	43.5	22.7	5.3	24.2	95.2	-	-	[4]
Busan, Korea	dust (urban)	4.2				12.6	19.1	4.5	21.9	11.8	-	-	[15]
Shijiazhuang, China	dust (industry)	2.4	1.1	1.4	1.6	5.7	7.6		38.7	9.5	-	-	[91]
Kathmandu, Nepal	dust (urban)	2.8				7	4.6		2.8	2.5	-	-	[81]
Palermo, Italy	dust (urban)	4	8.2	2.1	1.9	14	16.4		4	72	-	-	[92]
Bolgatanga, Ghana	dust (urban)	0.01	0.02	0.01	0.01	0.03	0.003		0	0.01	-	-	[93]
Taraba, Nigeria	dust (urban)					48.3	61.7		17.4	1.3	-	-	[94]
Baghdad, Iraq	dust (urban)	3.8	4.9		16.5	6.6	12.4		42.5	107.6	-	-	[73]
Kayseri, Turkey	Urban dust	0.95	1	2.8	2	5.2	20.2		190	111	-	-	[95]
Paris, France	dust (rural highway)			12									[96]
Sonora, Mexico	dust (urban)	17.1		1.7	0.9	8.1	62.5		11.5	126	-	-	[69]
Vellore, India	dust (urban)	1.3		0.6	0.4	3.6	79.4		601	39.1	-	-	[97]
Enugu, Nigeria	dust (urban)	2.3	0.5	83.5	171.9	129.3	22.7		0.9	16.3	0.5	-	[34]
Huainan, China	dust (industry)	2.3	1.3	0.4	1.5	4.2	13.7		596	180	-	-	[53]
							13		2.9	4.5			

: EF > 40; Extremely high enrichment;   : 20 < EF < 40; Very high enrichment;   : 5 < EF < 20; Significant enrichment;   : 2 < EF < 5; Moderate enrichment;   : EF < 2; Deficiency to minimal enrichment.

On the other hand, in the case of Zn, EF is the highest in the urban dust in the port area near to the Zn ore stockpile on empty land. This relationship indicates that the Mn and Zn ore-processing facility and ore stockpile in Donghae port presents a distinct point source. The EF results for urban dust in this study were significantly higher than those reported in other studies (Table 3). The average EF of Mn was 28.1 in the urban dust (port) sample and 140.9 in the urban dust (residence area) sample, which is substantially higher than that reported by Jeong (2020, EF = 1) [4], Wan (2016, EF = 1.1) [91], Varrica (2013, EF = 8.2) [92], and Hameed (2013, EF = 4.9) [73] in urban areas. The average EF of Zn is 119 in the urban dust (port) sample and 104 in the urban dust (residence area) sample. Our results for the EF values are significantly higher than those in industrial areas of China (Wan et al., 2016) [91], near highways in France [96], and urban areas in Mexico [69] and India [97]. Therefore, our results show that heavy metals, especially Mn and Zn ions, in urban dust and topsoil might severely impact biota and human health. Long-term exposure to Zn can lead to respiratory compression, high fever, chills, and gastroenteritis [98]. Mn toxicity occurs when excessive manganese is inhaled (or when drinking water contains abundant Mn) and results in neurotoxic symptoms such as muscle pain, tremors, and memory loss, which can lead to neuromotor disorders [99]. Cadmium is used for plastic plating and is classified as a Class 1 human carcinogenic substance by the International Cancer Institute (IARC). Long-term exposure to Cd dust can increase the risk of developing kidney stones composed of Ca and P [100]. Pb is one of the most important environmental pollutants, which is highly toxic even at low concentrations and can threaten human life due to rapid bioaccumulation and a long biological half-life when exposed [101,102]. Therefore, the high concentrations of some ions in dust and topsoil in this study area may adversely affect the health of residents. These observations confirm that the contamination of urban dust and topsoil in Donghae port should be a concern for local authorities, as these elements threaten both ecological and human health.

3.4. Contribution of Heavy Meatal Pollution to Urban Dust from the Pollution Source

The stable C isotope ratios ($\delta^{13}C$) in the urban dust (port) samples range from -23.8 to $-25.8‰$, except at the I-5 site ($-20.8‰$); urban dust (residence area) ranges from -23.5 to $-25.1‰$, and the topsoil samples from -24.3 to $-25.8‰$ (Figure 3). Urban dust (port) shows a heavy value of $-20.8‰$ at I-5, but the rest of the study area exhibits a similar range between urban dust (port) and topsoil, from -24.0 to $-25.0‰$. Among the pollutant sources, the stable C isotope ratios of Mn ore, cement, coke, Zn ore, coal, and control topsoil were -24.8, -19.9, -26.9, -24.2, -23.6, and $-25.1‰$, respectively, with a clear difference. The stable C isotope values of soils reflect the isotopic composition of the local vegetation, which in turn, depends on their photosynthetic pathways and land use [103]. However, the within-site $\delta^{13}C$ values in topsoil samples in the study area were smaller, such that there is no effect from local vegetation on the relative proportions of C_3 and C_4 plants. The $\delta^{13}C$ values in urban dust ranged from -23.5 to $-25.1‰$, except at I-5 ($-20.8‰$). Morera-Gomez et al. (2018) characterized the $\delta^{13}C$ of aerosols emitted by several sources of contamination in Cienfuegos: soot particles from the combustion of diesel ($\delta^{13}C$: $-26.3‰$), shipping ($\delta^{13}C$: $-25.7‰$), and power plants ($\delta^{13}C$: $-27.1‰$) [42]. The $\delta^{13}C$ value of urban dust in this study were enriched relative to these sources. In Mexico city, the $\delta^{13}C$ values in urban dust ($-17.0‰$) and $PM_{2.5}$ ($-22‰$) are more enriched [104], and are also more enriched, ranging from -16.4 to $-18.4‰$, in street dust in Japan [105], and more depleted, ranging from -26.4 to $-26.6‰$ of aerosol in France [106] (Figure 3). However, our results are similar to those from Kumasi street dust in Africa, which range from -23.9 to $-26.6‰$ [46]. We cannot easily explain the differences between the values for urban dust from our study and that from previous studies. This trend may be due to the concentration of black carbon, organic carbon, and inorganic carbon contained in the urban dust. The $\delta^{13}C$ value of black carbon is more depleted than that of TC because of the higher contribution of fossil fuels [106].

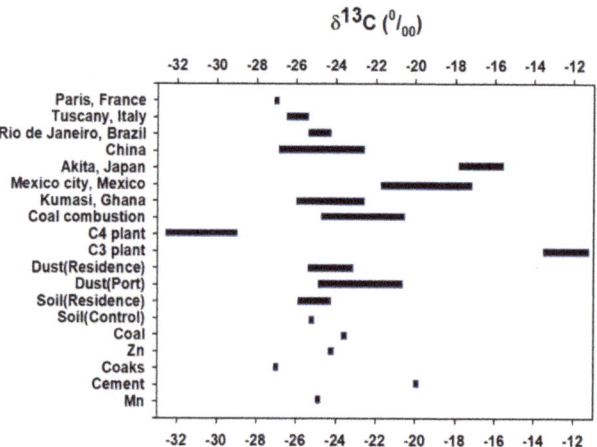

Figure 3. Comparison of $\delta^{13}C$ values between this study and literature reports, including coal-combustion [106], biomass burning from C_3 and C_4 plants [107,108] and various urban region: Kumasi, Ghana [46]; Mexico city, Mexico [104]; Akita, Japan [105]; several major cities in China [109]; Rio de Janeiro, Brazil [110]; Tuscany, Italy [111]; and Paris, France [112]).

The combustion of biomass and automobile fuels (gasoline, LPG, and diesel) can also contribute to the carbon content of urban dust. Previous studies have reported the typical $\delta^{13}C$ values associated with various fossil fuels, biomass, and their combustion products [45,82,84]. The $\delta^{13}C$ values in urban dust from the study area were out of range of the C_3 and C_4 plants [104,106]; also burning has not occurred in or near the study area for decades. Therefore, urban dust at each location in the study area are notably impacted by mixtures of the main sources (Mn ore, Zn ore, cement, cokes, coal, and topsoil) with different $\delta^{13}C$ values. The most negative $\delta^{13}C$ values were found at a coke stockpile, while the most enriched $\delta^{13}C$ values were found at a cement stockpile. The $\delta^{13}C$ values at site I-5 (port area) were ^{13}C-enriched relative to the other sites, which likely reflects different carbon sources. The location of site I-5 is close to the cement stockpile, where the $\delta^{13}C$ values are similar to those of cement source, such that there is a possible influence from cement. However, the $\delta^{13}C$ values at site I-4 (port area) had more negative values than the other sites, i.e., similar to the coke source, which had the most negative $\delta^{13}C$ value. The variations in the $\delta^{13}C$ of urban dust from the different locations may therefore reflect differences in the sources and/or intensity of pollution.

The Pb isotope signatures of urban dust (port) range from 0.864 to 0.889 for $^{207/206}Pb$ and 2.102 to 2.136 for $^{208/206}Pb$. The $^{207/206}Pb$ and $^{208/206}Pb$ ratios of urban dust (resident) range between 0.863 and 0.882, and 2.093 and 2.127, respectively. The $^{207/206}Pb$ and $^{208/206}Pb$ ratios of topsoil range between 0.869 and 0.891, and 2.107 and 2.139, respectively (Figure 4). Among the pollutant sources, the Pb stable isotope ratio of Mn ore, cement, coke, Zn ore, coal, and control topsoil is 0.911, 0.859, 0.874, 0.917, 0.836, and 0.774, respectively. In general, the results show that these source groups are notably different in terms of their Pb isotope compositions. The $^{207/206}Pb$ and $^{208/206}Pb$ ratios plotted in Figure 4 show a linear trend for all samples with an excellent regression coefficient ($R^2 = 0.89$), although a slightly better regression coefficient is obtained when only dust is considered ($R^2 = 0.92$, not shown in figure). The linear array is interpreted to illustrate mixing. The control topsoil has more radiogenic Pb isotope values, forming a restricted field that defines the lithologic Pb isotope signature for this region. The Pb isotope value of the pollution source sample does not overlap the soil sample, suggesting it may be an important component of the geogenic end-member. In contrast, urban dust, such as the topsoil sample, has a less radiogenic Pb value, which represents the isotopic imprint of a yet unknown anthropogenic end-member. In general, the characteristics of Pb isotopes, after the smelting of nonferrous metals, reflect the Pb isotope values in the ore before processing because the fractionation of Pb isotopes rarely occurs during the smelting process, or its effect is minimal. In general, the Zn concentrations in Zn ore are 4–10%, but when Zn ore is used as a raw material in Korea, the concentration is increased to 55–60% through flotation [67]. All of these materials are imported from Australia, Peru, and Mexico (http://www.kita.net accessed on 10 June 2021). In general, Zn ore from Central and South America is known to have $^{207/206}Pb$ values of 0.829 to 0.851, while Zn ore from Australia ranges from 0.909 to 0.970. For Australian Zn ore used in domestic Zn smelting facilities, $^{207/206}Pb$ was found to have a value of 0.929 to 0.956. The Pb isotope ratio of Zn ore in the study area falls within the range of the Pb isotope ratios of Australian Zn ore rather than those from Central and South America; furthermore, these ratios follow the characteristic Pb isotope line of large sulfide mines such as the Broken Hill mine in Australia. However, in the study area, the Pb isotope ratio in the urban dust sample was 0.864–0.891, which is different from the Pb isotope ratio of the Zn and Mn ore. These results indicate that Pb-induced pollutants in the urban dust are not only from Zn or Mn ore, but also from a wide variety of pollutants, such as cement, coke, Zn, and soil. The contribution rate was calculated using the C and Pb stable isotope ratio of the sample.

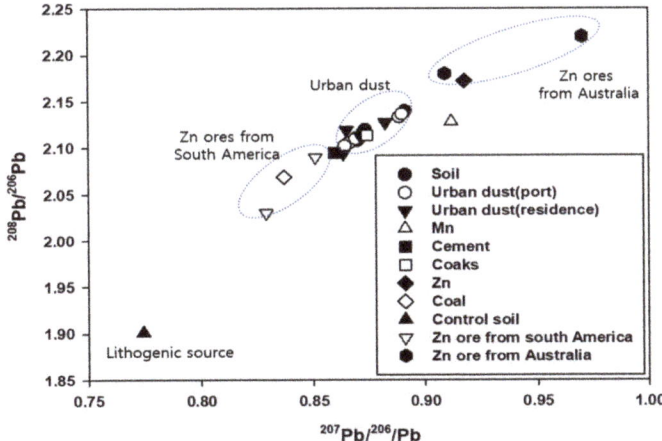

Figure 4. Relationship between $^{208}Pb/^{206}Pb$ and $^{207}Pb/^{206}Pb$ of soil and urban dust in Donghae port.

As a result of the evaluated contribution of pollutant sources on deposited dust through the Iso-source and SIAR models using the stable isotope ratios (^{13}C, $^{207/206}Pb$), we found that the largest contribution was derived from Mn (20.4%) and Zn (20.3%) from industrial factories (Figure 5). These results are consistent with the results of high concentrations of Mn and Zn in the urban dust mentioned above. In previous studies, Pb or C isotope ratios alone were used to trace pollution sources, but this is the first study to identify pollutants using both isotopes ratios.

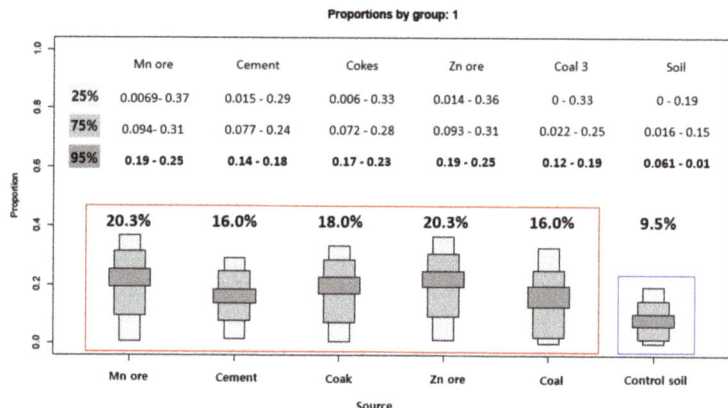

Figure 5. Average contribution of the different sources determined by Iso-source R to the soil and urban dust sample.

3.5. Application of Multi-Isotope Techniques as a Useful Indicator to Trace Pollutant Sources

This research combined the analysis of metal concentration with carbon and lead isotopes to characterize sources and source contributions for urban dust and soil in industrial complex areas near a port. Our results suggest that a stockpile of raw material and the operation of a steel factory in the Donghae port significantly influence the concentration levels of Mn, Zn, Cd, and Pb in the surrounding soil and urban dust. In this context, this study demonstrated that carbon and lead isotopes, combined with the analysis of metal concentrations, could more effectively trace the effects of anthropogenic pollutants related to urbanization on urban dust than the analysis of heavy metals alone.

Previous studies have developed numerous methods, such as metal concentration, metal ratios of some crustal elements, statistical analyses, and clustering analysis, to trace various types of environmental pollutions that are often difficult to identify. These methods are easy to use, but typically only offer general information on the source. In addition, this approach is restricted in its efficacy for determining the specific sources of pollutants and discriminating among them. In our results, when carbon or lead isotopes were used alone, it was difficult to distinguish between pollutants (Figures 3 and 4), but when carbon and lead were used together, pollutants could be distinguished (Figure 6). The source contribution analysis carry out herein shows that metal concentrations as well as C and Pb isotopes could be united to helpful quantify source contributions and supply a basis for pollution prevention. Furthermore, the application of an additional novel multi-isotope approach, such as Cd, Cu, and Zn as environmental tracers, could be important to identifying pollution sources, as well as for understanding the behavior or environmental pollution and contribution of urban dust in various environments. Finally, the establishment of a database on multi-isotopic composition would remarkably contribute to the identification and management of individual sources of heavy metal pollution.

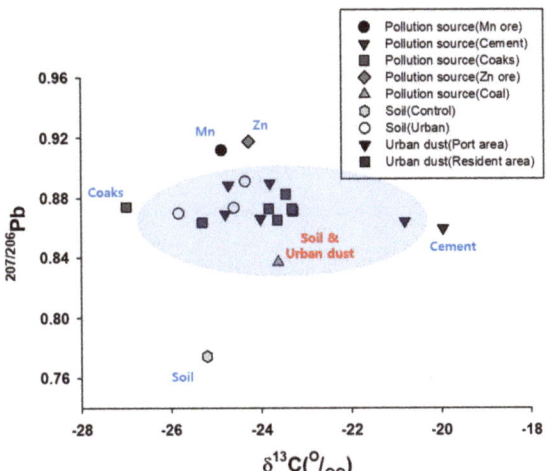

Figure 6. Scatter plot δ^{13}C vs. ^{207}Pb/^{206}Pb of soil and urban dust in Donghae port.

3.6. Implications for Environmental Management and Human Health

New ports are being built or existing ports are being expanded throughout the world to meet the increasing demands of the population and the requirements of industries [91]. This port activity has the potential to cause serious pollution problem for decades, over a large area. Port activities can have a negative effect of air quality in the surrounding areas due to various activities such as loading, transporting, and storing cargo. The particles derived from port and industrial activities are composed of a complex mixture of particles, among which the fine fraction may be resuspended by wind and thus cause a respiratory risk to human health [5,113]. This dust is highly bioaccessible through gastric and respiratory exposure pathways, leading to lethal disease. Hence, for the monitoring of pollution levels, identification of pollution sources, control of waste from point and non-point sources and estimation of pollution levels for future, regular observation and evaluation are required throughout the entire operation and construction phase of a port.

Urban and road dust runoff discharge into the ocean may also transfer a fairly large amount of nutrients. The availability of these nutrients beyond coastal ecosystem is also an important factor for algal blooms. Recently, such events have been reported in the world [114]. The local authorities in Donghae port are now investing significant efforts and resources in monitoring the local environment. Our results should help them design a more effective environmental management of air pollution in Donghae port.

4. Conclusions

The heavy metal pollution of urban dust in ports and residential areas was evaluated to obtain the relative contribution to pollution source. Most of the heavy metals in the study area were found in the range of variation of those reported in industrial complex areas, but some heavy metal such as Mn, Zn, Cd, and Pb presented 85~112-fold higher levels (EF > 100) than those of the control area, indicating significant contributions of these elements from anthropogenic sources. As a result of calculating the contribution of six major pollutant sources by Iso-source model, it was seen that Mn and Zn ore stockpiles contribute to more than 40% of urban dust. This suggests that both a stockpile of raw material and the operation of a steel factory in the Donghae port significantly influence the concentration levels of Mn, Zn, Cd, and Pb in the surrounding soil and urban dust. For the first time, C and Pb stable isotope ratios in urban dust were assessed to trace pollution sources in an industrial complex port area. This study provides appropriate guidance for further assessing the contributions of pollution sources in the study area, and could help to establish environmental strategies for the improvement of air quality and ecosystem. All of the above can be utilized by public health authorities and policymakers in Donghae port and in other areas with similar geo-environmental conditions.

Author Contributions: M.-S.K., conceptualization, resources, data curation, writing—original draft, and writing—review and editing; J.-Y.K., conceptualization; J.P. and S.-H.Y., formal analysis; S.S. and J.C., resources. All authors have read and agreed to the published version of the manuscript.

Funding: This study was supported by the National Institute of Environment Research (NIER, RP2016-167).

Conflicts of Interest: The authors declare no conflict of interest.

References

1. Kim, B.M.; Park, J.-S.; Kim, S.W.; Kim, H.; Jeon, H.; Cho, C.; Kim, J.-H.; Hong, S.; Rupakheti, M.; Panday, A.K.; et al. Source apportionment of PM10 mass and particulate carbon in the Kathmandu Valley, Nepal. *Atmos. Environ.* **2015**, *123*, 190–199. [CrossRef]
2. Squizzato, S.; Cazzaro, M.; Innocente, E.; Visin, F.; Hopke, P.K.; Rampazzo, G. Urban air quality in a mid-size city—PM2.5 composition, sources and identification of impact areas: From local to long range contributions. *Atmos. Res.* **2017**, *186*, 51–62. [CrossRef]
3. Li, F.; Jinxu, Y.; Shao, L.; Zhang, G.; Wang, J.; Jin, Z. Delineating the origin of Pb and Cd in the urban dust through elemental and stable isotopic ratio: A study from Hangzhou City, China. *Chemosphere* **2018**, *211*, 674–683. [CrossRef] [PubMed]
4. Jeong, H.; Choi, J.Y.; Lee, J.; Lim, J.; Ra, K. Heavy metal pollution by road-deposited sediments and its contribution to total suspended solids in rainfall runoff from intensive industrial areas. *Environ. Pollut.* **2020**, *265*, 115028. [CrossRef]
5. Davis, A.P.; Shokouhian, M.; Ni, S. Loading estimates of lead, copper, cadmium, and zinc in urban runoff from specific sources. *Chemosphere* **2001**, *44*, 997–1009. [CrossRef]
6. Lau, S.; Han, Y.; Kang, J.; Kayhanian, M.; Stenstrom, M.K. Characteristics of highway stormwater runoff in Los Angeles: Metals and polycyclic aromatic hydrocarbons. *Water Environ. Res.* **2009**, *81*, 308–318. [CrossRef]
7. Egodawatta, P.; Ziyath, A.M.; Goonetilleke, A. Characterising metal build-up on urban road surfaces. *Environ. Pollut.* **2013**, *176*, 87–91. [CrossRef]
8. Yu, Y.; Li, Y.; Li, B.; Shen, Z.; Stenstrom, M.K. Metal enrichment and lead isotope analysis for source apportionment in the urban dust and rural surface soil. *Environ. Pollut.* **2016**, *216*, 764–772. [CrossRef]
9. Harvey, P.J.; Rouillon, M.; Dong, C.; Ettler, V.; Handley, H.K.; Taylor, M.P.; Tyson, E.; Tennant, P.; Telfer, V.; Trinh, R. Geochemical sources, forms and phases of soil contamination in an industrial city. *Sci. Total Environ.* **2017**, *584–585*, 505–514. [CrossRef]
10. Gelly, R.; Fekiacova, Z.; Guihou, A.; Doelsch, E.; Deschamps, P.; Keller, C. Lead, zinc and copper redistributions in soils along deposition gradient from emissions of Pb-Ag smelter decommissioned 100 years ago. *Sci. Total Environ.* **2019**, *665*, 502–512. [CrossRef]
11. Kelepertzis, E.; Argyraki, A.; Chrastny, V.; Botsou, F.; Skordas, K.; Komarek, M.; Fouskas, A. Metal(loid) and isotopic tracing of Pb in soils, road and house dusts from the industrial area of Volos (central Greece). *Sci. Total Environ.* **2020**, *725*, 138300. [CrossRef]
12. Jeong, H.; Chio, J.Y.; Lee, J.; Ra, K. Investigations of Pb and Cu isotopes to trace contamination sources from the artificial Shihwa Lake in Korea. *J. Coast. Res.* **2020**, *95*, 1122–1127. [CrossRef]
13. Wong, C.S.C.; Li, X.; Thornton, I. Urban environmental geochemistry of trace metals. *Environ. Pollut.* **2006**, *142*, 1–16. [CrossRef]
14. Ali, M.U.; Liu, G.; Yousaf, B.; Ullah, H.; Abbas, Q.M.; Munir, M.A.M. A systematic review on global pollution status of particulate matter-associated potential toxic elements and health perspectives in urban environment. *Environ. Geochem. Health* **2019**, *41*, 1131–1162. [CrossRef]
15. Jeong, H.; Choi, J.Y.; Lim, J.; Shim, W.J.; Kim, Y.O. Characterization of the contribution of road deposited sediments to the contamination of the close marine environment with trace metals: Case of the port city of Busan (South Korea). *Mar. Pollut. Bull.* **2020**, *161*, 111717. [CrossRef]
16. Dytolw, S.; Gorka-Kostrubiec, B. Concentration of heavy metals in street dust: An implication of using different geochemical background data in estimating the level of heavy metal pollution. *Environ. Geochem. Health* **2021**, *43*, 521–535. [CrossRef]
17. McConnell, R.; Berhane, K.; Gilliand, F.; Molitor, J.; Thomas, D.; Lurmann, F.; Avol, E.; Gauderman, W.J.; Peters, J.M. Prospective study of air pollution and bronchitic symptoms in children with asthma. *Am. J. Respir. Crit. Care Med.* **2003**, *168*, 790–797. [CrossRef]
18. Pope, C.A.; Dockery, D.W. Health effects of fine particulate air pollution: Lines that connect. *J. Air Waste Manag. Assoc.* **2006**, *56*, 709–742. [CrossRef]
19. Dockery, D.W.; Stone, P.H. Cardiovascular risks from fine particulate air pollution. *N. Engl. J. Med.* **2007**, *3*, 511–513. [CrossRef]
20. Kumar, R.; Nagar, J.K.; Kumar, H.; Kushwah, A.S.; Meena, M.; Kumar, P.; Raj, N.; Singhal, M.K.; Gaur, S.N. Association of indoor and outdoor air pollutant level with respiratory problems among children in an industrial area of Delhi, India. *Arch. Environ. Occup. Health* **2007**, *62*, 75–80. [CrossRef]

21. Zhou, J.; Zhang, R.; Cao, J.; Chow, J.C.; Watson, J.G. Carbonaceous and ionic components of atmospheric fine particles in Beijing and their impact on atmospheric visibility. *Aerosol. Air. Qual. Res.* **2012**, *12*, 492–502. [CrossRef]
22. WHO. Health Effects of Particulate Matter. WHO Regional Office for Europe, Copenhagen. Available online: https://www.euro.who.int/__data/assets/pdf_file/0006/189051/Health-effects-of-particulate-matter-final-Eng.pdf (accessed on 10 June 2021).
23. WHO. WHO|WHO Releases Country Estimates on Air Pollution Exposure and Health Impact. Available online: https://www.who.int/news/item/27-09-2016-who-releases-country-estimates-on-air-pollution-exposure-and-health-impact (accessed on 10 June 2021).
24. Zahran, S.; Mielke, H.W.; McElmurry, S.P.; Filippelli, G.M.; Laidlaw, M.A.S.; Taylor, M.P. Determining the relative importance of soil sample locations to predict risk of child lead exposure. *Environ. Int.* **2013**, *60*, 7–14. [CrossRef]
25. Morera-Gomez, Y.; Santamaria, J.M.; Elustondo, D.; Lasheras, E.; Alonso-Hernandez, C.M. Determination and source apportionment of major and trace elements in atmospheric bulk deposition in a Caribbean rural area. *Atmos. Environ.* **2019**, *202*, 93–104. [CrossRef]
26. Li, H.-B.; Chen, K.; Juhasz, A.L.; Huang, L.; Ma, L.Q. Childhood lead exposure in an industrial town in China: Coupling stable isotope ratios with bioaccessible lead. *Environ. Sci. Technol.* **2015**, *49*, 5080–5087. [CrossRef]
27. Varrica, D.; Dongarrà, G.; Alaimo, M.G.; Monna, F.; Losno, R.; Sanna, E.; De Giudici, G.; Tamburo, E. Lead isotopic fingerprint in human scalp hair: The case study of Iglesias mining district (Sardinia, Italy). *Sci. Total Environ.* **2018**, *613–614*, 456–461. [CrossRef]
28. Franco-Uría, A.; López-Mateo, C.; Roca, E.; Fernández-Marcos, M.L. Source identification of heavy metals in pastureland by multivariate analysis in NW Spain. *J. Hazard. Mater.* **2009**, *165*, 1008–1015. [CrossRef]
29. Lu, X.; Wang, L.; Li, L.Y.; Lei, K.; Huang, L.; Kang, D. Multivariate statistical analysis of heavy metals in street dust of Baoji, NW China. *J. Hazard. Mater.* **2010**, *173*, 744–749. [CrossRef]
30. Sudheer, A.K.; Rengarajan, R. Atmospheric mineral dust and trace metals over urban environment in Western India during winter. *Aerosol. Air Qual. Res.* **2012**, *12*, 923–933. [CrossRef]
31. Zhao, H.; Li, X. Risk assessment of metals in road-deposited sediment along an urban-rural gradient. *Environ. Pollut.* **2013**, *174*, 297–304. [CrossRef] [PubMed]
32. Qiu, K.; Xing, W.; Scheckel, K.G.; Cheng, Y.; Zhao, Z.; Ruan, X.; Li, L. Temporal and seasonal variations of As, Cd and Pb atmospheric deposition flux in the vicinity of lead smelters in Jiyuan. *China. Atmos. Pollut. Res.* **2016**, *7*, 170–179. [CrossRef]
33. Zglobicki, W.; Telecka, M. Heavy metals in urban street dust: Health risk assessment (Lublin City, E Poland). *Appl. Sci.* **2021**, *11*, 4092. [CrossRef]
34. Ichu, C.R.; Ume, J.I.; Opara, A.I.; Ibe, F.C. Ecological risk assessment and pollution models of trace metal concentrations in road dust in parts of Enugu, Southeastern Nigeria. *J. Chem. Health Risks* **2021**, *11*, 135–151.
35. Al-Shidi, H.K.; Al-Reasi, H.A.; Sulaiman, H. Heayv metals levels in road dust from Muscat, Oman: Relationship with traffic voulmes, and ecological and health risk assessments. *Int. J. Environ. Health Res.* **2020**, *13*, 1–13.
36. Jeong, H.; Choi, J.Y.; Ra, K. Potentially toxic elements pollution in road deposited sediments around the active smelting industry of Korea. *Sci. Rep.* **2021**, *11*, 7238. [CrossRef]
37. Jeong, H.; Choi, J.Y.; Lim, J.; Ra, K. Pollution caused by potentially toxic elements present in road dust from indusrial areas in Korea. *Atmosphere* **2020**, *11*, 1366. [CrossRef]
38. Ma, S.X.; Peng, P.A.; Song, J.Z.; Zhao, J.P.; He, L.L.; Sheng, G.Y.; Fu, J.M. Stable carbon isotopic compositions of organic acids in total suspended particles and dusts from Guangzhou. *China Atmos. Res.* **2010**, *98*, 176–182. [CrossRef]
39. Masalaite, A.; Remeikis, V.; Garbaras, A.; Dudoitis, V.; Ulevicius, V.; Ceburnis, D. Elucidating carbonaceous aerosol sources by the stable carbon $\delta^{13}C_{TC}$ ratio in sizesegregated particles. *Atmos. Res.* **2015**, *158–159*, 1–12. [CrossRef]
40. Guo, Z.; Jiang, W.; Chen, S.; Sun, D.; Shi, L.; Zeng, G.; Rui, M. Stable isotopic compositions of elemental carbon in PM1.1 in north suburb of Nanjing Region, China. *Atmos. Res.* **2016**, *168*, 105–111. [CrossRef]
41. Dong, S.; Gonzalez, R.O.; Harrison, R.M.; Green, D.; North, R.; Fowler, G.; Weiss, D. Isotopic signatures suggest important contributions from recycled gasoline, road dust and non-exhaust traffic sources for copper, zinc and lead in PM_{10} in London, United Kingdom. *Atmos. Environ.* **2017**, *165*, 88–98. [CrossRef]
42. Morera-Gomez, Y.; Santamaria, J.M.; Elustondo, D.; Alonso-Hernandez, C.M.; Widory, D. Carbon and nitrogen isotopes unravels sources of aerosol contamination at Caribbean rural and urban coastal sites. *Sci. Total Environ.* **2018**, *642*, 723–732. [CrossRef]
43. Jung, C.C.; Chou, C.C.K.; Lin, C.Y.; Shen, C.C.; Lin, Y.C.; Huang, Y.T.; Tsai, C.Y.; Yao, P.H.; Huang, C.R.; Huang, W.R.; et al. C-Sr-Pb isotopic characteristics of PM2.5 transported on the East-Asian continental outflows. *Atmos. Res.* **2019**, *223*, 88–97. [CrossRef]
44. Gorka, M.; Zwolinska, E.; Malkiewicz, M.; Lewicka-Szczebak, D.; Jedrysek, M.O. Carbon and nitrogen isotope analyses coupled with palynological data of PM10 in Wroclawcity (SWPoland)-assessment of anthropogenic impact. *Isot. Environ. Health Stud.* **2012**, *48*, 327–344. [CrossRef] [PubMed]
45. Guo, Q.J.; Strauss, H.; Chen, T.B.; Zhu, G.X.; Yang, J.; Yang, J.X.; Lei, M.; Zhou, X.Y.; Petersa, M.; Xie, Y.F.; et al. Tracing the source of Beijing soil organic carbon: A carbon isotope approach. *Environ. Pollut.* **2013**, *176*, 208–214. [CrossRef] [PubMed]
46. Musa Bandowe, B.A.; Nkansah, M.A.; Leimer, S.; Fischer, D.; Lammel, G.; Han, Y. Cheimcal(C, N, S, black carbon, soot) and char and stable carbon isotope composition of street dusts from a major West African metropolis: Implication for source apportionment and exposure. *Sci. Total Environ.* **2019**, *655*, 1468–1478. [CrossRef]
47. Ault, W.U.; Senechal, R.G.; Erlebach, W.E. Isotopic composition as a natural tracer of lead in the environment. *Environ. Sci. Technol.* **1970**, *4*, 305–313. [CrossRef]

48. Komárek, M.; Ettler, V.; Chrastný, V.; Mihaljevič, M. Lead isotopes in environmental sciences: A review. *Environ. Int.* **2008**, *34*, 562–577. [CrossRef]
49. Kelepertzis, E.; Komárek, M.; Argyraki, A.; Šillerová, H. Metal(loid) Distribution and Pb Isotopic Signatures in the Urban Environment of Athens, Greece. *Environ. Pollut.* **2016**, *213*, 420–431. [CrossRef]
50. Han, L.F.; Gao, B.; Wei, X.; Xu, D.Y.; Gao, L. Spatial distribution, health risk assessment, and isotopic composition of lead contamination of street dusts in different functional areas of Beijing, China. *Environ. Sci. Pollut. Res.* **2016**, *23*, 3247–3255. [CrossRef]
51. Kumar, M.; Furumai, H.; Kurisu, F.; Kasuga, I. Tracing source and distribution of heavy metals in road dust, soil and soakaway sediment through speciation and isotopic fingerprinting. *Geoderma* **2013**, *211*, 8–17. [CrossRef]
52. Souto-Oliveira, C.E.; Babinski, M.; Araujo, D.F.; Andrade, M.F. Multi-isotopic fingerprints(Pb, Zn, Cu) applied for urban aerosol source apportionment and discrimination. *Sci. Total Environ.* **2018**, *626*, 1350–1366. [CrossRef]
53. Liu, Y.; Liu, G.; Yousaf, B.; Zhou, C.; Shen, X. Identification of the featured-element in fine road dust of cities with coal contamination by geochemical investigation and isotopic monitoring. *Environ. Int.* **2021**, *152*, 106499. [CrossRef]
54. Song, J.S.; Park, Y.G. *Health Effect Survey among Residents nearby Dong-Hae Harbor*; National Institute Environmental Research: Incheon, Korea, 2016; pp. 1–9, ISBN 11-1480523-002542-01.
55. EPA (1999) Determination of Trace Metals in Ambient Particulate Matter Using Inductively Coupled Plasma Mass Spectrometry (ICP/MS). Compendium of methods IO-3.5, EPA/625/R-96/010a. Available online: https://www.epa.gov/sites/production/files/2019-11/documents/mthd-3-5.pdf (accessed on 10 June 2021).
56. Kim, M.S.; Lee, W.S.; Kumar, K.S.; Shin, K.H.; Robarge, W.; Kim, M.S.; Lee, S.R. Effects of HCl pretreatment, drying, and storage on the stable isotope ratios of soil and sediment samples. *Rapid Commun. Mass Spectrom.* **2016**, *30*, 1575–1597. [CrossRef]
57. Rudnick, R.I.; Gao, S. Composition of the continental crust. In *The Crust*; Rudnick, R.L., Ed.; Elsevier: Amsterdam, The Netherlands, 2003; pp. 1–64.
58. Saeedi, M.; Li, L.Y.; Salmanzadeh, M. Heavy metals and polycyclic aromatic hydrocarbons: Pollution and ecological risk assessment in street dust of Tehran. *J. Hazard. Mater.* **2012**, *227–228*, 9–17. [CrossRef]
59. Yang, J.; Teng, Y.; Song, L.; Zuo, R. Tracing soures and contamination assessments of heavy metals in road and foliar dusts in a typical mining city, China. *PLoS ONE* **2016**, *11*, e0168528. [CrossRef]
60. Sutherland, R.A.; Tolosa, C.A. Multi-element analysis of road-deposited sediment in an urban drainage basin, Honolulu, Hawaii. *Environ. Pollut.* **2000**, *110*, 483–495. [CrossRef]
61. Yongming, H.; Peixuan, D.; Junji, C.; Posmentier, E.S. Multivariate analysis of heavy metal contamination in urban dusts of Xi'an, Cent, China. *Sci. Total Environ.* **2006**, *355*, 176–186. [CrossRef]
62. Stock, B.C.; Jackson, A.L.; Ward, E.J.; Parnell, A.C.; Phillips, D.L.; Semmens, B.X. Analyzing mixing systems using a new generation of Bayesian tracer mixing models. *PeerJ* **2018**, *6*, e5096. [CrossRef]
63. Seo, Y.H. Development of road dust source profile by a detailed chemical composition analysis of road dust. *J. Korean Soc. Environ. Admin.* **2010**, *16*, 43–52.
64. Duong, T.; Lee, B.K. Determining contamination level of heavy metals in road dust from busy traffic areas with different characteristics. *J. Environ. Manag.* **2011**, *92*, 554–562. [CrossRef]
65. Dietrich, M.; Wolfe, A.; Burke, M.; Krekeler, M.P.S. The first pollution investigation of road sediment in Gary, Indiana: Anthropogenic metals and possible health implications for a socieconomically disadvantaged area. *Environ. Int.* **2019**, *128*, 175–192. [CrossRef]
66. Argyraki, A. Garden soil and house dust as exposure media for lead uptake in the mining village of Stratoni, Greece. *Environ. Geochem. Health* **2014**, *36*, 677–692. [CrossRef] [PubMed]
67. Yu, S.M.; Kim, H.; Park, Y.M.; Park, K.W.; Park, J.J.; Kim, J.Y.; Seok, K.S.; Kim, Y.H. Characterization of lead pollution near zinc smelter facility in south Korea using lead stable isotopes. *J. Kor. Soc. Environ. Anal.* **2016**, *19*, 163–170.
68. Zhang, Z.; Song, X.; Wang, Q.; Lu, X. Cd and Pb contents in soil, plants, and grasshoppers along a pollution gradient in Huludao City, Northeast China. *Biol. Trace Elem. Res.* **2011**, *145*, 403–410. [CrossRef] [PubMed]
69. Meza-Figueroa, D.; O-Villanueva, M.; Parra, M.L. Heavy metal distribution in dusft from elementary schools in Hermosillo, Sonora, Mexico. *Atmos. Environ.* **2007**, *41*, 276–288. [CrossRef]
70. Yeung, Z.L.L.; Kwok, R.C.W.; Yu, K.N. Determination of multi-element profiles of street dust using energy dispersive X-ray fluorescenece (EDXRF). *Appl. Radiat. Isot.* **2003**, *58*, 339–346. [CrossRef]
71. Flett, L.; Krekeler, M.P.S.; Burke, M. Investigation of road sediment in an industrial corridor near low-income housing in Hamilton, Ohio. *Environ. Earth Sci.* **2016**, *75*, 1156–1166. [CrossRef]
72. Okorie, A.; Entwistle, J.; Dean, J.R. Estimation of daily intake of potentially toxic elements from urban street dust and the role of oral bioaccessibility testing. *Chemosphere* **2012**, *86*, 460–467. [CrossRef]
73. Hameed, A.; Al Mashhady, A. Heavy metal contaminations in Urban soil within Baghdad City, Iraq. *J. Environ. Prot.* **2013**, *4*, 73–82.
74. Hong, M.H.; Kang, D.G.; Paik, D.J.; Hwang, H.S.; Park, S.H. Effect of added magnesium on the coating properties of galvanized steel sheets. *Korean J. Met. Mater.* **2016**, *54*, 723–731. [CrossRef]
75. Yoon, S.Y.; Kim, U.J.; Kim, M.S.; Kim, M.S.; Park, J.M.; Shin, S.J. The analysis of inorganic compounds and water soluble ions in paper mill sludges from newspaper and printed paper. *J. Korean Tappi* **2014**, *46*, 30–34.

76. Adachi, K.; Yoshiaki, T. Characterization of heavy metal particle embedded in tire dust. *Environ. Int.* **2004**, *30*, 1009–1017. [CrossRef]
77. Acharya, C.; Kar, R.N.; Sukla, L.B. Studies on reaction mechanism of bioleaching of manganese ore. *Miner. Eng.* **2003**, *16*, 1027–1030. [CrossRef]
78. Hariprasad, D.; Dash, B.; Ghosh, M.K.; Anand, S. Mn recovery from medium grade ore using a waste cellulosic reductant. *Indian. J. Chem. Technol.* **2009**, *16*, 322–327.
79. Das, A.; Ghosh, S.; Mohanty, S.; Sukla, L.B. Advances in Manganese Pollution and Its Bioremediation. In *Environmental Microbial Biotechnology*; Springer: Berlin/Heidelberg, Germany, 2015; pp. 15–16.
80. Seiler, H.G.; Sigel, A.; Sigel, H. *Handbook on Metals in Clinical and Analytical Chemistry*; Marcell Dekker Inc.: New York, NY, USA, 1994.
81. Raj, S.P.; Ram, P.A. Determination and contamination assessment of Pb, Cd and Hg in roadside dust along Kathmandu-Bhaktapur road section of Arniko Highway, Nepa. *Res. J. Chem. Sci.* **2013**, *3*, 18–25.
82. Kushwaha, A.; Sanjay Kumar, N.H.; Rani, R. A critical review on speciation, mobilization and toxicity of lead in soil-microbe-plant system and bioremediation strategies. *Ecotoxicol. Environ. Saf.* **2018**, *147*, 1035–1045. [CrossRef]
83. Ullah, H.; Liu, G.; Yousaf, B.; Ubaid, M.; Abbas, Q. Combustion characteristics and retention-emission of selenium during co-firing of torrefied biomass and its blends with high ash coal. *Bioresour. Technol.* **2017**, *245*, 73–80. [CrossRef]
84. Yousaf, B.; Liu, G.; Abbas, Q.; Wang, R.; Imtiaz, M.; Zia-ur-Rehman, M. Investigating the uptake and acquisition of potentially toxic elements in plants and health risks associated with the addition of fresh biowaste amendments to industrially contaminated soil. *Land. Degrad. Dev.* **2017**, *28*, 2596–2607. [CrossRef]
85. Yuan, C.S.; Cheng, S.W.; Hung, C.H.; Yu, T.Y. Influence of operating parameters on the collection efficiency and size distribution of street dust during street scrubbing. *Aerosol Air. Qual. Res.* **2003**, *3*, 75–86. [CrossRef]
86. Patra, A.; Colvile, R.; Arnold, S.; Bowen, E.; Shallcross, D.; Martin, D.; Price, C.; Tate, J.; ApSimon, H.; Robins, A. On street observation of particulate matter movement and dispersion due to traffic on an urban road. *Atmos. Environ.* **2008**, *42*, 3911–3926. [CrossRef]
87. Kupiainen, K. Road dust from pavement wear and traction sanding. In *Monograph of Boreal Environment Research*; Finnish Environment Institute: Helsinki, Finland, 2007; p. 26.
88. Pacyna, J.M. *Trace Element Emission from Anthropogenic Sources in Europe*; Technical Report. 10/82; Norsk Institutt for Luftforskning: Kjeller, Norway, 1983; Volume 24781, p. 107.
89. Kowalczyk, G.S.; Gordon, G.E.; Rheingrover, S.W. Identification of atmospheric particulate sources in Washington, D.C., using chemical element balances. *Environ. Sci. Technol.* **1982**, *16*, 79–90. [CrossRef]
90. Wadge, A.; Hutton, M.; Peterson, P.J. The concentrations and particle size relationships of selected trace elements in fly ashes from U.K. coal-fired power plants and a refuse incinerator. *Sci. Total Environ.* **1986**, 13–27. [CrossRef]
91. Wan, D.; Han, Z.; Yang, J.; Yang, G.; Liu, X. Heavy metal pollution in settled dust associated with different urban functional areas in a heavily air polluted city I North Chin. *Int. J. Environ. Res. Public Health* **2016**, *13*, 1119. [CrossRef]
92. Varrica, D.; Bardelli, F.; Dongarra, G.; Tamburo, E. Speciation of Sb in airborne particulate matter, vehiclebrake linings, and brake pad wear residues. *Atmos. Environ.* **2013**, *64*, 18–24. [CrossRef]
93. Victoria, A.; Cobbian, S.J.; Dampare, S.B.; Duwiejuah, A.B. Heavy metals concentration in road dust in the Bolgatanga Municiplaith, Ghana. *J. Environ. Pollut. Hum. Health* **2014**, *2*, 74–80.
94. Kanu, M.O.; Meludu, O.C.; Oniku, S.A. Evaluation of heavy metal contents in road dust of Jalingo, Taraba State, Nigeria. *Jordan J. Earth Environ. Sci.* **2015**, *7*, 65–70.
95. Kartal, Ş.; Aydın, Z.; Tokalıoğlu, Ş. Fractionation of metals in street sediment samples by using the BCR sequential extraction procedure and multivariate statistical elucidation. *J. Hazard. Mater.* **2006**, *132*, 80–89. [CrossRef] [PubMed]
96. Pagotto, C.; Remy, N.; Legret, M.; Le Cloirec, P. Heavy metal pollution of road dust and roadside soil near a major rural highway. *Environ. Technol.* **2001**, *22*, 307–319. [CrossRef] [PubMed]
97. Jose, J.; Srimuruganandam, B. Investigation of road dust characteristics and its associated health risks from an urban environment. *Environ. Geochem. Health* **2020**, *42*, 2819–2840. [CrossRef]
98. Plum, L.M.; Rink, L.; Haase, H. The essential toxin: Impact of Zinc on human health. *Int. J. Environ. Res. Public Health* **2010**, *7*, 1342–1365. [CrossRef]
99. O'Neal, S.L.; Zheng, W. Manganese toxicity upon overexposure: A decade in review. *Curr. Environ. Health Rep.* **2015**, *2*, 315–328. [CrossRef]
100. Huff, J.; Lunn, R.M.; Waalkers, M.P.; Tomatis, L.; Infante, P.F. Cadmium-induced cancers in animals and in humans. *Int. J. Occup. Environ. Health* **2007**, *13*, 202–212. [CrossRef]
101. Yousaf, B.; Amina, L.G.; Wang, R.; Imtiaz, M.; Rizwan, M.S.; Zia-ur-Rehman, M.; Qadir, A.; Si, Y. The importance of evaluating metal exposure and predicting human health risks in urban-periurban environments influenced by emerging industry. *Chemosphere* **2016**, *150*, 79–89. [CrossRef]
102. Yousaf, B.; Liu, G.; Wang, R.; Imtiaz, M.; Zia-ur-Rehman, M.; Munir, M.A.M.; Niu, Z. Bioavailability evaluation, uptake of heavy metals and potential health risks via dietary exposure in urban-industrial areas. *Environ. Sci. Pollut. Res.* **2016**, *23*, 22443–22453. [CrossRef]
103. O'Leary, M.H. Carbon isotopes in photosynthesis. *BioScience* **1988**, *38*, 328–336. [CrossRef]

104. López-Veneroni, D. The stable carbon isotope composition of PM2.5 and PM10 in Mexico City Metropolitan Area air. *Atmos. Environ.* **2009**, *43*, 4491–4502. [CrossRef]
105. Kawashima, H.; Haneishi, Y. Effects of combustion emissions from the Eurasian continent in winter on seasonal δ^{13}C of elemental carbon in aerosols in Japan. *Atmos. Environ.* **2012**, *46*, 568–579. [CrossRef]
106. Widory, D. Combustibles, fuels and their combustion products: A view through carbon isotopes. *Combust. Theory Model.* **2006**, *10*, 831–841. [CrossRef]
107. Martinelli, L.A.; Camargo, P.B.; Lara, L.B.L.S.; Victoria, R.L.; Artaxo, P. Stable carbon and nitrogen isotopic composition of bulk aerosol particles in a C4 plant landscape of southeast Brazil. *Atmos. Environ.* **2002**, *36*, 2427–2432. [CrossRef]
108. Moura, J.M.S.; Martens, C.S.; Moreira, M.Z.; Lima, R.L.; Sampaio, I.C.G.; Mendlovitz, H.P.; Menton, M.C. Spatial and seasonal variations in the stable carbon isotopic composition of methane in stream sediments of eastern Amazonia. *Tellus* **2008**, *60B*, 21–31. [CrossRef]
109. Cao, J.J.; Chow, J.C.; Tao, J.; Lee, S.C.; Watson, J.G.; Ho, K.F.; Wang, G.H.; Zhu, C.S.; Han, Y.M. Stable carbon isotopes in aerosols from Chinese cities: Influence of fossil fuels. *Atmos. Environ.* **2011**, *45*, 1359–1363. [CrossRef]
110. Tanner, R.L.; Miguel, A.H. Carbonaceous aerosol sources in Rio de Janeiro. *Aerosol Sci. Technol.* **1989**, *10*, 213–223. [CrossRef]
111. Grassi, C.; Campigli, V.; Dallai, L.; Nottoli, S.; Tognotti, L.; Guidi, M. PM characterization by carbon isotope. In Proceedings of the European Aerosol Conference, Salzburg, Austria, 9–14 September 2007.
112. Widory, D.; Roy, S.; Le Moullec, G.; Cocherie, A.; Guerrot, C. The origin of atmospheric particles in Paris: A view through carbon and lead isotopes. *Atmos. Environ.* **2004**, *38*, 953–961. [CrossRef]
113. Gupta, A.K.; Gupta, S.K.; Patil, R.S. Environmental management plan for port and harbour projects. *Clean. Technol. Environ. Policy* **2005**, *7*, 133–141. [CrossRef]
114. Moreira González, A.; Abilio Comas, A.; Valle Pombrol, A.; Seisdedo, M. Bloom of Vulcanodinium rugosum linked to skin lesions in Cienfuegos Bay, Cuba. *Harmful Algae News* **2016**, *55*, 10–11.

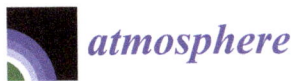

Article

Characteristics and Risk Assessment of 16 Metals in Street Dust Collected from a Highway in a Densely Populated Metropolitan Area of Vietnam

Van-Truc Nguyen [1], Nguyen Duy Dat [2,*], Thi-Dieu-Hien Vo [3,*], Duy-Hieu Nguyen [4], Thanh-Binh Nguyen [5], Ly-Sy Phu Nguyen [6,7], Xuan Cuong Nguyen [8,9], Viet-Cuong Dinh [10], Thi-Hong-Hanh Nguyen [11], Thi-Minh-Trang Huynh [12], Hong-Giang Hoang [13], Thi-Giang Huong Duong [1], Manh-Ha Bui [1] and Xuan-Thanh Bui [14,15]

1 Department of Environmental Sciences, Saigon University, Ho Chi Minh City 700000, Vietnam; nvtruc@sgu.edu.vn (V.-T.N.); huongduong@sgu.edu.vn (T.-G.H.D.); manhhakg@sgu.edu.vn (M.-H.B.)
2 Faculty of Chemical & Food Technology, Ho Chi Minh City University of Technology and Education, Ho Chi Minh City 700000, Vietnam
3 Faculty of Environmental and Food Engineering, Nguyen Tat Thanh University, Ho Chi Minh City 700000, Vietnam
4 College of Maritime, National Kaohsiung University of Science and Technology, Kaohsiung City 81157, Taiwan; andyhieuenv@gmail.com
5 Department of Marine Environmental Engineering, National Kaohsiung University of Science and Technology, Kaohsiung City 81157, Taiwan; ntbinh179@nkust.edu.tw
6 Faculty of Environment, University of Science, Ho Chi Minh City 700000, Vietnam; nlsphu@hcmus.edu.vn
7 Vietnam National University, Ho Chi Minh City 700000, Vietnam
8 Center for Advanced Chemistry, Institute of Research and Development, Duy Tan University, Da Nang 550000, Vietnam; nguyenxuancuong4@duytan.edu.vn
9 Faculty of Environmental Chemical Engineering, Duy Tan University, Da Nang 550000, Vietnam
10 Faculty of Environmental Engineering, Hanoi University of Civil Engineering, 55 Giai Phong, Hai Ba Trung, Hanoi 100000, Vietnam; cuongdv@nuce.edu.vn
11 Department of Civil Engineering, Vietnam Maritime University, Hai Phong 180000, Vietnam; honghanh.ctt@vimaru.edu.vn
12 Graduate Institute of Applied Geology, National Central University, Taoyuan 32000, Taiwan; tranghuynh44@gmail.com
13 Faculty of Health Sciences and Finance-Accounting, Dong Nai Technology University, Bien Hoa 810000, Vietnam; honggiangenv@gmail.com
14 Key Laboratory of Advanced Waste Treatment Technology, Vietnam National University Ho Chi Minh (VNU-HCM), Linh Trung Ward, Ho Chi Minh City 700000, Vietnam; bxthanh@hcmut.edu.vn
15 Faculty of Environment and Natural Resources, Ho Chi Minh City University of Technology (HCMUT), Ho Chi Minh City 700000, Vietnam
* Correspondence: datnd@hcmute.edu.vn (N.D.D.); vtdhien@ntt.edu.vn (T.-D.-H.V.)

Abstract: The present study focused on investigating the contamination and risk assessment for 16 metals in street dust from Ha Noi highway, Ho Chi Minh City. The results indicated that the concentrations of metals (mg/kg) were found, in decreasing order, to be Ti (676.3 ± 155.4) > Zn (519.2 ± 318.9) > Mn (426.6 ±113.1) > Cu (144.7 ± 61.5) > Cr (81.4 ± 22.6) > Pb (52.2 ± 22.9) > V (35.5 ± 5.6) > Ni (30.9 ± 9.5) > Co (8.3 ± 1.2) > As (8.3 ± 2.5) > Sn (7.0 ± 3.6) > B (5.7 ± 0.9) > Mo (4.1 ± 1.7) > Sb (0.8 ± 0.3) > Cd (0.6 ± 0.2) > Se (0.4 ± 0.1). The geo-accumulation index (I_{geo}) showed moderate contamination levels for Pb, Cd, Cu, Sn, Mo, and Zn. The enrichment factor (EF) values revealed moderate levels for Cd, Cu, Mo, and Sn but moderate–severe levels for Zn. The pollution load index of the heavy metals was moderate. The potential ecological risk (207.43) showed a high potential. Notably, 40.7% and 33.5% of the ecological risks were contributed by Zn and Mn, respectively. These findings are expected to provide useful information to decision-makers about environmental quality control strategies.

Keywords: metals; street dust; enrichment factor; geo-accumulation index; ecological risk; Vietnam

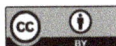

1. Introduction

Street dust, road dust, or urban street dust are names for dust on road surfaces. Street dust contains various metals deriving from many different sources, such as vehicle emissions, residential combustion, solid waste combustion, power plants, industrial activities, and city construction [1]. The presence of metals in the street dust may cause both adverse environmental effects and human health issues [2]. Metals associated with street dust are a current concern of scientists around the world. Many researchers have evaluated the levels of metals in street dust collected from various countries, for example China, Colombia, Iran, Jordan, Turkey, United Arab Emirates (UAE), Vietnam, etc. Most of these studies focused mainly on six to eight metals [3–12]. Some studies extended the list to more than eight metals [13–17]. The results showed that the concentration of metals fluctuates widely up to 8430 mg/kg [6]. Various methods were employed to determine the level of metal pollution in dust, for example the enrichment factor (EF) [4], geo-accumulation index (I_{geo}) [18–20], pollution load index (PLI) [3,21], and ecological risk assessment (ERA) [4,5,22–26]. The results all indicated significant potential risks of metals for human health as well as ecosystems.

The characteristics of street-dust metals and the related emission sources and risks have not received much attention in Vietnam, where there are many cities with high traffic density, dense population, and interwoven industrial zones. To the best of our knowledge, only three studies have been conducted to determine the street-dust metal levels in Vietnam. Firstly, Phi et al. [27] conducted monitoring of the concentration of six metals in street dust sampled at 163 locations from Hanoi, Vietnam. Secondly, the concentration of eight metals (Pb, Cu, Cr, Zn, Fe, Mn, K, and Ca), and the risk assessment for five metals (Cu, Pb, Cr, Zn, and Mn) from exposure to street dust from Highway No. 5 and Highway No. 18 in Northeast Vietnam were investigated by Phi et al. [28]. Thirdly, Dat et al. [12] measured the concentrations of eight metals (Pb, Cu, Cr, Zn, Mn, Ni, Cd, and Co) in street dust in Southern Vietnam. Information on the spatial distribution, potential emission sources, and risk assessments for multiple metals associated with the rapid urbanization and industrialization in Ho Chi Minh City is limited.

From the literature review, it was found that most studies focused on common metals (Cd, Co, Ni, Pb, Cr, Cu, Mn, and Zn). Recently, survey studies have been undertaken in cities with high traffic density and industrial development areas, such as Ho Chi Minh City [13,14]. The results showed that in addition to the metals mentioned above, many other metals were detected (Se, Sb, Mo, B, Sn, As, V, Ti, etc.) with relatively high concentrations. Measuring more elements results in a more complete assessment of pollution levels. Therefore, with the desire to provide a comprehensive view for policymakers on environmental pollution control strategies, this study investigated the spatial distribution and potential emission sources of 16 metals (Se, Cd, Sb, Mo, B, Sn, As, Co, Ni, V, Pb, Cr, Mn, Cu, Zn, and Ti) in the street dust collected from one of the main routes entering Ho Chi Minh City (Ha Noi highway). Possible sources and relationships between the metals were interpreted using multiple statistical analysis methods such as Pearson's correlation coefficient, principal component analysis (PCA), and hierarchical cluster analysis (HCA). In addition, we calculated the geo-accumulation index (I_{geo}), pollution load index (PLI), and enrichment factor (EF), to evaluate the levels of anthropogenic enrichment by metals. Finally, the potential ecological risk index (PER) was calculated.

2. Materials and Methods

2.1. Sampling Site

Ho Chi Minh (HCM) City is the biggest city in the Southeast of Vietnam (Figure 1a,b), with an area of 2095 km^2. It has a tropical climate (average annual precipitation of 1800 mm and temperature of 28 °C). There are two main seasons: the dry (December–April) and wet (May–November) seasons [29]. In recent years, Ha Noi highway has been the main thoroughfare (Figure 1c) connecting HCM city with Binh Duong and Dong Nai provinces, where there are many industrial zones.

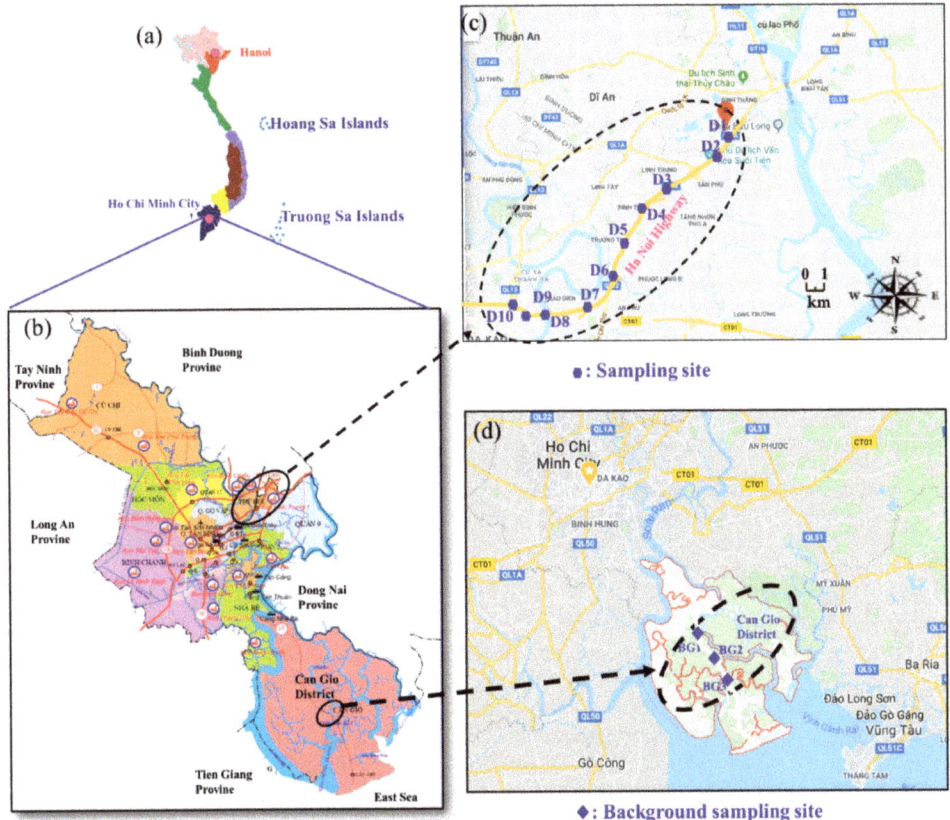

Figure 1. A regional map of Vietnam (**a**); Ho Chi Minh City (**b**); sampling sites on Ha Noi highway (**c**); background sampling sites in Can Gio District (**d**).

2.2. Sample Collection, Preparation, and Analytical Methods

A total of 13 samples were collected in this study, of which 10 were street-dust samples from Ha Noi highway (Figure 1c) and 3 were background soil samples from Rung Sac Street, Can Gio District (Figure 1d). Samples were collected during February 2020 using brushes, dustpans, and clean plastic. Each sample was collected over an approximate area of 2 m² adjacent to the street curb, and 500 g of the dust sample was collected into a polyethylene bag before shipping it to the lab for treatment and metals analysis [30]. In this study, background samples were collected in Can Gio District because no industrial zones are located in this area, and the population and traffic densities are low (Figure 1d). The samples were dried in ambient conditions to stabilize moisture and then sieved through a nylon sieve of 149 µm diameter. Finally, the samples were stored in a desiccator until further treatment for metals analysis. The locations of the sampling sites and the GPS coordinates are shown in Table S1.

In this study, the extraction procedures strictly followed those reported by Dat et al. (2021), which are presented in detail in the Supplementary Materials. Briefly, the dust samples were analyzed for extractable metals according to EPA Method 3051A [31] and Method 200.8, Revision 5.4 [32]. All reagents were of analytical grade (Merck) and purification was needed before digestion. Sixteen metals (Se, Cd, Sb, Mo, B, Sn, As, Co, Ni, V, Pb, Cr, Cu, Mn, Zn, and Ti) were quantified using inductively coupled plasma mass spectrometry (ICP-MS; model 7700x, Agilent, Santa Clara, CA, USA) with an ICP-MS-grade standard.

The metals were measured in triplicate for each sample and a blank test was conducted for every 10 samples. Blank samples were prepared and analyzed using the same procedure, showing concentrations below the method detection limit (MDL). QA/QC of the analytical method was ensured by analyzing the certificate reference material for urban particulates (SRM-1648a). The results indicated that the recoveries ranged from 90 to 120% for all metals. The MDLs of Se (20 µg/L), Cd (20 µg/L), Sb (20 µg/L), Mo (2 mg/L), B (2 mg/L), Sn (0.2 mg/L), As (20 µg/L), Co (0.2 mg/L), Ni (0.2 mg/L), V (2 mg/L), Pb (20 µg/L), Cr (0.2 mg/L), Cu (2 mg/L), Mn (2 mg/L), Zn (5 mg/L), and Ti (2 mg/L) were significantly lower than the concentrations of metals found in this study.

2.3. Degree of Contamination and Pollution Load Index

2.3.1. Geo-Accumulation Index (I_{geo})

We investigated the I_{geo} values to evaluate the contamination levels of the metals, computed according to Equation (1).

$$I_{geo} = \log_2 \left(\frac{C_n}{1.5 B_n} \right) \quad (1)$$

where C_n and B_n are the street-dust metal concentration of sample n and the background sample, respectively. The factor of 1.5 was applied to correct for potential background variation [12]. The risk was evaluated based on the criteria of seven grades, as presented in Table S2.

2.3.2. Enrichment Factor (EF)

The EF was computed to assess the degree of contamination. This was first carried out by Buat-Menard and Chesselet [33] for oceanic suspended matter, and then for heavy metals in street dust [19,25,34]. Table S2 shows the standard criteria for EFs, employed to evaluate the metals contamination. The EF was estimated based on Equation (2). The elements Fe [25,34–36], Al [37,38], and Mn [39,40] are common references (ref) when computing the EFs of toxic metals in environmental samples. In this study, we selected Fe to represent the reference element.

$$EF = \frac{(C_i/C_{Fe})_{Sample}}{(C_i/C_{Fe})_{Background}} \quad (2)$$

where EF is the enrichment factor and $(C_i/C_{Fe})_{Sample}$ and $(C_i/C_{Fe})_{Background}$ are the ratios of the metal concentration (C_i) to the concentration of Fe (C_{Fe}) in the street dust and background samples, respectively.

2.3.3. Pollution Load Index (PLI)

The pollution level of metals in street dust was evaluated via the PLI value calculated using Equations (3) and (4):

$$P_i = \frac{C_i}{C_b} \quad (3)$$

$$PLI = \sqrt[n]{P_1 \times P_2 \times P_3 \times \ldots .P_n} \quad (4)$$

where P_i is the pollution index for element i, C_i and C_b are the concentrations of element i and the background for element i, PLI is the pollution load index, and n is the number of metals analyzed in this study. The five categories of P_i and the four categories of PLI [41] are shown in Table S2.

2.4. Potential Ecological Risk (PER)

The PER index was first defined by Hakanson [42]. The PER represents the potential ecological risk factor of multiple metals, calculated [25,26,42] according to Equations (5) and (6):

$$E_i = T_i \times C_f^i \quad (5)$$

$$PER = \sum E_i \quad (6)$$

where E_i is the potential ecological risk index of metal i, T_i is the toxic response factor of each metal (i.e., Cu = Ni = Co = Pb = 5; Mn = Zn = Cr = 2; Cd = 30) [43], and C_f^i is the contamination factor of metal i. Detailed information on the five categories of E_i and four categories of PER can found in Table S3.

2.5. Data Analysis

Statistical analysis was carried out using OriginPro 2021 software (OriginLab Corporation, Northampton, MA, USA). Multivariate statistical analyses (i.e., Pearson's correlation, principal component analysis (PCA), and cluster analysis) were conducted to identify the potential sources of metals.

3. Results and Discussion

3.1. Basic Statistics of Metals Concentration

Figure 2a shows the box plot of the concentrations of the 16 metals from different sampling sites. In general, the metal concentrations (mg/kg) decreased in the order Ti (676.3 ± 155.4) > Zn (519.2 ± 318.9) > Mn (426.6 ± 113.1) > Cu (144.7 ± 61.5) > Cr (81.4 ± 22.6) > Pb (52.2 ± 22.9) > V (35.5 ± 5.6) > Ni (30.9 ± 9.5) > Co (8.3 ± 1.2) > As (8.3 ± 2.5) > Sn (7.0 ± 3.6) > B (5.7 ± 0.9) > Mo (4.1 ± 1.7) > Sb (0.8 ± 0.3) > Cd (0.6 ± 0.2) > Se (0.4 ± 0.1). Figure 2b shows the percentage contribution of the metals at different sampling points. Ti, Zn, and Mn were major contributors to the total metal concentration, accounting for about 35%, 23%, and 21%, respectively, while minor contributions were obtained from Se (0.02%), Cd (0.03%), and Sb (0.04%). In total, 93% of the samples collected on the highway had heavy metal concentrations in excess of their background concentrations. This result suggests a significant influence of anthropogenic sources on the concentrations of these metals [4,44].

In this study, Zn, Cu, Mn, Pb, Cr, and Ni contributed the most to the total metal concentration in the street-dust samples. The spatial distributions of six selected metals are shown in Figure 3. High values for Ni (55.7 mg/kg), Pb (93.5 mg/kg), Cr (123.6 mg/kg), Cu (289.4 mg/kg), and Mn (642.7 mg/kg) were also recorded at D4, and a high value for Zn (1062.7 mg/kg) was recorded at D3, a location close to high traffic density, a residential area, the university, and a supermarket. The highest value for heavy metals was recorded at locations D3 (Zn) and D4 (Ni, Pb, Cr, Cu, and Mn), while the minimum values for those metals were detected at D2 (Ni and Cr), and D9 (Pb, Cu, Mn, and Zn). At D4, high concentrations of metals were obtained because it is located near Thu Duc crossroads on Ha Noi highway, with high traffic density.

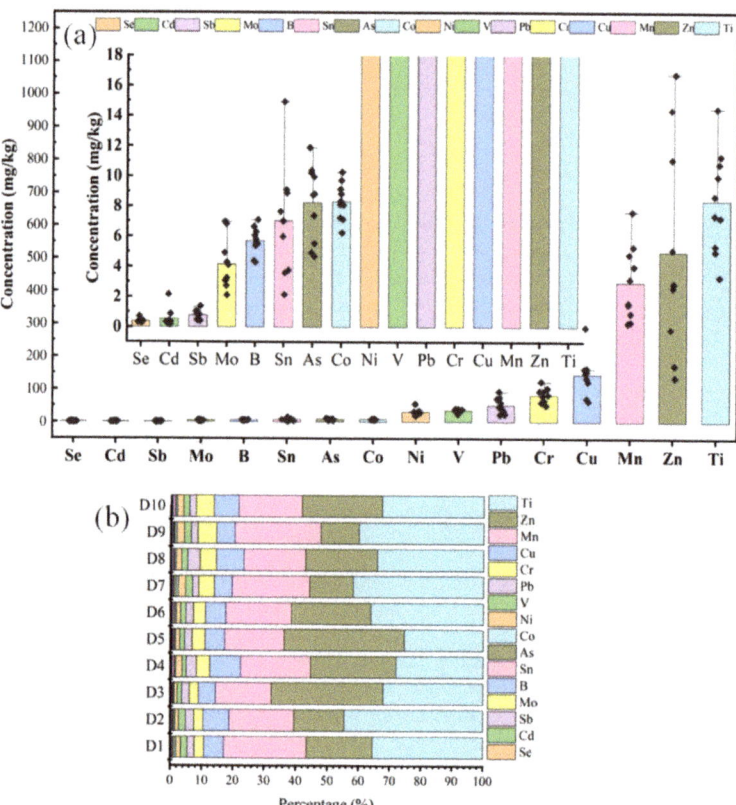

Figure 2. Average Concentrations of the metals (Se, Cd, Sb, Mo, B, Sn, As, Co, Ni, V, Pb, Cr, Mn, Cu, Zn, and Ti) in the sampling sites (black dots present the concentration values of metals at different sampling sites) (**a**) and the contributions of heavy metals at the sampling point (**b**).

In this study, the coefficients of variation (CV = S.D/mean value) were determined for 16 metals (Se, Cd, Sb, Mo, B, Sn, As, Co, Ni, V, Pb, Cr, Cu, Mn, Zn, and Ti). The CV values can be classified as low variability for CV < 0.2, moderate variability for $0.2 \leq CV < 0.5$, high variability for $0.5 \leq CV < 1.0$, and extremely high variability for $CV \geq 1.0$ [45]. In this study, the CV of Cd was 1.1, suggesting extremely high concentration variability. Relatively high CV values were also obtained for Zn and Sn (0.6 and 0.5). The CV values of Cu, Pb, Sb, Mo, Se, As, Ni, Cr, Mn, B, V, and Ti showed moderate variability, while the CV value of Co showed low variability. The high CV values of some of the elements showed a strong anthropogenic influence [4,41,46,47]. Detailed information on the mean, standard deviation, min, max, CV, and background concentrations of the 16 metals studied can be found in Table S4 in the Supplementary Materials.

In a comparison among the metals, high concentrations of Ti, Zn, Mn, Cu, Cr, and Pb and low concentrations of Sb, Cd, and Se were observed in this study (Table 1). The mean concentration of Ti (676.3 ± 155.4 mg/kg) in this study was significantly higher than that of 158.4 mg/kg reported from Asaluyeh County, Iran [17], but the value was significantly lower than those reported from Hefei, China (1522 mg/kg) [15], Xining City, China (1977.9 mg/kg) [14], and Nanchang City, China (3277.9 mg/kg) [4].

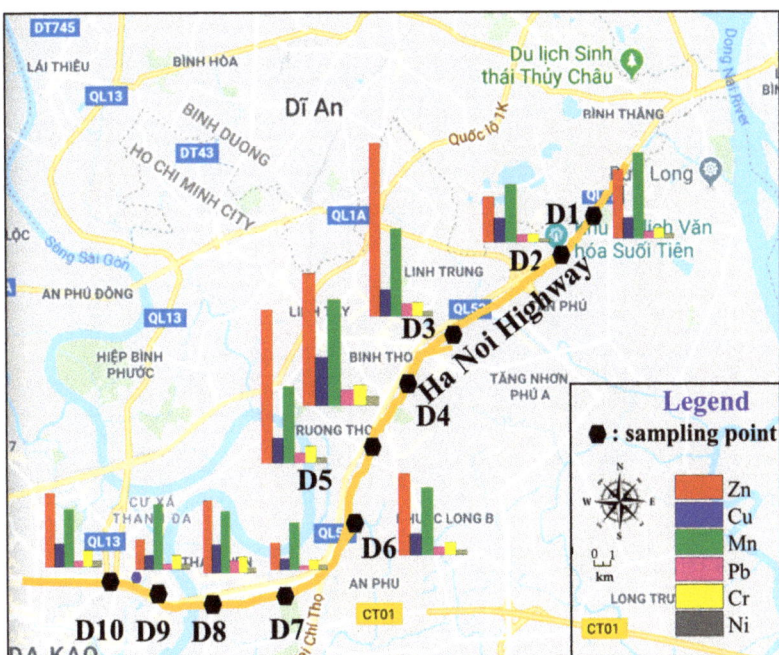

Figure 3. Spatial distribution of Zn, Cu, Mn, Pb, Cr, and Ni at sampling sites.

The average Zn concentration was 519.2 ± 318.9 mg/kg, with the highest Zn concentration found in sample D3 (1062.7 mg/kg), while the lowest level was measured in sample D9 (136.1 mg/kg). A high Zn level in street dust was also recorded by Shabbaj et al. [46] (487.5 mg/kg) and Bartholomew et al. [6] (8430.3 mg/kg). Bourliva et al. [47] and Idris et al. [48] showed that tire wear, brake wear, brake pads, lubricating oils, engine tires, diesel exhaust, and wear of machine parts were the potential emission origins of Zn in street dust. The Zn concentration (519 mg/kg) obtained in urban street dust was over 7.9-fold higher than the background level (71.27 mg/kg). A similar Zn level was found by Shabbaj et al. [46] in Jeddah (Saudi Arabia) (487.5 mg/kg). In addition, the Zn value reported in this study was much higher than those reported from Hanoi, Vietnam (369 mg/kg) [27], Urumqi, China (224.5 mg/kg) [49], the Petra region, Jordan (129 mg/kg) [9], and Lahore, Pakistan (67.9 mg/kg) [50]. On the other hand, our value was significantly lower than that from Jinhua, China (8430.3 mg/kg) [6].

The concentration of Cu (144.7 ± 61.5 mg/kg) was over 5.3-fold higher than the background level (27.1 mg/kg). The highest Cu concentration was observed in sample D4 (289.4 mg/kg) and the lowest level was reported in sample D9 (64.7 mg/kg). The mean value of the Cu concentration was higher than those previously reported from various sites worldwide. For instance, Cu concentrations of 51, 54.8, 64.9, 97.4, and 133.7 mg/kg were determined in street dust from Dezful, Iran [16], Xi'an China [3], Highway No. 5, Vietnam [28], Beijing, China [5], and Jinhua, China [6], respectively. This study found a Cu concentration lower than those documented in other sites, e.g., Ho Chi Minh, Vietnam (153.7 mg/kg) [12], and Tianjin, China (527.5 mg/kg) [13]. Copper in street dust may also originate from exhaust gases and lubricating oils [51], or be released from manhole cover metal, wear of tires and brake pads, and emissions from engine parts [21,52].

Table 1. Comparison of potentially toxic elements (mg/kg) in street dust from different sites worldwide.

Sampling Sites	Se	Cd	Sb	Mo	B	Sn	As	Co	Ni	V	Pb	Cr	Cu	Mn	Zn	Ti	References
Xi'an, China *	-	-	-	-	-	-	-	-	26.4	56.8	94.5	251.8	54.8	406	377	-	[3]
Nanchang City, China **	-	1.0	-	-	-	-	10.1	-	28.1	-	89.5	112.5	101.3	-	277.2	3277.9	[4]
Beijing, China *	-	0.5	-	-	-	-	4.1	-	40.8	-	62.3	99.5	97.4	536.3	255.9	-	[5]
Jinhua, China **	-	4.9	-	-	-	-	8.7	-	76.3	-	110.6	105.3	133.7	451	8430.3	-	[6]
Tianjin, China **	-	2.1	21.8	12.8	-	82.9	29.5	10.5	77.9	100.2	120.7	-	527.5	670.6	983.2	0.7	[13]
Xining City, China *	-	-	8.9	-	-	22.8	6.0	24.6	23.5	51.8	62.8	507.8	30.3	377.7	104.8	1977.9	[14]
Hefei, China **	-	-	1.6	-	-	1.2	2.0	7.2	28.6	31.4	0.9	139.3	41.6	240.5	130.1	1522	[15]
Urumqi, China **	-	1.2	-	-	-	-	-	10.9	43.3	-	53.5	54.3	94.5	926.6	294.5	-	[7]
Villavicencio, Colombia ***	-	0.04	-	-	-	-	-	-	1.3	-	20.7	18.7	47.7	164.1	118.1	-	[8]
Dezful, Iran ***	-	0.4	-	-	-	-	3	8	46	38	54	44	51	-	224	-	[16]
Asaluyeh County, Iran **	-	0.3	2.2	14.2	-	-	4.9	6.5	35.1	-	50.	37.3	121.3	252.7	518.5	158.4	[17]
Irbid-North Shooneh, Jordan ***	-	11.0	-	-	-	-	-	36.0	60.0	-	79.0	16.0	4.0	-	122.0	-	[9]
Konya, Turkey *	-	-	-	-	-	-	-	7	10	68	19	22	16	-	68	-	[10]
Abu Dhabi, UAE ***	-	0.5	-	-	-	-	0.2	-	0.3	-	50.1	306.3	-	-	173.0	-	[11]
Ho Chi Minh City, Vietnam **	-	0.5	-	-	-	-	-	7.9	36.2	-	49.6	102.4	153.7	393.9	466.4	-	[12]
Ho Chi Minh City, Vietnam **	0.4	0.6	0.8	4.1	5.7	7.0	8.3	8.3	30.9	35.5	52.2	81.4	144.7	426.6	519.2	676.3	This study

Note: "-" indicates data not available. The dust samples were analyzed by X-ray fluorescence spectrometry (*), ICP-MS (**), and atomic absorption spectroscopy (***).

The Cr mean concentration (81.4 mg/kg) exceeded the background level (27.1 mg/kg) by over 3.0 times. The highest Cr concentration was obtained in sample D4 (123.6 mg/kg), while the lowest value was observed in sample D2 (51.3 mg/kg). These values were higher than those previously reported from Asaluyeh County, Iran (37.3 mg/kg) [17], the Lagos metropolis, Southwestern Nigeria (41.3 mg/kg) [53], and Dezful, Iran (44 mg/kg) [16].

The value of the Pb concentration in street dust (52.2 mg/kg) was similar to the values reported by previous studies from Dezful, Iran (54 mg/kg) [16], Abu Dhabi–Al Ain National highway, UAE (50.1 mg/kg) [11], and Beijing, China (62.3 mg/kg) [5]. On the other hand, higher levels of Pb were also found in other studies, for instance, in Nanchang, China (89.5 mg/kg) [4], Xi'an, China (94.5 mg/kg) [3], Jinhua, China (110.6 mg/kg) [6], and Tianjin, China (120.7 mg/kg) [13].

The results of this study revealed that the mean Cd concentration (0.6 ± 0.2 mg/kg) in street dust was higher than for the background site (0.1 mg/kg). However, more than a few times higher Cd concentration was found in street dust samples in previous studies documented by Bartholomew et al. [6], Zhang et al. [13], and Alsbou and Al-Khashman [9]. The previous studies indicated that leakage of diesel fuel and lubricating oil were potential sources of Cd in street dust [54], and Wahab et al. [21] also revealed that Cd is one of the trace components in diesel fuel, car paints, and brake pads.

3.2. Heavy Metals Identification Resource

3.2.1. The Correlation Coefficient among the Heavy Metals in This Study

The Pearson's correlation coefficient could reveal the inter-element relationships that help to understand the transformation pathways of metals and their sources [25]. Egbueri et al. [24] suggested correlation coefficients in the range of 0.0–0.3 for poor, 0.4–0.6 for moderate, and 0.7–1.0 for strong correlations. A strong correlation between metal pairs would reveal a similar origin, such as the same sources [26]. The coefficients for inter-element correlation in street dust are presented in Figure 4a. Strong and significant ($p < 0.05$) correlations were obtained for various metal pairs, including: (a) Ti-V (r = 0.86), Ti-B (0.75), Ti-Mn (0.74), Ti-Pb (0.73); (b) Zn-Pb (0.77), Zn-Mn (0.77), Zn-Mo (0.72), Zn-Co (0.71); (c) Cu-Pb (0.91), Cu-Sn (0.89), Cu-Ni (0.8), Cu-Sb (0.82), Cu-Cr (0.76), Cu-Co (0.75), Cu-V (0.74); (d) Cr-Sn (0.9), Cr-Mo (0.87), Cr-Ni (0.86), Cr-Pb (0.73); (e) Pb-Sb (0.82), Pb-V (0.77), Pb-Sn (0.76), Pb-Co (0.71); (f) V-B (0.82), V-Co (0.79), V-Sb (0.71); (g) Ni-Sn (0.89), Ni-Mo (0.79), Ni-Sb (0.72); (h) Co-Sb (0.83), Co-Sn (0.83); (i) Sn-Mo (0.84), Sn-Sb (0.83); (j) Mo-Sb (0.75). Anthropogenic activities are well known as potential sources of metals in street-dust samples [23,55]. Processes including tire wear, brake wear, brake pads, diesel exhaust, lubricating oils, engine tires and wear of machine parts are possible sources of Zn, Pb, Ni, and Cr [47,48], while industrial processes, gas refineries, fuel combustion [56,57], and car paints are possible sources of Ni [21]. Lau et al. [58] showed that smelting industries produce a large number of heavy metals (e.g., Fe, Co, Mn, and V), and e-waste recycling could contribute large amounts of trace elements such as Pb and Cd to street dust.

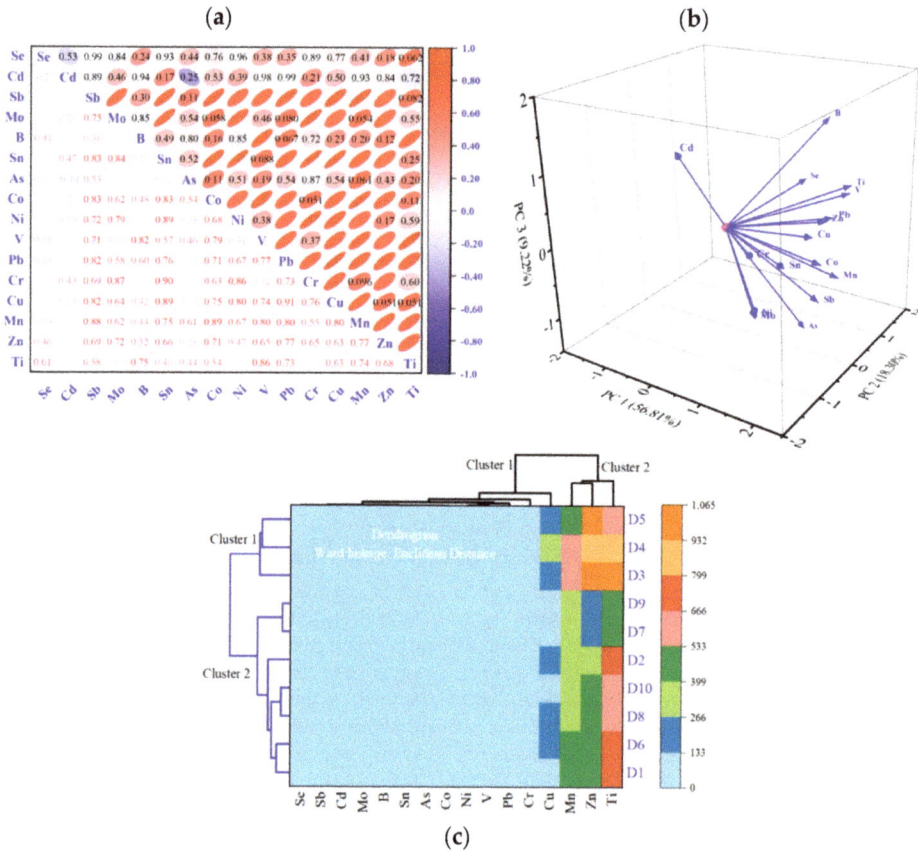

Figure 4. Analysis of sixteen metals in Ha Noi highway street dust: (**a**) Pearson correlation coefficients among the heavy metals; (**b**) results from PCA in 3-D space; (**c**) dendrogram results calculated using the Ward's method for cluster analysis.

3.2.2. Principal Component Analysis (PCA)

PCA is a widely applied multivariable statistical method to identify the potential sources of street-dust metals [26,59]. Figure 4b shows the rotated component matrix results for metals in street dust. Detailed information on the scree plot of the PCA and the results of the PCA for 16 metals in street dust from Ha Noi highway, HCM City, can be found in Figure S1 and Table S3. The Kaiser–Meyer–Olkin (KMO) value was 0.72, suggesting the suitability of the PCA method for this study. The PCA data displayed three main components with eigenvalues >1. The three principal components (PCs) obtained explained more than 84% of the variance of the data.

The component PC1 was dominated by Sb, Mo, Sn, As, Co, Ni, V, Pb, Cr, and Cu, accounting for 56.8% of the total variance. Sources of Cu, Pb, and Zn could be various anthropogenic activities (e.g., tire wear, brake wear, diesel exhaust, and wear of machine parts) [49,60,61]. Nickel (Ni) is used in battery and electronic manufacturing [2]. In addition, Hini et al. [49] indicated that Cr can be derived from the wearing and aging of tires and from tool manufacturing. The EF values of V (1.1), As (1.3), Ni (1.4), Sb (2.17), Cr (2.2), and Pb (2.8) were between 1 and 3, suggesting less enrichment of these metals. On the other hand, the EF values of Cu (3.9), Mo (4.2), and Sn (4.3) ranged between 3 and 5, suggesting a moderate enrichment level. Therefore, it is suggested that these metals (Sb, Mo, Sn, As, Ni, V, Pb, Cr, and Cu) might originate from vehicular and industrial activities. The result of the enrichment factor analysis showed that the EF value of Co (0.8 < 1) indicated a limited influence of human activity (i.e., no enrichment). The results of the PCA and the EF indicated that Co was of lithological (natural) origin, while other metals (i.e., Sb, Mo, As, Ni, Sn, V, Pb, Cr, and Cu) in street dust were of mixed origins (lithological and anthropogenic origins).

The PC2 component was characterized by high loading of Se, B, Mn, Ti, and Zn, contributing 18.3% to the total variance. The EF values of Se (0.95) and Mn (0.7) were lower than 1, thereby indicating that these metals showed limited enrichment and less impact from human activity. The EF values of B (2.02) and Ti (1.05) were between 1 and 3, demonstrating minor enrichment, and the EF value of Zn (5.28) ranged between 5 and 10, suggesting a moderate–severe level of enrichment. This means that Zn was caused by vehicular activities. The results of the PCA and the EF indicated that Se and Mn were of lithological (natural) origin, while the elements B, Ti, and Zn in street dust were of vehicular origin.

The PC3 component was dominated by Cd, and this factor contributed 9.2% to the total variance. Sources of Cd in street dust could be from diesel fuel, brake pads, and car paints [21]. In addition, the EF value of Cd (3.85) revealed moderate enrichment. This suggested that human activities may have influenced the concentration of Cd in street dust.

3.2.3. Cluster Analysis

Cluster analysis was used to reveal the differences between the potentially toxic elements and the differences among sampling sites for street-dust samples from the study area. The Euclidean distance method was used in the clustering of variables and row dendrograms. The results are represented as a heat map in Figure 4c. The top dendrogram shows the similarity between potentially toxic elements while the left dendrogram shows the clustering of the sampling sites. Two clusters of elements were identified: Mn, Zn, and Ti in cluster 1 and Se, Sb, Cd, Mo, B, Sn, As, Co, Ni, V, Pb, Cr, and Cu in cluster 2 (Figure 4c). The left dendrogram provides detailed information about the street-dust samples from which spatial differences were inferred. The cluster analysis results indicate two clusters of sampling sites: (1) D3, D4, and D5; (2) D1, D6, D8, D10, D2, D7, and D9, in terms of similarities (Figure 4c).

3.3. Pollution Indices

3.3.1. The Geo-Accumulation Index (I_{geo})

I_{geo} values were computed to assess the levels of accumulation of the metals in street dust (Figure 5a). The results show that Co, Se, Mn, Ti, and V were classified as uncontaminated, as the I_{geo} values of Co (-0.39 ± 0.22), Se (-0.25 ± 0.4), Mn (-0.1 ± 0.37), Ti (-0.08 ± 0.34), and V (-0.07 ± 0.25) were less than 0. The mean values of I_{geo} computed for As (0.15 ± 0.19), Ni (0.34 ± 0.38), B (0.87 ± 0.24), Sb (0.89 ± 0.59), and Cr (0.95 ± 0.4) belong to the uncontaminated-to-moderately-contaminated class. For Pb, Cd, Cu, Sn, Mo, and Zn, the I_{geo} values ranged from 1 to 2 (Pb (1.21 ± 0.67), Cd (1.37 ± 1.07), Cu (1.72 ± 0.61), Sn (1.79 ± 0.81), Mo (1.85 ± 0.56), and Zn (2 ± 0.99)), indicating a moderately contaminated level. Similar I_{geo} results for Pb, Cu, and Zn have been reported by Shahab et al. [18]. The mean I_{geo} value was the highest for Zn (2 ± 0.99) and increased in the following order: Co (-0.39 ± 0.22) < Se (-0.25 ± 0.4) < Mn (-0.1 ± 0.37) < Ti (-0.08 ± 0.34) < V (-0.07 ± 0.25) < As (0.15 ± 0.19) < Ni (0.34 ± 0.38) < B (0.87 ± 0.24) < Sb (0.89 ± 0.59) < Cr (0.95 ± 0.4) < Pb (1.21 ± 0.67) < Cd (1.37 ± 1.07) < Cu (1.72 ± 0.61) < Sn (1.79 ± 0.81) < Mo (1.85 ± 0.56) < Zn (2 ± 0.99), with higher I_{geo} values indicating greater levels of contamination. High I_{geo} values for Zn and Pb in the study can be linked to traffic activities. Among the 16 target metals, Zn was the biggest contributor to the potential ecological risk. The location exposed to the highest potential risk was D3.

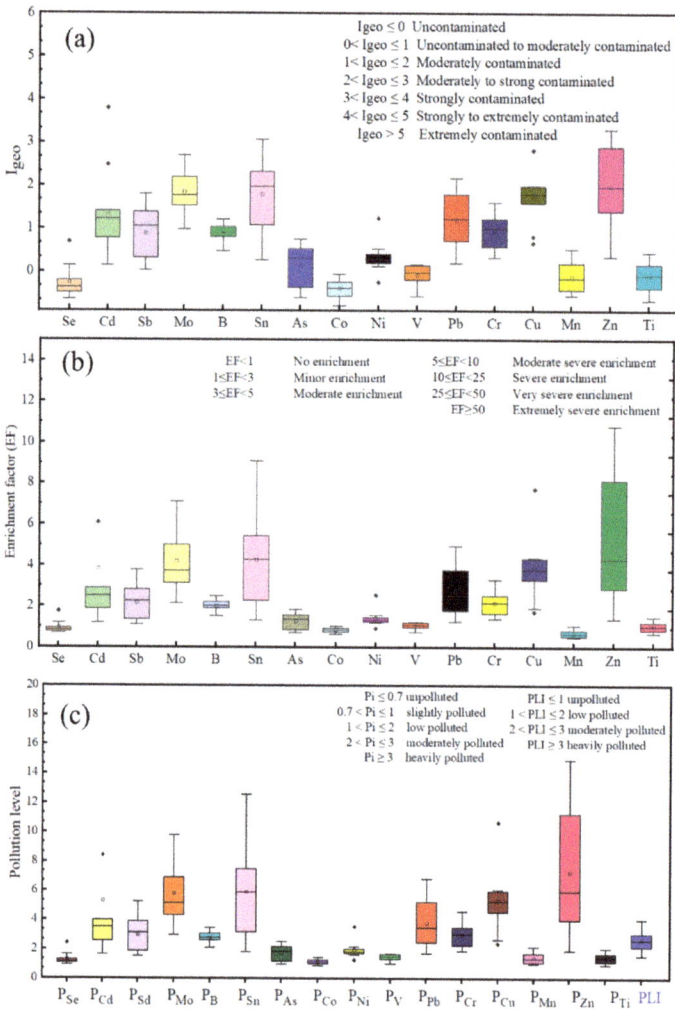

Figure 5. Box plots of enrichment factors (**a**), I_{geo} index values of heavy metals (**b**), and pollution levels of heavy metals (**c**) in this study (black dots present the outlier values).

3.3.2. Enrichment Factor (EF)

The EF values for each metal were determined to distinguish anthropogenic from natural sources and to evaluate the contamination level [62]. From Figure 5b, the mean values of the EF were ranked in the order Zn (5.28 ± 3.24) > Sn (4.27 ± 2.21) > Mo (4.21 ± 1.70) > Cu (3.86 ± 1.64) > Cd (3.85 ± 2.17) > Pb (2.75 >1.21) > Cr (2.18 ± 0.60) > Sb (2.17 ± 0.86) > B (2.02 ± 0.32) > Ni (1.42 ± 0.44) > As (1.27 ± 0.39) > V (1.05 ± 0.17) > Ti (1.05 ± 0.24) > Se (0.95 ± 0.32) > Co (0.84 ± 0.13) > Mn (0.70 ± 0.18). The mean values of the EF index of Mn (0.7), Co (0.84), and Se (0.95) were below 1, indicating that these elements were categorized as showing no enrichment. The EF values of Ti (1.05), V (1.05), As (1.27), Ni (1.42), B (2.02), Sb (2.17), Cr (2.18), and Pb (2.75) were between 1 and 3, thereby demonstrating minor enrichment. The EF values of Cd (3.85), Cu (3.86), Mo (4.21), and Sn (4.27) were between 3 and 5, revealing moderate enrichment by these elements. The EF value of Zn (5.28) ranged between 5 and 10, suggesting moderate–severe enrichment levels.

This suggests that in our sampling area, Cd, Cu, and Zn might be affected by anthropogenic activity. This indicates that human sources are very important [39].

3.3.3. Pollution Load Index (PLI)

A summary of the Pi and PLI values of the 16 target metals is shown in Figure 5c. The street-dust samples showed low pollution by Co (P_{Co} = 1.2), Se (P_{Se} = 1.3), V (P_V = 1.4), Mn (P_{Mn} = 1.4), Ti (P_{Ti} = 1.5), As (P_{As} = 1.7), and Ni (P_{Ni} = 2.0) and moderate pollution by B (P_B = 2.8), Sb (P_{Sb} = 3.0), and Cr (P_{Cr} = 3.0). The remaining elements, Pb (P_{Pb} = 3.8), Cd (P_{Cd} = 5.3), Cu (P_{Cu} = 5.3), Mo (P_{Mo} = 5.8), Sn (P_{Sn} = 5.9), and Zn (P_{Zn} = 7.3) were found to show heavy pollution. Kamani et al. [63] calculated the values of Pi for heavy metals in street dust in Tehran, Iran, obtaining values for Cd (P_{Cd} = 4.77), Pb (P_{Pb} = 4.78), Cu (P_{Cu} = 10.22), and Zn (P_{Zn} = 10.37), that indicated heavy pollution. Hayrat and Eziz [41] also revealed that dust samples from Korla, China were heavily polluted by Cr (P_{Cr} = 3.33), Cu (P_{Cu} = 5.81), Pb (P_{Pb} = 7.32), and Cd (P_{Cd} = 35.0), with the degree of pollution associated with anthropogenic activity. Another study conducted by Wahab et al. [21] in Malaysia presented the Pi values of metals in street dust in the Tunku Abdul Rahman road, Kuala Lumpur, where Zn (P_{Zn} = 3.94), Pb (P_{Pb} = 4.20), Cr (P_{Cr} = 5.78), and Cu (P_{Cu} = 8.43) showed high levels of pollution. The PLI values of metals in street dust fluctuate from 1.6 to 4.0, and an average value of 2.6 indicates moderate pollution (Figure 5c). Similar results have been reported by Dytłow and Górka-Kostrubiec [60] and Kabir et al. [22], who studied the toxic metals in street dust in Poland and Bangladesh.

3.4. Potential Ecological Risk (PER)

The PER data were calculated by summing the cumulative effects of all metals. The PER results for different locations are presented in Figure 6a. The mean level of the PER for the calculated metals in the street-dust samples was 207.43, and the values ranged from 111.17 to 431.53, suggesting a high potential ecological risk. Similarly, Kormoker et al. [61] found that the level of ecological risk from heavy metals (i.e., Cd, As, Pb, Cu, Ni, and Cr) in Lokhikol, Bangladesh was very high (PER = 270). Kamani et al. [63] conducted their study in the center of Tehran and revealed that the highest PER values were associated with bad traffic jams. The PER ranged from 81.93 to 508.2 with a mean value of 234.0, indicating a high level of potential ecological risk. Comparing the sampling sites, the highest PER value was at D4 and the lowest value was at D9. In this study, the average contribution of individual metals to the PER (Figure 6b) decreased in the following order for the elements: Zn (40.7%) > Mn (33.5%) > Cu (11.4%) > Cr (6.4%) > Pb > (4.1%) > Ni (2.4%) > Co (0.7%) > As (0.6%) > Cd (0.2%). The results suggest that Zn and Mn could be the main contributors to the ecological risk in our sampling area. Since Zn and Mn are known to be released from anthropogenic sources [48], it is necessary to control their emission to limit any threats to the ecosystem.

Figure 7 shows the relationship between the PER and the EF of nine metals (Cd, Co, Cr, Ni, Cu, Pb, As, Mn, and Zn). The R^2 values of Cu, Zn, and Mn were 0.9098, 0.8208, and 0.7563, respectively. This suggests that the EF values of Cu, Zn, and Mn were closely related to the PER. In contrast, no obvious correlation was found for Cd, Cr, Co, Ni, As, and Pb with regard to PER.

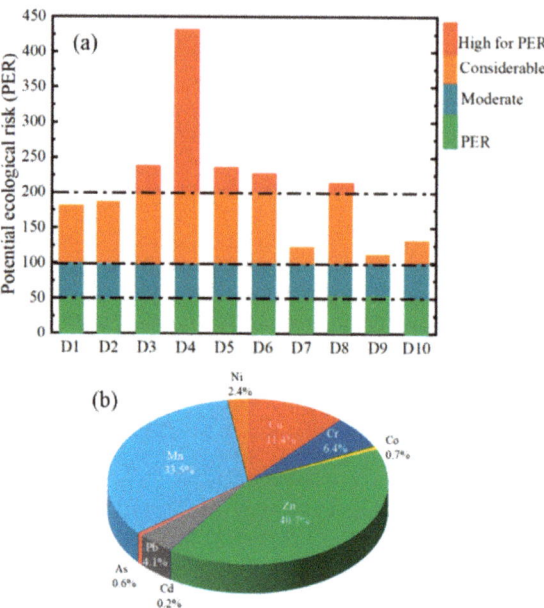

Figure 6. Spatial distribution of the potential ecological risk index: low (PER < 50), moderate (PER = 50–100), considerable (PER = 100–200), and high (PER > 200) (**a**) and percentage contribution of metals to ecological risk (**b**).

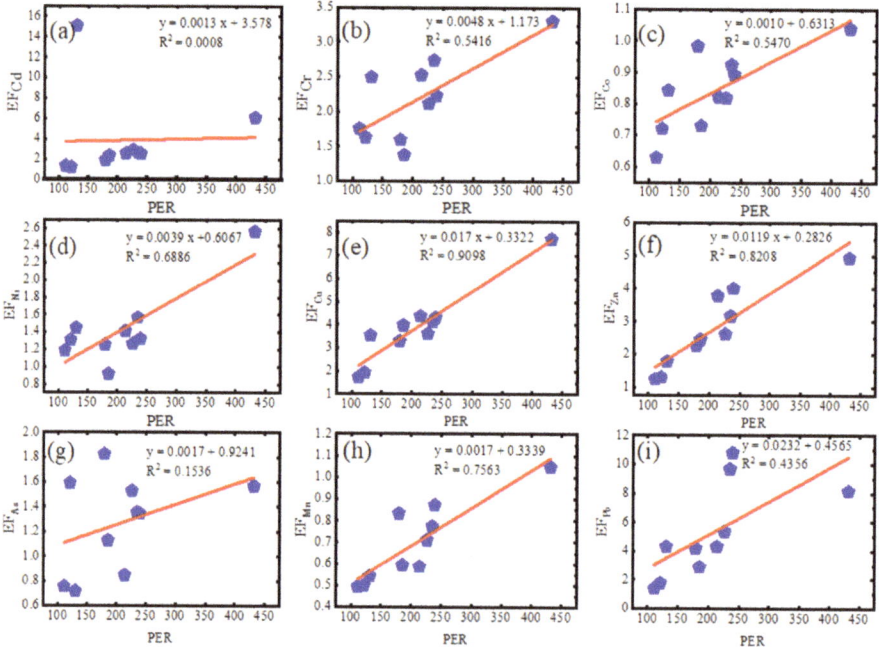

Figure 7. The relationship between the potential ecological risk index and enrichment factors: (**a**–**i**) show Cd, Co, Cr, Ni, Cu, Zn, As, Mn, and Pb results, respectively.

4. Conclusions

This study was conducted to evaluate the concentration of 16 metals (Se, Cd, Sb, Mo, B, Sn, As, Co, Ni, V, Pb, Cr, Cu, Mn, Zn, and Ti) in street dust from Ha Noi highway, HCM City. The mean concentrations of all metals were higher than the background values. Compared to the other metals, the highest concentration was observed for Ti (676.3 ± 155.4 mg/kg) and the lowest concentration for Se (0.4 ± 0.1 mg/kg). The metal concentrations decreased in the following order: Ti > Zn > Mn > Cu > Cr > Pb > V > Ni > Co > As > Sn > B > Mo > Sb > Cd > Se. The PCA and EF results revealed that Se, Mn, and Co were derived from a lithological (natural) origin, while most of the metals were significantly affected by anthropogenic activities, including industrial and vehicular sources. The PLI values of metals in street dust range from 1.6 to 4.0 and an average value of 2.6 indicates moderate pollution. We found that the value of PER (207.43) showed a high potential ecological risk. The results suggested that Zn (40.7%) and Mn (33.5%) could be the major contributors to the ecological risk. Although only a small number of samples were collected, the outcomes of this study will be useful for scientists to fill the information gap on the pollution of various metals in street dust from Vietnam, where there is a lack of available observational data. Furthermore, a large-scale survey including various areas with different characteristics is needed, as a future study, to better understand the pollution levels and emission sources of heavy metals in street dust.

Supplementary Materials: The following are available online at https://www.mdpi.com/article/10.3390/atmos12121548/s1, Figure S1: The scree plot of PCA; Table S1: Location and GPS coordinates of sampling (D) and background sites (BG); Table S2: The geo-accumulation index classification, standard criteria of enrichment factors, and pollution load index classification for the assessment of the pollution status of sampling sites; Table S3: The potential ecological risk index (Ei) and the potential ecological risk (PER) classification for ecological risk assessment; Table S4: Concentrations (mg/kg) of metals in street dust for the different sampling sites; Table S5: Results of principal component analysis for 16 heavy metals in street dust from Ha Noi highway, Ho Chi Minh City.

Author Contributions: Sampling, sample analysis, investigation, software, writing—original draft, writing—review and editing, V.-T.N.; data curation, conceptualization, methodology, writing—review and editing, D.-H.N., T.-B.N., L.-S.P.N., X.C.N., V.-C.D., T.-H.-H.N., T.-M.-T.H., H.-G.H., and T.-G.H.D.; supervision, conception, design of the methodology, writing—review and editing, N.D.D., T.-D.-H.V., M.-H.B., and X.-T.B. All authors have read and agreed to the published version of the manuscript.

Funding: This research was funded by Saigon University grant number [TĐ2020-57].

Institutional Review Board Statement: Not applicable.

Informed Consent Statement: Not applicable.

Data Availability Statement: The data presented in this study are available on request from the corresponding author.

Conflicts of Interest: The authors declare no conflict of interest. The funders had no role in the design of the study, in the collection, analyses, or interpretation of data, in the writing of the manuscript, or in the decision to publish the results.

References

1. Wei, X.; Gao, B.; Wang, P.; Zhou, H.; Lu, J. Pollution characteristics and health risk assessment of heavy metals in street dusts from different functional areas in Beijing, China. *Ecotoxicol. Environ. Saf.* **2015**, *112*, 186–192. [CrossRef] [PubMed]
2. Kabadayi, F.; Cesur, H. Determination of Cu, Pb, Zn, Ni, Co, Cd, and Mn in road dusts of Samsun City. *Environ. Monit. Assess.* **2010**, *168*, 241–253. [CrossRef] [PubMed]
3. Yu, B.; Lu, X.; Fan, X.; Fan, P.; Zuo, L.; Yang, Y.; Wang, L. Analyzing environmental risk, source and spatial distribution of potentially toxic elements in dust of residential area in Xi'an urban area, China. *Ecotoxicol. Environ. Saf.* **2021**, *208*, 111679. [CrossRef] [PubMed]
4. Chen, L.; Zhang, H.; Ding, M.; Devlin, A.T.; Wang, P.; Nie, M.; Xie, K. Exploration of the variations and relationships between trace metal enrichment in dust and ecological risks associated with rapid urban expansion. *Ecotoxicol. Environ. Saf.* **2021**, *212*, 111944. [CrossRef]

5. Men, C.; Liu, R.; Xu, L.; Wang, Q.; Guo, L.; Miao, Y.; Shen, Z. Source-specific ecological risk analysis and critical source identification of heavy metals in road dust in Beijing, China. *J. Hazard. Mater.* **2020**, *388*, 121763. [CrossRef] [PubMed]
6. Bartholomew, C.J.; Li, N.; Li, Y.; Dai, W.; Nibagwire, D.; Guo, T. Characteristics and health risk assessment of heavy metals in street dust for children in Jinhua, China. *Environ. Sci. Pollut. Res.* **2020**, *27*, 5042–5055. [CrossRef] [PubMed]
7. Wei, B.; Jiang, F.; Li, X.; Mu, S. Heavy metal induced ecological risk in the city of Urumqi, NW China. *Environ. Monit. Assess* **2010**, *160*, 33–45. [CrossRef]
8. Trujillo-González, J.M.; Torres-Mora, M.A.; Jiménez-Ballesta, R.; Zhang, J. Land-use-dependent spatial variation and exposure risk of heavy metals in road-deposited sediment in Villavicencio, Colombia. *Environ. Geochem. Health* **2019**, *41*, 667–679. [CrossRef]
9. Alsbou, E.M.E.; Al-Khashman, O.A. Heavy metal concentrations in roadside soil and street dust from Petra region, Jordan. *Environ. Monit. Assess.* **2018**, *190*, 48. [CrossRef]
10. Kariper, İ.A.; Üstündağ, İ.; Deniz, K.; Mülazımoğlu, İ.E.; Erdoğan, M.S.; Kadıoğlu, Y.K. Elemental monitoring of street dusts in Konya in Turkey. *Microchem. J.* **2019**, *148*, 338–345. [CrossRef]
11. Al-Taani, A.A.; Nazzal, Y.; Howari, F.M. Assessment of heavy metals in roadside dust along the Abu Dhabi–Al Ain National Highway, UAE. *Environ. Earth Sci.* **2019**, *78*, 1–13. [CrossRef]
12. Dat, N.D.; Nguyen, V.T.; Bui, X.T.; Bui, M.H.; Nguyen, L.S.P.; Nguyen, X.C.; Tran, A.T.K.; Ju, Y.R.; Nguyen, D.H.; Bui, H.N. Contamination, source attribution, and potential health risks of heavy metals in street dust of a metropolitan area in Southern Vietnam. *Environ. Sci. Pollut. Res.* **2021**, *28*, 50405–50419. [CrossRef]
13. Zhang, J.; Wu, L.; Zhang, Y.; Li, F.; Fang, X.; Mao, H. Elemental composition and risk assessment of heavy metals in the PM10 fractions of road dust and roadside soil. *Particuology* **2019**, *44*, 146–152. [CrossRef]
14. Zhang, M.; Li, X.; Yang, R.; Wang, J.; Ai, Y.; Gao, Y.; Zhang, Y.; Zhang, X.; Yan, X.; Liu, B. Multipotential toxic metals accumulated in urban soil and street dust from Xining City, NW China: Spatial occurrences, sources, and health risks. *Arch. Environ. Contam. Toxicol.* **2019**, *76*, 308–330. [CrossRef] [PubMed]
15. Ali, M.U.; Liu, G.; Yousaf, B.; Abbas, Q.; Ullah, H.; Munir, M.A.M.; Fu, B. Pollution characteristics and human health risks of potentially (eco) toxic elements (PTEs) in road dust from metropolitan area of Hefei, China. *Chemosphere* **2017**, *181*, 111–121. [CrossRef] [PubMed]
16. Sadeghdoust, F.; Ghanavati, N.; Nazarpour, A.; Babaenejad, T.; Watts, M.J. Hazard, ecological, and human health risk assessment of heavy metals in street dust in Dezful, Iran. *Arab. J. Geosci.* **2020**, *13*, 1–14. [CrossRef]
17. Abbasi, S.; Keshavarzi, B.; Moore, F.; Mahmoudi, M.R. Fractionation, source identification and risk assessment of potentially toxic elements in street dust of the most important center for petrochemical products, Asaluyeh County, Iran. *Environ. Earth Sci.* **2018**, *77*, 1–19. [CrossRef]
18. Shahab, A.; Zhang, H.; Ullah, H.; Rashid, A.; Rad, S.; Li, J.; Xiao, H. Pollution characteristics and toxicity of potentially toxic elements in road dust of a tourist city, Guilin, China: Ecological and health risk assessment. *Environ. Pollut.* **2020**, *266*, 115419. [CrossRef] [PubMed]
19. Alharbi, B.H.; Pasha, M.J.; Alotaibi, M.D.; Alduwais, A.K.; Al-Shamsi, M.A.S. Contamination and risk levels of metals associated with urban street dust in Riyadh, Saudi Arabia. *Environ. Sci. Pollut. Res.* **2020**, *27*, 18475–18487. [CrossRef]
20. Musa, A.; Hamza, S.; Kidak, R. Street dust heavy metal pollution implication on human health in Nicosia, North Cyprus. *Environ. Sci. Pollut. Res.* **2019**, *26*, 28993–29002. [CrossRef] [PubMed]
21. Wahab, M.I.A.; Abd Razak, W.M.A.; Sahani, M.; Khan, M.F. Characteristics and health effect of heavy metals on non-exhaust road dusts in Kuala Lumpur. *Sci. Total Environ.* **2020**, *703*, 135535. [CrossRef] [PubMed]
22. Kabir, M.H.; Kormoker, T.; Islam, M.S.; Khan, R.; Shammi, R.S.; Tusher, T.R.; Proshad, R.; Islam, M.S.; Idris, A.M. Potentially toxic elements in street dust from an urban city of a developing country: Ecological and probabilistic health risks assessment. *Environ. Sci. Pollut. Res.* **2021**, *28*, 57126–57148. [CrossRef]
23. Kabir, M.H.; Kormoker, T.; Shammi, R.S.; Tusher, T.R.; Islam, M.S.; Khan, R.; Omor, M.Z.U.; Sarker, M.E.; Yeasmin, M.; Idris, A.M. A comprehensive assessment of heavy metal contamination in road dusts along a hectic national highway of Bangladesh: Spatial distribution, sources of contamination, ecological and human health risks. *Toxin Rev.* **2021**, 1–20. Available online: https://www.tandfonline.com/doi/abs/10.1080/15569543.2021.1952436 (accessed on 16 November 2021). [CrossRef]
24. Egbueri, J.C.; Ukah, B.U.; Ubido, O.E.; Unigwe, C.O. A chemometric approach to source apportionment, ecological and health risk assessment of heavy metals in industrial soils from southwestern Nigeria. *Int. J. Environ. Anal. Chem.* **2020**, 1–19. Available online: https://www.tandfonline.com/doi/abs/10.1080/03067319.2020.1769615?journalCode=geac20 (accessed on 16 November 2021). [CrossRef]
25. Ghanavati, N.; Nazarpour, A.; De Vivo, B. Ecological and human health risk assessment of toxic metals in street dusts and surface soils in Ahvaz, Iran. *Environ. Geochem. Health* **2019**, *41*, 875–891. [CrossRef] [PubMed]
26. Roy, S.; Gupta, S.K.; Prakash, J.; Habib, G.; Baudh, K.; Nasr, M. Ecological and human health risk assessment of heavy metal contamination in road dust in the National Capital Territory (NCT) of Delhi, India. *Environ. Sci. Pollut. Res.* **2019**, *26*, 30413–30425. [CrossRef]
27. Phi, T.H.; Chinh, P.M.; Ly, L.T.M.; Thai, P.K. Spatial distribution of elemental concentrations in street dust of Hanoi, Vietnam. *Bull. Environ. Contam. Toxicol.* **2017**, *98*, 277–282. [CrossRef] [PubMed]

28. Phi, T.H.; Chinh, P.M.; Cuong, D.D.; Ly, L.T.M.; Van Thinh, N.; Thai, P.K. Elemental concentrations in roadside dust along two national highways in northern Vietnam and the health-risk implication. *Arch. Environ. Contam. Toxicol.* **2018**, *74*, 46–55. [CrossRef] [PubMed]
29. GSOVietnam. *General Statistics Office of Vietnam, Statistical Yearbook of Vietnam, Statistical Publishing House*; General Statistics Office of Vietnam: Hanoi, Vietnam, 2019.
30. Trojanowska, M.; Świetlik, R. Investigations of the chemical distribution of heavy metals in street dust and its impact on risk assessment for human health, case study of Radom (Poland). *Hum. Ecol. Risk. Assess.* **2019**, *26*, 1–20. [CrossRef]
31. USEPA. *SW-846 Test. Method 3051A: Microwave Assisted Acid Digestion of Sediments, Sludges, Soils, and Oils*; United States Environmental Protection Agency: Washington, DC, USA, 2007.
32. USEPA. *Method 200.8, Revision 5.4: Determination of Trace Elements in Waters and Wastes by Inductively Coupled Plasma—Mass Spectrometry*; United States Environmental Protection Agency: Washington, DC, USA, 1994.
33. Buat-Menard, P.; Chesselet, R. Variable influence of the atmospheric flux on the trace metal chemistry of oceanic suspended matter. *Earth Planet. Sci. Lett.* **1979**, *42*, 399–411. [CrossRef]
34. Khademi, H.; Gabarrón, M.; Abbaspour, A.; Martínez-Martínez, S.; Faz, A.; Acosta, J. Distribution of metal (loid) s in particle size fraction in urban soil and street dust: Influence of population density. *Environ. Geochem. Health* **2020**, *42*, 4341–4354. [CrossRef] [PubMed]
35. Fang, G.C.; Wu, Y.S.; Chang, S.Y.; Huang, S.H.; Rau, J.Y. Size distributions of ambient air particles and enrichment factor analyses of metallic elements at Taichung Harbor near the Taiwan Strait. *Atmos. Res.* **2006**, *81*, 320–333. [CrossRef]
36. Li, F.; Zhang, J.; Huang, J.; Huang, D.; Yang, J.; Song, Y.; Zeng, G. Heavy metals in road dust from Xiandao District, Changsha City, China: Characteristics, health risk assessment, and integrated source identification. *Environ. Sci. Pollut. Res.* **2016**, *23*, 13100–13113. [CrossRef] [PubMed]
37. Joshi, U.M.; Vijayaraghavan, K.; Balasubramanian, R. Elemental composition of urban street dusts and their dissolution characteristics in various aqueous media. *Chemosphere* **2009**, *77*, 526–533. [CrossRef]
38. Liu, E.; Yan, T.; Birch, G.; Zhu, Y. Pollution and health risk of potentially toxic metals in urban road dust in Nanjing, a mega-city of China. *Sci. Total Environ.* **2014**, *476*, 522–531. [CrossRef]
39. Zhou, L.; Liu, G.; Shen, M.; Hu, R.; Sun, M.; Liu, Y. Characteristics and health risk assessment of heavy metals in indoor dust from different functional areas in Hefei, China. *Environ. Pollut.* **2019**, *251*, 839–849. [CrossRef]
40. Cheng, Z.; Chen, L.-J.; Li, H.-H.; Lin, J.-Q.; Yang, Z.-B.; Yang, Y.-X.; Xu, X.-X.; Xian, J.-R.; Shao, J.-R.; Zhu, X.-M. Characteristics and health risk assessment of heavy metals exposure via household dust from urban area in Chengdu, China. *Sci. Total Environ.* **2018**, *619*, 621–629. [CrossRef]
41. Hayrat, A.; Eziz, M. Identification of the spatial distributions, pollution levels, sources, and health risk of heavy metals in surface dusts from Korla, NW China. *Open Geosci.* **2020**, *12*, 1338–1349. [CrossRef]
42. Hakanson, L. An ecological risk index for aquatic pollution control. A sedimentological approach. *Water Res.* **1980**, *14*, 975–1001. [CrossRef]
43. Vu, C.T.; Lin, C.; Nguyen, K.A.; Shern, C.-C.; Kuo, Y.-M. Ecological risk assessment of heavy metals sampled in sediments and water of the Houjing River, Taiwan. *Environ. Earth Sci.* **2018**, *77*, 388. [CrossRef]
44. Wang, G.; Xia, D.; Liu, X.; Chen, F.; Yu, Y.; Yang, L.; Chen, J.; Zhou, A. Spatial and temporal variation in magnetic properties of street dust in Lanzhou City, China. *Chin. Sci. Bull.* **2008**, *53*, 1913–1923. [CrossRef]
45. Pan, H.; Lu, X.; Lei, K. A comprehensive analysis of heavy metals in urban road dust of Xi'an, China: Contamination, source apportionment and spatial distribution. *Sci. Total Environ.* **2017**, *609*, 1361–1369. [CrossRef] [PubMed]
46. Shabbaj, I.I.; Alghamdi, M.A.; Shamy, M.; Hassan, S.K.; Alsharif, M.M.; Khoder, M.I. Risk assessment and implication of human exposure to road dust heavy metals in Jeddah, Saudi Arabia. *Int. J. Environ. Res. Public Health* **2018**, *15*, 36. [CrossRef]
47. Bourliva, A.; Christophoridis, C.; Papadopoulou, L.; Giouri, K.; Papadopoulos, A.; Mitsika, E.; Fytianos, K. Characterization, heavy metal content and health risk assessment of urban road dusts from the historic center of the city of Thessaloniki, Greece. *Environ. Geochem. Health* **2017**, *39*, 611–634. [CrossRef]
48. Idris, A.M.; Alqahtani, F.M.; Said, T.O.; Fawy, K.F. Contamination level and risk assessment of heavy metal deposited in street dusts in Khamees-Mushait city, Saudi Arabia. *Hum. Ecol. Risk Assess* **2020**, *26*, 495–511. [CrossRef]
49. Hini, G.; Eziz, M.; Wang, W.; Ili, A.; Li, X. Spatial distribution, contamination levels, sources, and potential health risk assessment of trace elements in street dusts of Urumqi city, NW China. *Hum. Ecol. Risk Assess.* **2019**, *26*, 2112–2128. [CrossRef]
50. Qadeer, A.; Saqib, Z.A.; Ajmal, Z.; Xing, C.; Khalil, S.K.; Usman, M.; Huang, Y.; Bashir, S.; Ahmad, Z.; Ahmed, S. Concentrations, pollution indices and health risk assessment of heavy metals in road dust from two urbanized cities of Pakistan: Comparing two sampling methods for heavy metals concentration. *Sustain. Cities Soc.* **2020**, *53*, 101959. [CrossRef]
51. Duong, T.T.T.; Lee, B.K. Determining contamination level of heavy metals in road dust from busy traffic areas with different characteristics. *J. Environ. Manag.* **2011**, *92*, 554–562. [CrossRef]

52. Dong, S.; Gonzalez, R.O.; Harrison, R.M.; Green, D.; North, R.; Fowler, G.; Weiss, D. Isotopic signatures in atmospheric particulate matter suggest important contributions from recycled gasoline for lead and non-exhaust traffic sources for copper and zinc in aerosols in London, United Kingdom. *Atmos Environ.* **2017**. Available online: https://kclpure.kcl.ac.uk/portal/en/publications/isotopic-signatures-in-atmospheric-particulate-matter-suggest-important-contribu-tions-from-recycled-gasoline-for-lead-and-nonexhaust-traffic-sources-for-copper-and-zinc-in-aerosols-in-london-united-kingdom(447f5aeb-b0b0-445b-b525-96602a3866fa).html (accessed on 16 November 2021). [CrossRef]
53. Taiwo, A.; Musa, M.; Oguntoke, O.; Afolabi, T.; Sadiq, A.; Akanji, M.; Shehu, M. Spatial distribution, pollution index, receptor modelling and health risk assessment of metals in road dust from Lagos metropolis, Southwestern Nigeria. *Adv. Environ.* **2020**, *2*, 100012. [CrossRef]
54. Men, C.; Liu, R.; Xu, F.; Wang, Q.; Guo, L.; Shen, Z. Pollution characteristics, risk assessment, and source apportionment of heavy metals in road dust in Beijing, China. *Sci. Total Environ.* **2018**, *612*, 138–147. [CrossRef] [PubMed]
55. Rahman, M.S.; Khan, M.D.H.; Jolly, Y.N.; Kabir, J.; Akter, S.; Salam, A. Assessing risk to human health for heavy metal contamination through street dust in the Southeast Asian Megacity: Dhaka, Bangladesh. *Sci. Total Environ.* **2019**, *660*, 1610–1622. [CrossRef] [PubMed]
56. Duong, T.T.; Lee, B.-K. Partitioning and mobility behavior of metals in road dusts from national-scale industrial areas in Korea. *Atmos Environ.* **2009**, *43*, 3502–3509. [CrossRef]
57. Peltier, R.E.; Lippmann, M. Residual oil combustion: Distributions of airborne nickel and vanadium within New York City. *J. Expo. Sci. Environ. Epidemiol.* **2010**, *20*, 342–350. [CrossRef] [PubMed]
58. Lau, W.K.Y.; Liang, P.; Man, Y.B.; Chung, S.S.; Wong, M.H. Human health risk assessment based on trace metals in suspended air particulates, surface dust, and floor dust from e-waste recycling workshops in Hong Kong, China. *Environ. Sci. Pollut. Res.* **2014**, *21*, 3813–3825. [CrossRef] [PubMed]
59. Shabanda, I.S.; Koki, I.B.; Low, K.H.; Zain, S.M.; Khor, S.M.; Bakar, N.K.A. Daily exposure to toxic metals through urban road dust from industrial, commercial, heavy traffic, and residential areas in Petaling Jaya, Malaysia: A health risk assessment. *Environ. Sci. Pollut. Res.* **2019**, *26*, 37193–37211. [CrossRef]
60. Dytłow, S.; Górka-Kostrubiec, B. Concentration of heavy metals in street dust: An implication of using different geochemical background data in estimating the level of heavy metal pollution. *Environ. Geochem. Health* **2021**, *43*, 521–535. [CrossRef] [PubMed]
61. Kormoker, T.; Proshad, R.; Islam, S.; Ahmed, S.; Chandra, K.; Uddin, M.; Rahman, M. Toxic metals in agricultural soils near the industrial areas of Bangladesh: Ecological and human health risk assessment. *Toxin Rev.* **2019**, 1–20. Available online: https://www.tandfonline.com/doi/abs/10.1080/15569543.2019.1650777 (accessed on 16 November 2021). [CrossRef]
62. Malakootian, M.; Mohammadi, A.; Nasiri, A.; Asadi, A.M.S.; Conti, G.O.; Faraji, M. Spatial distribution and correlations among elements in smaller than 75 μm street dust: Ecological and probabilistic health risk assessment. *Environ. Geochem. Health* **2021**, *43*, 567–583. [CrossRef] [PubMed]
63. Kamani, H.; Mahvi, A.H.; Seyedsalehi, M.; Jaafari, J.; Hoseini, M.; Safari, G.H.; Dalvand, A.; Aslani, H.; Mirzaei, N.; Ashrafi, S.D. Contamination and ecological risk assessment of heavy metals in street dust of Tehran, Iran. *Int. J. Environ. Sci. Technol.* **2017**, *14*, 2675–2682. [CrossRef]

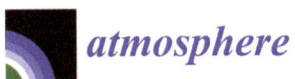

Article

Quantification and Characterization of Metals in Ultrafine Road Dust Particles

Suzanne Beauchemin [1,*], Christine Levesque [1], Clare L. S. Wiseman [2,3,4] and Pat E. Rasmussen [1,5]

1. Environmental Health Science and Research Bureau, Health Canada, 251 Sir Frederick Banting Driveway, Ottawa, ON K1A 0K9, Canada; christine.levesque@hc-sc.gc.ca (C.L.); pat.rasmussen@hc-sc.gc.ca (P.E.R.)
2. School of the Environment, University of Toronto, Toronto, ON M5S 3E8, Canada; clare.wiseman@utoronto.ca
3. Dalla Lana School of Public Health, University of Toronto, Toronto, ON M5T 3M7, Canada
4. Department of Physical and Environmental Sciences, University of Toronto (Scarborough), Toronto, ON M1C 1A4, Canada
5. Department of Earth and Environmental Science, University of Ottawa, Ottawa, ON K1N 6N5, Canada
* Correspondence: suzanne.beauchemin@hc-sc.gc.ca

Abstract: Road dust is an important source of resuspended particulate matter (PM) but information is lacking on the chemical composition of the ultrafine particle fraction (UFP; <0.1 µm). This study investigated metal concentrations in UFP isolated from the "dust box" of sweepings collected by the City of Toronto, Canada, using regenerative-air-street sweepers. Dust box samples from expressway, arterial and local roads were aerosolized in the laboratory and were separated into thirteen particle size fractions ranging from 10 nm to 10 µm (PM_{10}). The UFP fraction accounted for about 2% of the total mass of resuspended PM_{10} (range 0.23–8.36%). Elemental analysis using ICP-MS and ICP-OES revealed a marked enrichment in Cd, Cr, Zn and V concentration in UFP compared to the dust box material (nano to dust box ratio $\geq$ 2). UFP from arterial roads contained two times more Cd, Zn and V and nine times more Cr than UFP from local roads. The highest median concentration of Zn was observed for the municipal expressway, attributed to greater volumes of traffic, including light to heavy duty vehicles, and higher speeds. The observed elevated concentrations of transition metals in UFP are a human health concern, given their potential to cause oxidative stress in lung cells.

Keywords: road dust; street dust; metals; ultrafine particles; UFP; aerosolization; resuspension; incidental nanoparticles

Citation: Beauchemin, S.; Levesque, C.; Wiseman, C.L.S.; Rasmussen, P.E. Quantification and Characterization of Metals in Ultrafine Road Dust Particles. *Atmosphere* **2021**, *12*, 1564. https://doi.org/10.3390/atmos12121564

Academic Editors: Dmitry Vlasov, Omar Ramírez Hernández and Ashok Luhar

Received: 4 November 2021
Accepted: 24 November 2021
Published: 26 November 2021

Publisher's Note: MDPI stays neutral with regard to jurisdictional claims in published maps and institutional affiliations.

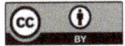

Copyright: © 2021 by the authors. Licensee MDPI, Basel, Switzerland. This article is an open access article distributed under the terms and conditions of the Creative Commons Attribution (CC BY) license (https:// creativecommons.org/licenses/by/ 4.0/).

1. Introduction

The chemical composition and contribution of ultrafine particles (UFP; <0.1 µm) to the toxicity of airborne particulate matter (PM) has yet to be fully characterized. Ambient air pollution has been associated with various adverse health effects such as respiratory and cardiovascular disease and lung cancer [1,2]. Air quality regulations have been established in many countries to limit the mass concentration of PM $\leq$ 10 µm aerodynamic diameter (PM_{10}), as well as PM $\leq$ 2.5 µm ($PM_{2.5}$). However, no regulation currently exists around the world for UFP due to a scarcity of data [3].

The penetration depth of PM into the respiratory system is largely determined by its size. PM_{10} is defined as the "thoracic" fraction, with 50% of particles small enough to penetrate beyond the larynx [4]. $PM_{2.5}$ represents the "respirable" particles capable of reaching the unciliated airways of the pulmonary region; this fine fraction can particularly affect those considered to be most vulnerable when exposed, including children and elders [2–4]. Ultrafine particles are of special concern due to their ability to reach the alveoli and be translocated into the blood stream. Upon entering systemic circulation, UFPs are easily distributed throughout the body and can accumulate in secondary organs such as the liver, brain and heart [5]. There is also evidence that UFP can be directly translocated to the brain via the olfactory pathway [6,7]. To better assess the potential impacts of UFP on health, more data on their concentration and composition in common sources of airborne PM, including road dust are essential.

Road dust contains particles from soils, eroded material from buildings and pavements, vehicle exhaust and non-exhaust emissions, de-icing salt and atmospheric deposition [8,9]. Resuspension of road dust represents a major source of PM_{10} in urban environments [10–14] but its contribution to airborne UFP remains ill-defined. According to the Air Quality Expert Group [3], combustion related to vehicular transport is one of the main sources of UFP in Europe. UFP arising from exhaust combustion have a short lifetime and are generally highest near intense traffic areas [12]. Vehicle non-exhaust emissions from frictional processes such as braking, tire wearing, and abrasion of road surface can also release UFP. While abrasion processes tend to emit coarser particles in brake and tire wear dust (>2.5 µm), UFP are also generated as a result of volatilization and re-condensation under higher temperature conditions characteristic of intense braking [8,11,15,16]. In laboratory tests using a brake dynamometer, the number of UFP released was at least three orders of magnitude higher than micron-size particles; a marked increase in UFP emissions occurred at around 300 °C, corresponding to the combustion of volatile organic compounds in the brakes [15]. In the last couple of decades, the implementation of stringent exhaust emission standards, along with improvements in engine technology, has resulted in a significant decline of automotive exhaust emissions. At the same time, the contribution of non-exhaust vehicle emissions, including nanoparticles, to ambient pollution has become an increasingly important issue to be considered in the context of air quality [11].

Compared to PM_{10} and $PM_{2.5}$, the chemical composition of UFP has been much less studied, largely due to challenges in collecting enough material for chemical analysis [17]. Airborne UFP contain a large fraction of organic compounds (up to 50%) [18]. The metal content of this fraction is also significant in urban environments. For instance, the mass concentration of the metal oxides of UFP measured in seven Californian cities was reported to range from 0.6% to 26% [19]. Metals and organic compounds have been identified as the main cause of the human toxicity of inhaled PM due to their ability to cause cellular oxidative stress by promoting electron transfer and inducing the production of reactive oxygen species (ROS) [20,21]. Trace elements, such as Pb, Zn, Cu, Cd, Cr, Ni, V and As, and ultratrace metals, such as Pt, Pd and Rh, released by vehicle exhaust or non-exhaust emissions (e.g., tires, brake pads) are typically elevated in urban road dust compared to the local background [22–25]. Of particular concern is the fact that these potentially toxic elements are even more enriched in the fine inhalable particles (PM_{10} or $PM_{2.5}$) compared to bulk road dust [9,14,26–30]. Similarly, enrichment in Cu, Zn, Sb, and Ti was observed in the nano-size fraction compared to the original bulk road dust (<100 µm) from Moscow [17].

In companion papers, Levesque et al. [31] and Wiseman et al. [14] recently evaluated the sources, concentrations and lung bioaccessibility of metals and metalloids in road dust samples collected by street-sweeping vehicles from expressways, arterial and local roads in Toronto (ON, Canada; 2.9 million inhabitants). These studies showed an enrichment in several metal(loid)s as particle size decreased: from the bulk road dust (<2 mm) to the dust box sweepings (<10 µm), and from the dust box sweepings to the fine fraction (<1.8 µm). The current study investigates the metal(loid) concentrations in UFP resuspended from a few key dust box sweepings representative of the three road types. The objectives of this study are to: (1) quantify the proportion of resuspendable UFP in a range of dust box sweepings, (2) determine metal(loid) concentrations in the nano-scale fractions; and (3) discuss the significance of the results for human health in view of selected relevant research studies. The overall goal is to advance our understanding of the metal composition of UFP and its potential implication for human health in an urban context.

2. Materials and Methods

2.1. Road Dust Samples

Road dust samples were collected in the fall of 2015 and the spring of 2016 by the city of Toronto using regenerative-air-street sweepers (see Wiseman et al. [28] for further details). Each sample represents a dust composite collected over many kilometers (from 6 to 45 km) and several hours. Samples from the dust box compartments of the street-sweeping vehicles were used in this study. Previous characterization of the dust box sweepings reported a measured median particle size diameter of 9.4 µm [28]. For the aerosolization and particle size fractionation experiments in the present study, a subset of six samples were selected from the 32 dust box samples characterized by Wiseman et al. [14]. The number of investigated samples was limited by the lengthy and time-consuming fractionation protocol. The samples were selected among different road types and areas in Toronto to represent a range of traffic volumes: two from local roads ("LR") from two different districts (<2500 vehicles day^{-1}; 30–50 km h^{-1}), three from arterial roads ("Art") within the same district (8000–40,000 vehicles day^{-1}; 40–60 km h^{-1}) and one from an expressway ("Ex") (>40,000 vehicles day^{-1}; 80–100 km h^{-1}). Samples were collected in three different community council areas (formerly called districts): (1) Toronto and East York (D1), which includes downtown and is the most densely populated; (2) Etobicoke York (D2); and (3) Scarborough (D4) [32]. The three arterial samples included in this study are from the same roads in Scarborough (D4), collected during consecutive weeks as part of the city's sweeping schedule (Art-D4-W1, -W2, -W3). Prior to particle size fractionation, the dust box sweepings were sieved < 56 µm to discard possible larger particles. Based on laser diffraction analysis, the median particle size diameter for the six sieved dust box samples ranged from 9.8 to 21.2 µm. These samples are referred to as "dust box" in this paper.

2.2. Particle Size Fractionation of the Resuspended Dust Box

The approach for aerosolization and particle size fractionation has been described by Levesque et al. [31]. Briefly, a fluidized bed aerosol generator (TSI Incorporated, model 3400 A) was used to resuspend the dust samples using a flow rate of 10 L/min and helium (He) as the carrier gas. The fluidized bed is composed of 100 µm bronze beads maintained in boiling action by the He flow to facilitate deagglomeration and resuspension of pre-existing fine particles in the dust. This approach has been selected because the particle size distribution of the produced aerosols is representative of the parental sample. The optimized breaking of aggregates by the boiling action of beads may overestimate the aerosol mass compared to natural road conditions but a conservative estimate is preferable for health risk assessment. A ½ inch cyclone at the top of the chamber prevents the dispersal of particles > 40 µm. After 1 h of stabilization, the aerosol generator was connected to a micro-orifice uniform deposit impactor (MSP Corp., MOUDI II^{TM} 125B) consisting of 13 impaction stages, which allows separation of the particles into size fractions ranging from 0.01 to 10 µm (aerodynamic diameter; Table 1). The dust was collected on Teflon filters (47 mm PTFE with polymethylpentene (PMP) support rings, Pall Corp.) for 2 to 4 h; each sample was run in triplicate [31]. Between each sample, the aerosol generator and the impactor were disassembled and washed with deionized water to avoid cross-contamination. Buoyancy-corrected gravimetric analysis of the Teflon filters prior to and after loading was performed inside Health Canada's "Archimedes M3^{TM}" Buoyancy-Corrected Gravimetric Analysis Facility as described in Rasmussen et al. [33].

Table 1. Impaction stages of the MOUDI II impactor, corresponding particle sizes collected on the filters and classes defined for the current study.

Nano MOUDI Nominal Cut-Point	Particle Size on Filter	Classes
nm	nm	
10,000	>10,000	-
5600	<10,000 >5600	Micron
3200	<5600 >3200	1–10 μm
1800	<3200 >1800	(PM_{10-1})
1000	<1800 >1000	
560	<1000 >560	Sub-micron
320	<560 >320	0.1–1 μm
180	<320 >180	($PM_{1-0.1}$)
100	<180 >100	
56	<100 >56	Nano
32	<56 >32	<100 nm
18	<32 >18	($PM_{0.1}$ or UFP)
10	<18 >10	

2.3. Element Analysis

Total element concentrations of the dust box samples were determined in triplicate using a 1 h ultrasonic dissolution in 45% HNO_3/0.8% HF and a solid to solution ratio of 2 mg: 6 mL [34]. Inductively coupled plasma—mass spectrometry (ICP-MS) or inductively coupled plasma—optical emission spectrometry (ICP-OES) was used for elemental determination, depending on the concentration level. Filters from the resuspension experiments (two to three replicates per size fraction) were characterized for total concentrations using the same method.

2.4. Quality Assurance

Considering that filter samples in the nano-scale fraction are characterized by negligible to small particle mass (<0.26 mg/filter), it was important to implement rigorous quality assurance measures throughout the study to evaluate the reliability of the results. The accuracy of the gravimetric analyses was assessed by weighing a series of filter blanks (n = 15, mean weight 0.01 mg). For a filter with dust mass loading below the mean filter blank weight, concentrations of elements were not calculated to avoid generating artificially high values. Procedural blanks, filter blanks and certified reference materials for indoor dust (NIST 2584), urban particulate matter (NIST 1648), soil (NIST 2711), road dust (BCR-723) and auto catalysts (NIST 2557) were included during acid digestion of the dust-loaded filters and ICP determination. QA/QC results for digestion recovery of reference materials and limits of detection for elements of interest for ICP analyses are given in Supplemental Information (Table S1). As reported by Levesque et al. [31], total element recoveries for NIST 2584 ranged between 80–120%. When considering other reference materials, the recoveries fell within the 70–130% range, except for Cr (<43%) in BCR-723 and NIST 1648, and Ti (<63%) for all materials (SI-Table S1). In the NIST 1648 reference material, chromium occurs dominantly as chromite; refractory minerals such as chromite are not fully dissolved by acid digestion [35,36]. Therefore, the ultrasonic HNO_3/HF digestion method used in this study might underestimate total Cr in road dust samples if a fraction was in the form of chromite. For loaded filters, negative ICP values lower than the mean value of all procedural blanks minus three standard deviations were treated as outliers and were discarded [37]. Negative values falling within the mean value for all procedural blanks minus three standard deviations were replaced by "0". Positive values smaller than the limit of detection (<LOD) were kept as is but were flagged [38]. Procedural blank and filter blank values within each batch were subtracted from the ICP readings. Fresh bronze beads were used for each sample. A blank resuspension run was conducted to assess the occurrence of possible dust contamination by the bronze beads. The initial results

were inconclusive, however, as loading masses on filters were <LOD. To investigate this further, the bronze beads were digested by aqua regia in triplicate for total element analysis by ICP-OES or ICP-MS. The beads contained on average: 87.3 wt.% Cu, 10.8 wt.% Sn, 193 mg Pb kg^{-1}, 36 mg Ni kg^{-1}, 34 mg Zn kg^{-1}, 11 mg Bi kg^{-1}, 11 mg As kg^{-1}, 1.8 mg Ag kg^{-1}, 1.3 mg Co kg^{-1}, and 1.0 mg Sb kg^{-1}. Concentrations of Cu, Sn, Pb, Ni, Bi and As in the bronze beads were higher than, or in the same range as, those from the road dust samples. Given the potential for cross-contamination, these elements were not included in the analyses of aerosolized dust.

2.5. Data Analysis

Given frequent missing or <LOD values in the nano-scale range, the MOUDI fractions were categorized into three classes (micron, sub-micron and nano size; Table 1) to facilitate descriptive statistical analyses. Median and inter quantile ranges (IQR) were preferred as a measure of dispersion rather than mean and standard deviation because they are less influenced by outliers and can be used with a large number of <LOD values [39,40]. The IQR is calculated as the difference between the 75th and the 25th percentile values and provides the central range where 50% of the data reside [39]. For a given element and class fraction considered, concentrations greater than the median + 3 IQR were individually re-examined and discarded as outliers (NIST/SEMATECH [41]) when justifiable reasons could be identified (e.g., too low dust mass close to the filter blank weight). Otherwise, they were kept as representative of the natural variation associated with such nano-scale environmental samples.

2.6. Statistical Analysis

Kruskal–Wallis non-parametric ANOVA was used to determine differences between medians for road types; critical differences between medians and distributions were then evaluated using the Wilcoxon–Mann–Whitney rank test with a significance set at $p < 0.05$ [42]. These statistical analyses were conducted using Analyze-it for Microsoft Excel 2016. Hierarchical agglomerative clustering (HAC) was performed to highlight similarities between elements in the nano-scale dust according to their inter-correlation distances. The analysis was completed on the standardized (Z-score normalization) dataset of all measured nano-size dust fractions. HAC was applied on the Spearman's correlation matrix transformed using the square root of $(1 - r^2)$, where r is the correlation between the standardized variables; the latter transformation converts correlations into metric distances [43]. The Ward criterion was chosen for merging clusters. HAC was carried out using the R v.4.0.0 packages [44].

3. Results and Discussion

3.1. Basic Properties of the Dust Box Samples

The organic C content of the studied dust box samples varied from 3.8 to 8.7 wt.% (Table 2). Major elements present in the dust box samples were Si, Fe, Mg, Al and S (Table 2). Si, Fe and Al are generally representative of crustal elements. In terms of trace elements, Zn, Cu, Pb and Cr were the most abundant in the dust box, with concentrations that were elevated compared to those previously reported for surficial soils from the same physiographic region (Table 2) [45]. The concentrations of Zn, Cu, Pb and Cr were also higher than those measured in street dust collected from residential areas in the less populated city of Ottawa (Table 2) [46]. Several studies have reported these metals as the most abundant trace elements in road dust due to their occurrence in brake pads (Cu, Cr, Pb, Zn), tire rubber (Zn, Pb) and vehicle fuel combustion residues (Zn as an additive; Pb, Cu as natural contaminants) [9,13,22,23,26,47]. Other sources for these metals are wind erosion from soils and industrial emissions [13]. The three arterial road samples collected within the same district but on different weeks (Art-D4-W1, -W2, -W3) had, overall, a comparable composition over time (Table 2).

Table 2. Mean pH, organic carbon content (OC) and concentrations ($n = 3$) of the main [a] elements in the six dust box samples analyzed in the present study, with comparative data from literature.

	Units	Art-D4-W1	Art-D4-W2	Art-D4-W3	Ex-D1-D	LR-D1-D	LR-D2-D	Soil [b]	Ottawa Dust [c]
pH		7.94	7.55	7.90	8.08	8.01	8.58	n.d. [d]	n.d.
OC [e]	wt.%	7.5	4.8	8.6	8.7	3.8	n.d.	n.d.	n.d.
Si	wt.%	7.23	7.84	8.97	12.02	8.05	9.45	n.d.	n.d.
Fe	wt.%	3.07	3.15	3.58	3.69	2.37	3.10	2.4	1.89
Ca	wt.%	n.d.	n.d.	n.d.	n.d.	n.d.	n.d.	1.5	9.68
Mg	wt.%	2.99	2.96	3.36	2.93	2.82	3.98	0.70	1.58
Al	wt.%	2.67	2.85	3.30	4.24	2.86	3.36	6.1	4.75
S	wt.%	1.17	1.33	1.09	0.32	0.38	0.39	n.d.	n.d.
Ti	mg kg^{-1}	1279	1437	1781	2045	1111	1332	4400	n.d.
Zn	mg kg^{-1}	1258	1112	1310	881	597	1051	41	112
Mn	mg kg^{-1}	1017	1113	1016	931	1183	1120	636	431
Sr	mg kg^{-1}	530	538	522	485	289	332	283	459
Ba	mg kg^{-1}	466	483	527	575	335	499	n.d.	576
Cu	mg kg^{-1}	235	219	254	235	129	194	16	66
Pb	mg kg^{-1}	192	227	171	107	156	131	23	39
Cr	mg kg^{-1}	168	173	173	221	120	223	48	43

[a] Other elements (As, B, Be, Bi, Cd, Ce, Co, La, Mo, Ni, Rb, Sb, Se, U, Tl, V, Zr) < 100 mg kg^{-1}; Ag < LOD of 2.12 mg kg^{-1}. [b] Element contents in surficial soils (A horizon) from the same physiographic region as Toronto (St. Lawrence lowlands) [45]. [c] Mean concentrations in street dust collected in Ottawa residential areas (dust fraction 100–250 µm; n = 45) [46]. [d] n.d.: not determined. [e] Organic carbon content estimated as loss on ignition (LOI)/1.724 [28].

3.2. UFP in Resuspended Road Dust Box Samples

Hereinafter, the term "resuspended PM$_{10}$" is used to refer to the aerosolized fraction of dust box with an aerodynamic particle diameter < 10 µm and >10 nm, based on the adopted MOUDI fractionation scheme (Table 1). Overall, for the six samples, most of the resuspendable mass of dust particles was found in the micron and sub-micron fractions: a median of 72 wt.% of the resuspended PM$_{10}$ was collected in the 1–10 µm fractions, while a median of 26 wt.% was recovered in the 0.1–1 µm sub-micron fractions (Figure 1). The <100 nm fractions accounted for around 2 wt.% of the resuspended PM$_{10}$ (min–max: 0.23–8.36 wt.%); 50% of the UFP population values ranged within 1.25 to 5.25 wt.% of resuspended PM$_{10}$ (Figure 1). Interestingly, dust from the downtown district (D1), including both the expressway or local road samples, contained the highest amount of very fine particles: >47 wt.% (median) of the resuspended PM$_{10}$ was retained in the sub-micron fraction and up to 7 wt.% (median) was recovered as nanoparticles (Figure 1). While the sample number examined does not support a statistical analysis of results on a per district basis, these results might reflect differences in UFP emissions as a function of traffic volume, intensity and type, including fleet composition, between the downtown core of Toronto and other less populated districts (D2 and D4). A long-term air monitoring study in downtown Toronto reported that non-tailpipe PM$_{2.5}$ emissions (soil/road dust resuspension, brake and tire wear) have increased since 2011 [48]. The authors explained the results with longer dry periods (greater accumulation of road dust) and the increases in the number of heavier vehicles on the roads, such as minivans, sport-utility vehicles and light trucks (greater friction on the road surface).

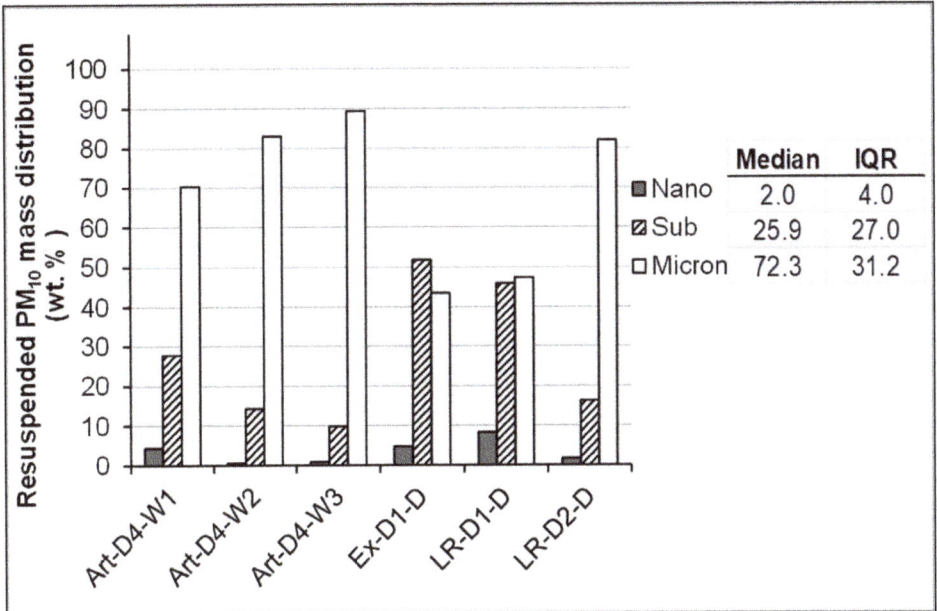

Figure 1. Distribution of the mass collected among the nano, sub-micron and micron classes of filters for each resuspended dust box sample, expressed as median % of the total resuspended PM_{10} (total mass recovered on filters < 10 µm >10 nm); inset overall median % of the total resuspended PM_{10} for all 6 samples, and inter quantile range (IQR).

The detailed size fractionation of UFP is presented in Table 3. While the variability was typically high between replicates within the same size fraction, the majority of UFP mass was generally found in the coarser UFP fractions. Of the total UFP mass, >65% was associated with the 32–100 nm fraction while <35% was measured on the 10–32 nm filters (Table 3).

3.3. Metals in UFP

This section does not include metals potentially impacted by cross-contamination (Cu, Sn, Pb, Ni, Bi and As) due to the bronze beads used for aerosolization (see discussion Section 2.4). In addition, Ag, Bi, Zr, B, Ce, Se and Si were not included in the statistical analysis because >50% of the values in the sub-micron and nano fractions were <LOD.

Compared to the dust box samples, the most notable enrichment in UFP was observed for Cd, Cr, Zn and V (nano/dust box ratio close to or >2; Figure 2). Fe and Ba also tended to accumulate in UFP, but to a lesser extent (nano/dust box ratio > 1.4). Ermolin et al. [17] also observed abnormally high Cd and Zn concentrations in UFP isolated from Moscow dust. This pattern of metal enrichment in UFP slightly differed from that of the sub-micron fraction of the same samples, which showed an additional marked enrichment in Mo and Sb (sub-micron/dust box ratio > 2; SI-Figure S1). In UFP, Mo and Sb median concentrations were <LOD. Several other studies have reported comparable metal enrichment in the fine road dust fractions for V, Cr and Mo ($PM_{2.5}$/bulk$_{<0.3mm}$ ratio > 5 in road dust from Shanghai [9]), Cd and Zn (PM_2/bulk$_{<2mm}$ ratio = 2 for highways in Spain [26]), Cr and Cd ($PM_{2.5}/PM_{10}$ ratio > 2 for road dust in Dongying, China [49]), and Zn and Sb ($PM_{2.5}$/bulk$_{<2mm}$ ratio $\geq$ 2 in urban dust, Italy [27]).

Table 3. Distribution of the recovered particle mass within the nano fractions and variability between replicates for each sample.

Sample	Size Fraction	Replicate 1	Replicate 2	Replicate 3	Median	Mean	±SD [a]	Fractions	Sum of Means
	nm			% of total nano mass				nm	% of total nano mass
Art-D4-W1	<18 >10	13	15	26	15	18	7		
	<32 >18	18	32	0	18	17	16	<32 >10	35
	<56 >32	25	39	28	28	30	8		
	<100 >56	44	14	46	44	35	18	<100 >32	65
Art-D4-W2	<18 >10	9	. [b]	6	6	7	4		
	<32 >18	8	.	13	13	11	10	<32 >10	18
	<56 >32	48	.	34	48	41	19		
	<100 >56	36	.	46	41	41	7	<100 >32	82
Art-D4-W3	<18 >10	2	2	28	2	11	15		
	<32 >18	9	18	0	9	9	9	<32 >10	20
	<56 >32	36	43	21	36	33	11		
	<100 >56	53	38	51	51	47	8	<100 >32	80
Ex-D1-D	<18 >10	9	0	26	9	11	13		
	<32 >18	0	0	28	0	9	16	<32 >10	21
	<56 >32	46	7	23	23	25	20		
	<100 >56	45	93	23	45	54	36	<100 >32	79
LR-D1-D	<18 >10	29	0	9	9	13	15		
	<32 >18	12	21	3	12	12	9	<32 >10	25
	<56 >32	38	37	62	38	46	14		
	<100 >56	21	42	25	25	29	11	<100 >32	75
LR-D2-D	<18 >10	15	0	.	8	8	11		
	<32 >18	6	5	.	5	5	1	<32 >10	13
	<56 >32	62	41	.	52	52	15		
	<100 >56	17	53	.	35	35	26	<100 >32	87

[a] SD: standard deviation; [b] ".": missing data.

The multivariate method of HAC was applied to the dataset of all nano-size fractions to regroup studied variables into subsets (clusters) according to their correlation-based similarities. The first group to form at the lowest value of the dissimilatory scale (Ba, V) has the highest similarity (Figure 3). As the dissimilatory scale values increase, the grouping becomes more heterogeneous, that is, group members' similarities decrease. High correlation or similarity between elements may reflect a common origin [18,27,48,50]. A non-exhaustive list of anthropogenic metal sources commonly associated with road dust is summarized in Table 4.

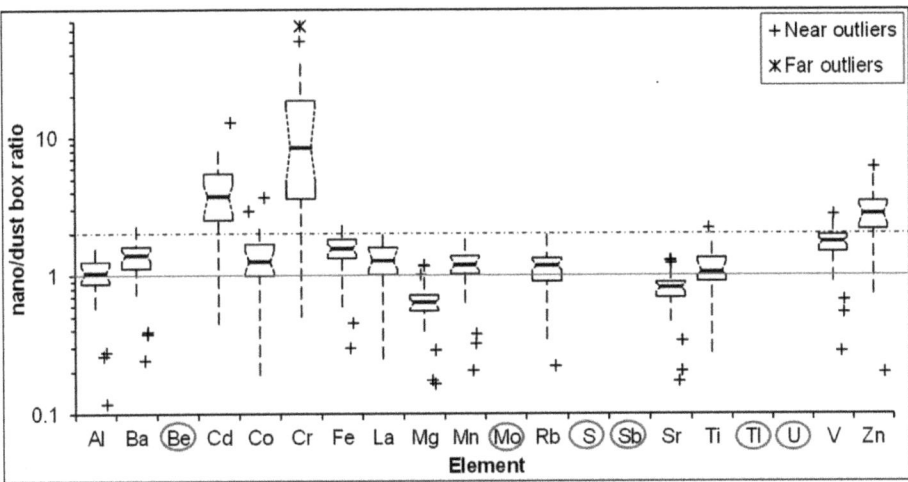

Figure 2. Ratios of element concentrations in the aerosolized nano fractions compared to the dust box considering all six road dust samples (nano/dust box ratio); each box plot shows the median within the 25th and 75th percentile box, dispersion extending 1.5 × IQR from each quartile, as well as near (>1.5 IQR) and far (>3 IQR) outliers. The 95% confidence interval for the median is plotted as a notch on the box. Elements circled in gray: not considered because >50% values < LOD; plain and dotted lines at nano/dust box ratio = 1 or 2 respectively: visual guidelines.

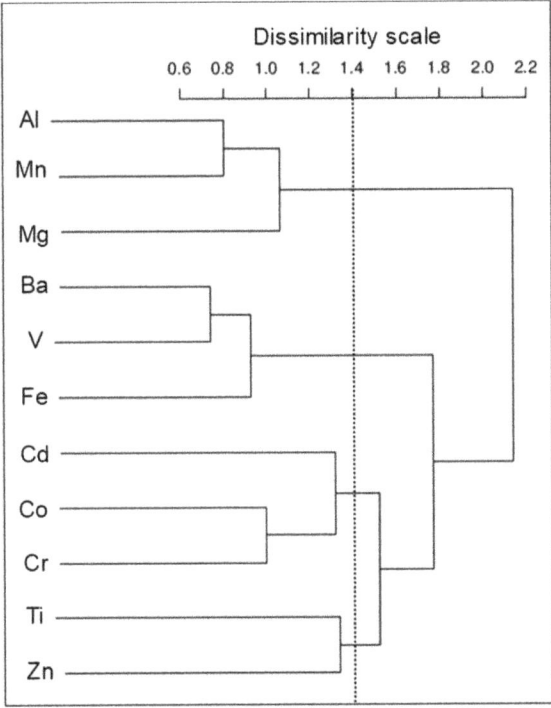

Figure 3. Dendrogram obtained by Spearman's correlation matrix-based HAC on the data set composed of key elements in all nano-scale dust fractions ($n = 35$).

Table 4. Anthropogenic sources for selected elements, other than mining, smelting and ore processing.

Sources [a]	Cd	Cr	Zn	V	Co	Ti	Ba	Fe	Al	Mg	Mn
brakes		x				x	x	x			
tires, rubber	x		x		x	x					
fossil fuel combustion (industrial, vehicle exhaust)	x	x	x	x	x						x
pigments, paints, plastic	x	x		x	x	x	x				
automobile parts, steel and alloys in transport	x	x		x	x			x	x	x	
galvanic protection	x		x								
cement	x	x					x				
asphalt (bitumen)				x				x			

[a] References—**Cd**: fossil fuel combustion, cement manufacture [51]; galvanic protection; and pigments in plastic, glass, ceramic [47]; metal sheets for automobile radiators, curing agent in rubber, production PVC [52]; **Cr**: brakes [9]; older pigments [47]; steel shiny plating, fossil fuel combustion, cement production [53]; **Zn**: galvanic protection [47]; Zn oxide as filler in tires [9,22,47]; fossil fuel combustion [54]; brake wear and burning of zinc thiophosphate stabilizer in motors and lubricating oils [55]; **V**: Alloy steel, combustion of crude oil residues in power plants and community-heating systems [51]; asphalt (bitumen) [8,56]; structural steel used in transport and manufacture of Ti-Al alloys for aerospace industry, catalyst for plastic production, use in lacquers and paints [57]; **Co**: electronic and electrical equipment, batteries, manufacturing rechargeable batteries, fossil fuel combustion, paints and primers, magnets, rubber and tire manufacturing, adhesives and sealants, alloys in automobile motor parts, plastic [58]; **Ti**: Fe, Ti, Cu and Ba measured in brake pads [8,22]; pigments in paint, plastic, glass [47]; Ti oxide as filler in rubber-based composites (tires) [59]; **Ba**: filler and extender in paints, plastics and rubber, heavy concrete production, use as alloy for iron production and as reducing agent during production of steel [60]; $BaSO_4$ is an abrasive and filler of the friction material in brake pads [9,22,61]; **Fe**, **Al**, **Mg**: Basic metal components in vehicles: frame, engines, body; lighter Al and Mg alloys often replacing steel in many components now (https://itstillruns.com/how-electric-cars-made-5006993.html; accessed on 18 June 2020); iron powder contained in brake pads [61]; **Mn**: used in some countries as a fuel additive [51].

Hereinafter, the dendrogram is interpreted by cutting the tree at a dissimilatory value of 1.4 to form four main clusters (Figure 3). The first cluster includes Al, Mn and Mg; all of which were not found to be enriched in UFP (Figure 2). The co-occurrence of Al, Mn and Mg in this cluster suggests a geogenic origin, as these elements are common constituents of soil minerals [50]. The second cluster groups Ba and V with Fe, which were all found to be moderately enriched in UFP. Steel and alloys used in various vehicle components are a possible common source of these metals (Table 4). Other potential sources for these elements include brake pads (Fe; Ba as a filler), pigments/filler in paints and catalysts used in plastic and rubber production (Ba, V; Table 4). Fossil fuel combustion is also a known source of V (Table 4). In Toronto, elevated concentrations of Ba and Fe, as well as Cu and Sb, in $PM_{2.5}$ sampled near major roads were previously attributed to brake wear [48]. In contrast, a recent study examining the elemental concentrations of bulk road dust (<2 mm) and dust box (median < 10 µm) collected in Toronto found that Ba concentrations in road dust were not elevated compared to soil background levels [14]. Ba was also not observed to significantly vary as a function of road type and corresponded to levels of traffic volume and predicted braking activity. While a moderate association was observed between Ba and Sb concentrations, suggesting that brake wear may be a source of Ba, Wiseman et al. [14] concluded that geogenic sources of Ba are likely to be comparatively more important. The third cluster relates Co and Cr with Cd at higher values on the dissimilatory scale. Both Cd and Cr had a nano/dust box ratio > 2, while Co was moderately enriched (median nano/dust box ratio = 1.3). In relation to road dust, Cr, Cd and Co may originate from fossil fuel combustion, pigments in paints or plastic, and various steel components from vehicles (Table 4). Cement may also be a source of Cd and Cr, while tires can release Cd- and Co-containing rubber particles via wear and tear processes during driving (Table 4). The fourth cluster is composed of Ti and Zn, linked at high values on the dissimilatory scale, indicating some similarity but lower correlation between these metals (r_s = 0.44; $p < 0.0066$; SI-Figure S2). Compared to dust box concentrations, UFP was enriched in Zn but not in Ti (Figure 2). Tires are a frequently reported source of Zn in road dust (Table 4), although other traffic-related sources such as brake wear can contribute to emissions of this element, especially for UFP [14,15]. TiO_2 and ZnO nanoparticles (NP) were observed in Shanghai $PM_{2.5}$ dust [9]. Nano- or micron-size particles of ZnO and TiO_2 are used as fillers or activators during the production of rubber-based composites [9,59]. Source apportionment studies in Toronto suggested local overnight industrial activity (metals processing), brake wear emissions and the combustion of lubricating oils containing Zn thiophosphate stabilizer to explain the Zn variation in airborne fine ($PM_{2.5}$) and ultrafine ($PM_{0.1}$) particles [55,61].

While metal enrichments in UFP and observed statistical associations between variables can help to clarify potential anthropogenic contributions, caution needs to be exercised in using trace elements as 'markers' to identify specific sources. The identification of specific elemental sources is hindered by the occurrence of multiple and overlapping sources for a given trace element, combined with the variability in chemical composition of automotive components between manufacturers. These limitations are reflected in Table 4 and have been previously discussed by Thorpe and Harrison [8] and Wiseman et al. [14]. Source identification is even more challenging in the case of UFP because they may be generated from thermal processes during which interactions with other sources or elements may occur. Therefore, complementary electron microscopic analysis would be needed to ascertain their origin with confidence.

3.4. Impact of Road Type on Key Metal Concentrations in UFP

Understanding the spatial variability of the chemical composition of UFP in specific environments provides insight into potential sources and health risks [18]. The impact of road type on metal concentrations in UFP was evaluated for the four metals with the greatest preferential accumulation in the nano-scale fractions (Cd, Cr, Zn and V; nano/dust box ratio close to or >2), after regrouping all resuspended nano fractions on the basis of major road type only (Figure 4). While these results should be interpreted with caution due to the limited number of dust box samples examined, the representativeness of each composite sample is reinforced by the strategy of sampling over many kilometers and several hours.

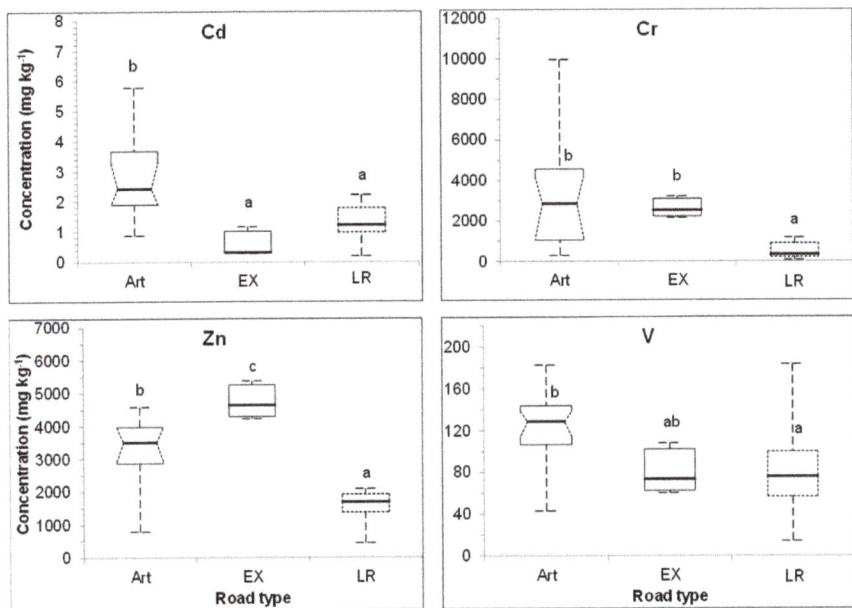

Figure 4. Concentrations of Cd, Cr, Zn and V in the nano fractions for each road type; each box plot shows the median within the 25th and 75th percentile box, dispersion from 5th to 95th percentile. The 95% confidence interval for the median is plotted as a notch on the box. For a given element, median concentrations labeled with the same letter are not statistically different based on Wilcoxon-Mann-Whitney rank test ($p > 0.05$). Fractionation was conducted in two to three replicates on each dust box and each replicate had 4 nano fractions (Art: $n = 31$; Ex: $n = 5$; LR: $n = 11$).

Among these four elements, Cr and Zn were the most abundant in UFP (Figure 4). Metal concentrations in UFP varied widely and the min–max ranges were (mg kg^{-1}): 60–11,228 (Cr); 259–5372 (Zn); 14–202 (V); 0.19–7.20 (Cd). The variation in Cd, Cr, Zn, and V concentrations in the nano-scale fractions was large for arterial roads (n = 31) and generally lower for expressways (n = 5) and local roads (except for V in LR; n = 11; Figure 4). Median concentrations of Cd, Cr, Zn and V in UFP from arterial road dust were significantly higher than those from local roads. Ultrafine particles from arterial roads containing two times more Cd, Zn and V and nine times more Cr than UFP from local roads (2.43 mg Cd kg^{-1}, 2846 mg Cr kg^{-1}, 3508 mg Zn kg^{-1}, 129 mg V kg^{-1} for Art vs. 1.22 mg Cd kg^{-1}, 329 mg Cr kg^{-1}, 1677 mg Zn kg^{-1}, 75 mg V kg^{-1} for LR; Figure 4). For UFP from the expressway, median concentrations of Cd and V (0.31 mg Cd kg^{-1} and 73 mg V kg^{-1}) were not significantly different from those measured in UFP from local roads (1.22 mg Cd kg^{-1} and 75 mg V kg^{-1}), and their median Cr concentration was comparable to that of arterial roads (respectively 2515 vs. 2846 mg kg^{-1}; Figure 4). Zn median concentration in UFP was the highest at the expressway with 4644 mg kg^{-1} compared to 3508 and 1677 mg kg^{-1} for arterial and local roads, respectively (Figure 4). In a related study in Toronto, the same trend was observed for Zn in dust box samples (median PM < 10 µm) [14].

Several factors, including seasonal effects, occurrence of industries, traffic pattern and intensity, can influence metal composition in dust [3,9,18,25,62]. Compared to arterial or local roads, expressways are characterized by heavier traffic with more heavy-duty commercial vehicles and higher speed, which can have an impact on contaminant release [55]. As discussed above, non-tailpipe traffic emissions related to the wear and tear of tires and brake components, as well as oil combustion, were identified as sources of Zn in airborne PM [8,15,16,22,55]. The UFP number concentration and particle size distribution emitted from road-tire friction or braking are influenced by various factors such as vehicle speed, vehicle weight, traffic pattern and frictional heat [8,11,16,63]. For example, slip events and harsh braking were associated with an increase in UFP concentrations released from tire wear [16]. High speed was also associated with a relative increase of finer particles (PM$_{2.5}$, which includes UFP) related to tire wear, likely due to the predominance of volatilization processes [16]. Likewise, an increase of concentrations in UFP from brake wear occurred at elevated temperature of the cast iron disc due to volatilization [15].

3.5. Implications for Human Health

3.5.1. Risk of Exposure to UFP and Their Oxidative Potential

In Toronto road dust, UFP constituted a small mass fraction of resuspended PM$_{10}$ (median 2 wt.%; Figure 1). However, toxicological studies generally agree that particle number and surface area are better metrics than mass to relate PM impact to health effects [18]. In terms of particle number concentration, UFP dominate in ambient air; in Europe, they account for >90% of airborne particles [3]. Considering that road vehicles are often the dominant sources of UFP in urban environments, populations living close to heavy-traffic roads are generally expected to be exposed to higher UFP concentration than those living in less traffic area [18,64]. The high number of UFP is of toxicological concern because the presence of high UFP numbers combined with their large surface area result in more particles accumulating in exposed lung cells, ultimately having an enhanced potential to induce adverse effects on target organs [5].

Our results indicate that communities living close to arterial roads would be exposed to UFP with higher concentrations of Cr, Cd, Zn and V compared to those living in less intense traffic areas (near local roads). Exposure to Zn-rich UFP from resuspended road dust would be the highest close to expressways. Transition metals are believed to play a direct role in the genotoxicity of PM by promoting the formation of ROS, which can lead to DNA damage [65]. The capacity of metals in UFP to cause oxidative stress and inflammation in the lung environment can be measured by various acellular oxidative potential (OP) assays [21]. A study in Toronto demonstrated that elements associated with non-tailpipe traffic emissions including Ba, Fe, Zn were moderately correlated with measured oxidative potential of PM$_{2.5}$ dust [48]. Likewise, elevated Fe and Ba concentrations in PM$_{10}$ from road emissions in London (UK) were associated with increased oxidative potential measured by depletion of glutathione [20]. In Birmingham (UK), various size fractions of airborne PM (<7 µm) collected at high-traffic locations displayed greater oxidative potential than comparable size-fraction PM sampled in areas with less traffic [65]. While the sampling location was generally a stronger determinant than particle size for the observed PM toxicity on the cells, it was noteworthy that the finest PM (<0.5 µm) caused a significantly greater release of pro-inflammatory mediators than the coarser fractions (0.5 to 7 µm), regardless of sampling locations. Wessels et al. [65] suggested that metal enrichment reported for UFP at high-traffic locations might explain their pro-inflammatory action.

3.5.2. Toxicity of Metals in UFP

Compared to the dust box samples, the enrichment in Cr, Cd, Zn, V and, to a lesser extent, Fe and Ba in UFP raises the question of potential toxic effects linked to exposures via the inhalation pathway. Cd and its compounds, as well as Cr (VI) and its compounds, have been classified as known carcinogens to humans (group 1, International Agency for Research on Cancer-IARC) based on strong evidence for increased risk of lung cancer [66]. Vanadium oxide is classified as a possible carcinogen (group 2B, IARC) and is a respiratory irritant [66]. Nanoparticles can lead to oxidative stress via two main modes of action: induction based on the dissolved species (high solubility like CuO and ZnO) vs. the nanoparticle itself (low solubility, e.g., $\alpha-Fe_2O_3$, Fe_3O_4, Al_2O_3) [67].

For the fine fraction (<1.8 µm) of these Toronto Road dust samples, the metal solubility/bioaccessibility in the lung environment was evaluated in a related study using ammonium citrate (pH 4.4) to simulate lysosomal fluid and Gamble's solution (pH 7.2) to simulate interstitial lung fluid [31]. At pH 4.4, the following bioaccessibility (% of total concentration) was reported for local road dust: Zn (78%) > Ba (56%) > Fe (35%) ≈ V (33%) > Cr (14%); Cd was <LOD. Metal bioaccessibilities were much lower in the Gamble's extracts (range for local road, arterial road and expressway): Ba (7 to 21%) > Zn (6 to 8%); Fe, V, Cr and Cd were <LOD. These in vitro bioaccessibility assays indicated that Zn would be the transition metal with the highest solubility following inhalation of these UFP. Given the high concentration of Zn in expressway UFP, combined with its high bioaccessibility, further research should address the potential inhalation toxicity of these UFP.

In addition to solubility, research on fairly homogeneous engineered NP (such as metal oxide nanomaterials) has shown that their capacity to induce oxidative and pro-inflammatory effects in the cells depends on their basic physico-chemical and mineralogical properties such as: size, crystalline structure, morphology, aspect ratio, surface area, catalytic nature, band gap energy level, composition, and surface coating [67–70]. In heterogeneous and complex media such as dust, metals occur as a mixture of various species with different properties. For example, a wide variety of Zn species were found in indoor dust and road dust, including distinct mineral phases (e.g., Zn oxide, Zn sulfide, Zn hydroxyl carbonate), Zn organic compounds (e.g., Zn phosphate), Zn sorbed on organic or Fe-, Mn-, Al-oxyhydroxide phases, and Zn-bearing silicates [71–73]. Likewise, a variety of Fe-bearing nanoparticles have been detected in street dust and vehicular emissions, including ferrihydrite, goethite, hematite, magnetite, maghemite, siderite, metallic Fe, wüstite, ferrohexahydrite and carbon/Fe agglomerates [9,74,75]. Understanding the mineralogical composition and speciation of metals in the nano-scale fraction of road dust is thus crucial to assess their solubility and potential toxicological impact. However, such studies are scarce and future research efforts should be oriented in that direction.

4. Conclusions

Resuspension of road dust is one of the major sources of airborne PM pollution in large cities. The literature has established elevated concentrations of key metals associated with vehicle emissions, and a tendency for metals to accumulate in the thoracic (PM$_{10}$) and respirable (PM$_{2.5}$) size fractions. Our study demonstrates that some of the transition metals, such as Cd, Cr, Zn and V, further concentrate into resuspendable UFP, a particle size fraction particularly relevant to human health concerns. The inhalation of UFP has the potential to cause oxidative stress in lung cells and transition metals play an active role in these toxicological responses. Much effort has been dedicated in the last 10 years to investigate the toxicological impact of engineered nanoparticles. However, important knowledge gaps still exist on the composition and toxicological impact of environmental UFP. To address the toxicological impact of metals in UFP, there is a need to advance our understanding of their contributing sources (natural vs. anthropogenic), their mineral phases/metal speciation, and their transformations resulting from thermal and chemical reactions during incidental release from vehicles, or from interactions with other road dust components (e.g., carbonaceous phase).

Supplementary Materials: The following are available online at https://www.mdpi.com/article/10.3390/atmos12121564/s1, Table S1: QA/QC for ICP measurements of certified reference materials; Figure S1: Ratios of element concentrations in the aerosolized sub-micron fractions compared to the dust box; Figure S2: Scatterplot matrix of Spearman's correlations between variables in UFP.

Author Contributions: Conceptualization, P.E.R. and C.L.S.W.; Data curation, S.B., C.L. and P.E.R.; Formal analysis, S.B.; Funding acquisition, P.E.R. and C.L.S.W.; Methodology, P.E.R. and C.L.; Visualization, S.B.; Writing—original draft, S.B.; Writing—review & editing, P.E.R., C.L. and C.L.S.W. All authors have read and agreed to the published version of the manuscript.

Funding: The project was supported by Health Canada's Chemicals Management Plan Nanotechnology Fund and the Natural Sciences and Engineering Research Council of Canada (NSERC Discovery Grants Program, RGPIN-2018-05966).

Data Availability Statement: Not applicable.

Acknowledgments: The authors thank Vesna Stefanovic-Briatico from the City of Toronto for coordinating the collection of the road dust sweepings, and Jianjun Niu for technical assistance in the laboratory. Mario Beauchemin (Natural Resources Canada, Ottawa; retired) is gratefully acknowledged for his contribution with hierarchical agglomerative clustering. The thorough internal reviews by Mary-Luyza Avramescu and Kathy Nguyen (Health Canada, Ottawa) were greatly appreciated.

Conflicts of Interest: The authors declare no conflict of interest.

References

1. WHO. *Preventing Disease through Healthy Environments: A Global Assessment of the Burden of Disease from Environmental Risks*; World Health Organization: Geneva, Switzerland, 2016; 147p, ISBN 978 92 4 156519 6.
2. WHO. *Ambient Air Pollution: A Global Assessment of Exposure and Burden of Disease*; World Health Organization: Geneva, Switzerland, 2016; 131p, ISBN 978 92 4 151135 3.
3. Air Quality Expert Group. *Ultrafine Particles (UFP) in the UK*; Prepared for the Department for Environment, Food and Rural Affairs; Scottish Government; Welsh Government; and Department of the Environment in Northern Ireland; Report No. PB14510; Department for Environment, Food and Rural Affairs: London, UK, 2018. Available online: https://uk-air.defra.gov.uk/library/reports.php?report_id=968 (accessed on 21 April 2020).
4. Brown, J.S.; Gordon, T.; Price, O.; Asgharian, B. Thoracic and respirable particle definitions for human health risk assessment. *Part. Fibre Toxicol.* **2013**, *10*, 12. [CrossRef]
5. Geiser, M.; Kreyling, W.G. Deposition and biokinetics of inhaled nanoparticles. *Part. Fibre Toxicol.* **2010**, *7*, 2–17. [CrossRef]
6. Sutunkova, M.P.; Katsnelson, B.A.; Privalova, L.I.; Gurvich, V.B.; Konysheva, L.K.; Shur, V.; Shishkina, E.V.; Minigalieva, I.A.; Solovjeva, S.N.; Grebenkina, S.V.; et al. On the contribution of the phagocytosis and the solubilization to the iron oxide nanoparticles retention in and elimination from the lungs under long-term inhalation. *Toxicology* **2016**, *363–364*, 19–28. [CrossRef]
7. Tian, L.; Shang, Y.; Chen, R.; Bai, R.; Chen, C.; Inthavong, K.; Tu, J. Correlation of regional deposition for inhaled nanoparticles in human and rat olfactory. *Part. Fibre Toxicol.* **2019**, *16*, 6. [CrossRef] [PubMed]
8. Thorpe, A.; Harrison, R.M. Sources and properties of non-exhaust particulate matter from road traffic: A review. *Sci. Total Environ.* **2008**, *400*, 270–282. [CrossRef]
9. Yang, Y.; Vance, M.; Tou, F.; Tiwari, A.; Liu, M.; Hochella, M.F., Jr. Nanoparticles in road dust from impervious urban surfaces: Distribution, identification, and environmental implications. *Environ. Sci. Nano* **2016**, *3*, 534–544. [CrossRef]
10. Lenschow, P.; Abraham, H.-J.; Kutzner, K.; Lutz, M.; Preu, J.-D.; Reichenbächer, W. Some ideas about sources of PM_{10}. *Atmos. Environ.* **2001**, *35* (Suppl. S1), S23–S33. [CrossRef]

11. Kumar, P.; Pirjola, L.; Ketzel, M.; Harrison, R.M. Nanoparticle emissions from 11 non-vehicle exhaust source—A review. *Atmos. Environ.* **2013**, *67*, 252–277. [CrossRef]
12. Pant, P.; Harrison, R.M. Estimation of the contribution of road traffic emissions to particulate matter concentrations from field measurements: A review. *Atmos. Environ.* **2013**, *77*, 78–97. [CrossRef]
13. Ramirez, O.; Sánchez de la Campa, A.M.; Amato, F.; Moreno, T.; Silva, L.F.; de la Rosa, J.D. Physicochemical characterization and sources of thoracic fraction of road dust in a Latin American megacity. *Sci. Total Environ.* **2019**, *652*, 434–446. [CrossRef]
14. Wiseman, C.L.S.; Levesque, C.; Rasmussen, P.E. Elemental sources and concentrations in thoracic-sized road dust fractions and their potential for resuspension. *Sci. Total Environ.* **2021**, *786*, 147467. [CrossRef] [PubMed]
15. Kukutschová, J.; Moravec, P.; Tomášek, V.; Matejka, V.; Smolík, J.; Schwarz, J.; Seidlerová, J.; Šafářová, K.; Filip, P. On airborne nano/micro-sized wear particles released from low-metallic automotive brakes. *Environ. Pollut.* **2011**, *159*, 998–1006. [CrossRef]
16. Kim, G.; Lee, S. Characteristics of tire wear particles generated by a tire simulator under various driving conditions. *Environ. Sci. Technol.* **2018**, *52*, 12153–12161. [CrossRef] [PubMed]
17. Ermolin, M.S.; Fedotov, P.S.; Ivaneev, A.I.; Karandashev, V.K.; Fedyunina, N.N.; Eskina, V.V. Isolation and quantitative analysis of road dust nanoparticles. *J. Anal. Chem.* **2017**, *72*, 520–532. [CrossRef]
18. Heal, M.R.; Kumar, P.; Harrison, R.M. Particles, air quality, policy and health. *Chem. Soc. Rev.* **2012**, *41*, 6606–6630. [CrossRef] [PubMed]
19. Cass, G.R.; Hughes, L.A.; Bhave, P.; Kleeman, M.J.; Allen, J.O.; Salmon, L.G. The chemical composition of atmospheric ultrafine particles. *Phil. Trans. R. Soc. Lond. A* **2000**, *358*, 2581–2592. [CrossRef]
20. Godri, K.J.; Harrison, R.M.; Evans, T.; Baker, T.; Dunster, C.; Mudway, I.S.; Kelly, F.J. Increased oxidative burden associated with traffic component of ambient particulate matter at roadside and urban background school sites in London. *PLoS ONE* **2011**, *6*, e21961. [CrossRef]
21. Bates, J.T.; Fang, T.; Verma, V.; Zeng, L.; Weber, R.J.; Tolbert, P.E.; Abrams, J.Y.; Sarnat, S.E.; Klein, M.; Mulholland, J.A.; et al. Review of acellular assays of ambient particulate matter oxidative potential: Methods and relationships with composition, sources and health effects. *Environ. Sci. Technol.* **2019**, *53*, 4003–4019. [CrossRef]
22. Apeagyei, E.; Bank, M.S.; Spengler, J.D. Distribution of heavy metals in road dust along an urban-rural gradient in Massachusetts. *Atmos. Environ.* **2011**, *45*, 2310–2323. [CrossRef]
23. Abdel-Latif, N.M.; Saleh, I.A. Heavy metals contamination in roadside dust along major roads and correlation with urbanization activities in Cairo, Egypt. *J. Am. Sci.* **2012**, *8*, 379–389.
24. Wiseman, C.L.S.; Hassan Pour, Z.; Zereini, F. Platinum group element and cerium concentrations in roadside environments in Toronto, Canada. *Chemosphere* **2016**, *145*, 61–67. [CrossRef] [PubMed]
25. Miazgowicz, A.; Krennhuber, K.; Lanzerstorfer, C. Metals concentrations in road dust from high traffic and low traffic area: A size dependent comparison. *Int. J. Environ. Sci. Technol.* **2020**, *17*, 3365–3372. [CrossRef]
26. Acosta, J.A.; Faz, A.; Kalbitz, K.; Jansen, B.; Martínez-Martínez, S. Heavy metal concentrations in particle size fractions from street dust of Murcia (Spain) as the basis for risk assessment. *J. Environ. Monit.* **2011**, *13*, 3087–3096. [CrossRef] [PubMed]
27. Padoan, E.; Romè, C.; Ajmone-Marsan, F. Bioaccessibility and size distribution of metals in road dust and roadside soils along a peri-urban transect. *Sci. Total Environ.* **2017**, *601–602*, 89–98. [CrossRef] [PubMed]
28. Wiseman, C.L.S.; Niu, J.; Levesque, C.; Chénier, M.; Rasmussen, P.E. An assessment of the inhalation bioaccessibility of platinum group elements in road dust using a simulated lung fluid. *Environ. Pollut.* **2018**, *241*, 1009–1017. [CrossRef]
29. Lanzerstorfer, C. Heavy metals in the finest size fractions of road-deposited sediments. *Environ. Pollut.* **2018**, *239*, 522–531. [CrossRef]
30. Lanzerstorfer, C.; Logiewa, A. The upper size limit of the dust samples in road dust heavy metal studies: Benefits of a combined sieving and air classification sample preparation procedure. *Environ. Pollut.* **2019**, *245*, 1079–1085. [CrossRef]
31. Levesque, L.; Wiseman, C.L.S.; Beauchemin, S.; Rasmussen, P.E. Thoracic fraction (PM_{10}) of resuspended urban dust: Geochemistry, particle size distribution and lung bioaccessibility. *Geosciences* **2021**, *11*, 87. [CrossRef]
32. Statistics Canada. Census Profile by Toronto Community Areas. 2016. Available online: https://www.toronto.ca/city-government/data-research-maps/neighbourhoods-communities/community-council-area-profiles/ (accessed on 15 April 2020).
33. Rasmussen, P.E.; Gardner, H.D.; Jianjun, J. Buoyancy-corrected gravimetric analysis of lightly loaded filters. *J. Air Waste Manag. Assoc.* **2010**, *60*, 1065–1077. [CrossRef]
34. Niu, J.; Rasmussen, P.E.; Chénier, M. Ultrasonic dissolution for ICP-MS determination of trace elements in lightly loaded airborne PM filters. *Intern. J. Environ. Anal. Chem.* **2013**, *93*, 661–678. [CrossRef]
35. Morrison, J.M.; Goldhaber, M.B.; Lee, L.; Holloway, J.M.; Wanty, R.B.; Wolf, R.E.; Ranville, J.F. A regional-scale study of chromium and nickel in soils of northern California, USA. *Appl. Geochem.* **2009**, *24*, 1500–1511. [CrossRef]
36. Huggins, F.E.; Huffman, G.P.; Robertson, J.D. Speciation of elements in NIST particulate matter SRMs 1648 and 1650. *J. Hazar. Mater.* **2000**, *74*, 1–23. [CrossRef]
37. Tabachnick, B.G.; Fidell, L.S. *Using Multivariate Statistics*, 2nd ed.; HarperCollins Publishers: New York, NY, USA, 1989.
38. Analytical Methods Committee. *What Should Be Done with Results below the Detection Limit? Mentioning the Unmentionable*; AMC Technical Brief. No. 5; Royal Society of Chemistry: London, UK, 2001. Available online: https://www.rsc.org/images/results-below-detection-limit-technical-brief-5_tcm18-214854.pdf (accessed on 26 September 2019).

39. Helsel, D.R. Less than obvious. Statistical treatment of data below detection limit. *Environ. Sci. Technol.* **1990**, *24*, 1767–1774. [CrossRef]
40. USEPA. *Guidance for Data Quality Assessment. Practical Methods for Data Analysis*; EPA QA/G-9. QA00 Update; United States Environmental Protection Agency: Washington, DC, USA, 2000. Available online: https://www.epa.gov/sites/production/files/2015-06/documents/g9-final.pdf (accessed on 15 October 2019).
41. NIST/SEMATECH. *e-Handbook of Statistical Methods*; Section 7.1.6; U.S. Department of Commerce: Washington, DC, USA, 2012. Available online: http://www.itl.nist.gov/div898/handbook/ (accessed on 26 September 2019).
42. Hart, A. Mann-Whitney test is not just a test of medians: Differences in spread can be important. *Br. Med. J.* **2001**, *323*, 391–393. [CrossRef]
43. Van Dongen, S.; Enright, A.J. Metric distances derived from cosine similarity and Pearson and Spearman correlations. *arXiv* **2012**, arXiv:1208.3145v1.
44. R Core Team. *A Language and Environment for Statistical Computing*; Version 4.0.0; Released 24 April 2020; R Foundation for Statistical Computing: Vienna, Austria, 2020. Available online: https://www.r-project.org/ (accessed on 2 June 2020).
45. McKeague, J.A.; Desjardins, J.G.; Wolynetz, M.S. *Minor Elements in Canadian Soils*; Land Resource Research Institute Contribution No. LRRI 27; Agriculture and Agri-Food Canada: Edmonton, AB, Canada, 1979; 75p.
46. Rasmussen, P.E.; Subramanian, K.S.; Jessiman, B.J. A multi-element profile of house dust in relation to exterior dust and soils in the city of Ottawa, Canada. *Sci. Total Environ.* **2001**, *267*, 125–140. [CrossRef]
47. Ciacci, L.; Reck, B.K.; Nassar, N.T.; Graedel, T.E. Lost by design. *Environ. Sci. Technol.* **2015**, *49*, 9443–9451. [CrossRef] [PubMed]
48. Jeong, C.-H.; Traub, A.; Huang, A.; Hilker, N.; Wang, J.M.; Herod, D.; Dabek-Zlotorynska, E.; Celo, V.; Evans, G.J. Long-term analysis of $PM_{2.5}$ from 2004 to 2007 in Toronto: Composition, sources, and oxidative potential. *Environ. Pollut.* **2020**, *263*, 114652. [CrossRef]
49. Kong, S.; Lu, B.; Ji, Y.; Zhao, X.; Bai, Z.; Xu, Y.; Liu, Y.; Jiang, H. Risk assessment of heavy metals in road and soil dusts within PM2.5, PM10 and PM100 fractions in Dongying city, Shandong Province, China. *J. Environ. Monit.* **2012**, *14*, 791–803. [CrossRef]
50. Padoan, E.; Malandrino, M.; Giacomino, A.; Grosa, M.M.; Lollobrigida, F.; Martini, S.; Abollino, O. Spatial distribution and potential sources of traces elements in PM_{10} monitored in urban and rural sites of Piedmont region. *Chemosphere* **2016**, *145*, 495–507. [CrossRef]
51. WHO. *World Health Organization Air Quality Guidelines for Europe*, 2nd ed.; CD ROM Version; World Health Organization: Geneva, Switzerland, 2000. Available online: https://www.euro.who.int/en/health-topics/environment-and-health/air-quality/publications/pre2009/who-air-quality-guidelines-for-europe,-2nd-edition,-2000-cd-rom-version (accessed on 12 October 2020).
52. Canadian Council of Ministers of the Environment (CCME). Canadian soil quality guidelines for the protection of environmental and human health: Cadmium (1999). In *Canadian Environmental Quality Guidelines*; Canadian Council of Ministers of the Environment: Winnipeg, MB, Canada, 1999.
53. Canadian Council of Ministers of the Environment (CCME). Canadian water quality guidelines for the protection of aquatic life: Chromium—Hexavalent chromium and trivalent chromium. In *Canadian Environmental Quality Guidelines*; Canadian Council of Ministers of the Environment: Winnipeg, MB, Canada, 1999.
54. Canadian Council of Ministers of the Environment (CCME). Canadian soil quality guidelines for the protection of environmental and human health: Zinc (2018). In *Canadian Environmental Quality Guidelines*; Canadian Council of Ministers of the Environment: Winnipeg, MB, Canada, 1999.
55. Dabek-Zlotorzynska, E.; Celo, V.; Ding, L.; Herod, D.; Jeong, C.-H.; Evans, G.; Hilker, N. Characteristics and sources of $PM_{2.5}$ and reactive gases near roadways in two metropolitan areas in Canada. *Atmos. Environ.* **2019**, *218*, 116980. [CrossRef]
56. WHO. *Asphalt (Bitumen)*; Concise International Chemical Assessment Document 59; World Health Organization: Geneva, Switzerland, 2004; ISBN 92 4 153059 6.
57. Canadian Council of Ministers of the Environment (CCME). Canadian soil quality guidelines for the protection of environmental and human health: Vanadium (1997). In *Canadian Environmental Quality Guidelines*; Canadian Council of Ministers of the Environment: Winnipeg, MB, Canada, 1999.
58. Canada. *Screening Assessment Cobalt and Cobalt-Containing Substances*; Cat. No.: EN14-273/2017E-PDF; Environment and Climate Change Canada: Gatineau, QC, Canada; Health Canada: Tunney's Pasture, ON, Canada, 2017. Available online: https://www.ec.gc.ca/ese-ees/default.asp?lang=En&n=DCEB359C-1 (accessed on 18 June 2020).
59. Datta, J.; Kosiorek, P.; Wloch, M. Effect of high loading of titanium dioxide particles on the morphology, mechanical and thermo-mechanical properties of the natural rubber-based composites. *Iran. Polym. J.* **2016**, *25*, 1021–1035. [CrossRef]
60. Canadian Council of Ministers of the Environment (CCME). Canadian soil quality guidelines for the protection of environmental and human health: Barium. In *Canadian Environmental Quality Guidelines*; Canadian Council of Ministers of the Environment: Winnipeg, MB, Canada, 2013.
61. Jeong, C.-H.; Wang, J.M.; Hilker, N.; Debosz, J.; Sofowote, U.; Su, Y.; Noble, M.; Healy, R.M.; Munoz, T.; Dabek-Zlotorynska, E.; et al. Temporal and spatial variability of traffic-related $PM_{2.5}$ sources: Comparison of exhaust and non-exhaust emissions. *Atmos. Environ.* **2019**, *198*, 55–69. [CrossRef]
62. Khan, R.K.; Strand, M.A. Road dust and its effect on human health: A literate review. *Epidemiol. Health* **2018**, *40*, e2018013. [CrossRef] [PubMed]

63. Nosko, O.; Vanhanen, J.; Olofsson, U. Emission of 1.3–10 nm airborne particles from brake materials. *Aerosol Sci. Technol.* **2017**, *51*, 91–96. [CrossRef]
64. Hata, M.; Zhang, T.; Bao, L.; Otani, Y.; Bai, Y.; Furuuchi, M. Characteristics of the nanoparticles in a road tunnel. *Aerosol Air Qual. Res.* **2013**, *13*, 194–200. [CrossRef]
65. Wessels, A.; Birmili, W.; Albrecht, C.; Hellack, B.; Jermann, E.; Wick, G.; Harrison, R.M.; Schins, R.P.F. Oxidant generation and toxicity of size-fractionated ambient particles in human lung epithelial cells. *Environ. Sci. Technol.* **2010**, *44*, 3539–3545. [CrossRef]
66. Carex Canada. *Priority Carcinogens*; Faculty of Health Sciences, Simon Fraser University: Vancouver, BC, Canada, 2020. Available online: https://www.carexcanada.ca (accessed on 15 October 2020).
67. Zhang, H.; Ji, Z.; Xia, T.; Meng, H.; Low-Kam, C.; Liu, R.; Pokhrei, S.; Lin, S.; Wang, X.; Liao, Y.-P.; et al. Use of metal oxide nanoparticle band gap to develop a predictive paradigm for oxidative stress and acute pulmonary inflammation. *ACS Nano* **2012**, *6*, 4349–4368. [CrossRef]
68. Jin, C.; Tang, Y.; Yang, F.G.; Li, X.L.; Xu, S.; Fan, X.Y.; Huang, Y.Y.; Yang, Y.J. Cellular toxicity of TiO_2 nanoparticles in anatase and rutile crystal phase. *Biol. Trace Elem. Res.* **2011**, *141*, 3–15. [CrossRef] [PubMed]
69. Bushell, M.; Beauchemin, S.; Kunc, F.; Gardner, D.; Ovens, J.; Toll, F.; Kennedy, D.; Nguyen, K.; Vladisavljevic, D.; Rasmussen, P.; et al. Characterization of commercial metal oxide nanomaterials: Crystalline phase, particle size and specific surface area. *Nanomaterials* **2020**, *10*, 1812. [CrossRef]
70. Boyadzhiev, A.; Avramescu, M.-L.; Wu, D.; Williams, A.; Rasmussen, P.; Halappanavar, S. Impact of copper oxide particle solubility on lung epithelial cell toxicity: Response characterization using global transcriptional analysis. *Nanotoxicology* **2021**, *15*, 380–399. [CrossRef]
71. Rasmussen, P.E.; Beauchemin, S.; Nugent, M.; Dugandzic, R.; Lanouette, M.; Chénier, M. Influence of matrix composition on the bioaccessibility of copper, zinc, and nickel in urban residential dust and soil. *Hum. Ecol. Risk Assess.* **2008**, *14*, 351–371. [CrossRef]
72. Barrett, J.E.S.; Taylor, K.G.; Hudson-Edwards, K.A.; Charnock, J.M. Solid-phase speciation of Zn in road dust sediment. *Mineral. Mag.* **2011**, *75*, 2611–2629. [CrossRef]
73. Beauchemin, S.; Rasmussen, P.E.; Mackinnon, T.; Chénier, M.; Boros, K. Zinc in house dust: Speciation, bioaccessibility, and impact of humidity. *Environ. Sci. Technol.* **2014**, *48*, 9022–9029. [CrossRef] [PubMed]
74. Gonet, T.; Maher, B.A. Airborne, vehicle-derived Fe-bearing nanoparticles in the urban environment: A review. *Environ. Sci. Technol.* **2019**, *53*, 9970–9991. [CrossRef] [PubMed]
75. Silva, L.F.O.; Pinto, D.; Neckel, A.; Oliveira, M.L.S. An analysis of vehicular exhaust derived nanoparticles and historial Belgium fortress building interfaces. *Geosci. Front.* **2020**, *11*, 2053–2060. [CrossRef]

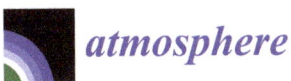

Article

Human Health Risk Assessment of Heavy Metals in the Urban Road Dust of Zhengzhou Metropolis, China

Muhammad Faisal [1], Zening Wu [1,2], Huiliang Wang [1,2,*], Zafar Hussain [1,3] and Muhammad Imran Azam [4]

[1] College of Water Conservancy Engineering, Zhengzhou University, Zhengzhou 450001, China; engineerfaisi@gs.zzu.edu.cn (M.F.); zeningwu@zzu.edu.cn (Z.W.); zafar775@yahoo.com (Z.H.)
[2] Zhengzhou Key Laboratory of Water Resource and Environment, Zhengzhou 450001, China
[3] Water Resources Section, Ministry of Planning, Development & Special Initiatives, Islamabad 44000, Pakistan
[4] Hydropower and Water Resources Section, Zeeruk International (PVT), Islamabad 44000, Pakistan; drimran@zeeruk.com
* Correspondence: wanghuiliang@zzu.edu.cn

Citation: Faisal, M.; Wu, Z.; Wang, H.; Hussain, Z.; Azam, M.I. Human Health Risk Assessment of Heavy Metals in the Urban Road Dust of Zhengzhou Metropolis, China. *Atmosphere* **2021**, *12*, 1213. https://doi.org/10.3390/atmos12091213

Academic Editors: Dmitry Vlasov, Omar Ramírez Hernández and Ashok Luhar

Received: 12 August 2021
Accepted: 15 September 2021
Published: 17 September 2021

Publisher's Note: MDPI stays neutral with regard to jurisdictional claims in published maps and institutional affiliations.

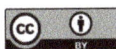

Copyright: © 2021 by the authors. Licensee MDPI, Basel, Switzerland. This article is an open access article distributed under the terms and conditions of the Creative Commons Attribution (CC BY) license (https:// creativecommons.org/licenses/by/ 4.0/).

Abstract: The goal of this research is to assess hazardous heavy metal levels in $PM_{2.5}$ fractioned road dust in order to quantify the risk of inhalation and potential health effects. To accomplish this, Inductively Coupled Plasma Mass Spectroscopy (ICP-MS) was used to determine concentrations of eight heavy metals (Cr, Cu, Ni, Zn, Cd, As, Pb, and Hg) in the $PM_{2.5}$ portion of road dust samples from five different land use areas (commercial, residential, industrial, parks, and educational) in Zhengzhou, China. The following were the average heavy metal concentrations in the city: Cr 46.26 mg/kg, Cu 25.13 mg/kg, Ni 12.51 mg/kg, Zn 152.35 mg/kg, Cd 0.56 mg/kg, As 11.53 mg/kg, Pb 52.15 mg/kg, and Hg 0.32 mg/kg. Two pollution indicators, the Pollution Index (PI) and the Geoaccumulation Index (I_{geo}), were used to determine the degree of contamination. Both PI and I_{geo} indicated the extreme pollution of Hg and Cd, while PI also ranked Zn in the extreme polluted range. The US Environmental Protection Agency (USEPA) model for adults and children was used to estimate health risks by inhalation. The results identified non-carcinogenic exposure of children to lead (HI > 0.1) in commercial and industrial areas. Both children and adults in Zhengzhou's commercial, residential, and park areas are exposed to higher levels of copper (Cu), lead (Pb), and zinc (Zn).

Keywords: geo-accumulation index; heavy metals; road dust; inhalation; resuspension; cancer

1. Introduction

Heavy metals pose a serious threat to human health, and their increasing presence in urban road dust warrants a health emergency. Studies reveal that the accumulation and spread of heavy metals in urban road dust is caused by both anthropogenic and natural factors [1]. Major anthropogenic sources of heavy metals include industrial, household and traffic emissions, while natural sources include soil particle deposition, resuspension, weathering, and erosion [2]. In general, urban areas are more vulnerable to heavy metal contamination compared to rural areas, given the population density and presence of diverse sources of pollution [3]. There has been a worldwide increase in pollutants owing to urban dust, which constitutes a genuine environmental and public health hazard [4].

Environmentalists believe that heavy metal contamination is a significant hazard to the environment [5], and during the previous two decades, a crisis happened with the increasing buildup and spread of heavy metals [6]. There is evidence that chronic deposition of metals in metropolitan environments can operate as a secondary pollution source, resulting in public health issues. Because of their weakened or underdeveloped immune systems, the elderly and children are generally considered the most vulnerable groups. Unintentional intake of road powder, most of which goes from dirty hands to nasal passages, can cause heavy metals to be transferred to the human body [7–9]. Exposure to high amounts of ambient particulates (PMs) can induce severe respiratory effects [10]. In prior research, the respiratory system has been found to be more easily and more seriously affected by $PM_{2.5}$ than other human body systems [11]. Children once again make up the group more susceptible to heavy metals, which can negatively influence their natural growth [12].

The resuspension of dust belonging to the fraction of $PM_{2.5}$ is predominantly a cause of exposure of humans to heavy metals [13,14]. Water-soluble heavy metals have been found to contribute significantly to $PM_{2.5}$ and PM_{10} emissions in a variety of locales, particularly in urban areas [15]. It has been reported in previous research that re-suspended dust is primarily responsible for the presence of PM_1, PM_{10}, and $PM_{2.5}$ fractions. Their traffic emission percentages were found to be 3%, 36%, and 14%, respectively [16]. Moreover, dust particles with sizes < 100 μm can re-suspend due to winds and the movement of vehicles [17]. This kind of resuspension is particularly dangerous as heavy traffic flows do not only move the road dust, but are also responsible for the emission of metals such as Cu, Zn, Fe, and Pb [18]. The situation becomes worse in the case of unmaintained vehicles, not fully meeting the requirements of road-worthiness as is the situation in most of the developing countries. Hence, the production level of $PM_{2.5}$ is increased significantly [19,20].

In urban areas, parks, leisure places, and city squares are the centers of recreational, sporting, and commercial activities. As the living standard and lifestyles in China are improving, people are now more conscious about their health and entertainment, and there is increased anthropogenic activity at such places. Industrial areas are considered even more polluted due to the emission of hazardous gases. So, the health of people who live around these places are affected by the poor quality of environment. The dust containing heavy metals makes its way to the human body through inhalation, resuspension, ingestion, and dermal contact, culminating into serious health issues. That is why it is important to assess and mitigate the pollution levels and their effects on human health.

The main focus of this study is the assessment of health risk caused by $PM_{2.5}$ fraction of road dust. For this purpose, samples were collected from 29 locations that included different functional areas, such as industrial, residential, parks, educational, and commercial areas of Zhengzhou city and the capital of the Henan province in China. The intention behind choosing these areas was to include every prospect of environment where normal human beings come in contact with road dust. In previous studies, mostly the biggest cities received the attention of researchers for road dust pollution analysis, and minor attention was paid to medium or small cities [21,22]. As a result, despite being an economic, educational, industrial, and transportation center in China's central plains, Zhengzhou was overlooked. The key aims of this research, which is concentrated on the Zhengzhou metropolitan area, are as follows: (1) to find out the heavy metal concentrations related to traffic emissions of fraction $PM_{2.5}$ from the road dust of different functional areas; (2) assessment of the pollution degree using pollution indices, and (3) health risk assessment using risk carcinogenic (CR), and Hazard Index (HI) methods for old adults and children [23,24].

2. Materials and Methods

2.1. Study Area Background

As shown in Figure 1, the capital of Henan Province, Zhengzhou (34°45′50.4″ N, 113°41′2.4″ E), located in the megalopolis of the Central Plain, is an important commercial, transport, and logistics hub of central China. The city lies at the foot of the Funiu Mountains on the northeastern side. To the west, it is adjacent to high lands; to the east, it is encompassed by intermediate and lower terrain [25].

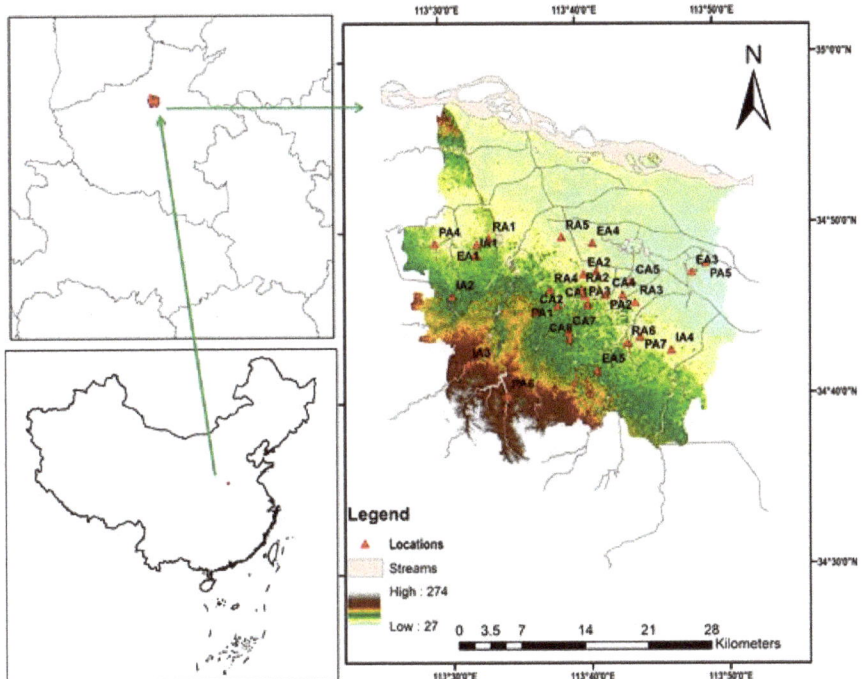

Figure 1. Study Area of Zhengzhou city.

The town has a moderate continental mountain climate in the northern zone. The yearly average temperature is 15.6 degrees Celsius, and the annual average precipitation is 542.15 mm. A monthly average temperature is 25.9 °C in the warmest month of August, while a monthly average temperature was 2.15 °C during the coldest month of January [26]. Despite the fact that there are four different seasons, the summers and winters are of significantly longer durations [27].

Zhengzhou's geographic location, natural resources, cultural glory, political prominence, administrative stature, historical splendor, and significance continue to draw an overwhelming number of visitors and inhabitants. In December 2019, the city's population was anticipated to be 10.350 million people [28]. It was also projected that the city had more than 4,500,000 authorized motor cars [29] and 3,000,000 un-registered automobiles [30]. Each of these features of urbanism contributes to an increase in carbon footprint and the emergence of environmental repercussions that are currently being observed in the city.

2.2. Sampling and Laboratory Analysis

2.2.1. Sample Collection

Twenty-nine locations were selected in Zhengzhou city that cover almost all the important places of different functional nature and the busiest roads, serving the maximum population (adults, patients, and children) of the city, comprising of those directly exposed to road dust pollution. Three samples of road dust were collected from each location: one sample from the center of the road, the second from the side of the road, and the third from the front of building areas near that road. In this way, eighty-seven samples in total were collected from twenty-nine locations, including five educational areas, four industrial areas, six residential areas, seven commercial areas, and seven park/leisure areas. A plastic brush was used to collect the road dust with the help of a pan and then collected into the plastic bags. The quantity of the dust samples was >150 g from one sampling point [31,32].

After that, all the samples were shifted to the laboratory for analysis and kept for at least one week for drying purposes [33].

2.2.2. PM$_{2.5}$ Preparation and Total Metal Concentration

For the preparation of PM$_{2.5}$, Teflon filters were used with a size of 47 mm to acquire the inhalable segment of the PM$_{2.5}$ of road dust [34]. Prior to this process, all the Teflon filters (47 mm) were dried out in a vacuum freeze dryer at 150 °C and kept for 6 h to fully remove the moisture contents, and then were conditioned at 25 °C for next 48 h. Afterwards, using an electronic microbalance, the blank filters were measured thrice and a flask with a size of 250 mL was used to pour road dust with particle sizes <53 μm. The road dust was pushed into the re-suspension chamber with the air pressure after its entry into the flask, and samples of dust were gathered through the outlets of PM$_{2.5}$ on Teflon filters (47 mm) for around a minute [35]. The filters contained PM$_{2.5}$ fractions that were separated from the outlets in the next step. Again, the weight was measured of all the filters thrice using electronic microbalance after the filtration of the PM$_{2.5}$ fraction. At the last step, the filters were folded halfway and stored at 20 °C by wrapping in the foil sheets of aluminum till the analysis was conducted.

Using the same technique employed in prior research studies [36], the total metal content was measured using Inductively Coupled Plasma Mass Spectroscopy (ICP-MS) subsequent aqua-regia digestion with the same approach as per earlier studies. In brief, Teflon filters holding the PM$_{2.5}$ proportion of samples of dust were composed of two equal portions, with each part digested with 5 mL of aqua-regia mixture. In order to analyze the samples using ICP-MS, they were diluted with 2 percent nitric acid (HNO$_3$) solution and then analyzed using a mass spectrometer.

2.2.3. Quality Control (QC)

In order to ensure the quality of the analysis, all samples were collected in triplicate, including the Standard Reference Material (SRM) and filter blanks. Acids with trace concentrations are deemed appropriate for analysis and digestion. Therefore, we used trace-grade acids (nitric acid and hydrochloric acid) instead of pure acids. The National Center of Standard Materials of China (NCSMC) provided the standard reference material (GBW07451), which was acquired by the institution, i.e., Zhengzhou university (ZZU). The analysis was carried out twice so as to ensure the precision of the spiked samples and aqua-regia digestion process. The recovery percentage was determined using spiked samples, SRM metal concentrations, and samples using the same method as prior studies [36]. The recoveries varied from (90% to 100.3%) and (80% to 130.2%) correspondingly from internal and SRM standards.

2.3. Pollution Level Assessment

The amount of heavy metal contamination in natural environmental samples including dust, soil, and water is determined using a number of methodologies. In this study, Pollution Index (PI) and Geoaccumulation Index (I$_{geo}$) were used to quantify the pollution degree of heavy metals in PM$_{2.5}$ fractioned road dust samples, and the conclusions were drawn. Because of the log function and constant factor of 1.5, the index of Geoaccumulation differs from various other pollution indices, and thus allows for the prevention of lithogenic effects that may be connected to variations in baseline levels [31]. However, the enrichment factor has been used to distinguish between the roles of natural and manmade sources of pollution [37]. For the purposes of computing the enrichment factor and Geoaccumulation Index, background values of (Cr, Ni, Cu, Zn, As, Cd, Pb, and Hg) in Zhengzhou city were obtained from a previous study [38], that are 64 mg/kg, 21 mg/kg, 14 mg/kg, 42 mg/kg, 8 mg/kg, 0.08 mg/kg, 18 mg/kg and 0.023 mg/kg, respectively.

2.3.1. GeoAccumulation Index (Igeo)

In the following study [39], Geoaccumulation Index (I_{geo}) was used to measure heavy metal pollution in sediments. This approach has been adopted by a large number of researchers for determining the degree of heavy metal pollution in road dust and soil [40–42]. Here is the I_{geo} equation to calculate it:

$$I_{geo} = \log_2 \frac{C_{HM}}{1.5 \times BV} \quad (1)$$

where C_{HM} = heavy metals concentration, BV = background value of metals.

2.3.2. Pollution Index (PI)

The following equation was used to calculate the pollution level that defines the Pollution Index [43]:

$$PI = \frac{C_n}{B_n} \quad (2)$$

where C_n = concentration of metal, B_n = background value of that metal.

Geoaccumulation Index (I_{geo}) and Pollution Index (PI) values and categories were classified in Table 1.

Table 1. Indexes classification for Geoaccumulation Index (I_{geo}) and Pollution Index (PI).

Index	Value	Category
Geo-accumulation Index (I_{geo})	$I_{geo} < 0$	Unpolluted
	I_{geo} 0–1	Unpolluted–moderately
	I_{geo} 1–2	Moderately
	I_{geo} 2–3	Moderately–strongly
	I_{geo} 3–4	Strongly
	I_{geo} 4–5	Strongly–extremely
	$I_{geo} > 5$	Extremely
Pollution Index (PI)	$PI \leq 1$	Low
	$1 < PI \leq 3$	Medium
	$PI > 3$	High

2.4. Health Risk Assessment

The buildup of hazardous metals in urban road dust has the potential to have a significant adverse effect on human health. By identifying the potential exposure, the level of risk to human health presented by hazardous metals may be quantified [24]. The breathing route has been assigned a significant place among the major routes of heavy metal exposure to human body [44]. The health hazards of $PM_{2.5}$ fractioned road dust samples were examined for old adults and children in this study using a two-step methodology devised by the researchers, which includes risk characterization and exposure assessment [12].

2.4.1. Exposure Assessment

The ongoing research has concentrated exclusively on exposure concentrations and inhalation exposure that were derived using the equation below [23,24].

$$MDI_{inh} = \frac{C \times R_{inh} \times EF \times ED}{PEF \times BW \times AT} \quad (3)$$

where MDI_{inh} = daily average intake dose of metals for inhalation, C = metal concentration, R_{inh} = inhalation rate, EF = exposure frequency, ED = exposure duration, PEF = particular emission factor, BW = body weight, and AT = average time.

2.4.2. Risk Assessment

The Hazards Index (HI), Hazards Quotient (HQ), and Carcinogenic Risk Index (CRI) were used to measure health risks for children and old adults. HQ and HI denote non-carcinogenic risk, but CRI denotes the chances of heavy metals being potentially carcinogenic in old adults and children. These parameters were calculated using the following equations:

$$HQ_i = \frac{MDI}{RFD} \quad (4)$$

$$HI = \sum HQ_i \quad (5)$$

$$CR_i = MDI \times SF \quad (6)$$

$$CR = \sum CR_i \quad (7)$$

where MDI = daily metals intake dose, RFD = reference dose, HQ_i = non-carcinogenic risk, HI = sum of hazard quotient, CR = carcinogenic risk, and SF = slope factor.

3. Results and Discussions

3.1. Heavy Metals in Road Dust

Except for Cr and Ni, all heavy metal mean concentrations were determined to be higher than corresponding background values [38]. The amounts of Hg and Cd were found to be 14 and 7 times higher, respectively, than respective background values. Anthropogenic activity, coal and oil burning, and metal refining can all be attributed for the substantially increased levels of Hg and Cd [45,46]. The mean, median, and minimum and maximum values of heavy metal concentrations are presented in Table 2.

Table 2. Heavy metal statistical values in (mg/kg).

Statistical Values	Cr	Ni	Cu	Zn	As	Cd	Pb	Hg
Background values [38]	64	21	14	42	8	0.08	18	0.02
Min	19.93	6.77	7.99	35.53	8.03	0.12	19.30	0.03
Max	94.78	28.23	63.26	1319.28	17.49	3.48	160.62	1.54
Mean	46.26	12.51	25.13	152.35	11.53	0.56	52.15	0.32
Median	40.96	12.38	22.08	113.45	11.11	0.45	43.16	0.14

The concentration of Zn was the highest among all the heavy metals, but it was lower than that of other major cities of China. Cr, Cu, Ni, Zn, Cd, and Pb concentrations in Zhengzhou were lower than all other cities of China used for the comparison, as presented in Table 3. As and Hg were the only two heavy metals whose concentrations in Zhengzhou were in the intermediate range compared to other cities. Their concentrations in Zhengzhou were higher than those of Beijing but lower than those of Baoji and Guangzhou [47,48]. The concentration of Hg was lower than in Baoji, but higher than in Beijing and Guangzhou [3,48]. In comparison to the background values of Zhengzhou, the concentration was considerably greater, requiring the serious response of regulators and other stakeholders to address the situation. Land use in Zhengzhou's counties had no discernible effect on mercury concentrations. This demonstrates the little effect on the propagation of mercury from road cleaning and sweeping systems and rainfall handling. The heavy metal mean concentrations in the samples were in the following order: Zn > Pb > Cr > Cu >Ni > As > Cd > Hg. It was found that the concentration of heavy metals was maximum in commercial areas, which can be attributed to increased traffic volumes and recreational activities. Additionally, the dense concentration of high-rise structures in a region can impair spontaneous aeration, culminating into increased levels of pollutants [49]. Consequently, the presence of high-rise structures in commercial areas may be responsible for the increased concentration of pollutants. When comparing residential regions to educational and commercial sectors, the zinc concentration was greater in residential areas [50].

The lowest concentrations of heavy metals were found in parks and recreation places, with the exception of As and Cd, which may be related to the distinct behaviors and properties of these metals. For Cr, the maximum concentration was seen in commercial areas, while the lowest concentration was observed in parks. In general, the risk of the presence of toxins was higher in commercial areas. As is evident from the examples of lead and copper, commercial zones had the heaviest loads, whereas parks had the lowest.

Table 3. Comparison of concentrations with other cities of China in (mg/kg).

City	Cr	Ni	Cu	Zn	As	Cd	Pb	Hg
Zhengzhou, China (Background values) [38]	64	21	14	42	8	0.08	18	0.02
Zhengzhou, China (Mean)	46.26	12.51	25.13	152.35	11.53	0.56	52.15	0.32
Beijing, China [3]	92.1	32.47	83.12	280.65	4.88	0.59	60.88	0.16
Beijing Park, China [51]	69.33	25.97	72.13	219.2	-	0.64	201.82	-
Baoji, China [47]	126.7	48.8	123.2	715.3	19.8	NA	433.2	1.1
Chengdu, China [50]	84.3	24.4	100	296	-	1.66	82.3	-
Guangzhou, China [48]	176.22	41.38	192.36	1777.18	20.05	2.14	387.53	0.22
Guiyang, China [52]	129.04	60.43	129.33	176.05	-	0.61	63.12	-
Nanjing, China [21]	126	55.9	123	394	13.4	1.1	103	0.12
Shanghai, China [53]	157	NA	NA	NA	8.73	1.24	246	0.16

The possible source of these heavy metals has been explained in Table 4.

Table 4. Possible sources of heavy metals of this study.

Metals	Possible Emission Source
Cr	Fuel and incineration of lubricants [2]
Ni	Tire abrasion and fuel combustion [54]
Cu	Brake wear, coal combustion, and brake pad [55]
Zn	Brake wear, lubricants, and tire abrasion [56]
Cd	Engine wear, lubricating oil, and brake wear [57]
As	Drinkable water, foods, and tobacco [58]
Pb	Fuel, motor oil combustion, brake wear [18]
Hg	Anthropogenic and natural sources [1]

3.2. Pollution Level Assessment

Numerous approaches for measuring the degree of metal contamination in dust and soil have been proposed. While assessing the degree of accumulation of heavy metals in the $PM_{2.5}$ portion of road dust, we utilized the Geoaccumulation Index (I_{geo}) and the Pollution Index (PI). I_{geo} and PI indices have been deemed well-established techniques for measuring the impacts of heavy metals on the environment by prior research and have been used in a range of applications [41].

3.2.1. Geoaccumulation Index (I_{geo})

Each of the eight metals had their Geoaccumulation Index (I_{geo}) computed, and the results can be seen in Table 5.

Table 5. Heavy metals' Geoaccumulation Index (I_{geo}) in road dust (mg/kg).

Geoaccumulation Index	Cr	Ni	Cu	Zn	As	Cd	Pb	Hg
Minimum	−2.26	−2.21	−1.39	−0.82	−0.57	−0.02	−0.48	−0.02
Maximum	−0.01	−0.15	1.59	4.38	0.54	4.85	2.57	10.02
Mean	−1.14	−1.38	0.07	0.91	−0.08	1.91	0.79	2.71

As per the Geoaccumulation Index (I_{geo}), the exposure of chromium (Cr), arsenic (As), and nickel (Ni) was determined to be minimal and within the range of being unpolluted. They were less than zero in their risk assessment values, demonstrating that the road dust of Zhengzhou was not contaminated with Cr, As, and Ni. Cu, Zn, and Pb contamination values were within the unpolluted to moderately polluted ranges. In the case of Cd and Hg, however, the levels of pollutants, owing to air deposition and road particle absorption, were quite high. The former was determined to be in the moderately contaminated category, whilst the latter was found to be in the moderate to severe polluted range, respectively. In the following order, the Igeo values decreased: Hg > Cd > Zn > Pb > Cu > As > Cr > Ni.

3.2.2. Pollution Index (PI)

The Pollution Index (PI) was computed for each of the eight factors under study, and Table 6 shows the resulting minimum, maximum, and mean values for each of the eight elements under research.

Table 6. Heavy metals' Pollution Index (PI) in road dust (mg/kg).

Pollution Index	Cr	Ni	Cu	Zn	As	Cd	Pb	Hg
Minimum	0.31	0.32	0.65	0.86	1.12	2.19	1.24	1.54
Maximum	1.33	1.08	3.97	16.86	1.81	25.77	5.74	48.12
Mean	0.72	0.59	1.79	3.62	1.43	7.15	2.89	14.25

Chromium (Cr) and nickel (Ni) pollution index values were lower than 1, i.e., 0.72 and 0.59, respectively, which indicated the low pollution or no pollution based on PI estimation. In the case of Copper (Cu), arsenic (As), and lead (Pb), the Pollution Index showed the values 1.79, 1.43, and 2.89, respectively and lies within the range ($1 < PI \leq 3$) of moderate pollution. Zinc (Zn), cadmium (Cd) and mercury (Hg) were in the range ($PI > 3$) of high pollution having values 3.62, 7.15 and 14.25, respectively. So, the concerned heavy metals were Zn, Cd, and Hg as per the Pollution Index (PI) estimation, similar to the Geoaccumulation Index (I_{geo}), with the exception of Zn.

3.3. Health Risk Assessment

For those with weak immune systems, including children and patients, harmful metal-laden road dust can be highly hazardous. Children and adults have inhalation exposure to the heavy metals investigated within $PM_{2.5}$ factionalized road dust samples collected from Zhengzhou. A United States Environmental Protection Agency (USEPA) health risk assessment technique was used to calculate children's and adults' health risks associated with the investigated metals, both non-carcinogenic and carcinogenic. The absence of local guideline values necessitated the use of the USEPA's model to compute health risks. The values from prior literature were used, as indicated in Table 7, to quantify health risks using the model. RFD values were: Cd (1.00×10^{-3}), Cr (2.86×10^{-5}), Cu (4.02×10^{-2}), Ni (2.06×10^{-2}), Pb (3.52×10^{-3}), Zn (3.00×10^{-1}), Hg (8.57×10^{-5}), and As (1.23×10^{-4}), while SF values were; As (1.51×10^{0}), Cd (6.30×10^{0}), Cr (4.20×10^{1}), Ni (8.40×10^{-1}), and Pb (8.50×10^{-3}). A carcinogenic and non-carcinogenic health risk Hazard Index (HI) and Hazard Quotient (HQ) was determined by using MDI_{inh} values for child and adult exposition to toxic metals via resettled road dust. In the current study, eight hazardous metals were chosen for non-carcinogenic and carcinogenic health risk evaluation.

Table 7. Carcinogenic and non-carcinogenic indices parameters.

Parameter	Factor	Values	Units
Average Time	AT	$365 \times ED$	Days
Bodyweight	BW (Child)	15	Kg
Bodyweight	BW (Adult)	70	Kg
Exposure duration	ED (Child)	6	Years
Exposure duration	ED (Adult)	24	Years
Exposure frequency	EF	180	Days/year
Dust inhalation rate	R_{Inh} (Child)	10	m^3/day
Dust inhalation rate	R_{Inh} (Adult)	20	m^3/day
Particular emission rate	PEF	1.36×10^9	m^3/kg

3.3.1. Non-Carcinogenic Risk

The samples of dust collected from distinct land-use areas were used to determine the HI values and HQs in different exposure routes. As per the evaluation made according to statistical data in Table 8, the sequence of the HI values of the all the heavy elements at risk in various functional domains is as follows: commercial > industrial > residential > educational > parks, for adults and children. Although the non-carcinogenic risk score of each heavy element was higher in magnitude for children, compared to those for adults in comparable functional domains, no statistically significant difference was detected between land-use areas. Children in industrial and commercial areas had the highest non-carcinogenic risk level, HI > 0.1, to all the heavy elements exposed to the human body by urban dust in diverse land use. Furthermore, even at low concentrations, lead (Pb) is harmful to human health because it interferes with the development of the brain system and other organs [59]. High amounts of lead in the bloodstream, additionally, can induce bone deformities [60], particularly in youngsters, and may also have a detrimental influence on the body's neurological system, kidneys, and brain tissues [12,52]. The people, particularly youngsters, chronically exposed to polluted commercial and industrial environments require special protection and healthcare. It shows that the HI geographical distribution trend of each heavy element is the same for adults and children. Since children are more vulnerable than adults, the HI for a given heavy element at a given concentration is higher in children than in adults [59]. Arsenic can be present in a variety of sources, including drinkable water, foods, and tobacco. Long-term inorganic arsenic exposure, which is most typically acquired by drinking water and food, has been linked to chronic arsenic poisoning. As per a World Health Organization study, arsenic in contaminated water is easily absorbed and might cause health problems based on its metabolic form [58].

Table 8. Hazard Index (HI) values of heavy metals in different land use areas.

Land Use Areas	Non-Carcinogenic	HI							
		Cr	Ni	Cu	Zn	As	Cd	Pb	Hg
Educational	Adult	9.12×10^{-3}	1.83×10^{-4}	4.07×10^{-4}	3.66×10^4	1.06×10^{-2}	9.90×10^{-4}	9.79×10^{-3}	1.03×10^{-2}
	Children	1.71×10^{-2}	4.15×10^{-4}	3.82×10^{-3}	3.41×10^{-3}	2.42×10^{-2}	1.75×10^{-3}	9.07×10^{-2}	1.04×10^{-2}
Residential	Adult	1.18×10^{-2}	1.86×10^{-4}	5.66×10^{-4}	3.92×10^{-4}	1.04×10^{-2}	5.80×10^{-4}	1.05×10^{-2}	1.56×10^{-2}
	Children	2.13×10^{-2}	4.15×10^{-4}	5.29×10^{-3}	3.65×10^{-3}	2.32×10^{-2}	1.02×10^{-3}	9.64×10^{-2}	1.54×10^{-2}
Parks	Adult	8.41×10^{-3}	1.64×10^{-4}	2.88×10^{-4}	2.25×10^{-4}	1.06×10^{-2}	5.41×10^{-4}	7.11×10^{-3}	7.96×10^{-3}
	Children	1.54×10^{-2}	3.67×10^{-4}	2.67×10^{-3}	2.08×10^{-3}	2.43×10^{-2}	9.58×10^{-4}	6.59×10^{-2}	7.87×10^{-3}
Commercial	Adult	1.56×10^{-1}	1.87×10^{-4}	7.44×10^{-4}	3.46×10^{-4}	9.22×10^{-3}	8.43×10^{-4}	1.36×10^{-2}	1.61×10^{-2}
	Children	2.85×10^{-2}	4.16×10^{-4}	6.93×10^{-3}	3.25×10^{-3}	2.08×10^{-2}	1.51×10^{-3}	1.25×10^{-1}	1.59×10^{-3}
Industrial	Adult	1.65×10^{-2}	2.81×10^{-4}	3.32×10^{-4}	3.17×10^{-4}	9.72×10^{-3}	5.16×10^{-4}	1.17×10^{-2}	9.77×10^{-3}
	Children	3.07×10^{-2}	6.32×10^{-4}	3.06×10^{-3}	2.92×10^{-3}	2.21×10^{-2}	9.11×10^{-4}	1.06×10^{-1}	9.64×10^{-3}

3.3.2. Carcinogenic Risk

The carcinogenic risk of heavy metals such as Cr, Ni, Cd, and As assessed in this study revealed that the risk of cancer for Ni, Cd, and As was negligible, with average cancer risk factors of 6.57×10^{-10}, 2.03×10^{-10}, and 9.66×10^{-10}, correspondingly, which fell below the lower range of threshold values 10^{-6} to 10^{-4} and are considered acceptable, as shown in Table 9. However, the higher value of As was a cause for concern and can lead to many harmful consequences such as severe damage (keratosis, leucomelanosis, and melanosis) [61]. In Zhengzhou, the cancer risk (Cr = 1.16×10^{-7}) posed to the population was possibly near to the lower limit value of 10^{-6}, while the samples collected from inside the industrial region exhibited a cancer risk of 8.57×10^{-7}. Carcinogenic elements are classified into five functional categories based on their hazard index values. The largest cancer health hazards are associated with Cr and Ni and are found in the industrial region, followed by commercial, residential or educational, and parks, which have comparable HI values. Furthermore, chromium is widely used to preserve metal surfaces and construction materials, including in electrolysis, cells, polymers, and fertilizers [50]. Thus, the development of educational and commercial buildings, as well as the usage of cells and polymers in residential areas, may account for the educational, commercial, and residential areas having higher carcinogenic values of chromium (Cr). As a result, the cancer risk associated with Cr exposure to people, particularly in industrial settings, should be given significant consideration. A comprehensive assessment of pollution risks for a city should also consider the health risks posed by certain toxins, such as polycyclic aromatic hydrocarbons ($PM_{2.5}$), other undetected heavy metals including Fe and Mn, or in somewhat high-pollution areas (such as mining areas), in addition to the risks posed by other pollutants.

Table 9. Carcinogenic Risk (CR) values of heavy metals in different land use areas.

Land Use Areas	Carcinogenic	CR			
		Cr	Ni	As	Cd
Educational	Adult	8.93×10^{-8}	6.31×10^{-10}	1.02×10^{-9}	2.90×10^{-10}
Residential	Adult	1.12×10^{-7}	6.25×10^{-10}	9.77×10^{-10}	1.71×10^{-10}
Parks	Adult	8.21×10^{-8}	5.55×10^{-10}	1.04×10^{-9}	1.60×10^{-10}
Commercial	Adult	1.53×10^{-7}	6.33×10^{-10}	8.86×10^{-10}	2.46×10^{-10}
Industrial	Adult	1.60×10^{-7}	9.61×10^{-10}	9.31×10^{-10}	1.50×10^{-10}

4. Conclusions

Heavy chemicals in road dust pose a serious health risk to people. The amounts of eight heavy metals in Zhengzhou metropolitan road dust and the level of harm to human health have been evaluated in the current study. With the exception of Ni and Cr, all heavy metal concentrations were determined to be greater than their background levels. The amounts of Hg and Cd were 14 and 7 times greater than their respective background levels, which shows high contamination. This alarming situation requires immediate action by all stakeholders. I_{geo} indicated a range of pollution categories, from strongly polluted (Cd and Hg) to unpolluted (Ni and Cr). PI produced almost similar results, placing Ni and Cr in the range of low pollution or no pollution and Cd, Zn, and Hg in the range of high pollution, whereas Zn pollution was not indicated by Igeo.

Analyzing non-carcinogenic risk factors, the largest for children was the exposure to Pb (HI > 0.1) in commercial and industrial areas among all the land-use areas under consideration. It was further divulged that that both children and adults in Zhengzhou's commercial, residential, and park areas were highly exposed to Cu, Pb, and Zn. The major source of these metals in such cases is vehicular exhaust. Northwestern Zhengzhou was found at the highest non-carcinogenic exposure risk to Cr and Ni from point sources. The cancer risk value of Cr was more likely to be at the lower limit of the threshold value, particularly in the industrial sector. As a result of the enhanced heavy metal concentrations in road dust as compared to background levels, it appears that the current situation is deteriorating, and people of the Zhengzhou metropolitan are at high risk of experiencing to these heavy metals.

Author Contributions: Conceptualization, M.F., Z.W. and H.W.; data curation, M.F.; formal analysis, M.F.; investigation, M.F.; methodology, M.F. and Z.W.; visualization, M.F.; writing—original draft preparation, M.F.; writing—review and editing, M.F., Z.W., H.W., Z.H. and M.I.A.; funding acquisition, Z.W.; project administration, Z.W. and H.W.; resources, Z.W.; software, Z.W. and H.W.; supervision, Z.W. and H.W.; validation, H.W. All authors have read and agreed to the published version of the manuscript.

Funding: This research was funded by National Natural Science Foundation of China, grant number 51879242 and 51739009.

Institutional Review Board Statement: Not applicable.

Informed Consent Statement: Not applicable.

Data Availability Statement: Not applicable.

Acknowledgments: The research was financially supported by the National Natural Science Foundation of China.

Conflicts of Interest: The authors affirm that they have no conflict of interest.

References

1. Faisal, M.; Wu, Z.; Wang, H.; Hussain, Z.; Shen, C. Geochemical Mapping, Risk Assessment, and Source Identification of Heavy Metals in Road Dust Using Positive Matrix Factorization (PMF). *Atmosphere* **2021**, *12*, 614. [CrossRef]
2. Ali, M.U.; Liu, G.; Yousaf, B.; Abbas, Q.; Ullah, H.; Munir, M.A.M.; Fu, B. Pollution characteristics and human health risks of potentially (eco)toxic elements (PTEs) in road dust from metropolitan area of Hefei, China. *Chemosphere* **2017**, *181*, 111–121. [CrossRef]
3. Men, C.; Liu, R.; Xu, F.; Wang, Q.; Guo, L.; Shen, Z. Pollution characteristics, risk assessment, and source apportionment of heavy metals in road dust in Beijing, China. *Sci. Total Environ.* **2018**, *612*, 138–147. [CrossRef]
4. Lanzerstorfer, C. Toward more intercomparable road dust studies. *Crit. Rev. Environ. Sci. Technol.* **2021**, *51*, 826–855. [CrossRef]
5. Huang, H.; Lin, C.; Yu, R.; Yan, Y.; Hu, G.; Li, H. Contamination assessment, source apportionment and health risk assessment of heavy metals in paddy soils of Jiulong River Basin, Southeast China. *RSC Adv.* **2019**, *9*, 14736–14744. [CrossRef]
6. Kastury, F.; Smith, E.; Juhasz, A. A critical review of approaches and limitations of inhalation bioavailability and bioaccessibility of metal(loid)s from ambient particulate matter or dust. *Sci. Total Environ.* **2017**, *574*, 1054–1074. [CrossRef] [PubMed]
7. Wiseman, C.L.; Levesque, C.; Rasmussen, P.E. Characterizing the sources, concentrations and resuspension potential of metals and metalloids in the thoracic fraction of urban road dust. *Sci. Total Environ.* **2021**, *786*, 147367. [CrossRef] [PubMed]
8. Zhu, X.; Yu, W.; Li, F.; Liu, C.; Ma, J.; Yan, J.; Wang, Y.; Tian, R. Spatio-temporal distribution and source identification of heavy metals in particle size fractions of road dust from a typical industrial district. *Sci. Total Environ.* **2021**, *780*, 146557. [CrossRef] [PubMed]
9. Gujre, N.; Rangan, L.; Mitra, S. Occurrence, geochemical fraction, ecological and health risk assessment of cadmium, copper and nickel in soils contaminated with municipal solid wastes. *Chemosphere* **2021**, *271*, 129573. [CrossRef]
10. Shakerkhatibi, M.; Seifipour, H.; Sabeti, Z.; Kahe, D.; Jafarabadi, M.A.; Benis, K.Z.; Hajaghazadeh, M. Correlation of ambient particulate matters (PM10, PM2.5) with respiratory hospital admissions: A case-crossover study in Urmia, Iran. *Hum. Ecol. Risk Assess. Int. J.* **2021**, *27*, 2184–2201. [CrossRef]
11. Khan, R.K.; Strand, M.A. Road dust and its effect on human health: A literature review. *Epidemiol. Health* **2018**, *40*, e2018013. [CrossRef]
12. Rahman, M.S.; Khan, M.; Jolly, Y.; Kabir, J.; Akter, S.; Salam, A. Assessing risk to human health for heavy metal contamination through street dust in the Southeast Asian Megacity: Dhaka, Bangladesh. *Sci. Total Environ.* **2019**, *660*, 1610–1622. [CrossRef] [PubMed]
13. Alves, C.; Evtyugina, M.; Vicente, A.; Vicente, E.; Nunes, T.; Silva, P.; Duarte, M.; Pio, C.; Amato, F.; Querol, X. Chemical profiling of PM10 from urban road dust. *Sci. Total Environ.* **2018**, *634*, 41–51. [CrossRef] [PubMed]
14. Chen, S.; Zhang, X.; Lin, J.; Huang, J.; Zhao, D.; Yuan, T.; Huang, K.; Luo, Y.; Jia, Z.; Zang, Z.; et al. Fugitive Road Dust PM2.5 Emissions and Their Potential Health Impacts. *Environ. Sci. Technol.* **2019**, *53*, 8455–8465. [CrossRef] [PubMed]
15. Chow, J.C.; Watson, J.; Lu, Z.; Lowenthal, D.H.; Frazier, C.A.; Solomon, P.A.; Thuillier, R.H.; Magliano, K. Descriptive analysis of PM2.5 and PM10 at regionally representative locations during SJVAQS/AUSPEX. *Atmos. Environ.* **1996**, *30*, 2079–2112. [CrossRef]
16. Amato, F.; Pandolfi, M.; Escrig, A.; Querol, X.; Alastuey, A.; Pey, J.; Perez, N.; Hopke, P. Quantifying road dust resuspension in urban environment by Multilinear Engine: A comparison with PMF2. *Atmos. Environ.* **2009**, *43*, 2770–2780. [CrossRef]

17. Zhao, H.; Shao, Y.; Yin, C.; Jiang, Y.; Li, X. An index for estimating the potential metal pollution contribution to atmospheric particulate matter from road dust in Beijing. *Sci. Total Environ.* **2016**, *550*, 167–175. [CrossRef]
18. Lough, G.C.; Schauer, J.J.; Park, J.-S.; Shafer, M.M.; DeMinter, J.T.; Weinstein, J.P. Emissions of Metals Associated with Motor Vehicle Roadways. *Environ. Sci. Technol.* **2005**, *39*, 826–836. [CrossRef]
19. Alshetty, V.D.; Kuppili, S.K.; Nagendra, S.S.; Ramadurai, G.; Sethi, V.; Kumar, R.; Sharma, N.; Namdeo, A.; Bell, M.; Goodman, P.; et al. Characteristics of tail pipe (Nitric oxide) and resuspended dust emissions from urban roads—A case study in Delhi city. *J. Transp. Health* **2020**, *17*, 100653. [CrossRef]
20. Lurie, K.; Nayebare, S.R.; Fatmi, Z.; Carpenter, D.O.; Siddique, A.; Malashock, D.; Khan, K.; Zeb, J.; Hussain, M.M.; Khatib, F.; et al. $PM_{2.5}$ in a megacity of Asia (Karachi): Source apportionment and health effects. *Atmos. Environ.* **2019**, *202*, 223–233. [CrossRef]
21. Liu, E.; Wang, X.; Liu, H.; Liang, M.; Zhu, Y.; Li, Z. Chemical speciation, pollution and ecological risk of toxic metals in readily washed off road dust in a megacity (Nanjing), China. *Ecotoxicol. Environ. Saf.* **2019**, *173*, 381–392. [CrossRef]
22. Han, N.M.M.; Latif, M.T.; Othman, M.; Dominick, D.; Mohamad, N.; Juahir, H.; Tahir, N.M. Composition of selected heavy metals in road dust from Kuala Lumpur city centre. *Environ. Earth Sci.* **2014**, *72*, 849–859. [CrossRef]
23. Rehman, A.; Liu, G.; Yousaf, B.; Rehman, M.Z.U.; Ali, M.U.; Rashid, M.S.; Farooq, M.R.; Javed, Z. Characterizing pollution indices and children health risk assessment of potentially toxic metal(oid)s in school dust of Lahore, Pakistan. *Ecotoxicol. Environ. Saf.* **2020**, *190*, 110059. [CrossRef]
24. Jayarathne, A.; Egodawatta, P.; Ayoko, G.A.; Goonetilleke, A. Assessment of ecological and human health risks of metals in urban road dust based on geochemical fractionation and potential bioavailability. *Sci. Total Environ.* **2018**, *635*, 1609–1619. [CrossRef]
25. The State Council on the General Planning of Zhengzhou City. Available online: http://www.gov.cn/zwgk/2010-08/23/content_1686432.htm (accessed on 23 October 2010).
26. Zhengzhou Local History Office. Available online: http://szb.zhengzhou.gov.cn/html/2012/zzgl_1219/57.html (accessed on 11 February 2016).
27. Zhengzhou Local History Office. Available online: http://szb.zhengzhou.gov.cn/zzgl/1142969.jhtml (accessed on 18 April 2014).
28. Zhengzhou Statistical Bulletin on National Economic and Social Development 2019. Available online: http://tjj.zhengzhou.gov.cn/tjgb/3112732.jhtml (accessed on 7 February 2021).
29. Zhengzhou Municipal Public Bureau. Available online: http://zzga.zhengzhou.gov.cn/jfgg/3460061.jhtml (accessed on 24 June 2020).
30. China Electric Vehicle Association. The Number of Electric Vehicles in Zhengzhou Has Exceeded 3 Million. Available online: http://www.ceva.org.cn/cn/viewnews/20191015/20191015102917.htm (accessed on 15 October 2019).
31. Othman, M.; Latif, M.T.; Matsumi, Y. The exposure of children to PM2.5 and dust in indoor and outdoor school classrooms in Kuala Lumpur City Centre. *Ecotoxicol. Environ. Saf.* **2019**, *170*, 739–749. [CrossRef] [PubMed]
32. Tian, S.; Liang, T.; Li, K. Fine road dust contamination in a mining area presents a likely air pollution hotspot and threat to human health. *Environ. Int.* **2019**, *128*, 201–209. [CrossRef] [PubMed]
33. Wang, Q.; Lu, X.; Pan, H. Analysis of heavy metals in the re-suspended road dusts from different functional areas in Xi'an, China. *Environ. Sci. Pollut. Res.* **2016**, *23*, 19838–19846. [CrossRef] [PubMed]
34. Ramírez, O.; de la Campa, A.M.S.; Amato, F.; Moreno, T.; Silva, L.; de la Rosa, J.D. Physicochemical characterization and sources of the thoracic fraction of road dust in a Latin American megacity. *Sci. Total Environ.* **2019**, *652*, 434–446. [CrossRef] [PubMed]
35. Kong, S.; Lu, B.; Ji, Y.; Zhao, X.; Bai, Z.; Xu, Y.; Liu, Y.; Jiang, H. Risk assessment of heavy metals in road and soil dusts within PM2.5, PM10 and PM100 fractions in Dongying city, Shandong Province, China. *J. Environ. Monit.* **2012**, *14*, 791–803. [CrossRef]
36. Kastury, F.; Smith, E.; Karna, R.R.; Scheckel, K.; Juhasz, A. Methodological factors influencing inhalation bioaccessibility of metal(loid)s in PM2.5 using simulated lung fluid. *Environ. Pollut.* **2018**, *241*, 930–937. [CrossRef]
37. Chen, H.; Lu, X.; Li, L.Y.; Gao, T.; Chang, Y. Metal contamination in campus dust of Xi'an, China: A study based on multivariate statistics and spatial distribution. *Sci. Total Environ.* **2014**, *484*, 27–35. [CrossRef] [PubMed]
38. Hangxin, C.; Kuo, L.; Min, L.; Ke, Y.; Fei, L.; Xiaomeng, C. Background and benchmark values of chemical elements in urban soils in China. *Geoscience Frontiers.* **2014**, *21*, 265. [CrossRef]
39. Müller, G. Index of Geo-Accumulation in Sediments of the Rhine River—ScienceOpen. Available online: https://www.scienceopen.com/document?vid=4b875795-5729-4c05-9813-64951e2ca488 (accessed on 1 April 2021).
40. Adimalla, N.; Wang, H. Distribution, contamination, and health risk assessment of heavy metals in surface soils from northern Telangana, India. *Arab. J. Geosci.* **2018**, *11*, 684. [CrossRef]
41. Faiz, Y.; Tufail, M.; Javed, M.T.; Chaudhry, M.; Siddique, N. Road dust pollution of Cd, Cu, Ni, Pb and Zn along Islamabad Expressway, Pakistan. *Microchem. J.* **2009**, *92*, 186–192. [CrossRef]
42. Trujillo-González, J.M.; Torres-Mora, M.A.; Keesstra, S.; Brevik, E.C.; Jiménez-Ballesta, R. Heavy metal accumulation related to population density in road dust samples taken from urban sites under different land uses. *Sci. Total Environ.* **2016**, *553*, 636–642. [CrossRef]
43. Lu, X.; Wang, L.; Lei, K.; Huang, J.; Zhai, Y. Contamination assessment of copper, lead, zinc, manganese and nickel in street dust of Baoji, NW China. *J. Hazard. Mater.* **2009**, *161*, 1058–1062. [CrossRef] [PubMed]
44. Hernández-Pellón, A.; Nischkauer, W.; Limbeck, A.; Fernandez-Olmo, I. Metal(loid) bioaccessibility and inhalation risk assessment: A comparison between an urban and an industrial area. *Environ. Res.* **2018**, *165*, 140–149. [CrossRef] [PubMed]

45. Al-Khashman, O.A. Determination of metal accumulation in deposited street dusts in Amman, Jordan. *Environ. Geochem. Health* **2007**, *29*, 1–10. [CrossRef] [PubMed]
46. Wang, G.; Xia, D.; Liu, X.; Chen, F.; Yu, Y.; Yang, L.; Chen, J.; Zhou, A. Spatial and temporal variation in magnetic properties of street dust in Lanzhou City, China. *Sci. Bull.* **2008**, *53*, 1913–1923. [CrossRef]
47. Lu, X.; Wang, L.; Li, L.; Lei, K.; Huang, L.; Kang, D. Multivariate statistical analysis of heavy metals in street dust of Baoji, NW China. *J. Hazard. Mater.* **2010**, *173*, 744–749. [CrossRef]
48. Huang, M.; Wang, W.; Chan, C.Y.; Cheung, K.C.; Man, Y.B.; Wang, X.; Wong, M.H. Contamination and risk assessment (based on bioaccessibility via ingestion and inhalation) of metal(loid)s in outdoor and indoor particles from urban centers of Guangzhou, China. *Sci. Total Environ.* **2014**, *479–480*, 117–124. [CrossRef] [PubMed]
49. Giyasov, B.; Giyasova, I. The Impact of High-Rise Buildings on the Living Environment. *E3S Web Conf.* **2018**, *33*, 01045. [CrossRef]
50. Li, H.-H.; Chen, L.-J.; Yu, L.; Guo, Z.-B.; Shan, C.-Q.; Lin, J.-Q.; Gu, Y.-G.; Yang, Z.-B.; Yang, Y.-X.; Shao, J.-R.; et al. Pollution characteristics and risk assessment of human exposure to oral bioaccessibility of heavy metals via urban street dusts from different functional areas in Chengdu, China. *Sci. Total Environ.* **2017**, *586*, 1076–1084. [CrossRef]
51. Du, Y.; Gao, B.; Zhou, H.; Ju, X.; Hao, H.; Yin, S. Health Risk Assessment of Heavy Metals in Road Dusts in Urban Parks of Beijing, China. *Procedia Environ. Sci.* **2013**, *18*, 299–309. [CrossRef]
52. Duan, Z.; Wang, J.; Xuan, B.; Cai, X.; Zhang, Y. Spatial Distribution and Health Risk Assessment of Heavy Metals in Urban Road Dust of Guiyang, China. *Nat. Environ. Pollut. Technol.* **2018**, *17*, 407–412.
53. Wang, J.; Chen, Z.; Sun, X.; Shi, G.; Xu, S.; Wang, D.; Wang, L. Quantitative spatial characteristics and environmental risk of toxic heavy metals in urban dusts of Shanghai, China. *Environ. Earth Sci.* **2009**, *59*, 645–654. [CrossRef]
54. Dehghani, S.; Moore, F.; Keshavarzi, B.; Beverley, A.H. Health risk implications of potentially toxic metals in street dust and surface soil of Tehran, Iran. *Ecotoxicol. Environ. Saf.* **2017**, *136*, 92–103. [CrossRef]
55. Pant, P.; Baker, S.J.; Shukla, A.; Maikawa, C.; Pollitt, K.G.; Harrison, R.M. The PM 10 fraction of road dust in the UK and India: Characterization, source profiles and oxidative potential. *Sci. Total Environ.* **2015**, *530–531*, 445–452. [CrossRef]
56. Hwang, H.-M.; Fiala, M.; Park, D.; Wade, T.L. Review of pollutants in urban road dust and stormwater runoff: Part 1. Heavy metals released from vehicles. *Int. J. Urban Sci.* **2016**, *20*, 334–360. [CrossRef]
57. Gope, M.; Masto, R.E.; George, J.; Hoque, R.R.; Balachandran, S. Bioavailability and health risk of some potentially toxic elements (Cd, Cu, Pb and Zn) in street dust of Asansol, India. *Ecotoxicol. Environ. Saf.* **2017**, *138*, 231–241. [CrossRef] [PubMed]
58. Chung, J.-Y.; Yu, S.-D.; Hong, Y.-S. Environmental Source of Arsenic Exposure. *J. Prev. Med. Public Health* **2014**, *47*, 253–257. [CrossRef] [PubMed]
59. Ackah, M. Soil elemental concentrations, geoaccumulation index, non-carcinogenic and carcinogenic risks in functional areas of an informal e-waste recycling area in Accra, Ghana. *Chemosphere* **2019**, *235*, 908–917. [CrossRef] [PubMed]
60. Mohmand, J.; Eqani, S.A.M.A.S.; Fasola, M.; Alamdar, A.; Mustafa, I.; Ali, N.; Liu, L.; Peng, S.; Shen, H. Human exposure to toxic metals via contaminated dust: Bio-accumulation trends and their potential risk estimation. *Chemosphere* **2015**, *132*, 142–151. [CrossRef] [PubMed]
61. Shil, S.; Singh, U.K. Health risk assessment and spatial variations of dissolved heavy metals and metalloids in a tropical river basin system. *Ecol. Indic.* **2019**, *106*, 105455. [CrossRef]

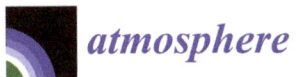

Article

Size-Segregated Elemental Profile and Associated Heath Risk Assessment of Road Dust along Major Traffic Corridors in Kolkata Mega City

Deepanjan Majumdar [1,*], Bratisha Biswas [2], Dipanjali Majumdar [1] and Rupam Ray [2]

1 Kolkata Zonal Centre, CSIR-National Environmental Engineering Research Institute, i-8, Sector C, EKDP, EM Bypass, Kolkata 700107, India; ds_majumdar@neeri.res.in
2 Asutosh College, University of Calcutta, 92 Shyamaprasad Mukherjee Road, Kolkata 700026, India; bratishabiswas@gmail.com (B.B.); rupamray14nov@gmail.com (R.R.)
* Correspondence: d_majumdar@neeri.res.in; Tel.: +91-33-24415999; Fax: +91-33-24417608

Abstract: Particle size distribution (PSD) of road dust has significant repercussions on atmospheric pollution by road dust resuspension. The PSD of road dust at a few major commercial, traffic, and residential sites in Kolkata mega city was analyzed in the size range of <28–2000 µm. Predominance of the coarse size range (212–600 µm followed by 106–212 µm) was observed. In size-segregated road dust, Fe (4.02–31.2 g kg^{-1}) dominated other elements and was followed by Mg (2.13–10.9 g kg^{-1}), Mn (79.2–601 mg kg^{-1}), Li (395.8–506.8 mg kg^{-1}), and others. Fine particles (<28 µm) had higher elemental concentrations than coarser ones. Cd and Li showed the highest degree of enrichment compared to the Earth's crust, but only Cd posed significant ecological risk due to its high ecological toxicity. Individual elements did not post significant non-cancer health risks, except for Li in children. However, the cumulative non-cancer risk from all toxic elements for children was almost four times higher than the acceptable level. Lifetime exposure to carcinogenic elements at the current level may pose 5 to 6 times higher cancer risk in the adult population than the acceptable risk of one in a million.

Keywords: air pollution; dry sieving; dust resuspension; human health risk; exposure; optical analysis; street dust

1. Introduction

Road dust is a complex mixture of particles of both natural and anthropogenic origins. The former is derived primarily from soil, plant, and animal kingdoms (e.g., mold spores, animal dander, pollen, pollen fragments) and atmospheric deposition. The latter comes from construction and demolition materials (asphalt, concrete, paint), road wear and tear, automobiles (tire and brake wear and tear, body rust, tailpipe exhaust, etc.), and industrial inputs [1–4].

Road dust shares a dynamic relationship with the ground-level atmosphere and gets resuspended in the air via the sweeping action of wind and vehicle movements on roads [5,6]. In a resuspension chamber study, Martuzevicius et al. [7] found that PM$_{2.5}$, PM$_{10}$, and PM$_{total}$ increased proportionally with increased airspeed from 8 m s^{-1} to 15 m s^{-1}. Dust particles with an aerodynamic diameter of about <1 µm to about 100 µm may become airborne, depending on their origin, physical characteristics, and ambient conditions [8]. The Urban Air Quality Management Strategy in Asia (URBAIR), based on the estimates of PM$_{10}$/TSP ratios for different sources, found that 20% of atmospheric PM10 came from road dust resuspension [9]. In Barcelona (Spain), Amato et al. [10] estimated that road dust accounted for 17% in PM$_{10}$, 8% of PM$_{2.5}$, and 2% of PM$_1$, implying that resuspension was responsible for 37%, 15%, and 3% of total traffic emissions, respectively, in PM$_{10}$, PM$_{2.5}$, and PM$_1$. It was estimated that annual total suspended particulates (TSP) emissions accounted for about 240,000 t y^{-1} in 2000 in urban and suburban Beijing. Traffic resuspended dust contributed more than 30% of atmospheric TSP [11]. In Kanpur (India), road dust emission was a significant source of air pollution, amounting to 25–50% of tailpipe emissions [12].

Particle size distribution (PSD) of road dust is of extreme importance as it governs mobility of particles in the association of attached pollutants and, together, govern air pollution potential of an area by resuspension [13,14]. In a study in Haidian District, Beijing, China, the median diameter of road dust (d_{50}) ranged from 100 to 200 µm [1]. Road dust from selected land-use types were predominantly fine particles (<250 µm, 60–75%), while grain size of 62–106 µm was the most abundant amongst eight size fractions, contributing 27 ± 5% and 38 ± 21% from college & residential and main traffic roads, respectively. Zafra et al. [15] reported that 82% of road dust vacuumed directly from the road surface was <1000 µm and 6.5% was <63 µm in Torrelavega (Northern Spain), while dust collected after sweeping was much finer, in which about 98% was of <1000 µ and 27% was under 63 µ. Vaze and Chiew [16] reported 10% and 15% contribution of vacuumed and swept road dust particles, respectively, in <100 µ road dust particles. Smaller particles with lower density, greater surface area per unit volume [17], and potential association with higher amounts of organics and pollutants are of particular concern [18,19]. A significant positive association between $PM_{2.5}$ in road dust and hospital admissions due to cardiovascular and respiratory complications have been reported [20,21]. Therefore, road dust has immense importance from environmental and health perspectives. Populations with specific occupations such as drivers, roadside hawkers, shop owners, workers in roadside offices, and traffic police personnel are particularly vulnerable due to their occupational exposure towards fine road dust and road dust-borne contaminants.

Kolkata is a megacity and one of the largest in the world in terms of population density of 24,252 persons per sq. km, underlining the importance of likely health risk from road dust resuspension [22]. In a recent study, it was reported that the only significant risk combination (hazard index) in Kolkata was lead (Pb) exposure to children via road dust and ingestion was the dominant risk pathway [23]. ADB [24] had reported that about 15% of the average contribution (ranging from 5% to 28% over various seasons) of road dust atmospheric $PM_{2.5}$ and about 60% of respirable particulate matter were contributed by road dust in Kolkata during 2003. A recent emission inventory study for Kolkata indicates that vehicle-induced road dust resuspension contributed about 15 kt y^{-1} of PM_{10} in 2015, i.e., 25% of the total estimated PM_{10} emission. Due to increasing vehicular movements, road dust is projected to contribute 41 kt yr^{-1}, i.e., about 48% of the total PM_{10} in 2030 [25]. Proper control of road dust may reduce the PM_{10} and $PM_{2.5}$ load of the air of Kolkata city by 7.5% and 2.3%, respectively [26].

Investigating the PSD of road dust vis a vis potential elemental signature at busy city locations is crucial to assess spatiotemporal variation in road dust and potential health risks. The PSD of road dust in Kolkata city has not been studied in detail yet. This study was designed to examine PSD of road dust at some significant commercial and densely populated areas in Kolkata, along with elemental loading in size-segregated road dust, keeping in view the potential effects of dust exposure on human health.

2. Materials and Methods

2.1. Background of the Study Area and Road Dust Sampling

The present population of the Kolkata Municipality area is more than 4.5 million, making it the third-largest city after Delhi and Mumbai in South Asia [22]. Due to issues like agglomeration, congested narrow roads, and construction and repairing activities, the city experiences substantial air pollution by particulates and is one of the non-attainment cities in India in terms of air pollution [27]. High emissions from the firing of smoking fuels in commercial eateries, use of adulterated fuels in two- and three-wheelers, lack of maintenance of vehicles, heavy traffic, congestion at traffic intersections, road encroachment by pavement dwellers and street hawkers, etc., lead to substantial air pollution in the city [28].

Locations selected for road dust collection were mainly busy traffic roads, feeder roads, and service roads made up of asphalt coats. Most of the chosen sites were lined by shops and other commercial establishments, while a few were near bus stands, petrol pumps, and other government offices (Table 1). The sites were classified into traffic, commercial, residential, traffic + commercial, and traffic + residential areas based on primary activities or major inhabitation types observed around the sites. The sampling sites are depicted in a map vis-a-vis the city roads and urban agglomerations (Figure 1). Road dust was collected from about 3–4 points over an approximately 8 m^2 area on asphalt city roads and turned into one composite sample per site. Road dust was collected using the 'Brush and Pan' method, which is the most common method of road dust collection reported in about 88% of reviewed studies worldwide that collected bulk road dust samples (n = 177) [29]. Road dust was collected by thorough brushing of deposited dust, in a way so as not to cause abrasion on the road surface, by an inert nylon brush, and then stored in sample containers after collection in a stainless steel pan. Thorough brushing was done on the sampling spots to ensure maximum recovery of all deposited particles, including fines. Gravels, leaves, visible fibers, broken twigs, if any, large construction materials, and other large particles (>3 mm) were discarded during collection. A total of 11 site-specific samples of road dust were collected.

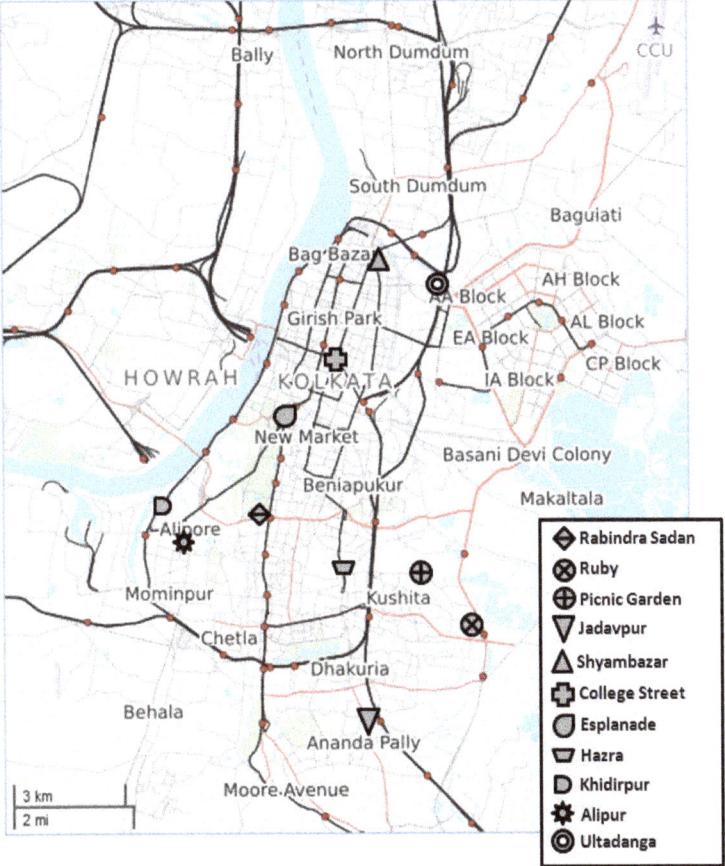

Figure 1. Road dust collection sites in Kolkata City (major road transport corridors are marked as dotted black bands).

Table 1. Summary of road dust collection sites.

Site Name	Site Coordinates	Details
		Commercial Area
Alipore	88.3363° N 22.5268° E	Semi-congested area; Asphalt Road; Court and Urban Local Body office nearby, a bus stop and a petrol pump are nearby
		Residential Area
Jadavpur	88.3707° N 22.4940° E	Asphalt Road; Low vehicular load; Railway station is within 500 m; A flyover is just adjacent; Local market is nearby
Picnic Garden	88.3884° N 22.5266° E	Semi-congested; Dotted by residences and small roads; Low vehicular road; Busy traffic square is nearby
		Traffic Area
College Street	88.36408° N 22.5774° E	Congested Area; Asphalt Road; High vehicular traffic; Presidency College and College Square are nearby
Ruby Square	88.4029° N 22.5135° E	Congested area; Asphalt Road; Heavy construction activity; Very high vehicular traffic; Gateway Hotel, a petrol pump are nearby; Small roadside food stalls that use biomass cookstoves
Ultadanga	88.3402° N 22.5927° E	Asphalt Road; Very high vehicular traffic; Circular rail station is nearby
		Traffic + Commercial Area
Rabindra Sadan	88.3451° N 22.5433° E	Wide Asphalt Road; Heavy vehicular traffic; Cinema Hall and Childrens' Museum are nearby
Hazra	88.34706° N 22.52372° E	Congested Area; Asphalt Road; Heavy vehicular traffic; Cancer Hospital, College and a big Park are nearby
Esplanade	88.3504° N 22.5647° E	Wide asphalt road; Heavy vehicular traffic; Mosque, a metro station, Income Tax Office, etc. are nearby; Large stores are also there in the vicinity
Shyambazar	88.3731° N 22.6006° E	Congested area; Asphalt Road; Very high vehicular traffic; Metro station is nearby; High commercial activity and surrounded by food stalls
Khidirpur	88.3268° N 22.5404° E	Congested Area; Asphalt Road; Traffic load is high; Commercial area, a bridge and a large market, etc. are nearby

2.2. Particle Size Distribution Analysis

Particle size distribution (PSD) analysis of road dust samples was undertaken using two different methods. A microcontroller-based electromagnetic sieve shaker (EMS-8, Electrolab, Electrolab India Pvt. Ltd., Navi Mumbai, India), having tri-dimensional movement integrating a vertical movement with a rotation, was used to segregate and determine PSD of road dust samples in 5 different cut-off sizes viz. > 2000 µm, 1000–2000 µm, 600–1000 µm, 212–600 µm, 106–212 µm, 63,106 µm, 45–63 µm, 28–45 µm, and $\leq$28 µm. Recovery of road dust samples from the series of sieves ranged from 98.1–98.8%. Each size portion of dust samples was weighed and stored in a refrigerator. Percentage distribution of particulates in each size range was calculated and recorded.

Segregated road dust samples in <106 µm size range was subjected to finer particle size distribution analysis in an Optical Particle Size Analyser (make: Sympatec, Clausthal-Zellerfeld, Germany) fitted with a HELOS (Helium-Neon-Laser for Optical Spectrometry) sensor in dry sample feed mode. Within each HELOS, the primary physical diffraction set-up is realized by deploying a parallel laser beam that yielded an optimum optical alignment to analyze extended spatial arrangements of particles. The analyzer was operated with a pressure of 3 bar, a vacuum of 10 mbar, a feed rate of 50%, a temperature control of 10–60 $\pm$ 0.1 °C in a measurement duration of 5 s.

2.3. Analysis of Elements

Analysis of elements in road dust was restricted to <106 μm particles due to higher health risks associated with fine particles amenable to resuspension in air [30–33]. Sieved and oven-dried samples (105 °C for 2 h before analysis; about 0.1 g) were digested with 10 mL concentrated HNO_3 in a microwave digester (Start MOD, Make M/s Milestone s.r.l., Sorisole, Italy). After digestion, samples were cooled and diluted to 50 mL by ultrapure water (MiliQ, Make M/s Millipore) and filtered through a 0.2 μm PTFE filter (M/s Millipore). Altogether, fourteen elements (Cd, Cr, Co, Pb, Mn, Ni, Sr, Zn, Fe, Mg, Li, Ti, Cu, Ba) were determined in road dust using Inductively Coupled Plasma-Optical Emission Spectrometry (ICP-OES, make: Teledyne Leeman Labs). A multi-point external calibration curve was prepared to estimate elements in extracted samples from a multi-element standard (M/s Accustandard) through serial dilutions. Calibration curves were prepared in two concentration ranges, the lower in μg L^{-1} range and higher one in mg L^{-1} range. Extracted samples were first analyzed against μg L^{-1} range and elements with concentrations beyond the μg L^{-1} range were again analyzed against the mg L^{-1} range calibration curve. No contamination was detected in reagent blanks.

2.4. Assessment of Elemental Pollution by Enrichment Factor and Other Indices

The enrichment factor (EF) approach was utilized to assess the degree of elemental pollution [34]. EF is defined mathematically as:

$$EF = \frac{\left(\frac{X_n}{R}\right)_{dust}}{\left(\frac{X_n}{R}\right)_{background}}$$

where, $(X_n/R)_{dust}$ and $(X_n/R)_{background}$ are the concentration ratios of element n and the normalizer R in the road dust and background material, respectively. Titanium (Ti) was used as the normalizer and average elemental concentrations in earth crust were used as background [35]. Ti was used as the reference element for geochemical normalization as: (1) Ti is naturally associated with earth crust, is stable, non-reactive, and inert standard element with respect to the physico-chemical parameters of the environment [36]; (2) Ti geochemistry is similar to many other trace elements; and (3) its crustal concentration is fairly stable and is negligibly added by anthropogenic activities which is an important criterion [37]. Degree of element pollution was classified into five categories [38]: (1) EF < 2 (depletion to minimal); (2) EF = 2–5 (moderate); (3) EF = 5–20 (significant); (4) EF = 20–40 (very high); and (5) EF > 40 (extremely high).

The Contamination Factor (C_f^i) provides a single pollution index of a given element and is quantified as the ratio of an element to the background concentration of the corresponding element [39]. The C_f^i is the ratio obtained by dividing the concentration of each element in road dust by the background values in the earth crust [35].

$$C_f^i = \frac{C_{element}}{C_{background}}$$

$C_{element}$ and $C_{background}$ are the measured concentrations of the element 'i' and the background concentrations, respectively. In this study, the average crustal concentration for elements [35] was used as a reference concentration. The degree of contamination (C_{deg}) is the sum of the contamination factors of measured elements that indicates the overall and extent of contamination of the study sites. It is estimated as follows [40].

$$C_{deg} = \sum_{i=1}^{n} C_f^i$$

The C_{deg} of the contamination may be classified based the scale ranging from <8 to >32 with classes such as <8, 8–16, 16–32, and >32 indicates low degree, moderate, considerate, and a very high degree of contamination, respectively [39,41].

The potential ecological risk index (RI), proposed by Hakanson [42], was calculated to assess the likely ecological risk levels of selected elements Hg, As, Cu, Cr, Zn, and Pb in four different fractions (<28, >28–<45, >45–<63, and >63–<106 µm) in road dust. RI was calculated using the following relationships [42,43].

$$RI = \sum_{i=1}^{n} E_i$$

where,

$$E_i = T_i f_i$$

$$f_i = C_i / B_i$$

where E_i is the potential ecological risk factor of element i, T_i is the element toxic factor, i.e., Cu = 5, Pb = 5, Cr = 2, Ni = 5, Cd = 30, and Zn = 1 [42,43], f_i is the element pollution factor of element i, which equals to the amount of element i in the sample (C_i) divided by its reference value (B_i) in earth crust. Levels of potential ecological risk assessment are <150, 150 ≤ RI <300, 300 ≤ RI < 600, and RI > 600 indicating low, moderate, severe, and serious ecological pollution level, respectively [42,44,45].

2.5. Human Health Risk Assessment

The population in an urban area is exposed to road dust daily. Exposure to the elements in the road dust can be potentially toxic and may pose considerable non-cancer and cancer health risks to the population of Kolkata. Pathways of human exposure to road dust can be ingestion (I_g), inhalation (I_h), or dermatological contact (D_m). The exposure (E) from chronic daily intake of potentially toxic elements (PTEs) through the above pathways has been calculated as per the following equations.

$$E_{ig} = \frac{C_i \times 10^6 \times R_{Ig} \times F_{exp} \times ED}{(BW_{avg} \times T_{avg})} \quad (1)$$

$$E_{ih} = \frac{C_i \times R_{Ih} \times F_{exp} \times ED}{(EF_p \times BW_{avg} \times T_{avg})} \quad (2)$$

$$E_{Dm} = \frac{C_i \times 10^6 \times SAF \times AF_{Dm} \times A_{skin} \times F_{exp} \times ED}{(BW_{avg} \times T_{avg})} \quad (3)$$

Cancer and Non-Cancer Risk Assessment

Integrated lifetime cancer risk or CR is estimated from Equation (4):

$$CR_i = E_{i(Ig)} \times SF_i \quad (4)$$

The non-cancer health hazard from exposure to PTEs has been estimated as hazard quotient, HQ as per Equation (5):

$$HQ = E_{i(Ih/Ig/Dm)} / RfD_i \quad (5)$$

RfD_i is a chronic exposure reference dose for PTE 'i', below which undesirable health complications are not expected.

The cumulative non-cancer health hazard from cumulative exposure to PTE 'i' is expressed as hazard index, HI, as per Equation (6):

$$HI = \sum_i HQ \quad (6)$$

The definition of various parameters and assumed values are presented in Table 2. [46–53].

Table 2. Definition of parameters and values for health risk assessment.

Parameter	Unit	Abbreviat-Ion	Assumptions for Health Risk Assessment
Ingestion Exposure	-	E_{Ig}	-
Inhalation Exposure	-	E_{Ih}	-
Dermatological Exposure	-	E_{Dm}	-
Observed concentration of element 'I' in road dust	-	C_i	-
Ingestion Rate	mg day^{-1}	R_{Ig}	Adult: 100; Children: 200
Inhalation rate	m^3 day^{-1}	R_{Ih}	20
Frequency of exposure	Days year^{-1}	F_{exp}	365
Exposure duration	Years	ED	Adult: 24; Children: 6
Average body weight	Kg	BW_{avg}	Adult: 60 kg; Children: 18 kg
Averaging time	Days	T_{avg}	(ED × F_{exp})
Particle Emission Factor	m^3 kg^{-1}	EF_P	1.36 × 10^9
skin adherence factor	mg cm^{-2}	SAF	Adult: 0.07; Children: 0.2
dermal absorption factor	-	AF_{Dm}	0.001
Area of skin	cm^{-2}	A_{skin}	Adult: 5700; Children: 2800
Carcinogenic Slope Factor of element 'I'	(mg kg^{-1} day^{-1})$^{-1}$	SF_i	*
reference dose for chronic exposure of element 'i'	(mg kg^{-1} day^{-1})	RfD_i	*

Average values adopted from published literature [48–57]. * Oral SF and RfD values of different exposure pathways for individual toxic elements are given in Section 3.4).

The chronic exposure reference dose and risk values for PTEs are adapted from Risk Assessment Information System of USEPA and other published literature [53,54]. PTEs with established RfDs were only selected for calculating the health risk index.

2.6. Statistical Analyses

To categorize the sites in clusters based on similarity in particle size distribution (<28–2000 μm and <106 μm size ranges analyzed by dry sieving and optical analysis, respectively). Cluster analysis was undertaken on particle size distribution data by Ward Method in Statistica Software (Dell Software, Round Rock, TX, USA, Version 13). Further, the average size distribution for all sites in <28–2000 μm and <106 size ranges of road dust particles were made to undergo distribution fitting separately via CDF (Cumulative Distribution Function) plot method by Statistica Software (Dell Software, Version 13). CDF plots display theoretical CDF of fitted distributions and empirical CDF based on sample data to determine data fitness to distributions. In the generated plots, N designates the number of non-missing observations.

3. Results and Discussion

3.1. Physical Attributes of Road Dust

PSD analysis of road dust by dry sieving technique revealed a predominance of 106–600 μm particles in all the samples in which the 212–600 μm size group had the highest share, followed by 106–212 and 63–106 μm size groups (Supplementary Figure S1). In Jadavpur, about 57.5% of road dust belonged to 212–600 μm diameter, followed by Esplanade (52.4%), and then Alipore, College Street Rabindra Sadan (48.0–49.6%). But at Khidirpur, the share of 212–600 μm particles was lower than the 106–212 and 63–106 μm size ranges, only 20%, the lowest amongst all. At Khidirpur, 106–212 μm particles had the highest share (about 23%), which was very closely followed by 212–600 and 63–106 μm ranges (19% and 20.5%, respectively). According to USDA (United States Department of Agriculture) classification, particles having a diameter in the range of 250–2000 μm (0.25–2.0 mm) are mainly medium and coarse sand particles, while particles from 50–250 μm (0.05 to 0.25 mm) range are various fine sand categories [55]. Particles of 1–2 mm diameter, categorized as very coarse sand, had a maximum share of about 6.8% at

Picnic Garden followed by Ultadanga, while the percentage of gravel (>2 mm) was highest at Picnic Garden (4%) but generally low in all others (0.05–2.4%). The average share of finer particles in the ranges of 45–63 μm, 28–45 μm, and <28 μm was highest at Khidirpur (8%), followed by Picnic Garden (5%), while the average share at all other sites was <5%. The above results implied the dominant presence of particles that matched size ranges designated to various types of sand.

More refined PSD analysis of segregated road dust (<106 μm) by optical particle size analysis went down to the estimation of the <4.5 μm size range, showcasing particles of concern from an air pollution perspective. The criteria air pollutant, PM_{10} (particles with <10 μm aerodynamic diameter), matched most closely to <11 μm range (PM_{11}) measured by the optical analyzer. This size group was most dominant at Picnic Garden (~23.4% of the 0–106 μm particle range), followed by College Street (18% of the 0–106 μm particle range), Khidirpur (~16% of the 0–106 μm particle range), Hazra and Esplanade (both ~14.3% of the 0–106 μm particle range) and others (Supplementary Table S1). About 50% of inhalable, thoracic, and respirable groups of dust designated for work environment corresponds to 100, 10, and 4 μm particles, respectively [56]. In the reported size groups in this study, the nearest corresponding size groups to the above groups were PM_{106}, PM_{11}, and $PM_{4.5}$. The actual share of the other criteria particulate air pollutants, i.e., $PM_{2.5}$ (particles with <2.5 μm aerodynamic diameter), could not be revealed by the optical PSD analysis. The nearest particle size group assessed was <4.5 μm. The $PM_{4.5}$ had the highest share at Picnic Garden (10.42%), followed by College Street, Khidirpur, Hazra (8.73%, 6.9%, and 6.2%, respectively) while the other sites had similar shares (4.5–5.7%). The non-cumulative particle size distribution resembles a normal distribution with negative skewness in <4.5–106 μm size range (Figure 2). Zafra et al. (2011) [15] reported that road dust and sediments collected from drains, bicycle lanes exhibited positively skewed log-normal distribution. Similar particle size distribution was also reported in road and gutter surface dust [57,58]. The optical size analysis 10, 16, 50, 84, 90, and 99 percentile contributions are given in Supplementary Figure S2. Picnic Garden had higher percentiles of smaller particles in every size range, indicating the finer nature of this road dust. Other critical physical characteristics like Volumetric Mean Diameter (VMD), Sauter Mean Diameter (SMD), surface area to volume ratio (S_v), and specific surface area (S_m) are also reported (Supplementary Table S2). Road dust at Picnic Garden had the highest S_v and S_m (0.51 and 1877.3) and correspondingly lowest VMD and SMD (32.58 and 11.79) that confirmed the finer nature of road dust at this site. The S_v, S_m, VMD, and SMD ranges were 0.28–0.44, 1038.2–1617, 35.46–48.3, and 13.69–21.32, respectively, at other sites.

The average particle size distribution was tested for distribution fitting by cumulative distribution function (CDF) plots in <28 μm–2 mm and <106 μ size ranges. It was found that the data did not fit very well to a normal distribution (Supplementary Figure S3a,b). Cluster analysis was performed amongst sites, separately for <28–2000 μm and <106 μm size ranges and site-wise cluster trees were developed to categorize sites with similar PSDs. The height of vertical lines in the branching dendrogram signifies the degree of difference between branches; the longer the line, more significant is the difference. In <28 μm–2000 μm, the branching dendrogram represented similarity amongst the site-groups of Khidirpur and Picnic Garden, Shyambazar and Hazra; Rabindra Sadan and Ruby Square; and Esplanade and Alipore. Khidirpur and Picnic Garden group was much different from other groups. Sites of Ultadanga, College Street, and Jadavpur each were outstanding (Figure 3a). In <106 μm size, Rabindra Sadan and Ruby Square; Shyambazar and Jadavpur; Hazra and Esplanade; Picnic Garden and College Street could be categorized as similar sites. The Picnic Garden and College Street group differed from the other three groups (Figure 3b).

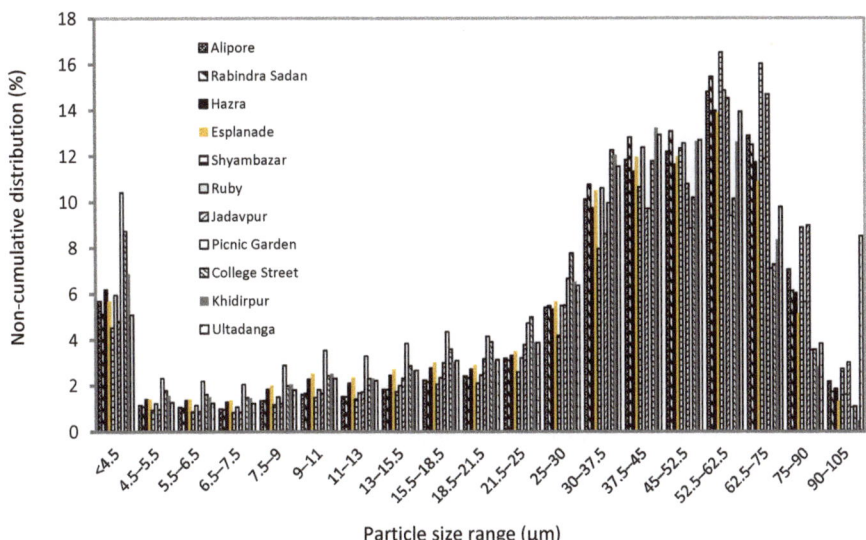

Figure 2. Non-cumulative distribution of road-dust (<106 μm size range) collected from different sites in Kolkata mega city.

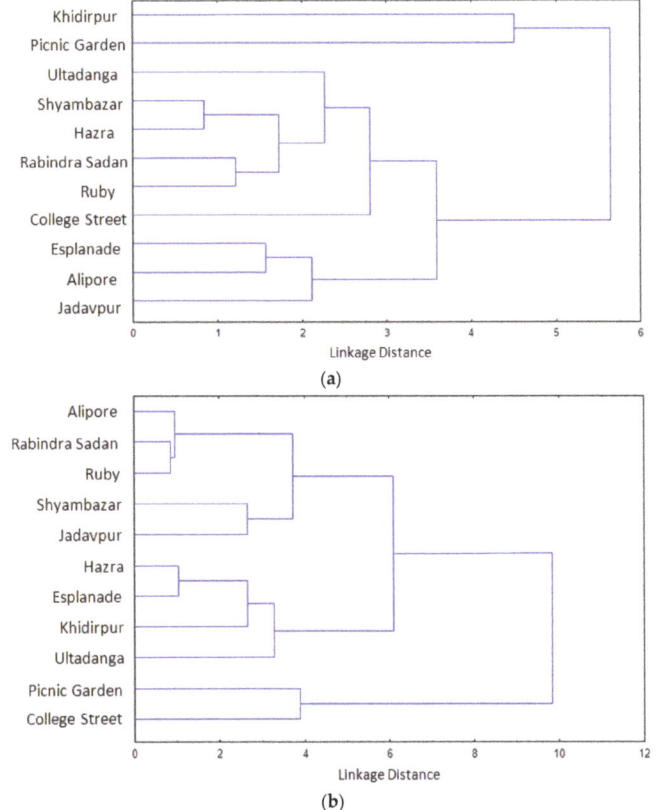

Figure 3. Tree clustering diagram depicting clustering of sites as per similarity in PSD of (**a**) road dust (<28–2000 μm size range) and (**b**) road dust (<106 μm size range).

3.2. Elemental Concentration in Road Dust

In size segregated road dust, Fe (4.02–31.2 g kg^{-1}) dominated other elements, including alkaline earth elements like Mg (2.13–10.9 g kg^{-1}), Mn (79.2–601 mg kg^{-1}), Li (395.8–506.8 mg kg^{-1}), followed by other detected elements above LOQ. The substantial presence of Li in Kolkata road dust may have to do with the presence of the sea at the Bay of Bengal within about 120 km from the city, implying the possibility of historical deposition of sea salt with Li on city roads, considering seawater is rich in Li [59]. Amongst the criteria elements (As, Ni, and Pb) earmarked in National Ambient Air Quality Standard (NAAQS) in India [60], Arsenic (As) was not detected in any sample. However, Ni and Pb were detected and ranged from 0.97–4.97 and 14.16–67.11 mg kg^{-1}, respectively, in various size groups (Supplementary Table S3). Amongst known toxic elements, Cr (8.1–143.9 mg kg^{-1}) recorded the maximum concentration, followed by Sr (9.2–66.3 mg kg^{-1}), Cd (0.83–5.1 mg kg^{-1}), Pb (0.97–6.15 mg kg^{-1}), and Co (2.44–11.0 mg kg^{-1}). Fe and Mg had a major share in total elemental load in all size groups ranging from 62.5%–64.9% and 27.6%–29.3%, followed by Ti, Li, Mn, Ba, and so on (Figure 4). In an earlier study at Kolkata city [61], Cd, Cr, Cu, Ni, Pb, and Zn in road dust were 3.12, 54, 44, 42, 536, and 159 mg kg^{-1}, respectively, in road dust of the <600 μm size range. In comparison, a recent study in the same city reported Fe, Cr, Mn, Co, Ni, Cu, Zn, Ba, Cd, and Pb concentrations in the ranges of 23.4–59.3 g kg^{-1}, 42–129, 503–1027, 8–18, 18–75, 28–279, 121–1258, 374–1643, 0.28–8.03, and 77–551 mg kg^{-1} in <53 μm road dust. In road dust in Bengaluru city in India, the same elements were reported in similar ranges (16.1–33.2 g kg^{-1}, 25–134, 258–621, 2–20, 9–192, 9–168, 43–617, 431–1921, 0.09–1.26, and 26–97 mg kg^{-1}, respectively) [23]. In a study on the presence of elements in road dust in Delhi, India, Cd, Cr, Cu, Ni, Pb, and Zn in <75 μm road dust were found to be 2.65, 148.8, 191.7, 36.4, 120.7, and 284.5 mg kg^{-1} [4]. The same study cited Indian soil background values as 0.9, 114, 56.5, 27.7, 13.1, 22.1 for Cd, Cr, Cu, Ni, Pb, and Zn, respectively [62,63].

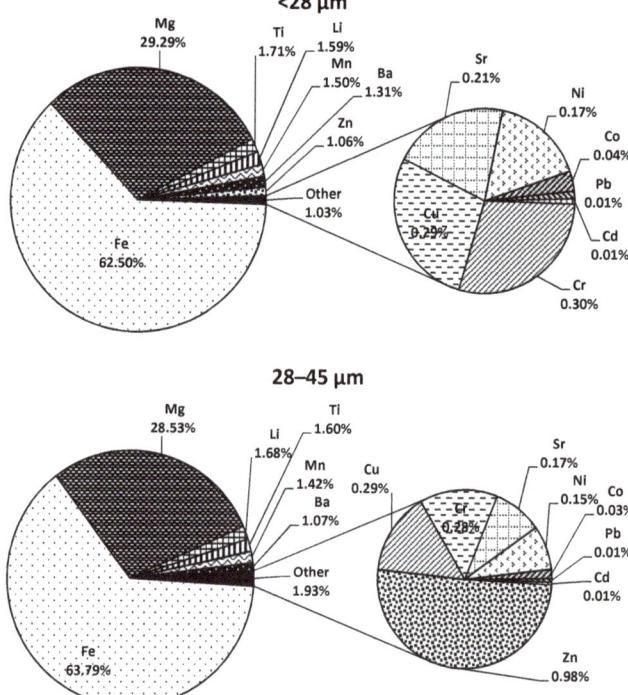

Figure 4. *Cont.*

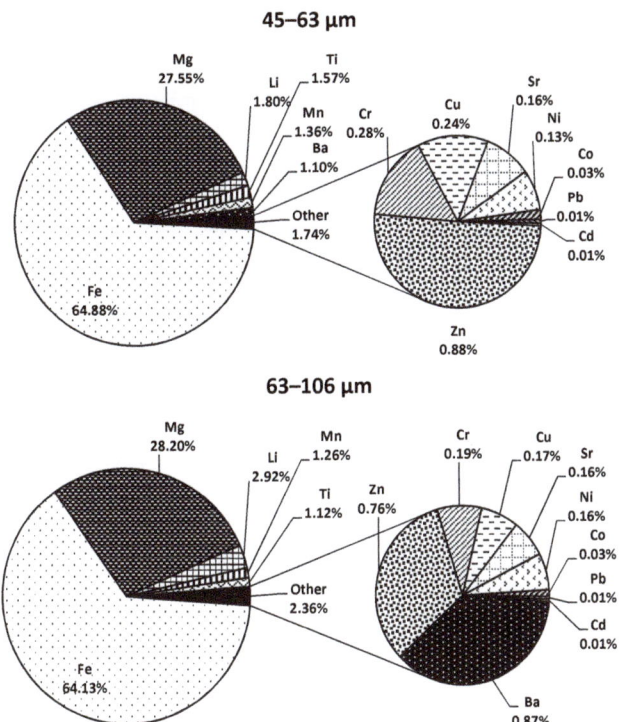

Figure 4. Percentage share of elements in road dust of various size groups.

With the exception of a few cases, <28 μm size group had a highest average concentration of the elements than larger size groups of >28–<45 μm, 45–<63 μm, and 63–<106 μm, while no wide variation in element concentration was apparent within each size group, as indicated by the coefficient of variation, CV (Table 3). Interestingly, the concentration of almost all elements except Li declined linearly, albeit to variable extents, with increasing particle size (Figure 5), indicating a higher association of elements in finer particles. The decreasing trends showed reasonably steep negative slopes with relatively high R^2 values (Supplementary Table S4). A substantial part of fine road dust is expected to get suspended in the air due to wind and vehicle movements [8]. Therefore, it is prudent to assess the potential ecological and health damages from likely exposure to elements attached to the finer dust.

Table 3. Average elemental concentration (mg kg^{-1}) in size-segregated road dust in Kolkata.

Parameter	Cd	Cr	Co	Pb	Mn	Ni	Sr	Zn	Fe	Mg	Li	Ti	Cu	Ba
<28 μm	2.68	71.27	9.11	3.53	402.19	38.85	66.32	297.16	14,736.23	8102.92	433.91	475.50	55.66	305.29
SD	0.47	17.49	0.72	0.63	66.02	7.89	4.45	45.02	3543.82	1304.46	20.32	76.35	44.34	78.11
CV (%)	17.62	24.54	7.85	17.74	16.42	20.30	6.71	15.15	24.05	16.10	4.68	16.06	79.65	25.59
>28–<45 μm	2.14	52.62	7.40	2.78	343.83	26.45	49.54	235.03	13,935.24	7380.53	452.82	420.64	38.63	225.50
SD	1.09	33.88	1.05	1.23	107.70	12.61	5.21	73.91	6170.33	1396.06	15.83	59.27	70.12	90.84
CV (%)	50.88	64.39	14.20	44.42	31.32	47.68	10.52	31.45	44.28	18.92	3.50	14.09	181.50	40.28
45–<63 μm	2.24	58.05	9.59	2.91	343.22	40.39	43.62	260.43	15,111.55	7572.23	468.99	375.60	63.00	341.24
SD	0.65	33.76	1.42	0.88	99.34	13.85	6.49	64.95	6404.68	1545.65	13.01	80.23	54.95	86.33
CV (%)	29.23	58.16	14.78	30.22	28.95	34.28	14.87	24.94	42.38	20.41	2.77	21.36	87.23	25.30
63–<106 μm	1.45	30.21	3.47	1.74	237.62	15.37	11.89	94.82	10,965.18	2749.98	502.46	188.52	11.08	66.87
SD	0.70	17.71	1.68	0.86	93.94	12.16	11.94	71.02	5192.17	2406.81	14.08	74.65	41.09	57.35
CV (%)	48.43	58.62	48.51	49.51	39.53	79.12	100.43	74.90	47.35	87.52	2.80	39.60	370.88	85.77

N.B. Average concentration in earth crust is adopted from Taylor, 1964.

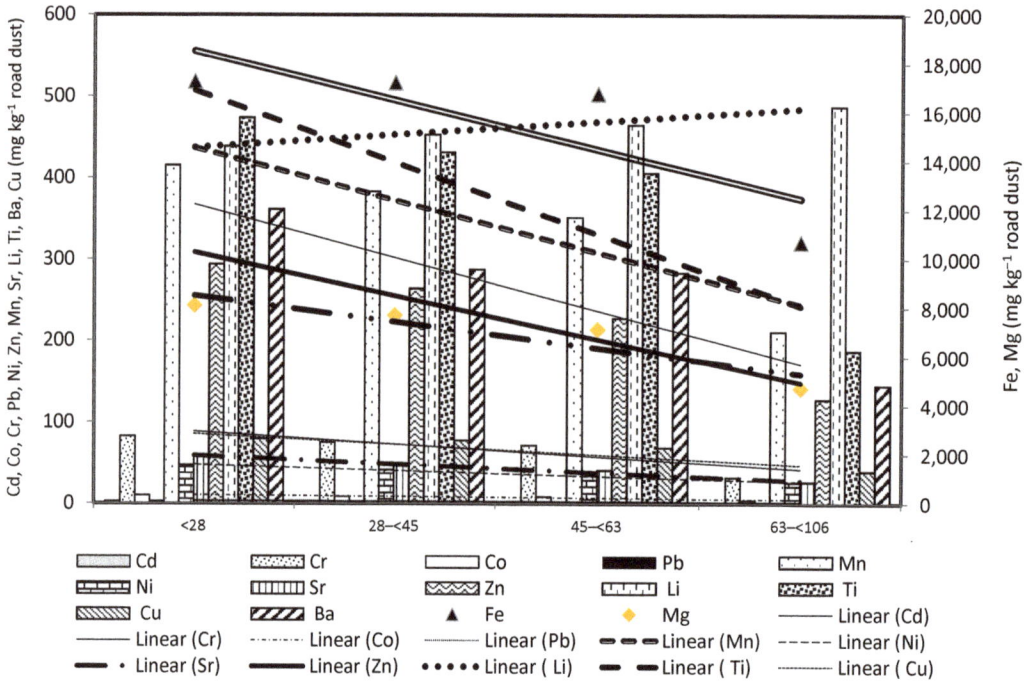

Figure 5. Decreasing trends in elemental concentration with increasing particle size.

3.3. Assessment of Elemental Pollution

The enrichment factors (EF) of elements in size segregated road dust revealed that Cd and Li had extremely high degree of enrichment. In contrast, the rest of the elements had significantly lower enrichment factors (Supplementary Table S5). Consequently, the degree of contamination in different size ranges was very high for Li (175 in <28 µm to 244 in 63–106 µm) followed by Cd (84 in 63–106 µm to 109 in 28–43 µm). Amongst other elements, Zn and Cu showed a moderate degree of contamination (Table 4). The ecological risk was (Ei) estimated for six elements (Cu, Pb, Cr, Ni, Cd, and Zn). Cd posed the highest ecological risk values, ranging from 125 to 760 in different size ranges. The rest of the elements showed low ecological risk, ranging from 0.79 for Pb to 22.48 for Cu (Supplementary Table S6). It is evident from the potential ecological risk index (Ri) that only Cd posed a significant ecological risk, with Ri ranging from 2518 in 63–106 µm to 3270 in 28–45 µm size range (Table 5).

Table 4. Degree of contamination (C_{deg}) of metals in different size groups in road dust in Kolkata.

Metals	C_{deg}			
	<28	28–43	43–63	63–106
Cd	**108.51**	**109.01**	**107.08**	**83.93**
Cr	6.61	6.01	6.46	3.23
Co	3.21	2.76	2.99	1.82
Pb	2.37	2.19	2.30	1.73
Mn	3.50	3.23	3.33	2.22
Ni	5.03	4.46	4.17	3.48
Sr	1.26	1.00	0.99	0.71
Zn	**33.54**	*30.16*	*29.28*	*18.23*
Fe	2.45	2.45	2.68	1.90
Mg	2.78	2.64	2.75	2.02
Mn	2.30	2.24	2.26	1.31
Li	**175.37**	**181.10**	**209.19**	**243.59**
Ti	0.66	0.61	0.64	0.33
Cu	11.55	11.29	10.26	5.62
Ba	6.80	5.41	6.00	3.41

$C_{deg} \leq 8$ (low degree of contamination indicated by no highlight), 8–16 (moderate degree of contamination indicated by light grey highlight), 16–32 (*considerable* degree of contamination *indicated by italics*), and >32 (very high degree of contamination indicated by boldface).

Table 5. Potential Ecological Risk Index (Ri) of individual elements in various size groups in Kolkata.

Metal	Ecological Risk * in Particulate Size Range			
	<28	28–45	45–63	63–106
Cu	57.75	56.44	51.31	28.09
Pb	11.86	10.95	11.51	8.63
Cr	13.22	12.01	12.92	6.47
Ni	25.14	22.31	20.83	17.41
Cd	**3255.15**	**3270.19**	**3212.35**	**2518.02**
Zn	33.54	30.16	29.28	18.23

* Elements in a particular size range posing highly strong potential ecological risk are marked with boldface. Rest are of low potential risk.

3.4. Health Risk Assessment

Non-cancer health hazards from chronic element exposure through road dust to adults and children via ingestion, inhalation, and dermal contact pathways was assessed for twelve potentially toxic elements (PTEs, namely, Cd, Cr, Co, Pb, Mn, Ni, Sr, Zn, Fe, Li, Cu, and Ba) found in the road dust of Kolkata. These twelve elements have well-established non-cancer health impacts. Four elements (Cd, Cr, Pb, and Ni) have established carcinogenic health impacts and established slope factors for oral uptake. The cancer risk from long-term exposure to adults has been assessed for these elements for ingestion exposure only. This risk assessment was carried out assuming that the soil model applies to road dust as well. Complete assimilation of taken-up elements into the bloodstream was also assumed.

Co is the most toxic one among the studied elements, followed by Cd, Li, Cr, and Pb respectively, indicated by very low RfD values for ingestion exposure. Other elements are comparatively less toxic. Cd has the highest carcinogenic potential exhibited by the highest slope factor, followed by Ni, Cr, and Pb, respectively. The health risk assessment results are presented in Table 6. Non-cancer health risks are indicated by estimated Hazard Quotients (HQs) for different exposure pathways, and carcinogenic risk values are indicated as estimated Cancer Risk (CR) values. It was observed in the HQs that for all elements that the most significant exposure pathway was ingestion. Non-cancer health hazards for all elements were high for the ingestion pathway, followed by dermal contact and the lowest via inhalation pathway in adults and children alike. Similar estimates have been reported in other risk assessment studies from road dust exposure [50,53,64]. They reported HQ from the ingestion pathway to be 10 and 100 times more than from dermal contact or the inhalation pathway respectively. The size range of settled road dust is generally >10 μm. Here, elements in road dust of <28–106 μm size range were studied. Particulates of >10 μm diameter are filtered through our nasal follicles while breathing and cannot enter human lungs or subsequently in the bloodstream. The non-cancer risk of road dust is negligible for the inhalation pathways for both adults and children. Children have a higher exposure to road dust than adults, as they spend more time outdoors. Children also have a higher hand-to-mouth interaction, especially during playtime, leading to even higher exposure than adults. Moreover, children with lower body weight experience a considerably higher weight normalized exposure. Consequently, children face a higher risk of non-cancer health impact from exposure to PTEs in road dust. The dermal contact pathway of exposure to Fe for children was observed to be considerable. In this study, HQs corresponding to individual elements have not exceeded unity, indicating that they do not pose significant non-cancer health risks for adults or children, except for ingestion exposure to Li in the case of children. The same from exposure to Li can still be considered 'of concern' for adults, while exposure to Fe, Cr, and Co can be regarded as 'of concern' for children.

The cumulative HI from all PTEs was estimated to be less than unity (0.58). Therefore, exposure from target PTEs in road dust may not pose a significant non-cancer health risk for the city population. However, the same for children was assessed as 3.8, almost four times the desired HI of unity. Thus, it can be concluded that children are more vulnerable to the PTEs in road dust and have a significant probability of suffering from non-cancer health complications. Here, it was assumed that the HIs for different PTEs are additive, and the synergistic or antagonistic effect of cumulative PTE exposure, if any, has not been considered.

Among the four carcinogenic elements, Cd, Ni, and Cr posed a significant cancer risk in more than acceptable limits, i.e., one in a million for the exposed city population. This assessment indicates that an inhabitant of Kolkata city has a 5 to 6 times higher risk of developing cancer upon lifelong exposure to the city road dust. In Kolkata, 1.4 million people, i.e., 31% of the total population, resides in the city slums, most of which are settled along the roadside walkway or footpath [65]. Their daily chores, including cooking, sleeping, leisure, etc., occur just adjacent to the city roads. Therefore, they may have a much-elevated exposure to the road dust and PTEs compared to the rest of the city population living in better housing. In addition, children residing in slum settlements are also highly vulnerable to non-cancer health effects, primarily via the ingestion pathway. Therefore, children would have a higher chance of developing cancer upon lifelong exposure to road dust if they continue to live in roadside slums.

Table 6. Cancer and non-cancer health risk indicators from exposure to PTEs present in road dust.

Parameter	Exposure Type	Cd	Cr	Co	Pb	Mn	Ni	Sr	Zn	Fe	Li	Cu	Ba
RfD (mg kg^{-1} day^{-1})	Ingestion	1.0×10^{-3}	3.0×10^{-3}	3.0×10^{-4}	3.5×10^{-3}	1.4×10^{-1}	2.0×10^{-2}	6.0×10^{-1}	3.0×10^{-1}	7.0×10^{-1}	2.0×10^{-3}	4.0×10^{-2}	2.0×10^{-1}
	Inhalation	-	2.8×10^{-5}	6.0×10^{-6}	3.5×10^{-3}	5.0×10^{-5}	2.6×10^{-3}	-	3.0×10^{-1}	7.0×10^{-2}	-	4.2×10^{-2}	-
	Dermal	-	7.0×10^{-5}	-	5.2×10^{-4}	1.8×10^{-3}	5.4×10^{-3}	-	6.0×10^{-2}	2.2×10^{-3}	-	1.2×10^{-2}	-
SF (mg kg^{-1} day^{-1})$^{-1}$		**1.5×10^{1}**	4.2×10^{-1}	-	8.5×10^{-3}	-	9.1×10^{-1}	-	-	-	-	-	-
HQ (Ingestion)	Adult	4.1×10^{-3}	3.6×10^{-2}	4.5×10^{-2}	1.5×10^{-3}	4.3×10^{-3}	3.0×10^{-3}	1.2×10^{-4}	1.3×10^{-3}	3.8×10^{-2}	3.8×10^{-1}	2.8×10^{-3}	2.3×10^{-3}
	Children	2.7×10^{-2}	2.4×10^{-1}	3.0×10^{-1}	1.0×10^{-2}	2.8×10^{-2}	2.0×10^{-2}	8.2×10^{-4}	8.9×10^{-3}	2.6×10^{-1}	**2.6**	1.9×10^{-2}	1.5×10^{-2}
HQ (Inhalation)	Adult	-	5.7×10^{-4}	3.3×10^{-7}	2.3×10^{-7}	1.8×10^{-3}	3.4×10^{-7}	-	2.0×10^{-7}	5.6×10^{-5}	-	4.0×10^{-7}	-
	Children	-	1.9×10^{-3}	1.1×10^{-3}	7.5×10^{-7}	5.9×10^{-3}	1.1×10^{-6}	-	6.5×10^{-7}	1.9×10^{-4}	-	1.3×10^{-6}	-
HQ (Dermal)	Adult	-	6.2×10^{-3}	-	4.1×10^{-5}	1.3×10^{-3}	4.5×10^{-5}	-	2.7×10^{-5}	4.9×10^{-2}	-	3.8×10^{-5}	-
	Children	-	2.9×10^{-2}	-	1.9×10^{-4}	6.2×10^{-3}	2.1×10^{-4}	-	1.2×10^{-4}	2.3×10^{-1}	-	1.8×10^{-4}	-
HI	Adult	4.1×10^{-3}	4.3×10^{-2}	4.5×10^{-2}	1.6×10^{-3}	7.3×10^{-3}	3.1×10^{-3}	1.2×10^{-4}	1.4×10^{-3}	8.7×10^{-2}	3.8×10^{-1}	2.9×10^{-3}	2.3×10^{-3}
	Children	2.7×10^{-2}	2.7×10^{-1}	3.0×10^{-1}	1.0×10^{-2}	4.0×10^{-2}	2.0×10^{-2}	8.2×10^{-4}	9.0×10^{-3}	4.8×10^{-1}	**2.6**	1.9×10^{-2}	1.5×10^{-2}
CR (oral) (10^{-6} population)	Adult	**6.1×10^{1}**	**4.6×10^{1}**	-	4.6×10^{-2}	-	**5.5×10^{1}**	-	-	-	-	-	-

RfD—Reference Dose for chronic exposure; SF—Oral Slope Factor; HQ—non-cancer hazard quotient; HI—non-cancer hazard index; CR—cancer risk. NB: boldface values indicate significant health risk; values in *italics* indicate heath risk *'of concern'*.

4. Conclusions

The nature and characteristics of road dust of Kolkata city have been studied for size distribution and elemental composition in various size ranges. Road dust collected from important traffic corridors of the city reveals its typical urban characteristics, despite site-to-site variation. The predominance of coarse particles (106–212 µm) and a comparatively lower share of fine particulates (<28 µm) in Kolkata road dust may be considered advantageous from and air pollution perspective, as coarser road dust would possibly have a lower residence in air. Road dust showed a strong presence of coarse dust with about 83–98% in the sand particle size range. The characteristic size distribution of road dust varied across various parts of the city as indicated by cluster analysis. Fe and Mg are the two primary elements dominating the metal composition of road dust with 92% contribution. Li followed by Cd in the different size ranges of road dust showed the highest enrichment compared to their abundance in earth crust. Zn showed high enrichment in fine (<28 µm) fraction, but Cd constitutes only about 0.01% of the metal composition of the road dust. However, owing to its low concentration in the earth's crust and high ecological risk, Cd in road dust of Kolkata is a concern.

Potentially harmful elemental content in the road dust of the city may pose considerable human health risk upon chronic exposure at the prevailing levels. Ingestion was estimated to be the most significant pathway for exposure for both adults and children. Exposure to an individual element does not indicate significant non-cancer health risk, except for exposure to Li for children. The cumulative non-cancer health risk is also not indicated to be significant for adults. However, the same is about four times higher than the acceptable level, indicating that children are at risk of non-cancer health impact from chronic exposure to toxic elements of the city road dust. The city inhabitants have a 5 to 6 times higher risk of developing cancer upon lifelong exposure due to the current level of three carcinogenic elements, namely, Cd, Ni, and Cr, in road dust. A sizable number of city populations residing in the roadside slums, including children, are even more vulnerable to the health impact of road dust exposure.

Regular road sweeping and cleaning remains an important option for local urban bodies in Kolkata to ensure city roads' cleanliness. Kolkata Municipal Corporation (KMC) has street sweeping as one of its primary activities [66], which needs to be fortified in terms of coverage and frequency, especially in areas with possibilities of substantial human exposure vis a vis population density. Deployment of vacuum-assisted road sweeping machines may be a pragmatic way forward for effective cleaning of city streets.

Supplementary Materials: The following are available online at https://www.mdpi.com/article/10.3390/atmos12121677/s1, Figure S1: Particle size distribution of road-dust samples (<28–>2000 µm size range) collected from different sites in Kolkata, Figure S2: Percentile of particle size distribution of road-dust (<106 µm) collected from different sites in Kolkata, Figure S3: Plot of empirical cumulative distribution function (CDF) of average particle size distribution of (a) road dust (<28–2000 m) (b) road dust (<106 m size range) against a normal distribution plot, Table S1: Summary of non-cumulative particle size distribution of road dust (<106 µm particle size range), Table S2: Volumetric mean diameter (VMD), Sauter Mean Diameter (SMD), surface area to volume ratio (Sv) and specific surface (Sm) area of road dust (<106 µm road dust), Table S3: Metal concentration (mg kg^{-1}) in size-segregated road dust at different sites in Kolkata, Table S4: Slope of decline in metal concentration with increasing particle size in size-segregated road dust, Table S5: Enrichment factors of metals and degree of pollution in road dust with respect to size range, Table S6: Range of Ecological Risk Values (Ei) of individual metals in different size groups in road dust of various sites in Kolkata.

Author Contributions: Conceptualization, D.M. (Deepanjan Majumdar); methodology, D.M. (Deepanjan Majumdar), D.M. (Dipanjali Majumdar) (elemental analysis and health risk assessment); software, D.M. (Deepanjan Majumdar), D.M. (Dipanjali Majumdar); validation, D.M. (Deepanjan Majumdar), D.M. (Dipanjali Majumdar); formal analysis, D.M. (Deepanjan Majumdar), D.M. (Dipanjali Majumdar), B.B.; investigation, D.M. (Deepanjan Majumdar), D.M. (Dipanjali Majumdar), B.B., R.R.; resources, D.M. (Deepanjan Majumdar), D.M. (Dipanjali Majumdar); data curation, D.M. (Deepanjan Majumdar), B.B., D.M. (Dipanjali Majumdar); writing—original draft preparation, D.M. (Deepanjan

Majumdar), D.M. (Dipanjali Majumdar); visualization, D.M. (Deepanjan Majumdar); supervision, D.M. (Deepanjan Majumdar); project administration, D.M. (Deepanjan Majumdar). All authors have read and agreed to the published version of the manuscript.

Funding: This research received no external funding, The APC charges are funded by CSIR-National Environmental Engineering Research Institute.

Informed Consent Statement: Not applicable.

Data Availability Statement: The data presented in this study are available on request from the corresponding author. The data are not publicly available due to institutional restrictions.

Acknowledgments: The Authors thank Director, CSIR-NEERI, for constant encouragement and support. The authors also thank Rita Mondal for her assistance during elemental analysis. This research did not receive any specific grant from funding agencies in the public, commercial, or not-for-profit sectors and was conducted using institutional resources of CSIR-NEERI. CSIR-NEERI Knowledge Resource Centre (KRC) number of the manuscript is CSIR-NEERI/KRC/2021/JUNE/KZC/2.

Conflicts of Interest: The authors declare no conflict of interest.

References

1. Zhao, H.; Li, X.; Wang, X.; Tian, D. Grain size distribution of road-deposited sediment and its contribution to heavy metal pollution in urban run-off in Beijing, China. *J. Hazard. Mater.* **2010**, *183*, 203–210. [CrossRef] [PubMed]
2. Majumdar, D.; Rajaram, B.; Meshram, S.; Rao, C.V.C. PAHs in Road Dust: Ubiquity, Fate, and Summary of Available Data. *Crit. Rev. Environ. Sci. Technol.* **2012**, *42*, 1191–1232. [CrossRef]
3. Kreider, M.L.; Panko, J.M.; McAtee, B.L.; Sweet, L.I.; Finley, B.L. Physical and chemical characterization of tyre-related particles: Comparison of particles generated using different methodologies. *Sci. Total Environ.* **2010**, *408*, 652–659. [CrossRef] [PubMed]
4. Suryawanshi, P.V.; Rajaram, B.S.; Bhanarkar, A.D.; Rao, C.V.C. Determining heavy metal contamination of road dust in Delhi, India. *Atmósfera* **2016**, *29*, 221–234. [CrossRef]
5. Jendritzki, G.; Grätz, A. Das Bioklima des Menschen in der Stadt. In *Stadtklima und Luftreinhaltung*; Helbig, A., Baumüller, J., Kerschgens, M.J., Eds.; VDI-Buch, Springer: Berlin/Heidelberg, Germany, 1999. [CrossRef]
6. Countess, R.; Barnard, W.; Claiborn, C.; Gillette, D.; Latimer, D.; Pace, T.; Watson, J. Methodology for Estimating Fugitive Windblown and Mechanically Resuspended Road Dust Emissions Applicable for Regional Air Quality Modeling. 2001. Available online: http://www.epa.gov/ttn/chief/conference/ei10/fugdust/countess.pdf (accessed on 2 March 2021).
7. Martuzevicius, D.; Kliucininkas, L.; Prasauskas, T.; Krugly, E.; Kauneliene, V.; Strandberg, B. Resuspension of particulate matter and PAHs from street dust. *Atmos. Environ.* **2011**, *45*, 310–317. [CrossRef]
8. Ghosh, M.K. An Analysis of Roadside Dust Fall in Bhilai-3 of Durg District Chhattisgarh, Central India and its Impact on Human Health. *Int. J. Res. Environ. Sci. Technol.* **2014**, *4*, 54–60.
9. Shah, J.; Nagpal, T. *Urban Air Quality Management Strategy in Asia URBAIR: Greater Mumbai Report*; World Bank: Washington, DC, USA, 1996.
10. Amato, F.; Pandolfi, M.; Escrig, A.; Querol, X.; Alastuey, A.; Pey, J.; Perez, N.; Hopke, P.K. Quantifying road dust resuspension in urban environment by multilinear engine: A comparison with PMF2. *Atmos. Environ.* **2009**, *43*, 2770–2780. [CrossRef]
11. Han, L.H.; Zhuang, G.; Cheng, S.; Wang, Y.; Li, J. Characteristics of resuspended road dust and its impact on the atmospheric environment in Beijing. *Atmos. Environ.* **2007**, *41*, 7485–7499. [CrossRef]
12. Sai Bhaskar, V.; Sharma, M. Assessment of fugitive road dust emissions in Kanpur, India: A note. *Transp. Res. Part D Transp. Environ.* **2008**, *13*, 400–403. [CrossRef]
13. Bian, B.; Zhu, W. Particle size distribution and pollutants in road-deposited sediments in different areas of Zhenjiang, China. *Environ. Geochem. Health* **2009**, *31*, 511–520. [CrossRef]
14. Zhao, H.; Yin, C.; Chen, M.; Wang, W. Risk assessment of heavy metals in street dust particles to a stream network. *Soil Sediment Contam.* **2009**, *18*, 173–183. [CrossRef]
15. Zafra, C.A.; Temprano, J.; Tejero, I. Distribution of the concentration of heavy metals associated with the sediment particles accumulated on road surfaces. *Environ. Technol.* **2011**, *32*, 997–1008. [CrossRef] [PubMed]
16. Vaze, J.; Chiew, H.S. Experimental study pollutant accumulation on an urban road surface. *Urban Water* **2002**, *4*, 379–389. [CrossRef]
17. Zhao, H.; Yin, C.; Chen, M.; Wang, W. Run-off pollution impacts of polycyclic aromatic hydrocarbons in street dusts from a stream network town. *Water Sci. Technol.* **2008**, *58*, 2069–2076. [CrossRef] [PubMed]
18. Andral, M.C.; Roger, S.; Montrejaud-Vignoles, M.; Herremans, L. Particle size distribution and hydrodynamic characteristics of solid matter carried by run-off from motorways. *Water Environ. Res.* **1999**, *71*, 398–407. [CrossRef]
19. German, J.; Svensson, G. Metal content and particle size distribution of street sediments and street sweeping waste. *Water Sci. Technol.* **2002**, *46*, 191–198. [CrossRef]

20. Kioumourtzoglou, M.A.; Coull, B.A.; Dominici, F.; Koutrakis, P.; Schwartz, J.; Suh, H. The impact of source contribution uncertainty on the effects of source-specific PM$_{2.5}$ on hospital admissions: A case study in Boston, MA. *J. Expo. Sci. Environ. Epidemiol.* **2014**, *24*, 365–371. [CrossRef]

21. Bell, M.L.; Ebisu, K.; Leaderer, B.P.; Gent, J.F.; Lee, H.J.; Koutrakis, P.; Wang, Y.; Dominici, F.; Peng, R.D. Associations of PM2.5 constituents and sources with hospital admissions: Analysis of four counties in Connecticut and Massachusetts (USA) for persons ≥65 years of age. *Environ. Health Perspect.* **2014**, *122*, 138–144. [CrossRef]

22. Kolkata Municipal Corporation. Basic statistics of Koltata Municipal Corporation. Available online: https://www.kmcgov.in/KMCPortal/jsp/BasicStatistics.jsp (accessed on 2 March 2021).

23. Chenery, S.R.N.; Sarkar, S.K.; Chatterjee, M.; Marriott, A.L.; Watts, M.J. Heavy metals in urban road dusts from Kolkata and Bengaluru, India: Implications for human health. *Environ. Geochem. Health* **2020**, *42*, 2627–2643. [CrossRef] [PubMed]

24. ADB. Air Quality Management. In *Strengthening Environmental Management at the State Level (Cluster): Component E—Strengthening Environmental Management at West Bengal Pollution Control Board (ADB TA 3423—IND)*; Final Report; Intercontinental Consultants and Technocrats Pvt. Ltd.: New Delhi, India; Ballofet International LLC: Fort Collins, CO, USA; Water & Power Consultancy Services (India) Ltd.: New Delhi, India, November 2005; Volume V.

25. Majumdar, D.; Purohit, P.; Bhanarkar, A.D.; Rao, P.S.; Rafaj, P.; Amann, M.; Sander, R.; Pakrashi, A.; Srivastava, A. Managing future air quality in megacities: Emission inventory and scenario analysis for the Kolkata Metropolitan City, India. *Atmos. Environ.* **2020**, *222*, 117135. [CrossRef]

26. Majumdar, D. How are the Two Most Polluted Metro-cities of India Combating Air Pollution? Way Forward after Lifting of COVID-19 Lockdown. *Aerosol Air Qual. Res.* **2021**, *21*, 200463. [CrossRef]

27. West Bengal Pollution Control Board. Air Action Plan. Available online: https://www.wbpcb.gov.in/air-action-plan (accessed on 2 March 2021).

28. Roy Chowdhury, I. Scenario of vehicular emissions and its effect on human health in Kolkata city. *Int. J. Humanit. Soc. Sci. Invent.* **2015**, *4*, 1–9.

29. Lanzerstorfer, C. Toward more intercomparable road dust studies. *Crit. Rev. Environ. Sci. Technol.* **2020**, *51*, 826–855. [CrossRef]

30. Charlesworth, S.; De Miguel, E.; Ordóñez, A. A review of the distribution of particulate trace elements in urban terrestrial environments and its application to considerations of risk. *Environ. Geochem. Health* **2011**, *33*, 103–123. [CrossRef] [PubMed]

31. Kennedy, N.J.; Hinds, W.C. Inhalability of large solid particles. *J. Aerosol Sci.* **2002**, *33*, 237–255. [CrossRef]

32. Li, H.; Zuo, X.J. Speciation and Size Distribution of Copper and Zinc in Urban Road Runoff. *Bull. Environ. Contam. Toxicol.* **2013**, *90*, 471–476. [CrossRef] [PubMed]

33. Zhao, H.; Li, X. Risk assessment of metals in road-deposited sediment along an urban–rural gradient. *Environ. Pollut.* **2013**, *174*, 297–304. [CrossRef]

34. Yuen, J.Q.; Olin, P.H.; Lim, H.S.; Benner, S.G.; Sutherland, R.A.; Ziegler, A.D. Accumulation of potentiallytoxic elements in road deposited sediments in residential and light industrialneighborhoods of Singapore. *J. Environ. Manag.* **2012**, *101*, 151–163. [CrossRef]

35. Taylor, S.R. Abundance of chemical elements in the continental crust: A new table. *Geochim. Cosmochim. Acta* **1964**, *28*, 1273–1285. [CrossRef]

36. Belhadj, H.; Aubert, D.; Dali Youcef, N. Geochemistry of major and trace elements in sediments of Ghazaouet Bay (western Algeria): An assessment of metal pollution. *C. R. Geosci.* **2017**, *349*, 412–421. [CrossRef]

37. Daskalakis, K.D.; O'Connor, T.P. Normalization and elemental sediment contamination in the Coastal United States. *Environ. Sci. Technol.* **1995**, *29*, 470–477. [CrossRef] [PubMed]

38. Sutherland, R.A.; Tolosa, C.A. Multi-element analysis of road-deposited sediment in an urban drainage basin, Honolulu, Hawaii. *Environ. Pollut.* **2000**, *110*, 483–495. [CrossRef]

39. Ogundele, L.T.; Owoade, O.K.; Hopke, P.K.; Olise, F.S. Heavy metals in industrially emitted particulate matter in Ile-Ife, Nigeria. *Environ. Res.* **2017**, *156*, 320–325. [CrossRef]

40. Islam, M.S.; Ahmed, M.K.; Raknuzzaman, M.; Habibullah-Al-Mamun, M.; Islam, M.K. Heavy metal pollution in surface water and sediment: A preliminary assessment of an urban river in a developing country. *Ecol. Indic.* **2015**, *48*, 282–291. [CrossRef]

41. Devanesan, E.; Suresh, G.M.; Selvapandiyan, M.; Senthilkumar, G.; Ravisankar, R. Heavy metal and potential ecological risk assessmentin sediments collected from Poombuhar to Karaikal coast of Tamil Nadu using energy dispersive X-ray fluorescence (EDXRF) technique. *Beni-Suef Univ. J. Basic Appl. Sci.* **2017**, *6*, 285–292. [CrossRef]

42. Hakanson, L. An ecological risk index for aquatic pollutioncontrol. A sedimentological approach. *Water Res.* **1980**, *14*, 975–1001. [CrossRef]

43. Lu, X.; Wu, X.; Wang, Y.; Chen, H.; Gao, P.; Fu, Y. Risk assessment of toxic metals in street dust from a medium-sized industrial city of China. *Ecotoxicol. Environ. Saf.* **2014**, *106*, 154–163. [CrossRef]

44. Ogunkunle, C.O.; Fatoba, P.O. Pollution loads and the ecological risk assessment of soil heavy metals around a mega cement factory in Southwest Nigeria. *Pol. J. Environ. Stud.* **2013**, *22*, 487–493.

45. Sun, Y.; Zhou, Q.; Xie, Q.; Liu, R. Spatial, sources and risk assessment of heavy metal contamination of urban soils in typical regions of Shenyang, China. *J. Hazard. Mater.* **2010**, *174*, 455–462. [CrossRef] [PubMed]

46. USEPA. Risk-Assessment Guidance for Superfund. Volume 1. Human Health Evaluation Manual. Part A. Interim Final. USEPA. 1989. Available online: https://www.lm.doe.gov/cercla/documents/fernald_docs/CAT/215579.pdf (accessed on 5 March 2021).

47. Van den Berg, R. *Human Exposure to Soil Contamination: A Qualitative Analysis towards Proposals for Humane Toxicological Intervention Values*; National Institute of Public Health and Environmental Protection: Bilthoven, The Netherlands, 1994.
48. Oomen, A.G.; Janssen, P.; Dusseldorp, A.; Noorlander, C.W. *Exposure to Chemicals via House Dust*; No. RIVM Report 609021064/2008; RIVM: Bilthoven, The Netherlands, 2008.
49. ICMR. Development of an Atlas of Cancer in India, a Project of National Cancer Registry Programme. Available online: https://www.ncdirindia.org/ncrp/ca/index.aspx (accessed on 16 August 2021).
50. Gope, M.; Masto, R.E.; George, J.; Balachandran, S. Tracing source, distribution and health risk of potentially harmful elements (PHEs) in street dust of Durgapur, India. *Ecotoxicol. Environ. Saf.* **2018**, *154*, 280–293. [CrossRef]
51. Najmeddin, A.; Moore, F.; Keshavarzi, B.; Sadegh, Z. Pollution, source apportionment and health risk of potentially toxic elements (PTEs) and polycyclic aromatic hydrocarbons (PAHs) in urban street dust of Mashhad, the second largest city of Iran. *J. Geochem. Explor.* **2018**, *190*, 154–169. [CrossRef]
52. Praveena, S.M.; Aris, A.Z. Status, source identification, and health risks of potentially toxic element concentrations in road dust in a medium-sized city in a developing country. *Environ. Geochem. Health* **2018**, *40*, 749–762. [CrossRef]
53. Jose, J.; Srimuruganandam, B. Investigation of road dust characteristics and its associated health risks from an urban environment. *Environ. Geochem. Health* **2020**, *42*, 2819–2840. [CrossRef]
54. RAIS (The Risk Assessment Information System). Chemical Toxicity Value. 2020. Available online: https://rais.ornl.gov/tools/rais_chemical_risk_guide.html (accessed on 5 March 2021).
55. USDA. Soil Mechanics Level—I, Module 3—USDA Textural Soil Classification, Study Guide, USDA, USA. 1987. Available online: https://www.nrcs.usda.gov/Internet/FSE_DOCUMENTS/stelprdb1044818.pdf (accessed on 2 March 2021).
56. WHO/SDE/OEH/99.14 Document. Available online: http://www.who.int/occupational_health/publications/en/oehairbornedust3.pdf (accessed on 18 February 2021).
57. Ball, J.E.; Jenks, R.; Aubourg, D. An assessment of the availability of pollutant constituents on road surfaces. *Sci. Total Environ.* **1998**, *209*, 243–254. [CrossRef]
58. Ellis, J.B.; Revitt, D.M. Incidence of heavy metals in street surface sediments: Solubility and grain size studies. *Water Air Soil Pollut.* **1982**, *17*, 87–100. [CrossRef]
59. Yang, S.; Zhang, H.; Ding, H.; He, P.; Zhou, H. Lithium Metal Extraction from Seawater. *Joule* **2018**, *2*, 1648–1651. [CrossRef]
60. Central Pollution Control Board, Delhi, India. 2009. Available online: https://cpcb.nic.in/uploads/National_Ambient_Air_Quality_Standards.pdf (accessed on 2 March 2021).
61. Chatterjee, A.; Banerjee, R.N. Determination of lead and other metals in a residential area of greater Calcutta. *Sci. Total Environ.* **1999**, *227*, 175–185. [CrossRef]
62. Kuhad, M.S.; Malik, R.S.; Singh, A.; Dahiya, I.S. Background levels of heavy metals in agricultural soils of Indo Gangetic plains of Haryana. *J. Indian Soc. Soil Sci.* **1989**, *3*, 700–705.
63. Gowd, S.; Reddy, S.; Govil, P.K. Assessment of heavy metal contamination in soils at Jajmau (Kanpur) and Unnao industrial areas of the Ganga Plain, Uttar Pradesh, India. *J. Hazard. Mater.* **2010**, *174*, 113–121. [CrossRef]
64. Jiang, Y.; Shi, L.; Guang, A.L.; Mu, Z.; Zhan, H.; Wu, Y. Contamination levels and human health risk assessment of toxic heavy metals in street dust in an industrial city in Northwest China. *Environ. Geochem. Health* **2017**, *40*, 2007–2020. [CrossRef]
65. Census of India. 2011. Kolkata City Population 2011–2021. Available online: https://www.census2011.co.in/census/city/215-kolkata.html (accessed on 2 March 2021).
66. Kolkata Municipal Corporation. Solid waste Management Department. Available online: https://www.kmcgov.in/KMCPortal/jsp/SolidWasteFAQs.jsp (accessed on 2 March 2021).

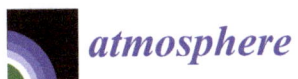

Article

Gross Alpha and Gross Beta Activity Concentrations in the Dust Fractions of Urban Surface-Deposited Sediment in Russian Cities

Mohamed Y. Hanfi [1,2,*], Ilia Yarmoshenko [3] and Andrian A. Seleznev [1,3]

1. Institute of Physics and Technology, Ural Federal University, Mira St 19, 620002 Ekaterinburg, Russia; sandrian@rambler.ru
2. Nuclear Materials Authority, Maadi, Cairo 520, Egypt
3. Institute of Industrial Ecology Ural Branch of Russian Academy of Sciences, S. Kovalevskoy St. 20, 620219 Ekaterinburg, Russia; ivy@ecko.uran.ru
* Correspondence: mokhamed.khanfi@urfu.ru

Citation: Hanfi, M.Y.; Yarmoshenko, I.; Seleznev, A.A. Gross Alpha and Gross Beta Activity Concentrations in the Dust Fractions of Urban Surface-Deposited Sediment in Russian Cities. *Atmosphere* **2021**, *12*, 571. https://doi.org/10.3390/atmos12050571

Academic Editors: Luhar Ashok and Omar Ramírez Hernández

Received: 1 April 2021
Accepted: 26 April 2021
Published: 28 April 2021

Publisher's Note: MDPI stays neutral with regard to jurisdictional claims in published maps and institutional affiliations.

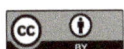

Copyright: © 2021 by the authors. Licensee MDPI, Basel, Switzerland. This article is an open access article distributed under the terms and conditions of the Creative Commons Attribution (CC BY) license (https:// creativecommons.org/licenses/by/ 4.0/).

Abstract: Studies of gross alpha and gross beta activity in road- and surface-deposited sediments were conducted in three Russian cities in different geographical zones. To perform radiation measurements, new methods were applied which allow dealing with low mass and low volume dust-sized (2–100 µm) samples obtained after the size fractionation procedure. The 2–10 µm fraction size had the highest gross beta activity concentration (GB)—1.32 Bq/g in Nizhny Novgorod and Rostov-On-Don, while the 50–100 µm fraction size was most prominent in Ekaterinburg. This can be attributed to the presence of radionuclides that are transferred through natural and anthropogenic processes. The highest gross alpha activity concentration (GA) in fraction sizes was found in Rostov-on-Don city within the 50–100 µm range—0.22 Bq/g. The fraction sizes 50–100 µm have a higher gross alpha activity concentration than 2–10 µm and 10–50 µm fraction sizes due to natural partitioning of the main minerals constituting the urban surface-deposited sediment (USDS). Observed dependencies reflect the geochemical processes which take place during the formation and transport of urban surface sediments. Developed experimental methods of radiation measurements formed the methodological base of urban geochemical studies.

Keywords: gross alpha activity; gross beta activity urban environment; sediment; size fraction

1. Introduction

There has been a variety of natural radionuclides in the aquatic and terrestrial ecosystems since Earth's creation. Radionuclides participate in environmental processes such as weathering, sedimentation, resuspension, etc. [1]. Consequently, many studies have measured radionuclide concentrations in various environmental matrices, such as the crust, rocks, sandy beaches, building materials, and the atmosphere [2–4].

Natural radionuclides in minerals and raw materials of natural origin are constantly emitted ionizing radiation that can be exposed to human beings and biota [3,5]. Naturally occurring radioactive materials (NORMs) have resulted from human activities that increase human exposure to Earth's crust radionuclides and can therefore be found in water, air, food, building materials, and the human body [4,6–8]. Radiation hazards are from external and internal exposure to these radioactive isotopes. External exposure is associated with direct gamma radiation emitted from the isotopes in the U and Th series, as well as from [40]K. Internal exposure is caused by the inhalation of inert radioactive gases radon [222]Rn, thoron [220]Rn, and short-lived radioisotopes of their progeny [9,10]. Some artificial radionuclides may be present in the environment (such as ^{137}Cs and ^{131}I), such as in Chernobyl [11,12] and due to nuclear weapons testing and nuclear accident. Monitoring of any release of radioactive materials to the environment is necessary for the protection of the environment; for example, if NORM content exceeds the typical background radiation levels, it is therefore essential to evaluate what precautions should be taken, if any. Additionally, it is suitable to identify the sources of radionuclides, the transportation into the environment, and their migration [13].

In the urban environment, processes such as weathering, soil erosion, as well as anthropogenic impacts on the surfaces produce essential amounts of sediment consisting of grained material of different origin [14,15]. Sediment can deposit in various urban landscape zones and form urban surface-deposited sediment (USDS) which play a significant role in shaping the urban environment [16].

Measuring the gross alpha and gross beta concentration in urban environmental compartments have become increasingly important due to concerns about radioactive environmental contamination through natural and anthropogenic activities resulting in human exposure [17,18]. The objective of the present work is to study the concentration of gross alpha and gross beta activity in size-fractionated samples obtained from the USDS in three Russian cities: Ekaterinburg, Rostov-On-Don, and Nizhny Novgorod. An essential feature of the applied measurements methods is the possibility to detect alpha and beta emitter content in samples of a small amount (mass and volume) of fractionated material.

2. Materials and Methods

2.1. Description of the Surveyed City

Description of Investigated Cities

The samples of USDS were collected in three Russian cities: Ekaterinburg, Nizhny Novgorod, and Rostov-on-Don [19]. These cities have a continental climate and are located in different geographical zones. The investigated cities are described in Table 1.

Table 1. Description of the investigated cities.

Parameter	Ekaterinburg	Nizhny Novgorod	Rostov-on-Don
Area	495 km^2	460 km^2	348.5 km^2
Population	1,468,833	1,259,013	1,130,305
Main rivers	Iset	Oka and Volga	Don
Latitudes and longitudes	56°50′ N, 60°35′ E	56°19 N, 44°00 E	47°14′ N, 39°42′ E
Temperature in July (night/day) °C	14/24	14/24	18/29
Temperature in January (night/day) °C	−15/−9	−11/−5	−5/−0.1
Climate	Temperate continental	Humid continental	Moderate continental, steppe
Geographical region	Eastern slope of the Middle Urals	Valley of the Volga and Oka rivers	Valley of the Don river
Geology	Ural Mountains	Alluvial river sediment	Alluvial river sediment
Main industries	Productions of machinery, metal processing, metallurgical production, chemical production.	Production of machinery and river shipping	Productions of machinery, river shipping, food industry.

2.2. Sampling Procedure

Approximately 1.5–2 kg of the representative samples of USDS were collected from the surfaces where they were deposited in relatively significant amounts. The samples were put into plastic vacuum bags directly after collection to prevent them from atmospheric moisture. The drying process was carried out under room temperature for one week. Then, two sieving process, decantation and filtration, were performed, which are referred to as wet sieving. Through these processes, the samples were sieved into small-sized fractions which represented dust-sized fractions (2–10 μm, 10–50 μm and 50–100 μm). Dry sieving for the remainder of the sample was used to fractionate into large-sized elements, which represented fine sand (100–250 µm and 250–1000 µm) and coarse sand (size > 1000 µm) size fractions. The separation by dry and wet sieving is described in Test Method WA 115.1-2017 [20,21].

2.3. Measurement of Gross Beta Activity

The method of GB measurements in solid sand and dust samples of low mass (1–10 g) was developed by [11]. For detecting the GB activities, a low background radiometer detector (BDPB-01) was utilized. A plastic scintillation detector with 60 mm diameter and a photomultiplier tube was inserted into a special plastic container. A lead stabilization system of the measuring path was used, which simultaneously enabled testing of the whole path when operating, to promote stability in the disclosure unit. The detection system was shielded by the lead to prevent any external radiation which would impact the beta measurements. The sieved fractions of each sample were weighed and settled in a planchet 2 cm in diameter and 0.6 cm in height. Before the detection of beta in the samples, an empty planchet was assessed for the same counting time using the detector to estimate the background count rate. This process was repeated where the average value of background count rate was 0.017 cpm for beta particles. The GB activity concentration (Bq g^{-1}) in the USDS size fractions was computed via the following formula:

$$A_\beta = \frac{I_c - I_{BG}}{\varepsilon(m) \cdot m} \quad (1)$$

where Ic represents the count rate of beta (s^{-1}), I_{BG} refers to the background beta count rate (s^{-1}), m is the weight of the fractionated sample (g) and the efficiency of detector identified with $\varepsilon(m)$ which depends on m (s^{-1}/Bq). The calibration of the detection system is described elsewhere [11].

2.4. Gross Alpha Measurement Method

The method of GA measurements in solid grained samples of low mass (about 5 g) was developed by [22]. First, the applied detectors are calibrated using a monazite sample with a known thorium activity concentration (190 ± 15% Bq/g). Twenty-four LR-115 (2.5 × 2.5 cm^2) detectors were exposed in direct contact with the monazite sample with a known thorium activity concentration (190 ± 15% Bq/g) for 40 min. After irradiation using the calibration source, the etching process began under standard procedures: a chemical NaOH solution with normality 2.5 N at 50 °C for 2 h [23–25].

After that, a spark counter was employed to register the alpha tracks density in LR-115 films. The calibration factors k, (track cm^{-2} min^{-1}/ Bq g^{-1}) for the LR-115 films was computed via Equation (2):

$$k = \frac{\rho_t}{A_m \, t} \quad (2)$$

For the GA measurements in the fractionated USDS samples, The LR-115 films (2.5 × 2.5 cm^2) were exposed in contact with the fractionated sample (approximately 5 g) and were placed in the hole with a 2 cm diameter for 90 days. During the exposure time, the samples were stored in an accumulation chamber ventilated with fresh air with a low radon concentration where the α particles were released from the radionuclides (238 U, 232 Th and their decay progenies) and formed alpha tracks on the LR-115 film. At the end of exposure time, the LR-115 films were collected and etched under the standard procedures mentioned above. After that, the spark counter was employed to register the alpha track density in LR-115 films. Unexposed LR-115 films were etched and counted via the spark counter to estimate the background alpha track density in the detectors. The GA activity concentration values were estimated by Equation (3) [26]:

$$A = \frac{\rho_t}{k \, t} \quad (3)$$

The uncertainty values were computed for the obtained results and found to be approximately 5% and 3% for GB and GA, respectively. Furthermore, the minimum detectable activity (MDA) values for LR-115 detectors can be computed as follows:

$$\text{MDA} = \frac{\sqrt{N_b} + 2.7}{T\varepsilon} \quad (4)$$

where N_b represents the number of background count rate, T is the exposure duration, and ε is the detector efficiency. The values of MDA were 0.03 Bq/g, obtained using the Curie standard method [27]. For SSNTDs, the MDA values depend only on the exposure period.

2.5. Chemical Analysis

The chemical analysis of the USDS fractionated samples was performed for other studies. The methods of the chemical analyses applied in these studies are described elsewhere [19,20].

The chemical analysis was conducted in the laboratory of the Institute of Industrial Ecology, UB RAS (Ekaterinburg, Russia). Certified methodologies and accreditation by the Russian System of State Accreditation Laboratories of the Institute of Industrial Ecology Chemical Analytical Center provided the quality control for the measurements. The solid fractionated sample was digested utilizing HNO_3, $HClO_4$, and HF, pure for analysis [28,29]. Then, the prepared sample solution was analyzed using inductively coupled plasma mass spectrometry (ICP-MS) to detect element concentrations, in particular, U and Th content.

3. Results

The descriptive statistics of gross alpha activity concentration (GA), gross beta activity concentration (GB), and uranium and thorium contents in the USDS dust fractions (2–10, 10–50 and 50–100 µm) of Ekaterinburg, Nizhny Novgorod, and Rostov-On-Don are presented in Table 2. As can be seen in Table 2, there is a tendency of variation of radioactive parameters depending on the USDS fractions and the city. The statistical significance of the difference was studied between radioactive parameters for the size fractions in the same city, as well as between the different cities. Due to a low number of measurements of GA which is associated with difficulties of measurements in low-volume samples, the tendencies obtained in GA are insignificant ($p > 0.1$). The dependencies of GB on the size fractions and geographical location are more reliable. The differences between the average GB values in Ekb and RND in size fraction 2–10 µm and 50–100 µm are significant, as is that between Ekb and NN in size fraction 50–100 µm ($p < 0.05$). Analysis of variances confirmed the size fraction and city of sampling as factors influencing the GB ($p < 0.05$).

It is clear that the highest values of GA in the investigated fractions were found in the fraction size 50–100 µm, while the lowest values were observed in the fraction size 2–10 µm for all studied cities. The GB activity concentrations reached the maximum values in the fraction size 50–100 µm for Ekaterinburg, and 2–10 µm for Nizhny Novgorod and Rostov-On-Don. Table 2 presents the chemical compositions obtained in the fraction size; the U and Th content values varied in between various fraction sizes in the investigated cities where the highest U and Th content average values were detected in Ekaterinburg within the fraction size 50–100 µm, and Rostov-On-Don within 10–50 µm, respectively. The minimum average values were recorded in Rostov-On-Don within 50–100 µm and in Ekaterinburg within 2–10 µm, respectively. The distribution of the radioactive parameters is plotted in Figure 1.

Table 2. Descriptive statistics for the gross alpha activity concentration (GA), gross beta activity concentration (GB), U content (ppm) and Th content (ppm) in the USDS size fractions (μm).

City	Descriptive Parameters	GA (Bq g^{-1})			GB (Bq g^{-1})			U (ppm)			Th (ppm)		
		2–10	10–50	50–100	2–10	10–50	50–100	2–10	10–50	50–100	2–10	10–50	50–100
Ekaterinburg	Athematic Mean	0.11	0.13	0.17	0.71	0.93	1.28	1.46	2.03	2.33	4.94	4.45	4.58
	Geometric mean	0.1	0.12	0.16	0.61	0.67	0.93	1.22	1.48	1.66	2.14	2.74	2.67
	SD	0.06	0.02	0.04	0.43	0.86	1.13	0.80	1.40	2.05	2.30	2.34	2.30
	Max	0.18	0.15	0.20	1.72	3.20	5.30	2.90	5.16	8.26	7.02	8.65	8.11
	Min	0.06	0.11	0.12	0.28	0.15	0.20	0.31	0.08	0.17	0.14	0.10	0.10
	n	3	4	4	10	23	24	12	14	14	12	14	14
Nizhny Novgorod	Athematic Mean	0.13	0.13	0.17	1.32	0.99	0.72	1.28	1.98	1.92	3.54	5.12	4.53
	Geometric mean	0.09	0.12	0.16	0.90	0.91	0.70	1.16	1.92	1.70	2.51	4.86	4.36
	SD	0.11	0.06	0.04	1.15	0.27	0.16	0.59	0.56	1.63	2.19	1.50	1.20
	Max	0.20	0.20	0.21	4.15	1.58	1.10	2.74	3.92	10.92	9.25	7.67	7.14
	Min	0.05	0.08	0.13	0.30	0.05	0.39	0.56	1.44	1.24	1.06	2.52	2.30
	n	2	4	3	12	32	35	22	34	34	22	34	35
Rostov On Don	Athematic Mean	0.15	0.19	0.22	0.95	0.90	0.69	1.52	1.94	1.97	4.64	7.45	7.35
	Geometric mean	0.14	0.18	0.20	0.88	0.85	0.65	1.45	1.93	1.96	3.84	7.39	7.23
	SD	0.04	0.07	0.11	0.33	0.33	0.23	0.51	0.21	0.22	2.89	0.95	1.33
	Max	0.18	0.26	0.37	1.69	2.34	1.24	2.79	2.33	2.59	9.78	8.96	10.04
	Min	0.10	0.12	0.14	0.21	0.36	0.40	0.67	1.59	1.49	1.08	5.45	4.11
	n	3	3	4	31	30	34	17	26	35	17	26	35

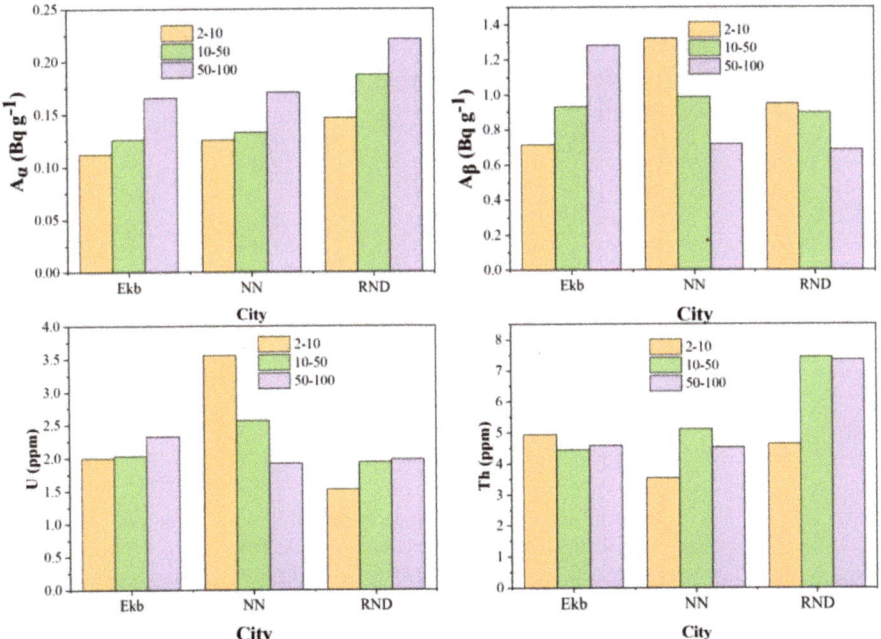

Figure 1. The variation of GA and GB within the fraction sizes 2-10, 10-50 and 50-100 μm in the investigated Russian cities.

4. Discussion

The detection of GA and GB in the urban environment is an indication of the presence of radionuclides in urban sediments [11]. As clarified from Figure 1, the GA and GB in Ekaterinburg within all fraction sizes had the same natural and anthropogenic origins. Figure 1 illustrates the influence of natural and anthropogenic factors which may be depicted by the results of the GA and GB. The chemical analysis illustrated that USDS contains uranium and thorium, which was higher in the fraction 50–100 μm than in the fractions 2–10 and 10–50 μm in the cities under study. Thus, the GA may be attributed to natural radionuclides in the environment such as uranium, radium, thorium and their decay products [30]. Increasing uranium and thorium content led to increases in the GA activity concentration in the USDS fractions. Moreover, the potassium-40, radium, and decay products were the main beta emitters in the urban sediments. Among the artificial products, agricultural fertilizer, which contains natural radionuclides, led to the increment of potassium (including isotope ^{40}K) content in USDS fractions [31,32].

The geology of the studied cities can impact the GA and GB in the various fraction sizes. In Ekaterinburg, the geological features are mainly established by the Ural Mountains, while the geologies of Nizhny Novgorod and Rostov-on-Don are related to the alluvial processes of rivers.

Furthermore, the presence of alpha and beta radioactivity can be explained by the migration and transportation of radionuclides from rocks and soils to the urban environment via various pathways such as rainwater, wind, and traffic emissions.

For instance, the correlation between radioactive components of fraction sizes in Ekaterinburg was studied via Pearson's correlation and is presented in Table 3. Strong correlation between GA and GB is obvious, as well between U content (0.99) and Th content (0.74) in the fraction size 2–10 μm. This means the GA and GB are contributed from the same natural and anthropogenic sources. For the fraction size 10–50 μm, the GA and GB were linked with the anthropogenic sources, where the GA changed with GB in opposite directions. The natural sources of fraction sizes 50–100 μm possessed radioactive components; however, the U and Th content changed in opposite direction with the GA.

Table 3. Pearson's correlation between radioactive components of fraction sizes in Ekaterinburg.

2–10	GA	GB	Th	U
GA	-			
GB	1 *	-		
Th	0.74	−0.14	-	
U	0.99	0.22	0.78	-
10–50	GA	GB	Th	U
GA	-			
GB	−0.98	-		
Th	0.38	−0.49	-	
U	0.31	−0.38	0.90	-
50–100	GA	GB	Th	U
GA	-			
GB	−0.60	-		
Th	−0.93	0.06	-	
U	−0.95	0.15	0.66	-

* 3 sample with GA is available.

The main industries in Ekaterinburg are the production of machinery, metal processing, metallurgical production, and chemical production. In Nizhny Novgorod, main industries are the production of machinery and river shipping. Finally, in Rostov-On-Don, productions of machinery, river shipping, and the food industry are dominant.

Domestic emissions, the weathering of facades and pavement surfaces, and the precipitation of previously suspended particles (atmospheric aerosols) are also sources of pollution in residential areas [33–37]. This shows that the GA and GB reflect the migration and transportation of radionuclides in the urban environment and potentially harmful elements through wind, traffic emissions, and industrial activities from one urban area to others and are closely linked to the examined fraction sizes.

5. Conclusions

New methods developed for the measurements of GA and GB in low mass and low volume samples of natural origin were applied to assess the radioactivity of the USDS. The results of the performed measurements were compared with early obtained measurements of the total U and Th concentrations in the same cities. The analysis allows us to draw the following conclusions:

1. Such natural radionuclides as U, Th, their decay products and ^{40}K present in the USDS;
2. Obtained values of GA and GB are generally associated with radionuclides of natural origin. The main sources of natural radioactivity in the urban environment are geological formations and building materials;
3. Natural radionuclides participate in the sedimentation processes and can be found in the sedimentation material in each city independently of climate, geographical location, and industrial development;
4. The radioactivity of fine sand and dust fractions can contribute to population radiation exposure in cases of significant resuspension of urban dust by wind and vehicles.

Author Contributions: Conceptualization, field sampling, methodology, writing—original draft preparation, M.Y.H., I.Y. and A.A.S.; methodology, writing—review and editing, M.Y.H. and I.Y. All authors have read and agreed to the published version of the manuscript.

Funding: The study was supported by Russian Science Foundation (grant No. 18-77-10024).

Institutional Review Board Statement: Not applicable.

Informed Consent Statement: Not applicable.

Data Availability Statement: Not Applicable.

Conflicts of Interest: The authors declare no conflict of interest.

References

1. Lin, W.; Chen, L.; Zeng, S.; Li, T.; Wang, Y.; Yu, K. Residual β activity of particulate Th as a novel proxy for tracking sediment resuspension in the ocean. *Sci. Rep.* **2016**, *6*, 27069. [CrossRef] [PubMed]
2. Ojovan, M.; Lee, W. Naturally Occurring Radionuclides. In *An Introduction to Nuclear Waste Immobilisation*; Elsevier: Amsterdam, The Netherlands, 2014; pp. 31–39. [CrossRef]
3. Lin, W.; Chen, L.; Yu, W.; Zeng, Z.; Lin, J.; Zeng, S. Radioactivity impacts of the Fukushima Nuclear Accident on the atmosphere. *Atmospheric Environ.* **2015**, *102*, 311–322. [CrossRef]
4. Liu, X.; Lin, W. Natural radioactivity in the beach sand and soil along the coastline of Guangxi Province, China. *Mar. Pollut. Bull.* **2018**, *135*, 446–450. [CrossRef] [PubMed]
5. Vives, J.; Aoyama, M.; Bradshaw, C.; Brown, J.; Buesseler, K.O.; Casacuberta, N.; Christl, M.; Duffa, C.; Impens, N.R.E.N.; Iosjpe, M.; et al. Science of the Total Environment Marine radioecology after the Fukushima Dai-ichi nuclear accident: Are we better positioned to understand the impact of radionuclides in marine ecosystems? *Sci. Total. Environ.* **2018**, *618*, 80–92. [CrossRef]
6. Huang, Y.; Lu, X.; Ding, X.; Feng, T. Natural radioactivity level in beach sand along the coast of Xiamen. *Mar. Pollut. Bull.* **2015**, *91*, 357–361. [CrossRef]
7. Trevisi, R.; Leonardi, F.; Risica, S.; Nuccetelli, C. Updated database on natural radioactivity in building materials in Europe. *J. Environ. Radioact.* **2018**, *187*, 90–105. [CrossRef]
8. Raghu, Y.; Ravisankar, R.; Chandrasekaran, A.; Vijayagopal, P.; Venkatraman, B. Assessment of natural radioactivity and radiological hazards in building materials used in the Tiruvannamalai District, Tamilnadu, India, using a statistical approach. *Integr. Med. Res.* **2015**. [CrossRef]
9. Khandaker, M.U. Radiometric analysis of construction materials using hpge gamma-ray spectrometry. *Radiat. Prot. Dosim.* **2012**, *152*, 33–37. [CrossRef] [PubMed]
10. Al-sewaidan, H.A. Journal of King Saud University—Science Natural radioactivity measurements and dose rate assessment of selected ceramic and cement types used in Riyadh, Saudi Arabia. *J. King Saud Univ. Sci.* **2019**, *31*, 987–992. [CrossRef]
11. Hanfi, M.Y.; Yarmoshenko, I.V.; Seleznev, A.A.; Zhukovsky, M.V. The gross beta activity of surface sediment in different urban landscape areas. *J. Radioanal. Nucl. Chem.* **2019**, *321*, 831–839. [CrossRef]

12. Buraeva, E.A.; Bezuglova, O.S.; Stasov, V.V.; Nefedov, V.S.; Dergacheva, E.V.; Goncharenko, A.A.; Martynenko, S.V.; Goncharova, L.Y.; Gorbov, S.N.; Malyshevsky, V.S.; et al. Geoderma Features of 137 Cs distribution and dynamics in the main soils of the steppe zone in the southern European Russia. *Geoderma* **2015**, *259–260*, 259–270. [CrossRef]
13. Izwan, M.; Adziz, A.; Siong, K.K. Determination of Gross Alpha and Gross Beta in Soil Around Repository Facility at Bukit Kledang, Perak, Malaysia. *AIP Conf. Proc.* **2018**, *1940*, 020009. [CrossRef]
14. Russell, K.L.; Vietz, G.J.; Fletcher, T.D. Global sediment yields from urban and urbanizing watersheds. *Earth-Sci. Rev.* **2017**, *168*, 73–80. [CrossRef]
15. Seleznev, A.A.; Yarmoshenko, I.V.; Malinovsky, G.P. Assessment of Total Amount of Surface Sediment in Urban Environment Using Data on Solid Matter Content in Snow-Dirt Sludge. *Environ. Process.* **2019**, *6*, 581–595. [CrossRef]
16. Yarmoshenko, I.; Malinovsky, G.; Baglaeva, E. A Landscape Study of Sediment Formation and Transport in the Urban Environment. *Atmosphere* **2020**, *11*, 1320. [CrossRef]
17. Alharbi, T. Simulation of α and β gross activity measurement of soil samples with proportional counters. *Appl. Radiat. Isot.* **2018**, *136*, 65–67. [CrossRef]
18. Hanfi, M.Y.; Yarmoshenko, I.; Seleznev, A.A.; Onishchenko, A.D.; Zhukovsky, M.V. Development of an appropriate method for measuring gross alpha activity concentration in low-mass size-fractionated samples of sediment using solid-state nuclear track detectors. *Radioanal. Nucl. Chem.* **2020**, *323*, 1047–1053. [CrossRef]
19. Seleznev, A.; Yarmoshenko, I.; Malinovsky, G.; Ilgasheva, E.; Baglaeva, E.; Ryanskaya, A.; Kiseleva, D.; Gulyaeva, T. Snow-dirt sludge as an indicator of environmental and sedimentation processes in the urban environment. *Sci. Rep.* **2019**, 1–12. [CrossRef] [PubMed]
20. Seleznev, A.; Rudakov, M. Some geochemical characterstics of puddle sediments from cities located in various geological, geographic, climatic, and industerial zones. *Carpathian J. Earth Environ. Sci.* **2018**, *14*, 95–106. [CrossRef]
21. MAIN ROADS Western Australia. *WA 115.1-2017 Particle Size and Particle Size Distribution*; MAIN ROADS Western Australia: East Perth, WA, Australia, 2017; p. 5.
22. Durrani, S.A.; Bull, R.K. *Solid State Nuclear Track Detection Principles, Methods and Applications*; Pergamon Press: Oxford, UK, 1985; ISBN 0080206050.
23. Fleischer, R.L.; Price, P.B.; Walker, R.M. *Nuclear Tracks in Solids*; Principles and applications; University of California Press: Berkeley, CA, USA, 1975; ISBN 9781137333438.
24. Oufni, L.; Taj, S.; Manaut, B.; Eddouks, M. Transfer of uranium and thorium from soil to different parts of medicinal plants using SSNTD. *J. Radioanal. Nucl. Chem.* **2010**, *287*, 403–410. [CrossRef]
25. Zhukovsky, M.; Onischenko, A.; Bastrikov, V. Radon measurements—Discussion of error estimates for selected methods. *Appl. Radiat. Isot.* **2010**, *68*, 816–820. [CrossRef] [PubMed]
26. Currie, L.A. Limits for Qualitative Detection and Quantitative Determination Application to Radiochemistry. *Anal. Chem.* **1968**, *40*, 586–593. [CrossRef]
27. Han, C.H.; Park, J.W. Analysis of the natural radioactivity concentrations of the fine dust samples in Jeju Island, Korea and the annual effective radiation dose by inhalation. *J. Radioanal. Nucl. Chem.* **2018**, *316*, 1173–1179. [CrossRef]
28. Vogel, C.; Hoffmann, M.C.; Taube, M.C.; Krüger, O.; Baran, R.; Adam, C. Uranium and thorium species in phosphate rock and sewage sludge ash based phosphorus fertilizers. *J. Hazard. Mater.* **2020**, *382*, 121100. [CrossRef] [PubMed]
29. Kücükömeroglu, B.; Kurnaz, A.; Keser, R.; Korkmaz, F.; Okumusoglu, N.T.; Karahan, G.; Sen, C.; Cevik, U. Radioactivity in sediments and gross alpha-beta activities in surface water of Firtina River, Turkey. *Environ. Geol.* **2008**, *55*, 1483–1491. [CrossRef]
30. NCRP. *Radiation Exposure of the U.S. Population from Consumer Products and Miscellaneous Sources*; NCRP: Bethesda, MD, USA, 1987.
31. Hanfi, M.Y.; Yarmoshenko, V.; Seleznev, A.A.; Malinovsky, G.; Ilgasheva, E.; Zhukovsky, M.V. Beta radioactivity of urban surface–deposited sediment in three Russian cities. *Environ. Sci. Pollut. Res.* **2020**, *27*, 1–7. [CrossRef]
32. IAEA. *Workplace Monitoring for Radiation and Contamination, Practical Radiation Technical*; IAEA: Vienna, Austria, 2004; p. 69.
33. Arslan, H. Heavy metals in street dust in bursa, turkey. *J. Trace Microprobe Tech.* **2001**, *19*, 439–445. [CrossRef]
34. Zereni, F.; Alt, F. (Eds.) *Palladium Emissions in the Environment*; Springer: Berlin/Heidelberg, Germany, 2006; ISBN 9783540292197.
35. Zereni, F.; Alt, F. (Eds.) New metal emission patterns in road traffic environments. *Environ. Monit. Assess.* **2006**, *117*, 85–98. [CrossRef] [PubMed]
36. Hjortenkrans, D.S.; Bergbäck, B.G.; Häggerud, A.V. Metal Emissions from Brake Linings and Tires: Case Studies of Stockholm, Sweden 1995/1998 and 2005. *Environ. Sci. Technol.* **2007**, *41*, 5224–5230. [CrossRef]
37. Winther, M.; Slento, E. (Eds.) *Heavy Metal Emissions for Danish Road Transport*; National Environmental Research Institute: Denmark, Roskilde, 2010; ISBN 9788770731706.

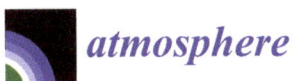

Article

Is the Urban Form a Driver of Heavy Metal Pollution in Road Dust? Evidence from Mexico City

Anahi Aguilera [1,2], Dorian Bautista-Hernández [2,*], Francisco Bautista [2], Avto Goguitchaichvili [3] and Rubén Cejudo [3]

[1] Posgrado en Ciencias Biológicas, Universidad Nacional Autónoma de México, Morelia 58341, Michoacán, Mexico; aaguilera@cieco.unam.mx
[2] Laboratorio Universitario de Geofísica Ambiental, Centro de Investigaciones en Geografía Ambiental, Universidad Nacional Autónoma de México, Morelia 58341, Michoacán, Mexico; leptosol@ciga.unam.mx
[3] Laboratorio Universitario de Geofísica Ambiental, Instituto de Geofísica Unidad Michoácan, Universidad Nacional Autónoma de México, Morelia 58341, Michoacán, Mexico; avto@geofisica.unam.mx (A.G.); ruben@igeofisica.unam.mx (R.C.)
* Correspondence: dobautistah@gmail.com

Citation: Aguilera, A.; Bautista-Hernández, D.; Bautista, F.; Goguitchaichvili, A.; Cejudo, R. Is the Urban Form a Driver of Heavy Metal Pollution in Road Dust? Evidence from Mexico City. *Atmosphere* **2021**, *12*, 266. https://doi.org/10.3390/atmos12020266

Academic Editor: Dmitry Vlasov

Received: 20 January 2021
Accepted: 14 February 2021
Published: 17 February 2021

Publisher's Note: MDPI stays neutral with regard to jurisdictional claims in published maps and institutional affiliations.

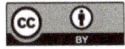

Copyright: © 2021 by the authors. Licensee MDPI, Basel, Switzerland. This article is an open access article distributed under the terms and conditions of the Creative Commons Attribution (CC BY) license (https://creativecommons.org/licenses/by/4.0/).

Abstract: Environmental pollution is a negative externality of urbanization and is of great concern due to the fact that it poses serious problems to human health. Pollutants, such as heavy metals, have been found in urban road dust; however, it is unclear whether the urban form has a role in its accumulation, mainly in cases where there is no dominant unique source. We collected 482 samples of road dust, we determined the concentrations of five heavy metals (Cr, Cu, Pb, Zn, and Ni) using inductively coupled plasma optical emission spectrometry (ICP-OES), and then we derived the pollution load index (PLI). After estimating the mostly anthropogenic origin of these pollutants based on global levels of reference, there were two main aims of this study. Firstly, to analyze the spatial correlation of heavy metals, and secondly, to identify the main factors that influenced the heavy metal concentrations in the road dust of Mexico City. We did this by using a spatial autocorrelation indicator (Global Moran's I) and applying ordinary least squares (OLS) and spatial regression models. The results indicated low levels of positive spatial autocorrelation for all heavy metals. Most variables failed to detect any relationship with heavy metals. The median strip area in the roads had a weak (significance level of 90%) but consistent positive relationship with Cr, Cu, Ni, Pb, and the PLI. The distance to the airport had a weak (significance level of 90%) and inverse relationship with Pb. Manufacturing units were associated with an increase in Cu (significance level of 95%), while the entropy index was associated with an increase in Ni (significance level of 95%).

Keywords: road dust; heavy metals; Mexico City; urban pollution; urban form

1. Introduction

The world is becoming increasingly urban. In the developing world, Latin America has already achieved this transition toward an urbanized society. For example, in Mexico, it is estimated that 80% of the population lives in urban areas [1]. The capital, Mexico City, along with its metropolitan area, concentrates around 17.5% of the country's population and has over 40,000 industries and 4 million vehicles that consume more than 40 million liters of fossil fuels per day, releasing, as a result, thousands of tons of pollutants into the urban environment [2]. Environmental pollution is one of the main negative externalities of huge urban agglomerations, especially in the developing context where weak institutions and planning efforts aggravate the problem [3].

Air pollution has attracted a great deal of attention, as it is considered one of the main causes of death in cities [4]; therefore, air pollution has been widely researched. Less attention has been paid to road dust pollution [5]; however, we assume that they are likely interlinked. Research reported that road dust is a sink for polluting emissions, which are deposited on the surface of streets, sidewalks, and windows [6]. At the same time, road dust is a source of pollutants of atmospheric particulate matter [7]. Studies found that urban structure factors, such as land use, industrial development, and building construction, worsened the pollution in urban areas [8,9]. From a social point of view, aspects such as tax revenue and education level are associated with a decrease in urban pollution [9]. In terms of country-level data, researchers have tested the environmental Kuznets curve (EKC) hypothesis, which states that the relationship between gross domestic product (GDP) per capita and different environmental indicators exhibit an inverted-U curve [10,11].

Heavy metals are some of the major pollutants found in road dust [12–14]. Due to their abundance, toxicity, persistence, and bioaccumulation, heavy metals can cause permanent damage to ecosystems and humans [15]. The severity of health problems due to heavy metal toxicity depends on several factors, such as the type and form of the element, the route and duration of exposure, and to a greater extent, the susceptibility of each person [16]. Low concentrations of non-essential heavy metals (As, Hg, Pb, Cr, and Cd) can be lethal to animals. In Mexico City, the median levels of lead in children's blood were found to be close to the reference level for public health interventions (5.0 µg/dL) [17]. Prenatal lead exposure has been associated with a decrease in child growth [18]. Even essential metals (Zn, Cu, and Ni), required for the proper function of different enzymes, can become toxic in high concentrations, inducing the generation of reactive nitrogen and oxygen species. This can result in the peroxidation of lipids, as well as the functional deterioration of DNA and proteins [19]. Nickel diminishes the protection that taurine provides against neurodegeneration [16].

The sources of heavy metals in road dust can be diverse. In some cities, the origins are very specific to major stationary emitting sources; for example, the smelting industry [13], e-waste recycling [20,21], and mining activities [22]. Natural processes may also be the cause of an increase in the concentrations of trace metals [23]. Using pollutant-tracing approaches, mobile sources of heavy metals have also been identified, such as vehicular emissions [24]. It is considered that Cu, Pb, Zn, and Cr are traffic-related metals [25–27]. The quantities emitted vary, but some metals can be linked to specific vehicle parts. For example, Cu emissions are generally related to brake abrasion [28,29]; Zn is mainly emitted by tire wear [25], as well as from diesel exhaust emissions [27]. Some Zn compounds are used as additives for motor oil [30]. In the case of Cr, this metal can originate from exhaust emissions [26]. Pb can come from brakes and the loss of lead wheel weights [27]; Cr and Pb have been reported to originate also from yellow street paint which contains lead chromate. Paint and pigments crack, peel, and turn to chalk, mobilizing metal particles into the urban environment [31,32]. Ni can come from mixed industrial/fuel-oil combustion [30].

In cities with an economy mostly related to the service sector, there are multiple small and scattered possible sources, which can be mobile or fixed. Therefore, it is vital to determine what characteristics of the urban form act as driving factors of heavy metal pollution in road dust to obtain a better understanding of the cycle in the city. This would bring insights to help plan measures that limit the exposure of the population to these pollutants.

This work goes beyond the description of heavy metals in urban road dust. To the best of our knowledge, this is the first attempt to make systematic statistical inferences regarding the characteristics of the urban form that could influence the concentration of heavy metals in urban road dust. In this paper, we respond to two main questions: (1) Is there a spatial correlation in the heavy metal contents of points sampled across Mexico City? (2) What are the main factors that explain the distribution and concentration of heavy metals in urban road dust? The first question is addressed by applying the Moran's I spatial correlation test to the heavy metal concentrations, and the second question by using linear regression models to analyze the relationship between heavy metals and the urban form.

2. Literature Review

There have been several approaches to evaluate the effects of the built environment on urban pollution, mainly in the air and taking the city as the unit of analysis. Liang et al. [9] in the Beijing–Tianjin–Hebei urban agglomeration, using a geographically weighted regression model, found that the rate of urbanization, the formation of metropolises, and the level of economic and industrial development, as well as building and road construction aggravate the environmental pollution (measured as an index for air, soil, and water pollution).

Predictors associated with a decrease in urban pollution include the industrial level, tax revenue, education level, and the use of the internet. Implementing taxes to protect the environment promotes the modernization of highly polluting industries, while an increase in resident incomes promotes a shift in the regional economy to low-pollution, knowledge-based industries. An improvement in the educational level drives environmental protection technology, improving the environmental quality.

Jung et al. [8], in Korea, applying a Bayesian spatial regression model, found that the total population, the commercial area, the industrial area, the total area, and the gross domestic product per person are factors associated with worse air pollution (nitrogen oxides, sulfur oxides, PM10, and PM2.5). Zhang et al. [33] in Calgary, Canada, using a land-use regression model, found that the main factors that increased the heavy metal concentrations in airborne particulate matter were industrial point sources.

Industrial and commercial zoning, as well as traffic indicators and population density, were also good predictors for most elements. In the case of specifically addressing the pollution by heavy metals in road dust, Alharbi et al. [14] compared the spatial distribution in two metropolitan cities (a typical corridor city and a compact city) of Saudi Arabia. They found that centrality was an important factor for determining the spatial distribution of heavy metals in road dust, which increased in concentration gradually toward the city center.

In Mexico City, research demonstrated that greenhouse gas emissions, caused by commuting, can be reduced by increasing the mix of residential and economic uses, as well as concentrating jobs near employment centers and economic activity corridors [34]. Studies determined that the sources of heavy metals in the urban road dust in Mexico City must be anthropogenic [35]. Therefore, we hypothesized that factors related to industrial land use, mixed land-use, and job density could be related to the concentrations of heavy metals associated with traffic, like Pb, Cu, and Zn. We hypothesized a negative association with the urban vegetation cover assuming a depuration effect.

3. Study Site

The Mexico City metropolitan area had a population of around 21,000,000 inhabitants in 2015 and was among the four largest urban agglomerations in the world [36]. The metropolitan area is formed by the urban areas of three states: Mexico City, the State of Mexico, and Hidalgo. Mexico City comprises mostly the central and south parts of the metropolitan area. The metropolitan area is located in a valley at 2240 m.a.s.l. The unique topography, with mountains surrounding the metropolis, results in thermal inversions preventing the dispersion of pollutants during the winter season from November to April.

Sierra del Ajusco's mountains in the southwest prevent the passage of the prevailing winds (northeast to southwest direction) and, thus, the dispersion of pollutants [37]. The land use geography in Mexico City is complex, but as a general description, Rodríguez-Salazar et al. [38] stated that the main industrial center, with a high population density, is located in the northern part of the city. The central part includes the historical and business center of the city, with high commercial activity.

The southern area has been dominated by residential and commercial activities. It was in the 1980s with the liberation of the economy that a process of absolute and relative deindustrialization related to the global economy began in the metropolis [39]. Factories were obligated to settle beyond the limits of Mexico City (formerly called the Federal

District) and the consolidation of light manufacturing began; overall, the tertiarization of the economy led to commercial and services activities beginning to dominate the economy in the city [40].

4. Materials and Methods

4.1. Data Collection

We collected 482 road dust samples associated with 482 sampling points for this study in a semi-grid pattern of approximately 1-km-wide squares across the urban area of Mexico City (Figure 1). The project was executed only within this political jurisdiction given that this was a project funded by the government. Thus, this sampling can be considered systematic, which covered the urban and peri-urban parts of the city. The collection of samples was done during the dry season in April and May (30 days) of 2017. The atmospheric conditions were stable; the temperature was between 15 and 20 °C, with winds in a north to south direction and speeds between 4 and 8 km/h [41]. During the sample collection campaign, there were no rains. All samples were collected under the same conditions: in a square meter of area on the pavement, below the sidewalk, the distance from the pedestrian area was between 0 and 1 m. All samples were taken in horizontal streets and without sedimentary traps (holes or potholes) to avoid biases. Because the sampling was systematic, the distance to the traffic lights was not considered. The urban road dust was sampled by brushing it from a 1 m^2 area at each point. The dust load in each sample point is defined as the amount of dust (<250 µm) per area of street space—in this case, 1 m^2—after the coarse material is removed [42,43]. Particles of less than 250 micrometers are most likely to adhere to hands and therefore be involuntarily ingested [44]. This particle size can be easily obtained in the laboratory using a sieve, which is very useful when analyzing a large number of samples.

The concentrations (mg/kg) of 14 elements were determined via inductively coupled plasma optical spectrometer (ICP-OES), which is a methodology used previously to this end [20,45,46]. However, only the most polluting metals identified in a previous study [47] were considered in the present work. Those elements were Chromium (Cr), Copper (Cu), Nickel (Ni), Lead (Pb), and Zinc (Zn). The concentrations were determined by digesting 0.4 g of each sample with 20 mL of concentrated HNO_3, using Teflon PFA beakers, in an ETHOS Easy microwave digestion system (Millestone Inc, Milan, Italy). The temperature was brought to 175 ± 5 °C in approximately 5 min and was kept for 4.5 min. After cooling, the digested samples were filtered with Whatman No. 42 paper, transferred into 50 mL flasks, and graduated with water type A (US-EPA method 3051A). Quality controls for the acid digestion method included reagent blanks and sample duplicates. The quality assurance and quality control (QA/QC) results showed no signs of contamination or loss in any of the analyzes. An Agilent Technologies 5100 ICP-OES (US: EPA method 6010C), sourced from Santa Clara, CA, USA, was used to analyze, in triplicate, the digestions and quality controls. A multi-elemental QCS-26R reference certified material was used (high purity brand) to prepare the calibration curve. The radiofrequency power (RF power) was 1.2 kW, the nebulization flow was 0.7 L/min, and the argon plasma flow was 12.0 L/min.

The pollution load index (PLI) was calculated as the geometric average of the Cr, Cu, Ni, Pb, and Zn results divided by their corresponding background value [48]. The contamination factors were obtained by dividing the concentrations of each heavy metal at each sampling point by the background value. We used the world background values for soils [49], which were obtained by determining heavy metal concentration in soils from places with the least anthropic disturbance possible. A PLI value close to 1 indicates that the heavy metal load was close to the naturally occurring level, while a PLI > 1 indicates contamination [48,50]. In Table 1, we can see the descriptive statistics of the dependent variables. The concentration of Pb in one sample was below the detection limit (Pb = 3.75 mg/kg). We took that limit as the Pb content in the sample because the statistical analysis requires numerical variables.

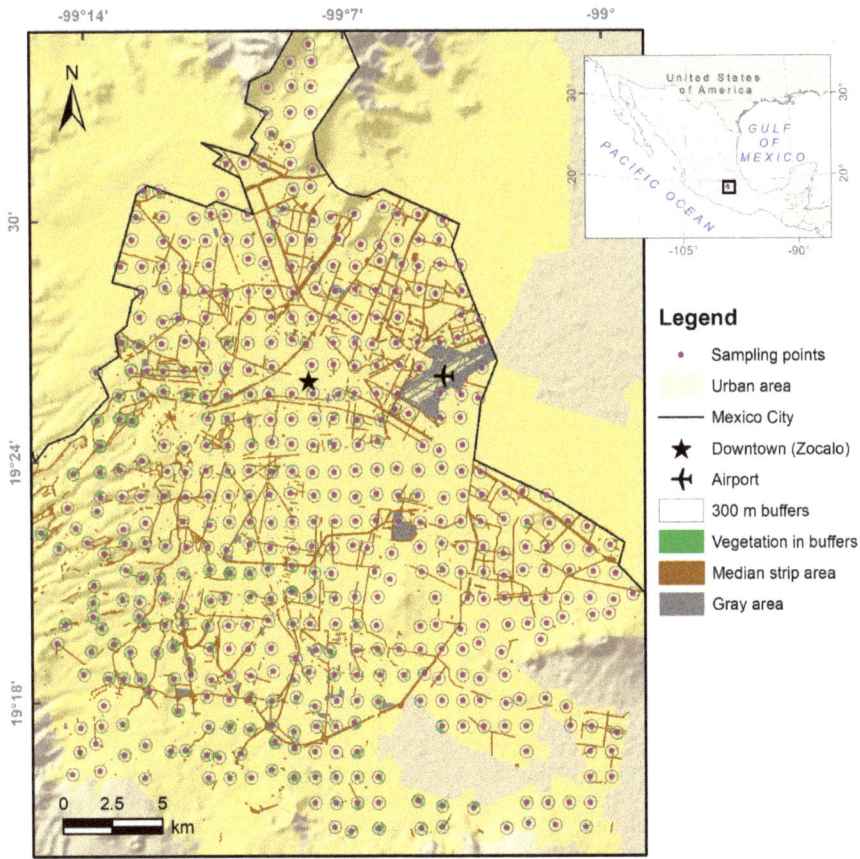

Figure 1. The study site and sampling point locations.

Table 1. The descriptive statistics of the heavy metal concentrations (mg/kg) in the 482 road dust samples.

Heavy Metal	Global [1] Background	Minimum	Maximum	Median	Mean	Standard Deviation
Cr	59.5	15.0	441.0	43.7	51.4	34.3
Cu	38.9	6.2	847.1	81.2	99.7	75.8
Ni	29	13.7	148.7	35.0	36.3	13.9
Pb	27	8.8	1907.8	101.2	128.2	134.6
Zn	70	18.7	4827.6	229.9	280.7	294.4
PLI [2]		0.3	6.3	2.0	1.9	0.8
Dust load [3]		5.4	173.3	43.0	46.4	23.2

Note: [1] Kabata-Pendias (2011); [2] unitless; [3] Amount of dust <250 μm in 1 m² of the street (g/m²).

Different explanatory variables were measured at each sampling point (Table 2). The population density was measured as inhabitants per hectare at the census tract level using the 2010 census data from the National Institute of Statistics and Geography [51]. The population density can determine the intensity of various socioeconomic activities that worsen air pollution [8]. Job density considered the number of jobs per hectare within the traffic analysis zone (TAZ) according to the 2017 Household Origin-Destination Survey [52]. Jobs were estimated according to the number of trips to work to a certain TAZ.

Table 2. Descriptive statistics of the covariates in the analysis. n = 482.

Covariate	Minimum	Maximum	Median	Mean	Standard Deviation
Population density (hab/ha)	0.0	443.1	132.4	139.8	81.1
Job density (jobs/ha)	4.2	349.7	30.0	43.9	50.7
Street intersections	0.0	162.0	38.0	45.4	29.2
Road surface (m^2)	2922.8	99,909.4	47,475.6	47,196.8	15,477.1
Distance to the airport (m)	803.2	25,424.3	12,792.8	12,571.7	5329.5
Distance to the city center (m)	633.9	24,361.9	10,304.1	10,977.3	5245.1
Manufacturing units	0.0	377.0	13.0	15.5	21.1
Potentially polluting units	0.0	24.0	1.0	1.4	2.7
Gray area (ha)	0.0	15.7	0.0	0.3	1.4
Entropy index	0.0	0.8	0.3	0.3	0.2
Vegetation (%)	0.0	65.6	5.5	10.0	11.9
Distance to vegetation (m)	0.0	329.3	22.0	40.2	48.2
Median strip area (m^2)	0.0	67,855.0	1498.0	4531.3	8161.5
Marginalization index	−1.4	1.3	−0.7	−0.7	0.5

Note: A minimum value of zero is expected when the covariate is not present at any of the road dust sampling points.

For the rest of the covariates, we considered a 300 m ring buffer around each sampling site. Street intersections were identified using the street network shapefiles from the official geostatistical framework [51], and, with the network analysis tool in ArcGis 10.0, we counted all intersections within the buffers. The road surface was estimated using this same layer. Street classification is not consistent between the municipalities of Mexico City; thus, for simplicity, we assumed three types of roads and their dimensions: local streets as 7 m wide, intermediate roads as 15 m wide, and highways as 25 m wide. We propose that this classification produces a conservative estimation of the road surface in each buffer.

Based on the 2014 urban geostatistical framework, we calculated the total area of polygons corresponding to large concrete surfaces, such as civil airfields, malls, markets, aviation tracks, and electrical substations. We called these surfaces "gray areas". The median strip area, which is usually covered with vegetation, was estimated using this same dataset, which has polygons explicitly categorized with this name, road median strip. The distance to the city center was calculated using the Euclidean distance (the straight line that connect two points assuming there are no obstacles in the space) from each sampling point to the historical center of downtown (also called Zócalo-Tenochtitlán).

The distance to the airport also considered the Euclidean distance to the Benito Juarez International Airport. The number of manufacturing units in each buffer was calculated based on those classified by the North American industry classification system in 2018. The number of potentially polluting units considered the economic units related to mining, construction, and pipelines in the National Statistical Directory of Economic Units (Directorio Nacional de Unidades Económicas, DENUE) [53].

We calculated the entropy index as a measure of the land-use mix, considering the relative percentages of different land-use types within an area. The entropy index varied from 0 to 1, with 0 indicating a homogeneous area with only one land-use type, and the mix level increasing as the index increases. Here, P^j is the percentage of each land-use type j in the area, and $k \geq 2$ is the number of land-use types j.

$$ENT = -\left[\sum_{j=1}^{k} P^j ln\left(P^j\right)\right]/ln(k) \qquad (1)$$

The entropy index was calculated using information from the publicly available urban data website "Portal de Datos de la Ciudad de México" [54]. Each land-use polygon was georeferenced as a data point, and information about the land use type and the area was provided. Thus, all polygons whose centroid lay within the 300 m buffer were considered in the estimation. There were 113 categories of land-use descriptions, and two categories were excluded (no zoning—"sin zonificación"—and existing uses—"usos existentes").

Then, the 111 categories were simplified to six general categories: (1) green areas, parks, open spaces, and agricultural areas; (2) residential; (3) office and commercial; (4) industrial; (5) mixed-use; and (6) institutional and public facilities. The official information did not provide concrete and clear definitions of the 111 initial categories; thus, a series of assumptions were made in the collapsing process. For example, land use corresponding to residential and low-scale retail was considered residential. It is very common that, in middle and low-income neighborhoods, small-scale retail coexists with residential uses.

Every original category that includes office and services, was counted in category 3. The mixed-use category included all polygons that were explicitly considered as this on the website as well as those centers of traditional towns and suburbs called "Centros de Barrio". Different land uses, such as residential, commercial, office, and open spaces, converge in these places. The column open area was used for those polygons lacking information about their area. Other corrections were made through a visual inspection on Google Earth for polygons with an important area within the buffer but not initially taken into account when their centroid was not within the buffer.

We calculated the mean normal difference vegetation index (NDVI) in each buffer zone from satellite images (March to May 2017) obtained from Planet Scope for Mexico City to estimate the urban vegetation. A supervised classification was made from the NDVI raster file in the QGIS version 3.4 software, using the "Semi-automatic Classification Plugin" tool. Two classes were determined: (1) vegetation, for the highest NDVI values (>0.6); and (2) no vegetation or the remainder of the urban area. Subsequently, the results of the classification were transformed into a shapefile to obtain the vegetation polygons and to calculate their area.

The vegetation polygons intersecting the buffers were summed up to obtain the total area of vegetation within each buffer. Finally, the total vegetation area was divided by the buffer surface and multiplied by 100 to obtain the percentage of vegetation present in each buffer, referred to here as "vegetation (%)". Another variable related to vegetation is the Euclidean distance from the sampling point to the closest vegetation polygon. Finally, as a measure of the socioeconomic characteristics, the index of marginalization was extracted at the census tract level for each sampling point. This index can have negative and positive values; the highest positive values correspond to the highest levels of marginalization [55].

We considered local variables as those related to characteristics of the immediate urban environment that surrounds the sample point. Examples of these are population density, percentage of vegetation, and the number of potentially polluting units. On the other hand, regional variables were those that characterize a sample with respect to a metropolitan point of reference. Examples are the distance from the city center, and the distance to the airport.

4.2. Spatial Autocorrelation

The univariate spatial autocorrelation was examined using Moran's I statistics for global measurements of spatial dependence [56]. The formula for standard correlation is expanded to incorporate a spatial weight matrix. Thus, its formula is defined as:

$$I = \frac{n}{S_o} \frac{\sum_{i=1}^{n} \sum_{j=1}^{n} w_{i,j} z_i z_j}{\sum_{i=1}^{n} z_i^2} \quad (2)$$

where n is the number of sample points indexed by i and j, Z_i is the deviation of an attribute (in this case, the heavy metal content) for point i from its mean, $W_{i,j}$ is the spatial weight between point i and j, while S_o is the aggregate of all spatial weights.

We defined neighbors as those spatial units within a specific distance threshold. For this analysis, we tested different thresholds of contiguity (1600, 5000, 10,000, and 15,000 m). All neighbors were weighted equally and then row standardized. This means that it depends on the number of neighbors to determine the final weight, as the larger the number, the lower the weights.

The range of Moran's I varies with the weights matrix, but it is usually expected to vary from −1 to 1. The sign corresponds to the type of autocorrelation, i.e., positive or negative. Values close to 1 indicate high spatial autocorrelation while values close to zero mean null spatial autocorrelation. The Moran's test for spatial autocorrelation uses the spatial weights matrix and tests the null hypothesis statement of 'no spatial autocorrelation'. In other words, the alternative hypothesis is if the Moran's I is greater than zero. Then, a p-value lower than 0.05 means there is strong evidence to reject the randomization null hypothesis in favor of an alternative hypothesis. We used the function "moran.test" of the R Project program to test the spatial autocorrelation. These results were compared with a Moran Monte Carlo permutations test and also using an inverse distance criterion to determine weights for neighbors. These results were relatively consistent with the moran.test function.

4.3. Regression Models

When two variables are close to a perfect linear combination of one another, it is called collinearity. Thus, when more than two variables are involved, it is called multicollinearity. This represents a problem when applying linear regression models given that it can result in unstable regression estimates with high standard errors. Variance inflation factors (VIF) measure how much the variance of the estimated regression coefficient is inflated by the existence of correlation among the predictor variables. The general rule of thumb is that VIFs exceeding 4 warrant further investigation, while VIFs exceeding 10 signify serious multicollinearity requiring correction. Thus, the variance inflation factor (VIF) was used to test the multicollinearity between the factors.

Ordinary least squares (OLS) regressions were tested for all response variables, i.e., the heavy metals contents. Due to a lack of normality evaluated through the Shapiro test, all covariates and dependent variables were log-transformed using a natural logarithm. Some variables with zero values were transformed using the natural logarithm of 1+x. An OLS model can be described in the form:

$$Y = \beta X + \varepsilon \quad (3)$$

where Y is the dependent variable, X is the independent variable, and β its coefficient. If we consider several covariates, then we have a vector of X and β. Finally, ε is the error term. Coefficients of log-log regression models can be interpreted in the following way, given a coefficient in the form "0.X". We expect about X increase in heavy metal content when the covariate increases by 10%.

After that, a spatial diagnostic of the OLS residuals was applied to select the appropriate spatial regression model for each of these dependent variables [57,58]. There are two main sources of spatial dependence: (1) spatial diffusion, which occurs when spatially proximate units are influenced by the behavior of their neighbors. This was modeled via a Lagrange multiplier spatial lag model (LMlag), estimated by the maximum likelihood; and (2) the geographic clustering of covariates, also called attributional dependence. This was modeled via a spatial error model (LMerror), estimated either with the maximum likelihood or with the generalized method of moments.

The Spatial lag model takes the form:

$$Y = \beta X + \rho W y + \varepsilon \quad (4)$$

Here, to the OLS equation it is added a W term that stands for the spatial weights matrix and the ρ coefficient.

In the case of the Spatial error model, this takes the form:

$$\varepsilon = \lambda W \varepsilon + v \quad (5)$$

We can see that this model is related to the error term, where W is also the spatial weights matrix, it is included the lambda coefficient and v is an uncorrelated additional error term.

Lagrange multiplier diagnostics for spatial dependence in R use the regression object and the object of neighbors and weights. In the case of the Spatial lag model, we test for a missing spatially lagged dependent variable, in other words, the null hypothesis is that rho = 0. In the case of the Spatial error model, the null hypothesis is that lambda (λ) = 0. The first step was to run the non-robust LMlag and LMerror diagnostic tests, the results of which can lead to three different paths: (1) if none of these diagnostic tests are statistically significant, then the OLS estimates are sufficient to model the dependent variable; (2) if only one of the diagnostics determined the presence of spatial dependence, the corresponding model was estimated; (3) if both diagnostic tests were significant, then both the robust LMlag and the robust LMerror diagnostics were tested, and the model with the largest value was used [58]. All the statistical analyses were done with the R Studio program, version 3.6.1.

5. Results

The median concentrations of the heavy metals were higher than the global background value in the soils, except for Cr. In the case of Ni, the median concentration is only 6 units above the global background level. Indeed, 91.5% of the samples had a pollution load index (PLI) greater than 1 (median=2) (see above Table 1). We propose that this is an important indication of the anthropogenic origin of the heavy metals found in the road dust from Mexico City. The dust load varied considerably from 5.4 to 173.3 g/m^2. As it is very difficult to control aspects related to the deposition of dust in the points of sampling, we decided to work with the heavy metal concentrations instead of the total heavy metal contents as dependent variables.

The mean concentrations of the heavy metals reported here are lower than those reported in a previous study in Mexico City (sampling in 2011) [35]. Even though there are not yet maximum permissible levels in urban road dust, the content of heavy metals in the samples is fortunately still lower than the closest regulation, i.e., the content of heavy metals in soils from residential areas. Therefore, it is important to continue monitoring for long-term fluctuations to avoid an increase in these pollutants and prove the good performance of the environmental policies.

5.1. Spatial Autocorrelation

Moran's I was significant for Cr only at a vicinity distance of 5000 m; however, the coefficient of autocorrelation was only 0.03. Therefore, a general pattern of clustering was not expected (Table 3). Cu had a significant Moran's I at all vicinity distances, but, again, the coefficient was very small. Moran's I for Ni became significant at a distance of 10,000 m and was even more significant at 15,000 m; however, the coefficient was only 0.01.

Contrary to Ni, Moran's I for Pb was significant at short distances (1600 and 5000 m), but, again, the coefficients were smaller than 0.1. Zn had a significant Moran's I at all distances, except at 5000 m, with the coefficient smaller than 0.1. Moran's I for the PLI was significant at all distances, and it was greater than 0.1 at 1600 m; hence, a general pattern of clustering could be expected at a short vicinity distance. The dust load had a significant Moran's I at all distances; thus, the coefficients (and consequently the autocorrelation) decreased as the distance increased.

As the global Moran's I was very close to 0 for all heavy metals, indicating low levels of positive spatial autocorrelation, it was not necessary to explore the local version of this index to identify any spatial clustering pattern. This is an initial sign that the local aspects are more relevant than any regional process in determining the concentrations of these metals.

Table 3. The global Moran's I and test of statistical significance at different vicinity distances (1600, 5000, 10,000, and 15,000 m).

Variable	1600 m	p-Value	5000 m	p-Value	10,000 m	p-Value	15,000 m	p-Value
Cr	0.05	0.07	0.03	0.00 ***	0.00	0.41	0.00	0.72
Cu	0.08	0.00 **	0.05	0.00 ***	0.02	0.00 ***	0.01	0.00 ***
Ni	0.00	0.11	0.02	0.06	0.01	0.01 *	0.01	0.00 ***
Pb	0.06	0.02	0.03	0.00 **	0.00	0.14	0.00	0.49
Zn	0.06	0.01 *	0.01	0.14	0.01	0.01 *	0.01	0.00 ***
PLI	0.13	0.00 ***	0.06	0.00 ***	0.02	0.00 ***	0.01	0.00 ***
Road dust load	0.18	0.00 ***	0.16	0.00 ***	0.10	0.00 ***	0.04	0.00 ***

* Significance at 95% confidence, ** 99% confidence, and *** 99.9% confidence.

In Table 4, we can see the p-values of the diagnostic tests of the OLS residuals. All non-robust tests were non-significant. In the case of the robust versions, for Cu, Ni, Zn, the PLI, and the dust load, the tests were also non-significant, which indicates that OLS is a suitable modeling approach. For Pb, the spatial error model was significant (alpha at 5%); thus, for this metal, the results of the spatial error regression model were analyzed.

Table 4. p-values of the diagnosis of the ordinary least squares (OLS) regression residuals.

Test	Cr	Cu	Ni	Pb	Zn	PLI	Dust Load
Lm (lag)	0.11	0.15	0.51	0.51	0.89	0.65	0.50
LM (error)	0.06	0.24	0.75	0.14	0.56	0.47	0.24
Robust LM (lag)	0.11	0.35	0.14	0.07	0.31	0.50	0.18
Robust LM (error)	0.06	0.65	0.17	0.02 *	0.24	0.38	0.10

* Significance at 95% confidence.

5.2. Factors Influencing the Heavy Metal Concentrations

The VIF indicators were below 4.3 for our vector of covariates, which indicates a low risk of multicollinearity that could bias the coefficient estimations. Overall, there were few significant relationships between the covariates and the heavy metal concentrations, including the road dust load (Table 5). Population density had a null association with all of the heavy metals, which indicates that the number of people in the surroundings of the sample point was not relevant to explain the presence of our dependent variables.

Table 5. Results of the ordinary least squares regressions.

Covariate	Cr			Cu			Ni			Pb		
	beta	p		beta	p		beta	p		beta	p	
Intercept	4.94	0.00	***	3.64	0.03	*	3.30	0.00	***	6.76	0.00	**
Population density (inhabitants/ha)	0.00	0.98		−0.03	0.40		−0.02	0.36		0.03	0.49	
Job density (jobs/ha)	−0.04	0.46		0.11	0.10	.	−0.01	0.76		0.04	0.61	
Street intersections	0.02	0.71		−0.06	0.49		0.02	0.63		0.01	0.93	
Road surface (m²)	−0.07	0.48		0.03	0.85		−0.07	0.35		−0.09	0.59	
Distance to the airport (m)	−0.06	0.38		0.05	0.57		0.10	0.06	.	−0.18	0.11	
Distance to the city center (m)	0.01	0.87		−0.04	0.71		0.02	0.79		−0.03	0.84	
Manufacturing units	0.04	0.34		0.10	0.04	*	0.02	0.37		0.07	0.27	
Potentially polluting units	0.08	0.12		−0.03	0.62		−0.02	0.58		0.00	0.96	
Gray area (ha)	0.00	0.97		0.08	0.45		0.05	0.43		−0.03	0.81	
Entropy index	0.02	0.93		-0.17	0.46		0.37	0.01	**	0.15	0.60	
Vegetation (%)	−0.01	0.82		−0.03	0.60		−0.05	0.10		−0.01	0.90	
Distance to vegetation (m)	−0.01	0.68		0.02	0.53		−0.03	0.21		0.01	0.84	
Median strip area (m²)	0.01	0.10	.	0.02	0.09	.	0.01	0.09	.	0.02	0.08	.
Marginalization index	−0.01	0.67		−0.01	0.80		0.01	0.80		−0.06	0.26	.
r²	−0.01			0.06			0.02			0.05		

Table 5. Cont.

Covariate	Zn		PLI		Dust Load		
	beta	p	beta	p	beta	p	
Intercept	2.98	0.07 .	0.59	0.62	8.13	0.00	***
Population density (inhabitants/ha)	−0.02	0.59	-0.01	0.77	−0.01	0.81	
Job density (jobs/ha)	0.08	0.22	0.04	0.43	−0.16	0.01	**
Street intersections	−0.11	0.16	-0.02	0.69	0.09	0.25	
Road surface (m^2)	0.23	0.09 .	0.00	0.98	−0.30	0.02	*
Distance to the airport (m)	0.03	0.76	−0.01	0.84	−0.06	0.44	
Distance to the city center (m)	−0.03	0.78	−0.01	0.86	−0.03	0.79	
Manufacturing units	0.08	0.10	0.06	0.08 .	−0.04	0.43	
Potentially polluting units	−0.03	0.65	0.00	0.99	0.12	0.05 .	
Gray area (ha)	0.05	0.60	0.03	0.69	−0.01	0.91	
Entropy index	−0.15	0.51	0.04	0.79	0.39	0.07 .	
Vegetation (%)	−0.04	0.43	−0.03	0.46	−0.13	0.00	**
Distance to vegetation (m)	0.03	0.37	0.01	0.84	0.01	0.77	
Median strip area (m^2)	0.01	0.21	0.01	0.04 *	0.01	0.28	
Marginalization index	−0.04	0.29	−0.02	0.41	0.02	0.51	
r^2	0.07		0.04		0.10		

beta is the slope; p represents the p-value; . Significance at 90% confidence, * 95% confidence, ** 99% confidence, and *** 99.9% confidence.

Job density had a weak positive association (significance level of 90%) with Cu. However, there was not any significant relationship with the rest of the metals. Our initial expectation was that in places with high job density, the heavy metal concentrations would be high due to an increased number of trips to work and, therefore, increased levels of polluting emissions. Thus, the association found between job density and Cu supports our initial hypothesis since the emission of this metal from vehicles has been associated with tire wear and brake abrasion [29] With the dust load, job density had a significant inverse association (significance level of 99%). We could expect about a 1.6% increase in the dust load when the job density decreased by 10%. This could be explained if we consider that employment centers in Mexico City are related to tertiary types (offices and commerce) that are not necessarily highly polluting activities. These workplaces tend to be better cared for and cleaner than lower-class areas.

The street intersections variable was not significant with any metal. The initial expectation was that this variable could represent the emissions of heavy metals due to car braking, with the higher the number of street intersections representing higher braking frequency. However, the braking emissions are likely not large enough to be detected through street intersections.

The road surface had a weak positive relationship with Zn (significance level of 90%). The emissions of Zn from vehicles have been associated with the combustion of lubricating oil [30], tire wear [25], and diesel exhaust emissions [27]. Therefore, this result supports the expectation that the road surface is a suitable proxy variable for traffic flow as a determinant of Zn in the road dust. On the other hand, there was a significant inverse association between the road surface and the dust load (significance level of 95%). We could expect about a 3% increase in the dust load when the road surface decreased by 10%. These surfaces are likely maintained and cleaned as brigades of cleaning workers sweep the larger roads.

The distance to the airport had a positive but weak relationship with Ni (significance level of 90%). Higher concentrations of this metal were found further away from the airport; therefore, the airport might not be an important source of this metal. An inverse weak association (significance level of 90%) was found for Pb and the distance to the airport in the spatial error model (Table 6). The coefficient tells us that we could expect about a 2% increase in the Pb content when the distance to the airport decreased by 10%. Our hypothesis is that tire wear in the aircraft take-off and landing could emit dust particles containing Pb. In the case of the distance to the city center, there was a null association with the other heavy metals.

Table 6. Spatial error model results for Pb.

Covariate	Pb	
	beta	p
Intercept	7.12	0.00
Population density (inhabitants/ha)	0.03	0.41
Job density (jobs/ha)	0.03	0.68
Street intersections	0.01	0.88
Road surface (m^2)	−0.10	0.56
Distance to the airport (m)	−0.19	0.08
Distance to the city center (m)	−0.05	0.68
Manufacturing units	0.08	0.19
Potentially polluting units	0.00	0.96
Gray area (ha)	−0.01	0.94
Entropy index	0.17	0.54
Vegetation (%)	0.00	0.95
Distance to vegetation (m)	0.01	0.87
Median strip area (m^2)	0.02	0.08
Marginalization index	−0.06	0.20
AIC	757.01	

Note: AIC (Akaike Information Criterion), lower AIC value suggest a better fit.

Manufacturing units had a positive significant association with Cu with an alpha level of 5%. We could expect about a 1% increase in Cu when manufacturing units increased by 10%. It is very likely that behind this variable there are a variety of chemical processes in the manufacturing; therefore, there could be several sources of Cu from these processes as well as traffic-related emissions. The relationship with PLI was also positive but less significant (significance level of 90%). Potentially polluting units failed to show any association with the heavy metals. This means that possible major pollutant units were not properly identified with our variable. Thus, other alternatives must be tackled in future research such as the use of other classification schemes to differentiate potentially polluting units from the whole census of economic units. Only in the case of the dust load was there a positive significant association at the 90% significance level. Thus, these units are associated with an increase in dust, but are not associated with an increase in the heavy metal content.

The gray area variable also failed to detect any association with the heavy metals. Our initial expectation was that this variable could be related to heavy metals due to the polluting emissions of activities related to large concrete surfaces (markets, aviation tracks, and electrical substations). The null association of the gray areas could be due to the huge diversity of activities considered in the covariate. The entropy index had a positive relationship at the alpha level of 5% with Ni. We could expect about a 4% increase in Ni when the entropy index increased by 10%. A high entropy index means a similar proportion of the six land uses considered; thus, these places could have a variety of potential sources of Ni together, such as sites of fuel combustion.

There was also a weak positive relation (alpha level of 10%) of the entropy index with the dust load. The difficulty in obtaining a clear relationship between the land-use covariates and heavy metal contents in urban dust in México City could be related to the tertiary-oriented economy. We assume that mobile sources of traffic emissions would be more relevant but also more difficult to trace. In the case of air pollution, industrial point emissions have been identified as the source of pollution, such as in the studies of Zhang et al. [33] in Alberta, Canada, and Jung et al. [8] in Korea, where commercial and industrial areas were associated with increased particulate matter pollution.

The percentage of vegetation in the buffer and the distance to the closest vegetation spot failed to show any association with the heavy metal content. In the case of the former, there was a significant negative association (significance level of 99%) with the dust load, which indicates that vegetated areas tended to have less dust but not necessarily a higher heavy metal content. The median strip area had a weak (significance level of 90%) but consistent positive relationship with Cr, Cu, Ni, Pb, and PLI. This led us to hypothesize that these areas may act as sinks of pollution in the roads, acting as places of heavy metal accumulation. For example, during the sweeping of the road, the dust may be dumped there. The positive relationship between the median strip area and Pb remained for the spatial error model at the alpha level of 10% (Table 6).

Initially, we considered the median strip area part of the vegetation area because it frequently has a vegetation cover. After testing the initial models, the previous vegetation area covaried positively with Pb and Cr. That result was unexpected, and we therefore decided to separate the components of the vegetation covariation and, finally, identified that only the median strip area was positively related to Cr, Pb, Zn, and the PLI. It will be important to untangle the relationship between heavy metals and the median strip area to define the best way to manage such areas. It is important to clarify that covariates of urban form do not necessarily represent specific detailed sources of heavy metals. They represent general characteristics (places) of the urban environment where these pollutants could be being emitted or places of concentration (sinks of pollution (from other mobile or fixed sources of pollution)).

Finally, there was no differential exposition to heavy metals according to the socioeconomic status of households, as we found a null association with the marginalization index. The good news is that road dust is not an important source of exposure to Pb for those in low-income areas, as they are at higher risk of developing health problems [59]. However, attention should be paid to keep the streets clean, because marginalized areas tended to be dustier than middle-income and affluent areas.

The study of the relationships between the urban form and heavy metals is incipient; further investigation is needed to develop a conceptual framework that guides the development of more robust models. The present study is an exploratory analysis in this sense, and we tested the group of covariates that we considered the most relevant. Although some of these variables did not show any association, the inclusion was supported by a deep reflection of what we considered could be the route of heavy metals in the urban environment.

The study of temporal variation in the short term is also important to design better sampling processes that minimize and control the effects of potential confounding factors. For example, natural cleaning mechanisms, such as rain and air currents, and the different practices of street sweeping. From a methodological point of view, we propose to test smaller buffers, which might be at 100 or 150 m around the sampling points, since the characteristics of the immediate surroundings are very important. A better characterization of the urban form might also benefit from more consistent and refined publicly available data regarding the urban environment. The characterization of the local urban environment is key to devising the sampling strategy. Further research lines also include the application of other modeling approaches and inter-city comparisons to test if the phenomena studied here present similar behavior in cities of different sizes and economic conditions. Furthermore, we suggest the inclusion of covariates related to atmospheric processes as well as covariates with more detailed georeferenced data about emission sources.

6. Conclusions

According to the global Moran's I, there were low levels of positive spatial autocorrelation in all the heavy metals analyzed. We interpret this as an indication of the greater relevance of the local aspects over regional processes as determinants of the heavy metal content in urban road dust. Any mapping exercise based on statistical interpolation would not be reliable. A lack of major unique sources of these pollutants could also cause a lack of spatial autocorrelation. In our regression exercise, the most striking finding was that the median strip area in urban roads had a weak but consistent positive relationship with Cr, Cu, Ni, Pb, and the Pollution Load Index. Other significant positive relationships were found for Cu with the manufacturing units, and Ni with the entropy index. More disaggregated indicators would be relevant to unveil the nature of these associations.

Certain variables failed to show any association with the heavy metals, such as the population density, street intersections, distance to the city center, gray area, distance to vegetation, and marginalized areas. Other variables that failed to be associated with heavy metals but showed an association with the dust load were the potentially polluting units (significance level of 90%) and vegetation (significance level of 99%), positive in the former and negative in the latter. The job density (significance level of 99%) and road surface (significance level of 95%) significantly reduced the dust load as well. For Pb, the spatial error model showed the correct specification, unlike the other metals where OLS was found to be appropriate. In this model, distance to the airport had a weak (significance level of 90%) and an inverse association with Pb. This presents an important suggestion to consider this place as a potential source of this metal in urban dust.

Thus, we can conclude that some features of the urban form, as described above, are important drivers of heavy metal pollution in the road dust. A better understanding of how road dust pollution is associated with the urban form will be important to design measures that mitigate the exposure of people to those pollutants.

Author Contributions: A.A.: data cleaning, calculations, statistical analysis, wrote the manuscript. D.B.-H.: original idea, data cleaning, calculations, statistical analysis, directed the research, trained the student, and wrote the final version of the manuscript. F.B.: project coordinator, coordinated the chemical analyzes, proposed the idea, and revised the previous texts. A.G.: project coordinator, reviewed the final version of the manuscript. R.C.: collected the urban dust samples and prepared them for analysis. All authors have read and agreed to the published version of the manuscript.

Funding: This research was funded by grant number 283135 SEP-CONACYT.

Institutional Review Board Statement: Not applicable.

Informed Consent Statement: Not applicable.

Data Availability Statement: The data about heavy metal content in the sampling points presented in this study are available on request from the corresponding author. This data are not publicly available due to belong to the funding agency. The rest of the data comes from publicly available datasets. This data can be found here: https://www.inegi.org.mx/programas/ccpv/2010/; http://en.www.inegi.org.mx/programas/eod/2017/default.html#Microdata (accessed 28 October 2020).

Acknowledgments: We are grateful to Gutiérrez-Ruiz, M.E., Ceniceros-Gómez, A.E., López-Santiago, N.R. for support in the chemical analysis of the dust samples. We would like to thank the four anonymous reviewers for their valuable feedback in the review process.

Conflicts of Interest: We declare no conflicts of interest.

References

1. CONAPO; SEDESOL. Catálogo Sistema Urbano Nacional 2012. Available online: http://www.conapo.gob.mx/work/models/CONAPO/Resource/1539/1/images/PartesIaV.pdf (accessed on 16 February 2021).
2. Molina, L.T.; Madronich, S.; Gaffney, J.S.; Apel, E.; De Foy, B.; Fast, J.; Ferrare, R.; Herndon, S.; Jimenez, J.L.; Lamb, B.; et al. An overview of the MILAGRO 2006 Campaign: Mexico City emissions and their transport and transformation. *Atmos. Chem. Phys.* **2010**, *10*, 8697–8760. [CrossRef]
3. Dash, D.P.; Behera, S.R.; Rao, D.T.; Sethi, N.; Loganathan, N. Governance, urbanization, and pollution: A cross-country analysis of global south region. *Cogent Econ. Finance* **2020**, *8*, 1742023. [CrossRef]
4. WHO. The Power of Cities: Tackling Noncommicable Diseases and Road Traffic Injuries. Switzerland. 2019. Available online: https://www.who.int/ncds/publications/tackling-ncds-in-cities/en/ (accessed on 16 February 2021).
5. Aguilera, A.; Bautista, F.; Goguitchaichvili, A.; Garcia-Oliva, F. Health risk of heavy metals in street dust. *Front. Biosci.* **2021**, *26*, 327–345. [CrossRef]

6. Safiur Rahman, M.; Khan, M.D.H.; Jolly, Y.N.; Kabir, J.; Akter, S.; Salam, A. Assessing risk to human health for heavy metal contamination through street dust in the Southeast Asian Megacity: Dhaka, Bangladesh. *Sci. Total Environ.* **2019**, *660*, 1610–1622. [CrossRef]
7. Zhao, H.; Shao, Y.; Yin, C.; Jiang, Y.; Li, X. An index for estimating the potential metal pollution contribution to atmospheric particulate matter from road dust in Beijing. *Sci. Total Environ.* **2016**, *550*, 167–175. [CrossRef]
8. Jung, M.C.; Park, J.; Kim, S. Spatial relationships between urban structures and air pollution in Korea. *Sustainability* **2019**, *11*, 476. [CrossRef]
9. Liang, L.; Wang, Z.; Li, J. The effect of urbanization on environmental pollution in rapidly developing urban agglomerations. *J. Clean. Prod.* **2019**, *237*, 117649. [CrossRef]
10. Selden, T.M.; Song, D. Environmental Quality and Development: Is There a Kuznets Curve for Air Pollution Emissions? *J. Environ. Econ. Manage.* **1994**, *27*, 147–162. [CrossRef]
11. Cole, M.A. Development, Trade, and the Environment: How Robust is the Environmental Kuznets Curve? *Environ. Dev. Econ.* **2004**, *8*, 557–579. [CrossRef]
12. Aguilera, A.; Bautista, F.; Gogichaichvili, A.; Gutiérrez-Ruiz, M.E.; Ceniceros-Gómez, A.E.; López-Santiago, N.R. Spatial distribution of manganese concentration and load in street dust in Mexico City. *Salud Publica Mex.* **2020**, *62*, 147–155. [CrossRef]
13. Aguilera, A.; Armendariz, C.; Quintana, P.; García-Oliva, F.; Bautista, F. Influence of Land Use and Road Type on the Elemental Composition of Urban Dust in a Mexican Metropolitan Area. *Polish J. Environ. Stud.* **2019**, *28*, 1535–1547. [CrossRef]
14. Alharbi, B.H.; Pasha, M.J.; Al-Shamsi, M.A.S. Influence of Different Urban Structures on Metal Contamination in Two Metropolitan Cities. *Sci. Rep.* **2019**, *9*, 4920. [CrossRef]
15. Men, C.; Liu, R.; Xu, F.; Wang, Q.; Guo, L.; Shen, Z. Pollution characteristics, risk assessment, and source apportionment of heavy metals in road dust in Beijing, China. *Sci. Total Environ.* **2018**, *612*, 138–147. [CrossRef]
16. Jan, A.T.; Azam, M.; Siddiqui, K.; Ali, A.; Choi, I.; Haq, Q.M.R. Heavy metals and human health: Mechanistic insight into toxicity and counter defense system of antioxidants. *Int. J. Mol. Sci.* **2015**, *16*, 29592–29630. [CrossRef] [PubMed]
17. Tamayo y Ortiz, M.; Téllez-Rojo, M.M.; Hu, H.; Hernández-Ávila, M.; Wright, R.; Amarasiriwardena, C.; Lupoli, N.; Mercado-García, A.; Pantic, I.; Lamadrid-Figueroa, H. Lead in candy consumed and blood lead levels of children living in Mexico City. *Environ. Res.* **2016**, *147*, 497–502. [CrossRef]
18. Liu, Y.; Peterson, K.E.; Montgomery, K.; Sánchez, B.N.; Zhang, Z.; Afeiche, M.C.; Cantonwine, D.E.; Ettinger, A.S.; Cantoral, A.; Schnaas, L.; et al. Early lead exposure and childhood adiposity in Mexico city. *Int. J. Hyg. Environ. Health* **2019**, *222*, 965–970. [CrossRef]
19. Kim, J.J.; Kim, Y.S.; Kumar, V. Heavy metal toxicity: An update of chelating therapeutic strategies. *J. Trace Elem. Med. Biol.* **2019**, *54*, 226–231. [CrossRef] [PubMed]
20. Leung, A.O.; Duzgoren-Aydin, N.S.; Cheung, K.C.; Wong, M.H. Heavy metals concentrations of surface dust from e-waste recycling and its human health implications in southeast China. *Environ. Sci. Technol.* **2008**, *42*, 2674–2680. [CrossRef]
21. Lin, M.; Gui, H.; Wang, Y.; Peng, W. Pollution characteristics, source apportionment, and health risk of heavy metals in street dust of Suzhou, China. *Environ. Sci. Pollut. Res.* **2017**, *24*, 1987–1998. [CrossRef]
22. Tapia, J.S.; Valdés, J.; Orrego, R.; Tchernitchin, A.; Dorador, C.; Bolados, A.; Harrod, C. Geologic and anthropogenic sources of contamination in settled dust of a historic mining port city in northern Chile: Health risk implications. *PeerJ* **2018**, *6*, e4699. [CrossRef] [PubMed]
23. Bañuelos, S.; Ajwa, H.A. Trace elements in soils and plants: An overview. *J. Environ. Sci. Health A* **1999**, *34*, 951–974. [CrossRef]
24. Taşpınar, F.; Bozkurt, Z. Heavy metal pollution and health risk assessment of road dust on selected highways in Düzce, Turkey. *Environ. Forensics* **2018**, *19*, 298–314. [CrossRef]
25. Budai, P.; Clement, A. Spatial distribution patterns of four traffic-emitted heavy metals in urban road dust and the resuspension of brake-emitted particles: Findings of a field study. *Transp. Res. D Transp. Environ.* **2018**, *62*, 179–185. [CrossRef]
26. Gunawardena, J.; Ziyath, A.M.; Egodawatta, P.; Ayoko, G.A.; Goonetilleke, A. Mathematical relationships for metal build-up on urban road surfaces based on traffic and land use characteristics. *Chemosphere* **2014**, *99*, 267–271. [CrossRef] [PubMed]
27. Świetlik, R.; Trojanowska, M.; Strzelecka, M.; Bocho-Janiszewska, A. Fractionation and mobility of Cu, Fe, Mn, Pb and Zn in the road dust retained on noise barriers along expressway-A potential tool for determining the effects of driving conditions on speciation of emitted particulate metals. *Environ. Pollut.* **2015**, *196*, 404–413. [CrossRef]
28. Amato, F.; Alastuey, A.; Karanasiou, A.; Lucarelli, F.; Nava, S.; Calzolai, G.; Severi, M.; Becagli, S.; Gianelle, V.L.; Colombi, C.; et al. AIRUSE-LIFE+: A harmonized PM speciation and source apportionment in five southern European cities. *Atmos. Chem. Phys.* **2016**, *16*, 3289–3309. [CrossRef]
29. Sternbeck, J.; Sjödin, A.; Andréasson, K. Metal emissions from road traffic and the influence of resuspension—results from two tunnel studies. *Atmos. Environ.* **2002**, *36*, 4735–4744. [CrossRef]
30. Viana, M.; Kuhlbusch, T.A.J.; Querol, X.; Alastuey, A.; Harrison, R.M.; Hopke, P.K.; Winiwarter, W.; Vallius, M.; Szidat, S.; Prévôt, A.S.H.; et al. Source apportionment of particulate matter in Europe: A review of methods and results. *J. Aerosol Sci.* **2008**, *39*, 827–849. [CrossRef]
31. Lee, P.K.; Chang, H.J.; Yu, S.; Chae, K.H.; Bae, J.H.; Kang, M.J.; Chae, G. Characterization of Cr (VI)–Containing solid phase particles in dry dust deposition in Daejeon, South Korea. *Environ. Pollut.* **2018**, *243*, 1637. [CrossRef]

32. Legalley, E.; Krekeler, M.P.S. A mineralogical and geochemical investigation of street sediment near a coal-fired power plant in Hamilton, Ohio: An example of complex pollution and cause for community health concerns. *Environ. Pollut.* **2013**, *176*, 26–35. [CrossRef]
33. Zhang, J.J.Y.; Sun, L.; Barrett, O.; Bertazzon, S.; Underwood, F.E.; Johnson, M. Development of land-use regression models for metals associated with airborne particulate matter in a North American city. *Atmos. Environ.* **2015**, *106*, 165. [CrossRef]
34. Muñiz, I.; Sanchez, V. Urban Spatial Form and Structure and Greenhouse-gas Emissions From Commuting in the Metropolitan Zone of Mexico Valley. *Ecol. Econ.* **2018**, *147*, 353–364. [CrossRef]
35. Delgado, C.; Bautista, F.; Gogichaishvili, A.; Cortés, J.L.; Quintana, P.; Aguilar, D.; Cejudo, R. Identificación de las zonas contaminadas con metales pesados en el polvo urbano de la Ciudad de México. *Rev. Int. Contam. Ambient.* **2019**, *35*, 81–100. [CrossRef]
36. UN DESA. World Urbanization Prospects. The 2018 Revision. New York. 2019. Available online: http://www.demographic-research.org/volumes/vol12/9/ (accessed on 16 February 2021).
37. Vallejo, M.; Jáuregui-Renaud, K.; Hermosillo, A.G.; Márquez, M.F.; Cárdenas, M. Efectos de la contaminación atmosférica en la salud y su importancia en la ciudad de México. *Gac. Med. Mex.* **2003**, *139*, 57–63.
38. Rodríguez-Salazar, M.T.; Morton-Bermea, O.; Hernández-Álvarez, E.; Lozano, R.; Tapia-Cruz, V. The study of metal contamination in urban topsoils of Mexico City using GIS. *Environ. Earth Sci.* **2011**, *62*, 899. [CrossRef]
39. Pradilla, C.E. Zona Metropolitana del Valle de México: Neoliberalismo y contradicciones urbanas. *Sociologias* **2016**, *18*, 54–89.
40. Delgado, J. El patrón de ocupación territorial de la Ciudad de Mexico al año 2000. In *Estructura Territorial de la Ciudad de México*; Terrazas, O., Preciat, E., Eds.; CDMX: Plaza y Valdez, Mexico, 1988.
41. CONAGUA. Servicio Meteorológico Nacional (2017). Resumen Mensual de Temperatura y Lluvias 2017. 2017. Available online: https://smn.conagua.gob.mx/es/climatologia/temperaturas-y-lluvias/resumenes-mensuales-de-temperaturas-y-lluvias (accessed on 2 February 2021).
42. Gunier, R.B.; Jerrett, M.; Smith, D.R.; Jursa, T.; Yousefi, P.; Camacho, J.; Hubbard, A.; Eskenazi, B.; Bradman, A. Determinants of manganese levels in house dust samples from the CHAMACOS cohort. *Sci. Total Environ.* **2014**, *497*, 360–368. [CrossRef]
43. Amato, F.; Pandolfi, M.; Moreno, T.; Furger, M.; Pey, J.; Alastuey, A.; Bukowiecki, N.; Prevot, A.S.H.; Baltensperger, U.; Querol, X. Sources and variability of inhalable road dust particles in three European cities. *Atmos. Environ.* **2011**, *45*, 6777–6787. [CrossRef]
44. Jadoon, W.A.; Khpalwak, W.; Chidya, R.C.G.; Abdel-Dayem, S.M.M.A.; Takeda, K.; Makhdoom, M.A.; Sakugawa, H. Evaluation of Levels, Sources and Health Hazards of Road-Dust Associated Toxic Metals in Jalalabad and Kabul Cities, Afghanistan. *Arch. Environ. Contam. Toxicol.* **2018**, *74*, 32–45. [CrossRef]
45. Li, N.; Han, W.; Tang, J.; Bian, J.; Sun, S.; Song, T. Pollution Characteristics and Human Health Risks of Elements in Road Dust in Changchun, China. *Int. J. Environ. Res. Public Health* **2018**, *15*, 1843. [CrossRef]
46. Sobhanardakani, S. Ecological and Human Health Risk Assessment of Heavy Metal Content of Atmospheric Dry Deposition, a Case Study: Kermanshah, Iran. *Biol. Trace Elem. Res.* **2019**, *187*, 602–610. [CrossRef]
47. Aguilera, A.; Bautista, F.; Gutiérrez-Ruiz, M.; Ceniceros-Gómez, A.E.; Cejudo, R.; Goguitchaichvili, A. Assessment of pollution, sources, and human health risk from heavy metal analyses in street dust of Mexico City. (In review).
48. Tomlinson, D.L.; Wilson, J.G.; Harris, C.R.; Jeffrey, D.W. Problems in the assessment of heavy-metal levels in estuaries and the formation of a pollution index. *Helgol. Meeresunters.* **1980**, *33*, 566–575. [CrossRef]
49. Kabata-Pendias, A. *Trace Elements in Soils and Plants*, 4th ed.; CRC Press: Boca Raton, FL, USA; Taylor and Francis Group, LLC: New York, NY, USA, 2010. [CrossRef]
50. Rastegari Mehr, M.; Keshavarzi, B.; Moore, F.; Sharifi, R.; Lahijanzadeh, A.; Kermani, M. Distribution, source identification and health risk assessment of soil heavy metals in urban areas of Isfahan province, Iran. *J. Afr. Earth Sci.* **2017**, *132*, 16–26. [CrossRef]
51. INEGI. Censo General de Población y Vivienda. Mexico. 2010. Available online: https://www.inegi.org.mx/programas/ccpv/2010/ (accessed on 16 February 2021).
52. INEGI. Origin-Destination Survey in Households of the Metropolitan Zone of the Valley of Mexico (EOD). 2017. Available online: http://en.www.inegi.org.mx/programas/eod/2017/default.html#Microdata (accessed on 28 October 2020).
53. INEGI. Instituto Nacional De Estadística y Geografía. 2018. Available online: www.inegi.gob.mx (accessed on 16 February 2021).
54. Gobierno de la Ciudad de México. Portal de Datos Abiertos de la CDMX Retrieved March 15. 2020. Available online: https://datos.cdmx.gob.mx/explore/dataset/uo-de-suelo/table/ (accessed on 25 February 2020).
55. CONAPO. Indice de Marginacion por AGEB Urbana 2000–2010 [WWW Document]. Available online: http://www.conapo.gob.mx/es/CONAPO/Datos_Abiertos_del_Indice_de_Marginacion (accessed on 8 June 2020).
56. Moran, P.A.P. Notes on Continuous Stochastic Phenomena. *Biometrika* **1950**, *37*, 17–23. [CrossRef] [PubMed]
57. Anselin, L. *Exploring Spatial Data with GeoDaTM: A Workbook, Revised Version*; Center for Spatially Integrated Social Science: Santa Barbara, CA, USA, 2005.
58. Darmofal, D. *Spatial Analysis for the Social Sciences*; Cambridge University Press: Cambridge, UK, 2015.
59. UN DESA. World Population Prospects 2019. United Nations. Department of Economic and Social Affairs. World Population Prospects 2019. Available online: http://www.ncbi.nlm.nih.gov/pubmed/12283219 (accessed on 16 February 2021).

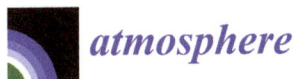

Article

A Landscape Study of Sediment Formation and Transport in the Urban Environment

Ilia Yarmoshenko *, Georgy Malinovsky, Elena Baglaeva and Andrian Seleznev

Institute of Industrial Ecology UB RAS, 620219 Ekaterinburg, Russia; georgy@ecko.uran.ru (G.M.); sem@ecko.uran.ru (E.B.); sandrian@rambler.ru (A.S.)
* Correspondence: ivy@ecko.uran.ru

Received: 27 October 2020; Accepted: 1 December 2020; Published: 6 December 2020

Abstract: Background: Sediment deposition in the urban environment affects aesthetic, economic, and other aspects of city life, and through re-suspension of dust, may pose serious risks to human health. Proper environmental management requires further understanding of natural and anthropogenic factors influencing the sedimentation processes in urbanized catchments. To fill the gaps in the knowledge about the relationship between the urban landscape and sedimentation, field landscape surveys were conducted in the residential areas of the Russian cities of Ekaterinburg, Nizhniy Novgorod, Rostov-on-Don, Tyumen, Chelyabinsk, and Murmansk. Methods: In each city, six elementary urban residential landscapes were chosen in blocks of multi-story apartment buildings typical for Russian cities. The method of landscape survey involved delineating functional segments within the elementary landscapes and describing each segment according to the developed procedure during a field survey. Results: The complexity of sedimentation processes in the urban environment was demonstrated. The following main groups of factors have significant impacts on sediment formation and transport in residential areas in Russian cities: low adaptation of infrastructure to a high density of automobiles, poor municipal services, and bad urban environmental management in the course of construction and earthworks. Conclusion: A high sediment formation potential was found for a considerable portion of residential areas.

Keywords: urban sediment; urban landscape; sediment transport; municipal service; earthworks; environmental management

1. Introduction

A growing proportion of the planet's population now resides in urban areas, and urbanization has become one of the key drivers of environmental processes in the Anthropocene [1–3]. Further enlargement of cities and urban agglomerations has been a significant trend in recent decades [4]. Geochemical transformation in the urban environment consists of modifications to the mineral and elemental composition and physicochemical properties of the urban soil [5–7], changes in the volume of the surface stormwater runoff [8], redistribution of pollutants [9,10], and forming geochemical barriers [11,12], among others. Given the complex interactions of nature, people, and the technosphere in cities, the development of a scientific basis for urban environmental management is a priority for humanity at the present stage of global development. Proper management of cities should ensure that they are ecologically, economically, and socially more sustainable places to live in the future [13,14].

Studies conducted in different regions demonstrated that contemporary sedimentation processes play a significant role in shaping the urban environment. Unlike natural landscapes, an intense anthropogenic impact on exposed surfaces supplies significant amounts of sedimentary material in the urban environment. As a result, the typical yield of sedimentation material in urban watersheds exceeds the rate of this process in natural and agricultural landscapes by an order of magnitude [15,16].

Due to their own physicochemical characteristics and the ability to carry various organic and inorganic toxicants, sediments deposited in streets and roads are characterized as a non-point source of pollution. Sediment deposition in urban areas has received considerable attention in recent years due to the ease of sampling of sediment material, and its potential to act as a proxy for urban pollution and an indicator of emissions of potentially harmful elements [17,18]. Many authors have noted elevated concentrations of heavy metals in road and sidewalk sediment [19–21]. Recently, contamination with microplastics [22] and organic compounds [23] was observed in urban wetland sediment samples.

The urban sedimentary system is a significant part of global waste and pollution transport, thereby changing the chemical composition and mineral content of streams, rivers, seas, and oceans [24–26].

Re-suspension of road dust by the wind or traffic-induced turbulence is an important source contributing to particulate atmospheric pollution [27,28]. Various pollutants present in urban sediment and suspended PM may pose serious risks to human health. Exposure to PM has been linked to increased mortality, and a wide range of diseases in several organ systems—in particular, cardiovascular and pulmonary diseases [29–31].

Particles of biological origin may be suspended in the air as attached to dust particles [32,33]. Evidence for the potential environmental sources of bacterial and viral species associated with airborne PM was provided in microbiome surveys in Beijing [34]. Acosta-Martínez et al. [35] reviewed studies of the microbial characteristics of wind-eroded sediments and distinguished microorganisms predominant in dust-sized sediment prone to removal by longer-range suspended transport and those more likely to be locally redistributed by saltation flux. Gardner et al. [36] suggested that dust-borne microorganisms can only affect human health if a combination of factors coincides with pathogenesis—in particular, inhalation of a substantial amount of dust occurs. Human exposure to environmental microbiota, including potentially opportunistic microbes carried indoors by dirt attached to shoes, was demonstrated in Finland [37].

Hong et al. [38] independently studied health effects of $PM_{2.5}$ (combination of biomass smoke, industrial emissions, and vehicular exhaust gas) and $PM_{10-2.5}$ (combination of sea salt, fugitive agricultural emissions, windblown crustal dust, and road dust) in British Columbia, Canada, and found statistically significant associations between the coarse fraction and non-accidental mortality during the spring season. Hong et al. [38] concluded that springtime road dust is of particular interest for health risk assessment in colder climates where snow can collect materials over the winter months.

Besides the health effects, sediment deposition in the urban environment affects aesthetic, economic, and other aspects of city life. Sedimentation is accompanied by the accumulation of dirt and dust over the urban surfaces, which reduce the quality of the urban environment. A high level of sediment accumulation in the urban landscape causes a negative perception of the environment by citizens. The negative aesthetic effects include the deterioration of the appearance of residential areas and objects of the urban landscape, buildings, vehicles, etc. Regular sediment supply increases costs for municipal services such as cleaning and stormwater system maintenance [11,39–41]. Siltation of stormwater systems, compaction of urban soils, lower fertility of the topsoil, etc., affect the urban infrastructure [10,42,43]. The accumulation of solid substances on street and sidewalks increases the wear and tear of vehicles, clothes, and shoes [44,45]. As dust deposits on insulators, pollution control is required to prevent electricity line outages [46].

In natural and agricultural systems, sedimentation starts with the detachment of soil particles due to soil erosion caused by wind, rainfall, and water flow. The rate of soil erosion is strongly dependent upon soil type, vegetation, and such topographic characteristics as slope, land use, etc. [35,47]. Part of eroded soil is deposited in different sub-areas of a catchment before it reaches the catchment outlet [47–49]. Sediment storage in catchments causes a discrepancy between estimates of catchment sediment erosion and sediment yield [48,50]. Sediment budget and the ratio of sediment yield to total surface erosion (sediment delivery ratio) characterize catchment sediment cascades [49–51]. Quantification of the sedimentary cascade, including the internal dynamics of sediment supply, transport, and storage in various catchments, may be performed through analysis of sediment connectivity between different landscape compartments, which has become a key interdisciplinary concept in the study of processes acting both in natural and human-impacted hydro-geomorphic systems [8,51–53]. As sediment connectivity is hardly measurable, indices and classification schemes (high/moderate/low) have been proposed for the investigation of connectivity drivers [51,53]. Study of connectivity within a catchment may be performed by means of a field survey of erosion, transport, and deposition signs that can be visually observed (rills, local deposits, splash pedestals, flow lines, etc.) [54].

Some specific factors have to be considered in studies of erosion, sedimentation, and anthropogenic-derived sediment deposition in urban environments [11,44]. The sources of nearly all sediments in urban areas are engineering materials and urban soils exposed to erosion [44]. Large proportions of urban areas are fully protected by the impermeable cap provided by buildings, roads, and other structures [44]. Runoff from impervious onto pervious surfaces produces concentrated flow paths and increases lateral connectivity in the urban landscape [8,41]. Urban pervious surfaces are potentially more erodible than is natural due to concentrated runoff, bare soil (e.g., construction and landscaping), and unstable slope conditions (e.g., earthworks) [12,55]. Construction is considered as a major source of sediment supply in the urban environment [56,57]. Accelerated erosion due to construction-related activities was observed in Korea [58], China [59], the USA [57,60], Brazil [61], and other countries. Mechanical sediment removal (extraction) by human activity (street sweeping, cleaning out of the stormwater network, sediment control at construction sites, etc.) is another specific feature of the urbanized landscape [60,62,63]. Comparing the urban sediment budget and natural catchment conditions, Russel et al. [41] concluded that urban catchments have specific extraction fluxes, higher hillslope erosion, less storage, and higher transport capacities than natural sediment cascades. Generally, sediment yields in urban catchments increase by an order of magnitude in a period of development and then remain higher than in natural and agricultural landscapes [16].

Historically, such terms as "street dirt," "street dust," "road dust," and "road deposited sediment" were used to define urban sediment as an object to control or study in different situations. The term "street dirt" was used in the context of street cleaning [62]. The term "road dust" implies fine, fugitive, and respirable material and can be applied in studies of dust suspended in the air [64]. However, this term is not appropriate for urban sediment that has shown to be composed of a full range of particle sizes [11,65]. Road-deposited sediment has become an important environmental sampling medium for assessing anthropogenic metal levels [19,66]. The term "urban sediment" refers to urban environmental sedimentology and it is applied in a broader manner to mean any sediments present within the urban environment [11,18].

The urban environment is considered as a separate landscape type that has been formed as a result of human activities and further develops under the influences of natural, human, and socio-cultural factors. The urban landscape accommodates natural (biotic and abiotic) and artificial components, such as buildings, engineering, and transport structures. The study of landscape heterogeneity was shown to be beneficial to evaluate various natural and anthropogenic processes in the urban areas, e.g., PM pollution [67,68], biodiversity [69,70], heat island effect [71], social behavior [69,72], and ecosystem services [73]. Like other urban-related processes, sediment formation, transport, and surface deposition are closely linked to landscape properties such as geomorphology, landscape connectivity, land cover, and land use [47,50–52,74,75].

The intrinsic heterogeneity of urban landscapes has been taken into account only in a few studies of the urban sediment. Russell et al. [76] considered the following land cover categories within the urban and sub-urban catchments in Melbourne: roofs, impervious areas, grass surfaces, gravel surfaces, and areas with low sediment connectivity. Land cover mapping for nine street-scale stormwater catchments (average area about 1700 m^2) was undertaken, using aerial imagery and field inspection. In the study based on the coarse-grained sediment sampling, it was obtained that most of the sediment was supplied by impervious surfaces and small-scale construction areas [12]. Construction sites and unpaved roads were identified as two major contributors to fugitive dust emission in Nanjing, China [77]. In Stockholm, Sweden, the dust load varies between streets and is dependent on pavement surface properties [64]. A study of the peri-urban catchment in Coimbra, Portugal pointed out that most of the catchment sediment is derived from small parts of the catchment subject to the constructional activity or active landscape change [78].

To summarize, we can say that a comprehensive understanding of the complex interactions of natural and anthropogenic factors in the sedimentation processes in heterogeneous urbanized catchments has not yet been achieved. In particular, it is important to analyze different parts of the urban landscape as potential sources and sinks of urban sediment, to estimate the total value and variability of urban sediment deposition over residential areas, to assess large-scale sediment connectivity, to reveal anthropogenic factors specific in different regions, etc. The aim of this study is to fill the gaps in the knowledge about the relationship between the urban landscape and sedimentation processes. The factors influencing the processes of sediment supply, its further wash off, sediment migration, and the accumulation of urban sediment in residential areas were qualitatively studied by means of landscape surveys in large Russian cities. The novelty of this research is associated with the potential to reveal significant micro-landscape characteristics and factors by applying high spatial resolution field study.

2. Experiments

2.1. Descriptions of the Studied Cities

The study was conducted in six Russian cities located in different climatic and geographical zones (Table 1 and Figure 1). The southernmost city was Rostov-on-Don (47°14′ N); the northernmost was Murmansk (68°58′ N). The average January and July temperatures in the surveyed cities range from −15 to −3 and from 12.8 to 23.4 °C, respectively. Of the six cities surveyed, four have populations of more than 1 million people. The most populated is Ekaterinburg (about 1.5 million people), while 0.3 million people live in the least populated, Murmansk. All the cities are the administrative centers of their regions and play significant socio-economic roles. Ekaterinburg, Chelyabinsk, Nizhniy Novgorod, and Rostov-on-Don are major centers of industry, transport, and engineering. In Murmansk, the main economic focus is associated with the seaport (ship repair, fishing, fish processing); Tyumen is largely oriented towards oil refining. Three cities lie in the valleys of large rivers (Nizhniy Novgorod, Rostov-on-Don, and Tyumen), two cities (Ekaterinburg and Chelyabinsk) are located in the foothills of the Ural Mountains, and one city (Murmansk) occupies hills along a sea bay.

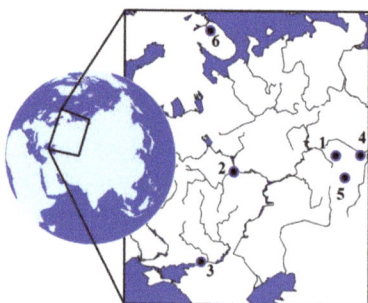

1 – Ekaterinburg, 2 – Nizhniy Novgorod, 3 – Rostov-on-Don, 4 – Tyumen, 5 – Chelyabinsk, 6 – Murmansk

Figure 1. The locations of cities studied.

The municipalities' budgets for the year 2018 ranged from 26.5 to 46.2 thousand rubles (approximately 400–750 USD) per citizen. The relatively large size of the city budget of Murmansk is due to its location in the Arctic region and high transport expenses. Among the other cities, the largest budget in 2018 was in the city of Tyumen, whose economy is related to the oil and gas industry. In other cities, the per capita budget was 20–30% less.

Table 1. Characteristics of cities studied.

City, Population, ×10³	Cars, ×10³/Cars Per 10³ People (2017)	Coor-Dinates	Average Jan/Jul Temp., °C	Average Precipitation Summer Months/Year, mm	Climate Zone	Geographical Region	General Relief	Industries	Municipal Budget in 2018 Per Capita, ×10³ RUB
Ekaterinburg 1480	446.5/302	56°50′ N 60°35′ E	−12.6 /19.0	213/501	Temperate continental	Eastern slope of the Middle Urals	Floodplain terraces along the river, hilly plains, low mountains	Machinery, metallurgy, research and development.	27.2
Nizhniy Novgorod 1260	352/276	56°19′ N 44°00′ E	−8.9 /19.4	224/648	Humid continental	Valley of the Volga and Oka rivers	Floodplains and hilly plains	Machinery, river shipping	26.5
Rostov-on-Don 1130	319.2/285	47°14′ N 39°42′ E	−3.0 /23.4	127/596	Moderate continental, steppe	Valley of the Don river	Floodplain terraces along the river	Machinery, river shipping, food industry	29.2
Tyumen 770	279/363	57°09′ N 65°32′ E	−15.0 /18.8	204/485	Temperate continental	Valley of the Tura river	Floodplain terraces along the river	Metal processing, machinery, oil processing, gas-fired power plants	34.7
Chelyabinsk 1200	320.4/269	55°09′ N 61°24′ E	−14.1 /19.3	186/430	Temperate	Eastern slope of the South Urals	Floodplain terraces along the river, hilly plains	Ferrous and non-ferrous metallurgy, chemical industry, machinery, coal-fired power plants	29.4
Murmansk 292	96.5/330 *	68°58′ N 33°05′ E	−10.1 /12.8	201/547	Subarctic climate	The Kola Peninsula, bank Kola Bay	Low mountains along sea bay	Seaport, ship repair, fishing, fish processing	46.2

* Data for Murmansk oblast.

2.2. Description of the Surveyed Sites

Multi-story apartment buildings are the main type of residential development in all cities. The residential districts consist of microrayons, which were the primary structural element of urban residential area construction in the former Soviet Union (Figure 2). The development of microrayons was mainly made up of blocks of apartment buildings of the same type. A group of apartment buildings (part of a block) with a common front yard and courtyard (back yard) including an adjacent part of a street was chosen as an elementary urban residential landscape (EURL). Such decomposition of the urban residential district, where EURL represents the minimal urban landscape element (micro-landscape), reflects typical apartment block development in Russia.

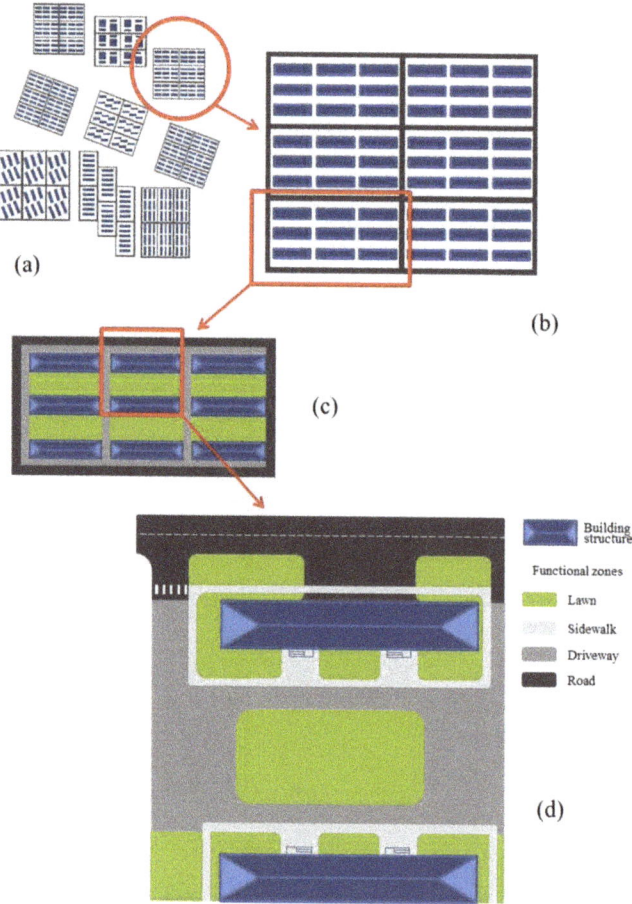

Figure 2. Typical structure of a residential area in a Russian city. (**a**) City's residential area; (**b**) Microrayon; (**c**) Block of buildings; (**d**) EURL.

A two-stage, semi-random procedure was used to select sites for the field landscape survey in each city. In the first stage, 30 typical EURLs were selected in different geographical areas associated with various historical periods of city development. Then six sites were chosen randomly from the list of 30 EURLs in each city.

2.3. Method of the Field Landscape Survey

Preliminary site plans were created based on city maps, satellite images, and street view images available on Google maps and Yandex maps services. The field surveys of the selected sites were performed in accordance with the developed protocol. In the first step, the preliminary site plan was split into disjointed segments providing particular functions or services within the EURL. The segments were assigned to one of the main functional zones:

- Road (a section of the street road network connecting residential areas, and public and industrial areas of the city);
- Green zone, including areas with pervious cover: lawns, flower beds, and playgrounds with a grass cover;
- Sidewalks and adjacent pedestrian paths;
- Vehicle zone (driveways connecting courtyard spaces with the road network, parking spaces, and illegal parking places that are areas of other functional zones illegally used for parking).

Additionally, sports grounds and communal service zones can be found in the EURLs.

The front yard and adjacent street, which are supposed to experience significant loads from vehicles and people, are considered as external parts of the EURL. A courtyard area separated from the street was considered as an internal part of the elementary urban landscape. As a rule, the courtyard is isolated by residential buildings, a fence, driveways, or landscape units. Each segment can be assigned to either the external or internal parts of the EURL.

After the site segmentation, the following characteristics and indicators were analyed for each segment during field inspection:

- Functional purpose (functional zone);
- Association with external or internal parts of the EURL;
- Type of surface cover, paving (asphalt, gravel, grass, etc.);
- Percentage of disturbed surface cover (expert's evaluation);
- Overall technical condition of the paving and infrastructure element (five-point expert's evaluation);
- Quality of the cleaning (five-point expert's evaluation);
- The number of parked cars;
- The number of parking spaces;
- Presence and type of earthworks, construction, and landscaping works;
- Slope gradient (yes/no);
- Local depressions(yes/no);
- Causes of soil erosion and sediment formation;
- Visual signs of external sources of sediment entry.

For some characteristics and indicators, the classification schemes were developed by applying five-point evaluations by experts basing on the visual observations during a field study.

For segments related to the green functional zone, the projective cover of trees, the projective cover of grasses, the type of vegetation (wild plants, lawn grass, ornamental plants), and insolation within the site segments were also evaluated.

A special questionnaire was developed that includes the site address and coordinates, segment ID marked on the site plan, date and time of the survey, and a formalized description of the main characteristics of the segment. The questionnaire was filled out for each site segment at each site. Expert grades were assigned by the agreement of two experts. To achieve consistency in the expert assessments in different cities, the field surveys were carried out by the same researchers according to the same procedure.

3. Results

Field surveys of 36 sites in six cities were performed in warm seasons 2017–2019 (Ekaterinburg—August 2017, Nizhniy Novgorod—August 2018, Rostov-on-Don—October 2018, Tyumen—July 2019, Chelyabinsk—August 2019, Murmansk—August 2019). The average area of a site excluding buildings was 7900 m^2, the minimum area was 1500 m^2, and the maximum area was 17,600 m^2. Buildings occupied an additional 2400 m^2 on average. At each site, 14 segments on average were delineated. A schematic division of a site into segments is presented in Figure 3. The average area for the segments was approximately 560 m^2; 75% of the segments had areas of more than 135 m^2.

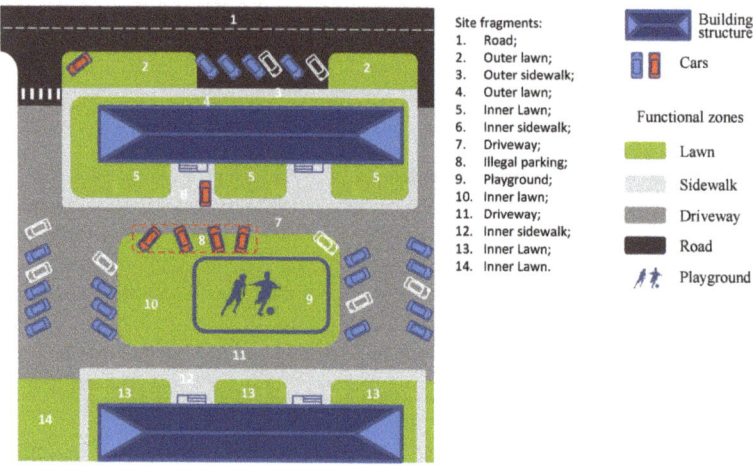

Figure 3. Schematic division of an elementary urban residential landscape (EURL) into segments and functional zones.

3.1. Functional Zones

Division of the EURL area by functional zones is presented in Figure 4. An average of 18% of the residential area is related to the roads, from 13% in Rostov-on-Don to 26% in Tyumen. On average, the green zone occupies 53% of the area of the site excluding the road network. The smallest contribution of the green zone to the area was 42% in Tyumen; the largest was 63% in Ekaterinburg. The average area of the vehicle zone (Figure S1), including driveways, parking, and illegal parking places is 35%, from 29% in Ekaterinburg to 42% in Rostov-on-Don. On average, 59% of the area of a site belongs to the courtyard space.

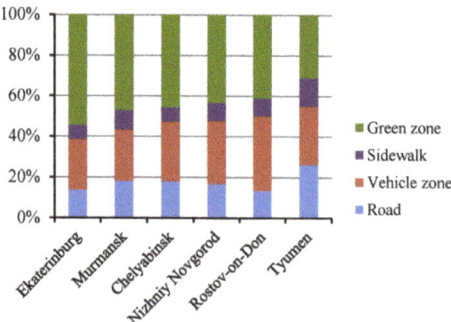

Figure 4. The division of residential quarters into the main types of functional zones.

3.2. Motor Transport

On average, 64 parking spaces determined by visual signs of parked vehicles were recorded at each site, of which 40 parking spaces were occupied by cars during the survey; 80% of the cars were parked in the courtyard. This constitutes 2.9 parking spaces, from 2.2 in Chelyabinsk to 3.8 in Ekaterinburg, per 100 m^2 of the area of the courtyards, driveways, and parking spaces (the vehicle zone of the courtyards) (Figure 5). In the daytime, when the survey was carried out, there was an average of 1.1 parking spaces and 0.7 cars per 100 m^2 of the courtyard area. The minimum number of cars was in Chelyabinsk (0.5), and the maximum in Tyumen (0.8).

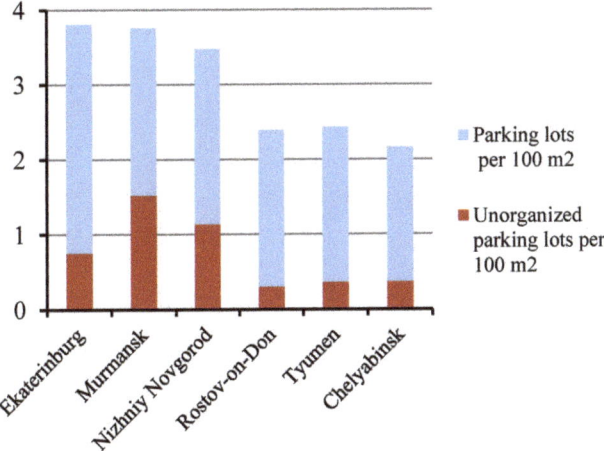

Figure 5. The numbers of proper and illegal parking places per 100 m^2 of the motor transport infrastructure zone of the EURL internal part.

Of the approximately 2300 parking spaces, 487 (21%) are illegal parks on the lawns, sidewalks, and playgrounds (Figure S2). The number of illegal parking places varies significantly by city (Figure 5), from 11% in Tyumen to 36% in Murmansk. One car parked on the lawn disturbs soil in an area of approximately 27 m^2. Illegal parking places occupy about 8% of the green area, sports and children's playgrounds, and sidewalks; in Murmansk and Nizhniy Novgorod—about 14%; in Ekaterinburg, Chelyabinsk, and Tyumen—from 4 to 6%.

3.3. Soils

Soils at the sites are mainly represented by technosols. Natural landscapes within residential areas are almost never found. Soils of natural origin are preserved in separate places with complex topography and elevation, for example, in Murmansk. The upper soil layers are represented by artificial lawn soils, peat, etc., formed as a result of landscaping.

3.4. Disturbed Cover

According to the survey results, the majority of the surfaces in residential areas are disturbed by natural and anthropogenic factors. Areas with visual signs of erosion and mechanical disturbance, bare ground, and paving in poor condition were assigned to the damaged surface cover category. In general, 24% of surfaces in the residential areas of all the cities together are disturbed. Assessment of the condition of surfaces showed that the total proportions of disturbed cover were 27% and 16% in the inner courtyards and the external parts of the sites, respectively. The damaged cover was the possible source of the urban sediment in 319 segments of the urban landscape, which is 2/3 of all those examined.

As can be seen in Figure 6b, the smallest proportion of damaged cover was found in Ekaterinburg—12%. In other cities, except Rostov-on-Don, it did not exceed 30%, and in Rostov-on-Don, more than 40% of EURL surfaces had disturbed cover. In all cities except Ekaterinburg and Murmansk, the largest share of damaged surfaces refers to the disturbed lawn cover. The contribution of the green zone to the total area of damaged cover in Rostov-on-Don reached 90%, while in other cities it was below 70%. The vehicle zones (illegal parking places and disturbed areas of driveways and parking lots) make up the majority of the disturbed cover for Ekaterinburg and Nizhniy Novgorod (Figure S3). In all cities, the portion of damaged cover areas was higher in courtyards than in external parts of the EURLs (Figure 6a).

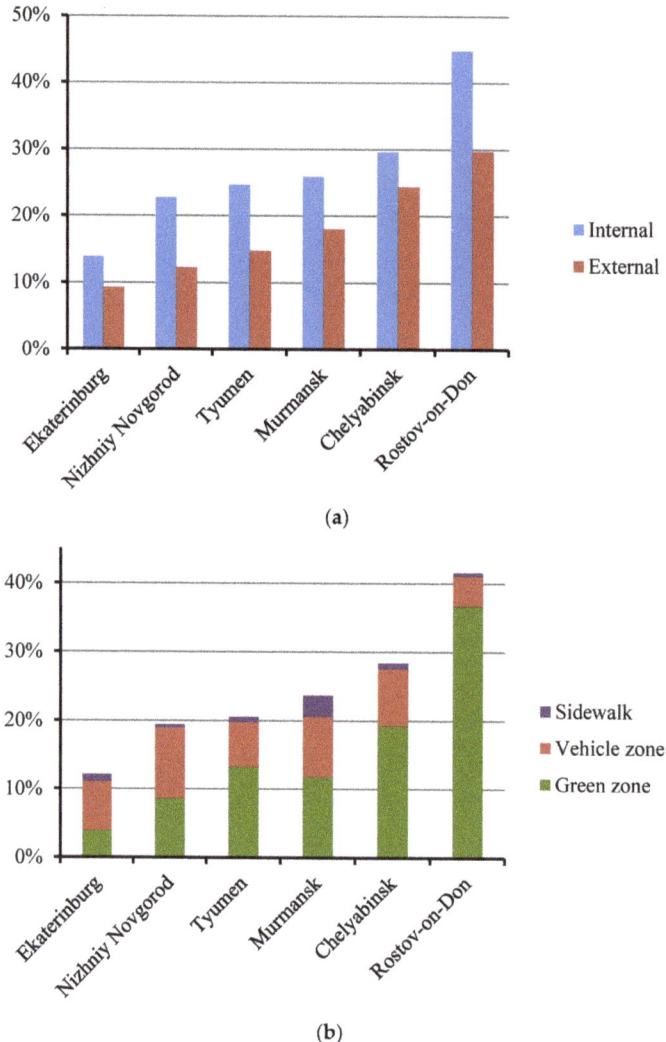

Figure 6. (a) Disturbed cover areas in courtyards and external parts of EURLs; (b) the share of disturbed cover areas on the site (excluding the area of roads), and the contribution of the main functional zones to the total area of damaged cover.

3.5. Vegetation

The lowest grass projective cover in lawns was found in Rostov-on-Don—only 16% (Figure 7a), where the bare soil in lawns was partly associated with the arid summer of steppe climate. The largest projective cover was found in Tyumen (68%). In other cities, projective coverage was in the range of 54–60%. In Tyumen, the largest area of lawns with high projective cover was observed: 27% of the total area of lawns had grass cover of more than 75%, whereas in Rostov-on-Don almost two-thirds of lawns had projective grass cover of less than 25%. In other cities, more than 50% of the lawn area had projective grass cover of more than 50%. The projective grass cover does not depend on the type of vegetation (wild specimens, lawn grass, and ornamental plants). In Tyumen, each type of vegetation makes a significant contribution to the total projective grass cover of green areas. In Chelyabinsk and Murmansk, the greatest contribution is associated with wild species of grass. In Nizhniy Novgorod, the wide use of a cultivated variety of grass was observed. An example of the contribution of low grass projective cover to soil erosion and sediment formation in the urban environment is presented in Figure S4.

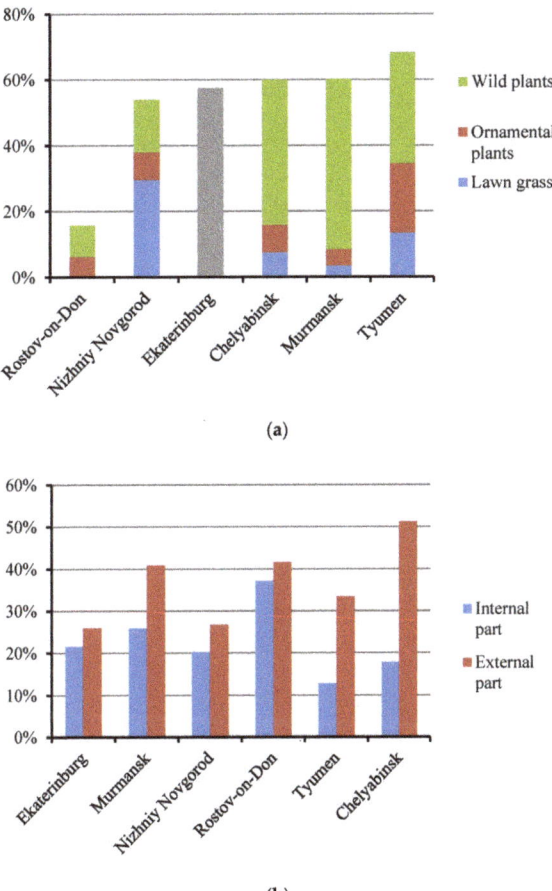

Figure 7. (a) Projective grass cover in lawns, taking into account the contributions of wild plants, lawn grass, and ornamental plants. In Ekaterinburg, the study was conducted according to another scheme. (b) Projective tree canopy cover of external and internal parts of the EURL.

According to a rough assessment of the insolation of lawns, it was found that approximately a third of the lawns can be attributed to areas with low insolation (the shadows of buildings and trees). In these areas, projective coverage is on average 14% lower than in areas with less shadowing.

The average tree canopy cover was 26% of the total area excluding buildings and roads (Figure 7b). In Rostov-on-Don, the largest projective coverage of trees was observed—38%, and the smallest in Tyumen—21%. In all cities, the coverage of the external part of the EURL was higher than in the courtyard (Figure 7b).

3.6. Cleaning and Technical Condition

To characterize the quality of cleaning and the technical condition, expert grades were qualitatively divided into two categories, satisfactory and low quality. Low quality of cleaning was demonstrated by the presence of large amounts of debris, communal waste, broken glass, cigarette butts, and leaf fragments (Figure S5 left). Observations show that under poor quality cleaning, urban sediment accumulates on surfaces, near curbs, and in relief depressions. The share of low-quality grades of cleaning varies significantly by city—from 40% in Nizhniy Novgorod to 80% in Rostov-on-Don. Lower quality of cleaning at pervious paving was observed in all cities (Figure 8a).

The quality of cleaning impervious ground surfaces is considered separately (Figure 8b). For this characteristic, the difference between cities is even greater: from 5% to 81% of areas with poor cleaning in Nizhniy Novgorod and Rostov-on-Don, respectively. Poorly cleaned driveways and parking places in yards make the greatest contributions; more than 50% of all impervious areas in Rostov-on-Don and Chelyabinsk have poor cleaning quality.

An expert assessment of the technical condition of the street, and of front and back yard infrastructure, showed that on average 59% of the areas, excluding the roads, are in unsatisfactory condition. The major visual signs of the unsatisfactory technical condition are as follows. On lawns: low projective grass cover, insufficient mowing, weed overgrowth, lawn damage by vehicles, earthwork with storage of excavated soil on lawns, and lack of restoration or landscaping. On driveways, parking places, and sidewalks: damaged asphalt or other paving, damage or lack of curbs, earthworks with storage of the excavated soil on the pavement, the presence of a large number of depressions with the formation of puddles and deposits of high thickness (Figure S5 right). In all cities, a large contribution to negative grades (<4) of technical condition relates to the green zones, on average 46%. In all cities except Tyumen and Rostov-on-Don, the contribution of driveways was quite large as well—10 to 15% (Figure 8c). In some cities (Murmansk, Chelyabinsk, Ekaterinburg) sidewalks make an additional contribution to the surface area with unsatisfactory technical condition. In general, 84% of the green zones area was in unsatisfactory technical condition (negative grades). About 32% and 22% of the areas of driveways and sidewalks, respectively, were associated with the unsatisfactory condition.

3.7. Earthworks and Construction on Sites

One of the most intense sources of surface contamination by sediment is earth and construction work. Under such activities, the destruction of surfaces, the storage of building materials, and piles of excavated soil without proper shelter occur. In some cases, proper restoration after completion of the earthwork was not undertaken in a timely way (delayed restoration, Figure S6). In total, various works affected 43 site segments (out of 484). Observed earthworks and construction included installing communications cables, sewage works, installing electricity cables, landscaping, road resurfacing, etc. Of all the cases of earthworks and construction documented at the sites, the storage of construction materials and waste on site occurred in 13 site segments (30%), and proper restoration was not carried out in 20 cases (47%). At 20 of the 36 sites, the consequences of such works associated with the formation and transfer of sediment were observed (55%). In total, earthworks and construction in residential areas affects about 9% of the territory. The largest number of segments with the delayed restoration was found in Ekaterinburg (Figure 9). In Tyumen, such sites were not identified at all.

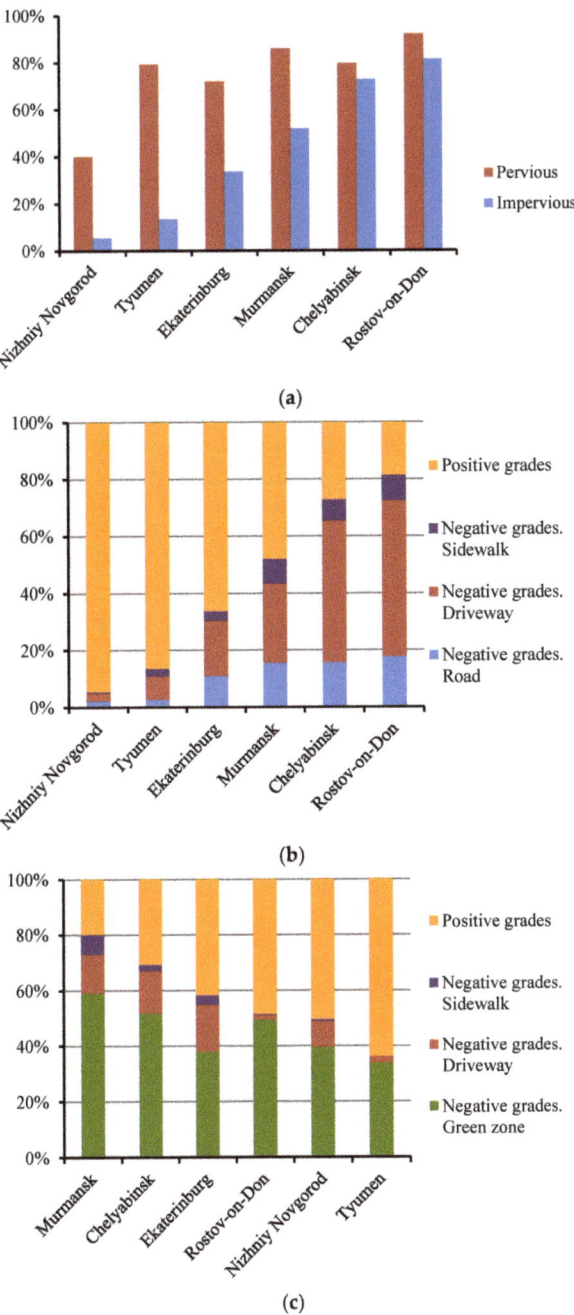

Figure 8. Grades of cleaning quality and technical condition. (**a**) Negative grades of cleaning in segments with pervious and impervious surfaces; (**b**) quality of cleaning by functional zones with impervious surfaces; (**c**) contributions of the main functional zones to the negative grades of the technical condition.

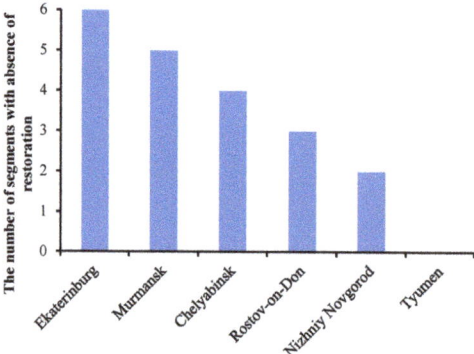

Figure 9. The number of segments with delayed restoration after earthworks and construction.

3.8. Gradient

Assessment of the gradient in the surveyed sites showed that on average 56% of the urban landscape has a visible slope and visual signs of stormwater runoff. The smallest proportion of areas with a registered gradient within sites was observed in Nizhniy Novgorod (34%), the largest was in Murmansk (81%), and it was 53–59% in other cities. The presence of the gradient could be associated with the features of the natural landscape and the architectural solutions. In Murmansk, residential neighborhoods are integrated into the existing mountainous terrain of the Murmansk bay region. In Nizhniy Novgorod, the landscape of residential areas is mostly flat, though some of the residential areas are also located on a hilly shore.

3.9. Sediment Formation and Transport

Where the soil erosion or mechanical destruction due to automobile impact occurred, segments were considered as places of sedimentation formation. As can be seen in Figure 10, the proportion of segments that were sources of sediment material was at least 60% of segments surveyed in all cities. In Murmansk and Chelyabinsk, more than 90% of the segments were sources of sediment. The smallest share of such segments was found in Ekaterinburg (61%).

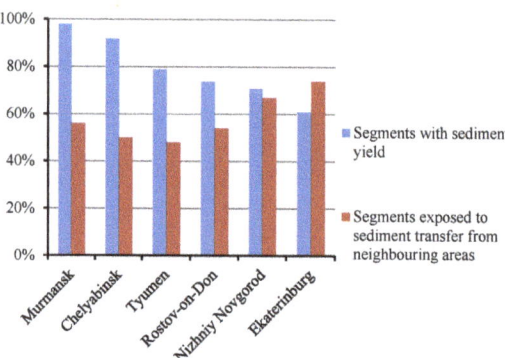

Figure 10. The proportions of site segments that were sources of sediment yield and the proportions of segments contaminated due to transfer from neighboring areas.

Sediment connectivity in the urban micro-landscape is characterized by the presence of sediment transfer between neighboring segments of the EURL. As can be seen in Figure 10, at least 48% of the segments were polluted with material transferred from adjacent areas. The maximum proportion of site segments with sediment supply due to transfer from neighboring areas was also found in Ekaterinburg (74%). In total, 430 of 484 site segments (80%) were subject to sediment formation or sediment transport that resulted in pollution of the urban environment with urban sediment.

The transport of deposited sediments together with the removal of degraded soil from places of illegal parking on the wheels of cars to the courtyards, driveways, and streets was noted at 26 of the 36 sites. The vehicles provide transport for sediment in both directions, from courtyards to roads and from roads to courtyards. Another factor of sediment connectivity in the urban landscape is the organization of runoff over landscape and equipment with a drainage system. According to the results of the surveys, courtyards are mostly designed to provide surface runoff without water stagnation. The flow of water is intentionally directed from courtyards to streets, which are usually equipped with municipal drainage systems. Among 36 surveyed sites, considerable water stagnation was observed at one site, and courtyard drainage systems were found at two sites.

4. Discussion

Field surveys of the urban residential environment conducted in six Russian cities revealed factors that significantly impact sediment formation, transport, and sediment surface deposition in residential areas.

4.1. Motor Transport

The landscape survey showed that significant portions of residential blocks, including courtyards, are occupied by motor vehicles. Intensive motorization is a feature of the socio-economic development of the last few decades in Russia. The Russian car parks amounted to 52.4 million units in 2019 with a growth of about 50% in the last decade. Intensive motorization gave rise to a number of urban problems. The city road networks were not designed for the increased traffic, which was also observed in many cities around the world during similar periods of development. Attempts to solve this problem by increasing the role of public transport have not yet yielded the expected results in Russian cities.

The second problem is the lack of parking spaces for an increasing number of cars. Unlike in low-rise residential areas in other regions of the world, parking problems exist not only "near the office," but also "near homes" in blocks of mid and high-rise buildings during non-working-hours. The survey results confirmed that the high density of automobiles increases sediment formation. By blocks of apartment buildings, not only are roadsides and designated asphalt areas used for parking, but any available piece of land that is not fenced is used as well. Car owners aggressively occupy lawns, sidewalks, playgrounds, and sports grounds.

In three cities—Ekaterinburg, Murmansk, and Nizhniy Novgorod—the largest number of cars per 100 m^2 of vehicle infrastructure area (driveways and parking places) inside yards was observed—3.7 parking places, of which 1.1 were illegal. It can be concluded that in the cities of Ekaterinburg, Murmansk, and Nizhniy Novgorod, the existing vehicle zone is almost completely occupied by private vehicle units. In these cities, the landscape experiences the maximum vehicle load—one car per 27 m^2 of the transport infrastructure (driveways and parking) of the yard. In the cities of Rostov-on-Don, Tyumen, and Chelyabinsk, there is one vehicle per 43 m^2 of vehicle zone of the internal part of the EURL. In these cities, the number of cars parked on lawns, sidewalks, and playgrounds is 3.3 times less (per 100 m^2 of the vehicle zone of the courtyard). At the same time, the number of cars parked within the vehicle zone is almost the same in both groups of cities, 2–2.5 parking spaces per 100 m^2 of the vehicle zone. It can be assumed that in Rostov-on-Don, Tyumen, and Chelyabinsk, a large proportion of cars are located outside the courtyards in legal parking spaces.

Estimates showed that one car illegally parked on a lawn or sidewalk occupies an area of about 27 m^2, taking into account the area necessary for driving. Lawns and sidewalks, places that do not have special cover, are mechanically damaged by the wheels of illegally parked cars. Every fifth car in the courtyard is fully or partially parked on a lawn, sidewalk, or playground. To ensure proper conditions for all the cars currently used in yards, an increase in the area of the vehicle zone by about 30% is required.

4.2. Management—Technical Condition

Poor technical condition of the landscape infrastructure increases the potential for the sediment formation. Attributes of the unsatisfactory technical condition of sidewalks, lawns, curbs, asphalt surfacing of driveways, building structures, and other elements were observed in all cities. These structures are exposed to weathering and the impacts of vehicles, and supply destructive products to the environment. The low technical condition of the green zones contributes to the negative assessment of the urban landscape in all cities as well. The technical condition of the vehicle zones in courtyards is unsatisfactory in most cities.

The technical condition of infrastructure varies significantly across the cities. The reasons for such differences are not precisely established and only to some extent may be related to the size of the municipal budget and climatic conditions.

4.3. Management—Vegetation

The total area occupied by green zones in cities is relatively high, and more than 50% of the area of courtyard spaces belongs to green zones. The presence of large pervious areas allocated for vegetation helps to solve the problem of surface water drainage, which plays an important role in the surface transport of solid sediment and runoff.

The grass cover is the major characteristic of lawns and other pervious surfaces in relation to protection against erosion and mechanical destruction. Given the low average projective grass cover (less than 60% in five cities), the low proportion (about 50%) of lawns with high projective cover, the rare use of cultivated varieties of lawn grasses, and the high proportion of lawns in low light conditions, the quality of lawns in Russian cities was assessed as unsatisfactory. Low projective grass cover and poor technical conditions of the green zone reduce the potential positive effect of green spaces.

4.4. Management—Cleaning

Unsatisfactory cleaning in considerable portions of residential areas leads to low extraction and high deposition of sediment on surfaces with suitable conditions. It turned out that the greatest difference between the cities was observed in the expert assessments of the quality of cleaning, especially on impervious surfaces. Despite the lowest municipal budget per capita, the best cleaning quality was noted in Nizhniy Novgorod. A characteristic feature of all the cities surveyed was the low quality of cleaning of a significant portion of the lawns and other elements of the green zone compared to paved surfaces.

4.5. Earthworks

Approximately 9% each of the green zones and the vehicle zones in the surveyed cities are affected by earthworks and construction. The main factors that pollute the environment with sediment during works are the placement of building materials and excavated soil on the ground and the lack of timely and proper restoration. The disposal of the excavated soil and building materials on the ground without shelter makes the soil and materials susceptible to wash off by runoff and to mechanical transfer on car wheels and biological transport by pedestrians.

The negative impact of earthworks and construction on the environment takes place due to the insufficient application of the principles and standards of environmental management. The introduction of such principles into companies involved in any works in the urban environment is not inspired by municipal authorities.

4.6. Sediment Production

The area of disturbed cover may be considered as an integral factor influencing sediment production in urban areas. This parameter summarizes the area with low projective grass cover, lack of grass cover on pervious surfaces, and poor technical condition of paving. The present study found that about 24% of the surfaces of residential areas are potential sources of solid sediment supply. Assuming erosion of 1 mm/year/m^2 of disturbed surfaces on land with a soil density of 2000 kg/m^3, sediment supply (all size fractions) in the city may be roughly estimated as 0.5 kg/year/m^2. This estimate corresponds to the range of sediment yield in urban areas made in [16]. According to observations, for individual segments with high vehicle load, the layer of soil removed annually may be even larger. In this case, the rough assessment of sediment yield may reach a few kg/year/m^2. Earlier, the amount of solid sedimentation material deposited in the urban environment was estimated from the accumulation of solid sediment in snow-dirt sludge in Ekaterinburg [65]. Snow-dirt sludge is a material formed as a result of the mixing of snow and urban sediment through the actions of vehicles' wheels and pedestrians' feet. The total amount of urban sediment deposited in residential land use areas in Ekaterinburg was estimated as 320,000 t or 3.2 kg/m^2 [65]. This estimate corresponds to the rough assessment of the present study—a few kg/year/m^2.

According to an assessment of sediment supply potential, the greater prevalence for sedimentation was observed in the internal courtyard parts of the urban landscape than in the external parts. The courtyard is characterized by a larger disturbed cover area, worse technical condition, lower quality of cleaning, and a larger area of green zones, on which these negative factors are more pronounced. It is also necessary to mention illegal parking on lawns as another negative factor. Higher sediment supply potential of courtyards is to some extent related to principles of responsibilities division between municipal authorities and owners of residential buildings in the Russian Federation.

4.7. Connectivity, Sediment Transport

In the framework of the present study, it is possible to qualitatively assess the sediment connectivity in the EURL by the number of segments exposed to contamination due to sediment transfer from neighboring areas. The sediment connectivity in the EURL can be considered as high, since about half of the segments have a significant gradient and half of the segments are contaminated due to sediment transport. In some cities, the number of segments contaminated due to migration is approximately equal to or greater than the number of segments in which sediment is produced. The largest numbers of segments subject to supply from neighboring areas were observed in the cities of Ekaterinburg and Nizhniy Novgorod, in which the largest number of parked cars per unit area of EURL was recorded. Thus, it can be assumed that motor transport plays an active role in migration and increasing landscape connectivity in the urban environment in addition to sediment wash off. Taking into account the directions of traffic flow and stormwater runoff, the sediment cascade is formed; it carries sediment outside the courtyards into the road network. The connection of the elements of the urban landscape into a single sediment cascade, which forms the urban landscape catena, is determined both by the slope gradient and mechanical sediment transport.

4.8. Representativeness of the Study

The total area surveyed in six cities was about 370,000 m^2 (including the area of residential buildings), which is approximately equal to the area of a small town such as Monte Carlo. At the same time, this area does not exceed 0.5% of the total residential area in Ekaterinburg alone. The representativeness of this study is enhanced by the fact that the most typical residential blocks of each city were considered when choosing the sites. The total perimeter of the site segments, i.e., the approximate route covered by the researchers during the surveys, which was about 50 km, also characterizes the size of the study.

During the Soviet era, standardized construction methods and regulatory approaches were applied throughout the country, which contributed to the homogeneity of the urban landscape in different cities. After the collapse of the USSR and changes in socio-economic policies, tenants of municipal housing were allowed to privatize their units with responsibility for managing adjacent courtyards. Homeowners of flats in multi-household residences cooperatively hire service organizations that maintain entire blocks of houses. The state partly continues to control and regulate the municipal service sphere, promoting common standards. Thus, the urban landscape remains relatively homogeneous and the results of the landscape surveys in the six cities can be considered representative for all major cities in Russia.

The study included cities located in various climatic zones. For urban studies in Russia, it is important to reflect the change in climatic conditions from south to north and from west to east. In the current study, the first vector is represented by the axis Rostov-on-Don–Nizhniy Novgorod–Murmansk, and the second, Nizhniy Novgorod–Ekaterinburg/Chelyabinsk–Tyumen. When comparing the survey results in different cities, it is necessary to take into account the effects of local climatic factors.

A landscape survey of Russian cities was carried out in the warm season. When analyzing the data obtained, it is necessary to take into account the significant seasonality of meteorological conditions in Russia. In all the cities surveyed, in winter the temperature is below zero degrees Celsius. In all cities except Rostov-on-Don, months-long snow cover is established. In the winter period, factors affecting sedimentation processes are significantly modified. Some aspects of sedimentation processes in an urban environment in the winter were presented in recent works [65,79].

It is appropriate to develop a model of a typical EURL for a Russian city. Table 2 shows the main parameters of EURL model according to the results of the present study, which are partly demonstrated in Figure 3 as well. By consecutively stacking the model units of external and internal parts of the elementary landscape to model blocks, microrayons, and an entire city, such a model can be used for various purposes in land use studies, estimates of sediment yield, and sediment accumulation at various scales. In particular, modeling of the sediment yield and dust dispersion in the urban environment may be performed by applying some specific coefficients in different segments. Such coefficients should take into account both the natural processes and the anthropogenic activity's influence on the sedimentation. The EURL model can be used to verify the results of urban research that can be performed using remote sensing methods as well.

Table 2. Characteristics of the typical EURL in a large Russian city.

Parameter	Value
Total area	10,000 m^2
Areas of road/front yard green zone/internal courtyard/buildings,%	14/17/46/23
Areas of green and sidewalks zones/vehicle zone in internal courtyard, %	57/43
Number of segments at the site/the average area of the segment	14/560 m^2
Number of parking spaces in internal/external parts	50/13
Number of illegal parking in internal/external parts	12/1
Area of segments with unsatisfactory technical condition	59%
Area of segments with impervious cover with poor cleaning	60%
Area of lawns with projective grass cover less than 50%	50%
Tree canopy cover (excluding the area of buildings and roads)	26%
Area affected by earthworks and construction	9%
Area of impervious cover/lawn/disturbed cover (roads and buildings excluded), %	38/38/24
Segments connectivity: probability of solid sediment transfer from neighbouring segments to the given one	0.5

4.9. Limitations of the Study

There are several of limitations and sources of uncertainty that could be taken into account to evaluate the obtained results. The study was conducted within the residential areas of the cities, and other land uses were not considered. At the same time, industrial and commercial land uses occupy a significant proportion of the urban territories and contribute to the urban sediment supply. Sediment formation and transport in the city, as a complex system, has to be studied in all specific urban landscapes. The field observations in this study were based in part on expert assessments of some landscape characteristics and indicators that are not free from subjectivity. While attempts to achieve the consistency of results of the field observations in different cities were undertaken, difficulties likely will arise when comparing with the work of other researchers in other regions of the world.

The urban landscape in this study was intentionally considered as a constant, non-dynamic system. This is not true. Two types of temporal variation of the urban landscape should not be missed for a more comprehensive understanding of the natural and anthropogenic influences on the sediment cascade. The first one is seasonality, which is a significant modifying factor. In the case of the northern cities, the snow cover interacts with urban sediment and inevitably transforms the erosion, transport, and depositional processes during cold winters [79]. Seasonality is an important factor determining an increase in surface runoff and sediment transport during the springtime melt [80]. In this study, the observations were made during the summer and early autumn, when soil erosion is not hidden by snow cover, and sediment transport is not restrained. It could be taken into account that the characteristics of recognized influencing factors may change throughout the year. The second type consists of permanent changes to the urban landscape and land cover in course of time. In order to study the effects of the long-term transformation of urban areas, repetitive monitoring for several years is required.

5. Conclusions

According to the results of the present study, the formation of sediment in the urban environment is a complex process involving the interaction of various natural and anthropogenic physical processes. The life cycle of the urban sediment starts with soil erosion and mechanical destruction and continues with the removal of degraded soil by wind, runoff, car wheels, and pedestrians. Significant storage of surface sediment in the urban environment may occur due to low removal rate. The following main groups of factors have significant impacts on sediment supply, transport, and deposition in residential areas of Russian cities: low adaptation of residential areas' infrastructure to the high density of automobiles, unsatisfactory municipal services, and bad environmental management in the course of construction and earthworks. The significant impact of motor vehicles in the urban environment includes mechanical sediment transport that sharply increases the sediment connectivity within the urban landscape. Results of the study approve negative trends in urban sedimentation caused by the mismatch between the current level of urban planning and management and the needs of residents in a high-quality environment in growing cities that can arise in different regions of the world.

Supplementary Materials: The following are available online at http://www.mdpi.com/2073-4433/11/12/1320/s1. Figure S1: Example of a vehicle zone (all photos were taken during the field survey). Figure S2: Examples of illegal parking on lawns and playgrounds. Figure S3: Examples of disturbed cover from illegal parking (left) and damaged driveway (right). Figure S4: Example of low grass projective cover. Figure S5: Examples of segments with negative grades of cleaning (left) and technical condition (right). Figure S6: Example of delayed restoration after earthwork.

Author Contributions: Conceptualization, I.Y. and A.S.; methodology, I.Y. and G.M.; formal analysis, I.Y. and G.M.; field study, I.Y., G.M., E.B., and A.S.; data curation, G.M.; writing—original draft preparation, I.Y. and G.M.; writing—review and editing, E.B. and A.S.; visualization, I.Y. and G.M.; supervision, I.Y.; project administration, A.S.; funding acquisition, A.S. All authors have read and agreed to the published version of the manuscript.

Funding: The study was supported by Russian Science Foundation (grant number 18-77-10024).

Conflicts of Interest: The authors declare no conflict of interest.

References

1. Chin, A.; Beach, T.; Luzzadder-Beach, S.; Solecki, W.D. Challenges of the "Anthropocene". *Anthropocene* **2017**, *20*, 1–3. [CrossRef]
2. Ford, J.R.; Price, S.J.; Cooper, A.H.; Waters, C.N. An assessment of lithostratigraphy for anthropogenic deposits. *Geol. Soc. Lond. Spec. Publ.* **2014**, *395*, 55–89. [CrossRef]
3. Waters, C.N.; Zalasiewicz, J.; Summerhayes, C.; Barnosky, A.D.; Poirier, C.; Galuszka, A.; Cearreta, A.; Edgeworth, M.; Ellis, E.C.; Ellis, M.; et al. The Anthropocene is functionally and stratigraphically distinct from the Holocene. *Science* **2016**, *351*, aad2622. [CrossRef]
4. Gerten, C.; Fina, S.; Rusche, K. The Sprawling Planet: Simplifying the Measurement of Global Urbanization Trends. *Front. Environ. Sci.* **2019**, *7*, 140. [CrossRef]
5. Kosheleva, N.E.; Vlasov, D.V.; Korlyakov, I.D.; Kasimov, N.S. Contamination of urban soils with heavy metals in Moscow as affected by building development. *Sci. Total Environ.* **2018**, *636*, 854–863. [CrossRef]
6. Tresch, S.; Moretti, M.; Le Bayon, R.-C.; Mäder, P.; Zanetta, A.; Frey, D.; Stehle, B.; Kuhn, A.; Munyangabe, A.; Fliessbach, A. Urban Soil Quality Assessment—A Comprehensive Case Study Dataset of Urban Garden Soils. *Front. Environ. Sci.* **2018**, *6*, 136. [CrossRef]
7. Konstantinova, E.; Minkina, T.; Sushkova, S.; Konstantinov, A.; Rajput, V.D.; Sherstnev, A. Urban soil geochemistry of an intensively developing Siberian city: A case study of Tyumen, Russia. *J. Environ. Manag.* **2019**, *239*, 366–375. [CrossRef]
8. Poeppl, R.E.; Keesstra, S.D.; Maroulis, J. A conceptual connectivity framework for understanding geomorphic change in human-impacted fluvial systems. *Geomorphology* **2017**, *277*, 237–250. [CrossRef]
9. Chambers, L.G.; Chin, Y.-P.; Filippelli, G.M.; Gardner, C.B.; Herndon, E.M.; Long, D.T.; Lyons, W.B.; MacPherson, G.L.; McElmurry, S.P.; McLean, C.E.; et al. Developing the scientific framework for urban geochemistry. *Appl. Geochem.* **2016**, *67*, 1–20. [CrossRef]
10. Muthusamy, M.; Tait, S.; Schellart, A.; Beg, M.N.A.; Carvalho, R.F.; de Lima, J.L.M.P. Improving understanding of the underlying physical process of sediment wash-off from urban road surfaces. *J. Hydrol.* **2018**, *557*, 426–433. [CrossRef]
11. Taylor, K. Urban environments. In *Environmental Sedimentology*; Perry, C., Taylor, K., Eds.; Wiley-Blackwell: Hoboken, NJ, USA, 2007; pp. 190–222.
12. Russell, K.L.; Vietz, G.J.; Fletcher, T.D. Urban sediment supply to streams from hillslope sources. *Sci. Total Environ.* **2019**, *653*, 684–697. [CrossRef] [PubMed]
13. Pickett, S.T.A.; Cadenasso, M.L.; Grove, J.M.; Boone, C.G.; Groffman, P.M.; Irwin, E.; Kaushal, S.S.; Marshall, V.; McGrath, B.; Nilon, C.H.; et al. Urban ecological systems: Scientific foundations and a decade of progress. *J. Environ. Manag.* **2011**, *92*, 331–362. [CrossRef] [PubMed]
14. Platt, R.H. The ecological city: Introduction and overview. In *The Ecological City: Preserving and Restoring Urban Biodiversity*; Platt, R.H., Rowntree, R.A., Muick, P.C., Eds.; University of Massachusetts Press: Amherst, MA, USA, 1994; pp. 1–17.
15. Chin, A. Urban transformation of river landscapes in a global context. *Geomorphology* **2006**, *79*, 460–487. [CrossRef]
16. Russell, K.L.; Vietz, G.J.; Fletcher, T.D. Global sediment yields from urban and urbanizing watersheds. *Earth Sci. Rev.* **2017**, *168*, 73–80. [CrossRef]
17. Taylor, K.G.; Owens, P.N. Sediments in urban river basins: A review of sediment–contaminant dynamics in an environmental system conditioned by human activities. *J. Soils Sediments* **2009**, *9*, 281–303. [CrossRef]
18. Seleznev, A.A.; Yarmoshenko, I.V.; Malinovsky, G.P. Urban geochemical changes and pollution with potentially harmful elements in seven Russian cities. *Sci. Rep.* **2020**, *10*, 1668. [CrossRef]
19. Sutherland, R.A. Lead in grain size fractions of road-deposited sediment. *Environ. Pollut.* **2003**, *121*, 229–237. [CrossRef]
20. Padoan, E.; Romè, C.; Ajmone-Marsan, F. Bioaccessibility and size distribution of metals in road dust and roadside soils along a peri-urban transect. *Sci. Total Environ.* **2017**, *601–602*, 89–98. [CrossRef]
21. Adamiec, E.; Jarosz-Krzemińska, E. Human Health Risk Assessment associated with contaminants in the finest fraction of sidewalk dust collected in proximity to trafficked roads. *Sci. Rep.* **2019**, *9*, 16364. [CrossRef]
22. Townsend, K.R.; Lu, H.-C.; Sharley, D.J.; Pettigrove, V. Associations between microplastic pollution and land use in urban wetland sediments. *Environ. Sci. Pollut. Res.* **2019**, *26*, 22551–22561. [CrossRef]

23. Marshall, S.; Sharley, D.; Jeppe, K.; Sharp, S.; Rose, G.; Pettigrove, V. Potentially Toxic Concentrations of Synthetic Pyrethroids Associated with Low Density Residential Land Use. *Front. Environ. Sci.* **2016**, *4*, 75. [CrossRef]
24. Froger, C.; Ayrault, S.; Evrard, O.; Monvoisin, G.; Bordier, L.; Lefèvre, I.; Quantin, C. Tracing the sources of suspended sediment and particle-bound trace metal elements in an urban catchment coupling elemental and isotopic geochemistry, and fallout radionuclides. *Environ. Sci. Pollut. Res.* **2018**, *25*, 28667–28681. [CrossRef] [PubMed]
25. Zhu, Y.; Huang, L.; Li, J.; Ying, Q.; Zhang, H.; Liu, X.; Liao, H.; Li, N.; Liu, Z.; Mao, Y.; et al. Sources of particulate matter in China: Insights from source apportionment studies published in 1987–2017. *Environ. Int.* **2018**, *115*, 343–357. [CrossRef] [PubMed]
26. Owens, P.N.; Blake, W.H.; Gaspar, L.; Gateuille, D.; Koiter, A.J.; Lobb, D.A.; Petticrew, E.; Reiffarth, D.; Smith, H.; Woodward, J. Fingerprinting and tracing the sources of soils and sediments: Earth and ocean science, geoarchaeological, forensic, and human health applications. *Earth Sci. Rev.* **2016**, *162*, 1–23. [CrossRef]
27. Alves, C.A.; Evtyugina, M.; Vicente, A.M.P.; Vicente, E.D.; Nunes, T.V.; Silva, P.M.A.; Duarte, M.; Pio, C.; Amato, F.; Querol, X. Chemical profiling of PM10 from urban road dust. *Sci. Total Environ.* **2018**, *634*, 41–51. [CrossRef] [PubMed]
28. Chen, S.; Zhang, X.; Lin, J.; Huang, J.; Zhao, D.; Yuan, T.; Huang, K.; Luo, Y.; Jia, Z.; Zang, Z.; et al. Fugitive Road Dust PM2.5 Emissions and Their Potential Health Impacts. *Environ. Sci. Technol.* **2019**, *53*, 8455–8465. [CrossRef] [PubMed]
29. Landrigan, P.J.; Fuller, R.; Acosta, N.J.R.; Adeyi, O.; Arnold, R.; Basu, N.; Baldé, A.B.; Bertollini, R.; Bose-O'Reilly, S.; Boufford, J.I.; et al. The Lancet Commission on pollution and health. *Lancet* **2018**, *391*, 462–512. [CrossRef]
30. Cohen, A.J.; Brauer, M.; Burnett, R.; Anderson, H.R.; Frostad, J.; Estep, K.; Balakrishnan, K.; Brunekreef, B.; Dandona, L.; Dandona, R. Estimates and 25-year trends of the global burden of disease attributable to ambient air pollution: An analysis of data from the Global Burden of Diseases Study 2015. *Lancet* **2017**, *389*, 1907–1918. [CrossRef]
31. WHO. *Review of Evidence on Health Aspects of Air Pollution–REVIHAAP Project: Final Technical Report*; The WHO European Centre for Environment and Health: Bonn, Switzerland, 2013.
32. Alghamdi, M.A.; Shamy, M.; Redal, M.A.; Khoder, M.; Awad, A.H.; Elserougy, S. Microorganisms associated particulate matter: A preliminary study. *Sci. Total Environ.* **2014**, *479–480*, 109–116. [CrossRef]
33. Groulx, N.; Urch, B.; Duchaine, C.; Mubareka, S.; Scott, J.A. The Pollution Particulate Concentrator (PoPCon): A platform to investigate the effects of particulate air pollutants on viral infectivity. *Sci. Total Environ.* **2018**, *628–629*, 1101–1107. [CrossRef]
34. Qin, N.; Liang, P.; Wu, C.; Wang, G.; Xu, Q.; Xiong, X.; Wang, T.; Zolfo, M.; Segata, N.; Qin, H.; et al. Longitudinal survey of microbiome associated with particulate matter in a megacity. *Genome Biol.* **2020**, *21*, 55. [CrossRef] [PubMed]
35. Acosta-Martínez, V.; Van Pelt, S.; Moore-Kucera, J.; Baddock, M.C.; Zobeck, T.M. Microbiology of wind-eroded sediments: Current knowledge and future research directions. *Aeolian Res.* **2015**, *18*, 99–113. [CrossRef]
36. Gardner, T.; Acosta-Martinez, V.; Calderón, F.J.; Zobeck, T.M.; Baddock, M.; Van Pelt, R.S.; Senwo, Z.; Dowd, S.; Cox, S. Pyrosequencing Reveals Bacteria Carried in Different Wind-Eroded Sediments. *J. Environ. Qual.* **2012**, *41*, 744–753. [CrossRef]
37. Hui, N.; Parajuli, A.; Puhakka, R.; Grönroos, M.; Roslund, M.I.; Vari, H.K.; Selonen, V.A.; Yan, G.; Siter, N.; Nurminen, N.; et al. Temporal variation in indoor transfer of dirt-associated environmental bacteria in agricultural and urban areas. *Environ. Int.* **2019**, *132*, 105069. [CrossRef] [PubMed]
38. Hong, K.Y.; King, G.H.; Saraswat, A.; Henderson, S.B. Seasonal ambient particulate matter and population health outcomes among communities impacted by road dust in British Columbia, Canada. *J. Air Waste Manag. Assoc.* **2017**, *67*, 986–999. [CrossRef]
39. Sevilla, A.; Rodríguez, M.L.; García-Maraver, Á.; Zamorano, M. An index to quantify street cleanliness: The case of Granada (Spain). *Waste Manag.* **2013**, *33*, 1037–1046. [CrossRef]
40. Yuen, J.Q.; Olin, P.H.; Lim, H.S.; Benner, S.G.; Sutherland, R.A.; Ziegler, A.D. Accumulation of potentially toxic elements in road deposited sediments in residential and light industrial neighborhoods of Singapore. *J. Environ. Manag.* **2012**, *101*, 151–163. [CrossRef]

41. Russell, K.L.; Vietz, G.J.; Fletcher, T.D. A suburban sediment budget: Coarse-grained sediment flux through hillslopes, stormwater systems and streams. *Earth Surf. Process. Landf.* **2019**, *44*, 2600–2614. [CrossRef]
42. Butler, D.; Davies, J.W. *Urban. Drainage*, 3rd ed.; Spon Press: London, UK, 2011.
43. Murakami, M.; Fujita, M.; Furumai, H.; Kasuga, I.; Kurisu, F. Sorption behavior of heavy metal species by soakaway sediment receiving urban road runoff from residential and heavily trafficked areas. *J. Hazard. Mater.* **2009**, *164*, 707–712. [CrossRef]
44. Knox, E.G.; Bouchard, C.E.; Barrett, J.G. Erosion and Sedimentation in Urban Areas. In *Agronomy Monographs*; American Society of Agronomy; Crop Science Society of America; Soil Science Society of America: Madison, WI, USA, 2015; pp. 179–197.
45. Hewett, C.J.M.; Simpson, C.; Wainwright, J.; Hudson, S. Communicating risks to infrastructure due to soil erosion: A bottom-up approach. *Land Degrad. Dev.* **2018**, *29*, 1282–1294. [CrossRef]
46. Volpov, E.; Kishcha, P. An advanced technique for outdoor insulation pollution mapping in the israel electric company power grid. *IEEE Trans. Dielectr. Electr. Insul.* **2017**, *24*, 3539–3548. [CrossRef]
47. Jain, M.K.; Kothyari, U.C. Estimation of soil erosion and sediment yield using GIS. *Hydrol. Sci. J.* **2000**, *45*, 771–786. [CrossRef]
48. Bhattarai, R.; Dutta, D. Estimation of Soil Erosion and Sediment Yield Using GIS at Catchment Scale. *Water Resour. Manag.* **2006**, *21*, 1635–1647. [CrossRef]
49. Fryirs, K. (Dis) Connectivity in catchment sediment cascades: A fresh look at the sediment delivery problem. *Earth Surf. Process. Landforms* **2012**, *38*, 30–46. [CrossRef]
50. Walling, D.E. The sediment delivery problem. *J. Hydrol.* **1983**, *65*, 209–237. [CrossRef]
51. Wohl, E.; Brierley, G.; Cadol, D.; Coulthard, T.J.; Covino, T.; Fryirs, K.A.; Grant, G.; Hilton, R.G.; Lane, S.N.; Magilligan, F.J.; et al. Connectivity as an emergent property of geomorphic systems. *Earth Surf. Process. Landf.* **2018**, *44*, 4–26. [CrossRef]
52. Mahoney, D.T.; Fox, J.F.; Al Aamery, N. Watershed erosion modeling using the probability of sediment connectivity in a gently rolling system. *J. Hydrol.* **2018**, *561*, 862–883. [CrossRef]
53. Heckmann, T.; Cavalli, M.; Cerdan, O.; Foerster, S.; Javaux, M.; Lode, E.; Smetanová, A.; Vericat, D.; Brardinoni, F. Indices of sediment connectivity: Opportunities, challenges and limitations. *Earth Sci. Rev.* **2018**, *187*, 77–108. [CrossRef]
54. Borselli, L.; Cassi, P.; Torri, D. Prolegomena to sediment and flow connectivity in the landscape: A GIS and field numerical assessment. *Catena* **2008**, *75*, 268–277. [CrossRef]
55. Ferreira, C.S.S.; Walsh, R.P.D.; Ferreira, A.J.D. Degradation in urban areas. *Curr. Opin. Environ. Sci. Health* **2018**, *5*, 19–25. [CrossRef]
56. Santikari, V.P.; Murdoch, L.C. Effects of construction-related land use change on streamflow and sediment yield. *J. Environ. Manag.* **2019**, *252*, 109605. [CrossRef] [PubMed]
57. Perez, M.A.; Zech, W.C.; Donald, W.N.; Turochy, R.; Fagan, B.G. Transferring Innovative Erosion and Sediment Control Research Results into Industry Practice. *Water* **2019**, *11*, 2549. [CrossRef]
58. Yoon, B.; Woo, H. Sediment Problems in Korea. *J. Hydraul. Eng.* **2000**, *126*, 486–491. [CrossRef]
59. Yan, H.; Ding, G.; Feng, K.; Zhang, L.; Li, H.; Wang, Y.; Wu, T. Systematic evaluation framework and empirical study of the impacts of building construction dust on the surrounding environment. *J. Clean. Prod.* **2020**, *275*, 122767. [CrossRef]
60. Perez, M.A.; Zech, W.C.; Donald, W.N.; Fang, X. Design Methodology for the Selection of Temporary Erosion and Sediment Control Practices Based on Regional Hydrological Conditions. *J. Hydrol. Eng.* **2016**, *21*, 05016001. [CrossRef]
61. Ercoli, R.F.; Matias, V.R.S.; Zago, V.C.P. Urban Expansion and Erosion Processes in an Area of Environmental Protection in Nova Lima, Minas Gerais State, Brazil. *Front. Environ. Sci.* **2020**, *8*, 52. [CrossRef]
62. Pitt, R.E.; Williamson, D.; Voorhees, J.; Clark, S.; Harrisburg, P.S. Review of Historical Street Dust and Dirt Accumulation and Washoff Data. *JWMM* **2005**. [CrossRef]
63. Zafra, C.A.; Temprano, J.; Tejero, I. Particle size distribution of accumulated sediments on an urban road in rainy weather. *Environ. Technol.* **2008**, *29*, 571–582. [CrossRef]
64. Gustafsson, M.; Blomqvist, G.; Järlskog, I.; Lundberg, J.; Janhäll, S.; Elmgren, M.; Johansson, C.; Norman, M.; Silvergren, S. Road dust load dynamics and influencing factors for six winter seasons in Stockholm, Sweden. *Atmos. Environ. X* **2019**, *2*, 100014. [CrossRef]

65. Seleznev, A.A.; Yarmoshenko, I.V.; Malinovsky, G.P. Assessment of Total Amount of Surface Sediment in Urban Environment Using Data on Solid Matter Content in Snow-Dirt Sludge. *Environ. Process.* **2019**, *6*, 581–595. [CrossRef]
66. Hong, N.; Guan, Y.; Yang, B.; Zhong, J.; Zhu, P.; Ok, Y.S.; Hou, D.; Tsang, D.C.; Guan, Y.; Liu, A. Quantitative source tracking of heavy metals contained in urban road deposited sediments. *J. Hazard. Mater.* **2020**, *393*, 122362. [CrossRef] [PubMed]
67. Guo, L.; Luo, J.; Yuan, M.; Huang, Y.; Shen, H.; Li, T. The influence of urban planning factors on PM2.5 pollution exposure and implications: A case study in China based on remote sensing, LBS, and GIS data. *Sci. Total Environ.* **2019**, *659*, 1585–1596. [CrossRef] [PubMed]
68. Fan, S.; Li, X.; Dong, L. Field assessment of the effects of land-cover type and pattern on PM10 and PM2.5 concentrations in a microscale environment. *Environ. Sci. Pollut. Res.* **2018**, *26*, 2314–2327. [CrossRef] [PubMed]
69. Cook, E.M.; Hall, S.J.; Larson, K.L. Residential landscapes as social-ecological systems: A synthesis of multi-scalar interactions between people and their home environment. *Urban. Ecosyst.* **2011**, *15*, 19–52. [CrossRef]
70. Cadenasso, M.L.; Pickett, S.T.A.; Schwarz, K. Spatial heterogeneity in urban ecosystems: Reconceptualizing land cover and a framework for classification. *Front. Ecol. Environ.* **2007**, *5*, 80–88. [CrossRef]
71. Ziter, C.D.; Pedersen, E.J.; Kucharik, C.J.; Turner, M.G. Scale-dependent interactions between tree canopy cover and impervious surfaces reduce daytime urban heat during summer. *Proc. Natl. Acad. Sci. USA* **2019**, *116*, 7575–7580. [CrossRef]
72. Zhang, A.; Xia, C.; Chu, J.; Lin, J.; Li, W.; Wu, J. Portraying urban landscape: A quantitative analysis system applied in fifteen metropolises in China. *Sustain. Cities Soc.* **2019**, *46*, 101396. [CrossRef]
73. Rioux, J.-F.; Cimon-Morin, J.; Pellerin, S.; Alard, D.; Poulin, M. How Land Cover Spatial Resolution Affects Mapping of Urban Ecosystem Service Flows. *Front. Environ. Sci.* **2019**, *7*, 93. [CrossRef]
74. Bogdan, S.-M.; Pătru-Stupariu, I.; Zaharia, L. The Assessment of Regulatory Ecosystem Services: The Case of the Sediment Retention Service in a Mountain Landscape in the Southern Romanian Carpathians. *Procedia Environ. Sci.* **2016**, *32*, 12–27. [CrossRef]
75. Apitz, S.E. Conceptualizing the role of sediment in sustaining ecosystem services: Sediment-ecosystem regional assessment (SEcoRA). *Sci. Total Environ.* **2012**, *415*, 9–30. [CrossRef]
76. Russell, K.L.; Vietz, G.J.; Fletcher, T.D. Urban catchment runoff increases bedload sediment yield and particle size in stream channels. *Anthropocene* **2018**, *23*, 53–66. [CrossRef]
77. Cui, M.; Lu, H.; Etyemezian, V.; Su, Q. Quantifying the emission potentials of fugitive dust sources in Nanjing, East China. *Atmos. Environ.* **2019**, *207*, 129–135. [CrossRef]
78. Ferreira, C.S.S.; Walsh, R.P.D.; Blake, W.H.; Kikuchi, R.; Ferreira, A.J.D. Temporal Dynamics of Sediment Sources in an Urbanizing Mediterranean Catchment. *Land Degrad. Dev.* **2017**, *28*, 2354–2369. [CrossRef]
79. Seleznev, A.; Yarmoshenko, I.; Malinovsky, G.; Ilgasheva, E.; Baglaeva, E.; Ryanskaya, A.; Kiseleva, D.; Gulyaeva, T. Snow-dirt sludge as an indicator of environmental and sedimentation processes in the urban environment. *Sci. Rep.* **2019**, *9*, 17241. [CrossRef] [PubMed]
80. Seleznev, A.A.; Teterin, A.F.; Yarmoshenko, I.V. Meteorological conditions of surface sediment runoff formation during spring snowmelt in urban environment. *Bull. Tomsk Polytech. Univ. Geo Assets Eng.* **2020**, *331*, 7–16. [CrossRef]

Publisher's Note: MDPI stays neutral with regard to jurisdictional claims in published maps and institutional affiliations.

© 2020 by the authors. Licensee MDPI, Basel, Switzerland. This article is an open access article distributed under the terms and conditions of the Creative Commons Attribution (CC BY) license (http://creativecommons.org/licenses/by/4.0/).

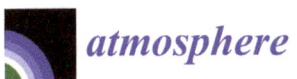

Article

SCAMPER Monitoring Platform to Measure PM_{10} Emission Rates from Unpaved Roads in Real-Time

Dennis R. Fitz * and Kurt Bumiller

Center for Environmental Research and Technology, College of Engineering, University of California, Riverside, CA 92507, USA; kurt@kurtbumiller.com
* Correspondence: dfitz@cert.ucr.edu

Abstract: The SCAMPER method for measuring PM_{10} emission rates from roadways was used to evaluate mitigation methods for public unpaved roads and a treated mine haul road. The SCAMPER method uses a small trailer to measure PM_{10} concentrations behind a vehicle at a point that is representative of the mean PM_{10} concentration in the vehicle's wake. This concentration multiplied by the frontal area has been shown to be a reasonable estimate of the emission rate in units of grams per meter traveled. On public roads it was towed by a 2006 Ford Expedition and on a mine haul road it was towed behind both the Expedition and an earth mover weighing over 150 tons fully loaded. Since the SCAMPER is capable of measuring emission rates on both paved and unpaved roadways, a direct comparison of the effectiveness of mitigation methods with respect to a similar paved road was possible.

Keywords: PM_{10}; road dust; fugitive dust; particulate matter; unpaved roads; emission factors

Citation: Fitz, D.R.; Bumiller, K. SCAMPER Monitoring Platform to Measure PM_{10} Emission Rates from Unpaved Roads in Real-Time. *Atmosphere* **2021**, *12*, 1301. https://doi.org/10.3390/atmos12101301

Academic Editors: Dmitry Vlasov, Omar Ramírez Hernández and Ashok Luhar

Received: 28 August 2021
Accepted: 28 September 2021
Published: 6 October 2021

Publisher's Note: MDPI stays neutral with regard to jurisdictional claims in published maps and institutional affiliations.

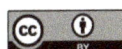

Copyright: © 2021 by the authors. Licensee MDPI, Basel, Switzerland. This article is an open access article distributed under the terms and conditions of the Creative Commons Attribution (CC BY) license (https://creativecommons.org/licenses/by/4.0/).

1. Introduction

Particulate matter less than 10 μm aerodynamic diameter (PM_{10}) has been implicated as being responsible for a wide variety of adverse health effects that have been shown in epidemiological studies to contribute to premature deaths [1]. For this reason concentration standards have been promulgated by many governments to protect the health of its citizens. These standards are routinely exceeded in many urban areas. In order to formulate effective mitigation approaches, the sources of the PM must be accurately known. Receptor modeling has shown that PM_{10} of geologic origin is often a significant contributor to the PM_{10} concentrations in areas that are in non-attainment and a significant portion of this geologic material has been estimated to originate from paved roads [2]. While unpaved roads are less common in urban areas, the nature of their road surface could lead to potentially large emission rates of geologic material and these roads are often found in many parts of the western United States. In addition, construction and other industrial activities sometimes use unpaved roadways, often used by heavy duty vehicles.

Since emissions from roadways cannot, by their nature, be measured directly, they must be calculated from the characteristics of a line source plume. This has been done using dispersion modeling [3–5], receptor modeling [6] a combination of dispersion and receptor modeling [7,8], tracer studies [9–11], measuring the flux of PM_{10} through a horizontal plane downwind of the source [12–17] and measurement of PM_{10} concentrations near the wheel or in the wake of a vehicle [18–22]. Using flux measurements the U.S. Environmental Protection Agency (EPA) in document AP-42 has derived empirical equations for estimating particulate emissions from both paved and unpaved roads using metrics such as surface silt and moisture content, mean vehicle weight, and mean speed [23,24].

For industrial unpaved roads the EPA equation for the PM_{10} emission rate in units of grams (g) per Vehicle Kilometer Traveled (VKT) is:

$$E = 423 * (s/12)^{0.9} * (W/3)^{0.45} \text{ g/VKT} \tag{1}$$

For public unpaved roads the EPA equation for the PM_{10} emission rate in units of g/VKT is:

$$E = 507 * (s/12) * (S/30)^{0.5} / (M/0.5)^{0.2} \text{ g/VKT} \quad (2)$$

where:

$E = PM_{10}$ emission factor g/VKT

s = surface material silt (silt defined as dry material passing through a 200 mesh screen) content (%)

W = mean vehicle weight in U.S. tons

M = surface material moisture content (%)

S = mean vehicle speed (miles per hour)

In many cases default values are used for these metrics, which can lead to large uncertainties.

We have previously reported the development and evaluation of SCAMPER (System for the Continuous Aerosol Measurement of Particle Emissions from Roads), a mobile real-time method that samples in the vehicle's wake on paved roads to determine PM_{10} emission rates [25,26]. Other mobile methods that sample PM_{10} near the vehicle's wheel, require the use of particle diluters so that the concentrations do not exceed the upper limit of the optical sensors used. This adds a great deal of complexity to the sampling system, which is generally integrated into the test vehicle. Since the SCAMPER samples in the vehicle's wake, the PM is much diluted and concentrations, even on unpaved roads, remain within the sensor's limits. In addition, it is much easier to move the system from one vehicle to another.

In the following we discuss the use of SCAMPER in measuring the emission rates from unpaved roads. While the AP-42 equation estimates PM_{10} emissions from unpaved roads using independent variables, the SCAMPER approach directly measures emissions and does not depend on these variables. In addition, a large amount of emission data may be easily collected. The data from the unpaved roads we report here was used to evaluate the effectiveness of surface treatments on public roadways and a mine haul road. We also showed that the measurement equipment can be attached to heavy duty vehicles, in this case 150 tons, to determine PM emission rates from any type of vehicle. This is the first time that mobile methods have been reported in measuring the PM_{10} emission rates from such heavy duty vehicles.

2. Materials and Methods

2.1. SCAMPER Description

The SCAMPER determines PM emission rates from roads by measuring the PM concentrations in front of (mounted on the hood) and behind the vehicle (mounted on a small open trailer) using optical sensors with a 1 s time resolution. As a first approximation, the concentration difference between the two (in mg m^{-3}) is multiplied by the vehicle's frontal area (m^2) to obtain an emission factor in units of mg m^{-1}. The system and its validation has previously been described [25,26]. Briefly, the SCAMPER includes five major components:

1. Tow vehicle and Trailer: A 2006 Ford Expedition was used to tow a small (3.1 m wide by 2 m long) open flatbed trailer. The trailer was fitted with a 1 m hitch extension to place the rear sampling inlet 3 m behind the tow vehicle at a height of 0.8 m above the ground on the centerline of the trailer. This position was found to give PM_{10} concentrations that were representative of the mean concentration of PM_{10} in the wake of the tow vehicle [24].
2. PM_{10} Sensors: Thermo Systems Inc. (Shoreville, MN, USA) Model 8520 DustTrak™ optical PM sensors with PM_{10} inlets.
3. Isokinetic Sampling Inlets: A custom made inlet where the inlet speed is matched to the air speed by a PC that monitors the static air pressure and adjusts the inlet pressure to match it by controlling a vacuum pump (mounted on the trailer). This

condition creates a no-pressure-drop inlet; therefore, the sampled air stream has the same energy as the ambient air stream.
4. Global Positioning System: Garmin (Kansas City, MO, USA) Map76 GPS to determine vehicle speed and location.
5. Data Collection System: A laptop PC was used to collect GPS and DustTrak™ data at 1s intervals in addition to controlling the inlet vacuum pumps.

2.2. Public Unpaved Road PM_{10} Emission Measurements

Field measurements of PM_{10} emission rates were made on two different Arizona state highways, State Routes SR 88 and SR 288. The SCAMPER test vehicle was operated at speeds consistent with safe operation and that observed of other vehicles. The segment of SR88 between mile point 220.1 and mile point 227.5 (12 km) was treated with Envirotac II Acrylic copolymer (Environmental Products and Applications, Inc., La Quinta, CA, USA) at a rate of 1.1 Lm^{-2}. To the west the road was paved and to the east it was unpaved gravel. The section between mile points 226.5 and 227.5 was treated two years before the measurement study and the section between mile points 220.1 and 226.5 was treated five months before. The SCAMPER testing was conducted from Tortilla Flats, AZ (GPS coordinates 33.5268 by −111.3896) eastbound on paved road to mile point 220.1 (GPS coordinates 33.5383 by −111.3258) where the road transitioned from paved to treated gravel. The treated section ended at mile point 227.5 (GPS coordinates 33.5483 by −111.2563) and the SCAMPER vehicle continued eastward on untreated gravel until reaching GPS coordinates 33.5829 by −111.22143 (10 km) where it turned around and headed westbound back to Tortilla Flats.

The segment of SR 288 between mile points 274.7 and 280.5 (9 km) was treated the year before the study by milling 15 cm of the base material that had just been treated with SS-1 low setting emulsion (McAsphalt Industries Limited, Toronto ON, Canada) followed by an application of their CRS II emulsified liquid at a rate of 1.6 L m^{-2} and then overlain with 14 kg m^{-2} of 1 cm stone chips. The road was untreated gravel on both sides of the treated section. The SCAMPER test route consisted of a circuit starting on the south approximately 0.4 km from the treated section (GPS coordinates of 33.7468 by −110.9624), covering the treated section (GPS coordinates 33.7496 by −110.9650 at the southern end and 33.7879 by −110.9714 at the northern end) and continued north on the gravel for another 0.4 km (GPS coordinates of 33.7935 by −110.9719).

2.3. Mine Haul Road PM_{10} Emission Measurements

The mine haul road was located near the Cricket Mountains in Utah. It was generally straight and approximately eight km long. The native soil of the road had been treated with a dust suppressant. The SCAMPER was used in its normal configuration (Ford Expedition tow vehicle) for measuring PM_{10} emissions during all of the first day of sampling and all but one roundtrip on the second day of sampling. The average speed was 72 ± 4 km/h. A frontal area of 3.66 m^2 was used for the Ford Expedition and the estimated weight is 2.5 tons. After completing four round trips on the second day of sampling, the SCAMPER equipment was installed on the haul vehicle (see Figure 1) for all subsequent testing. The average speed was 53 ± 5 km/h. The frontal area of the haul vehicle was estimated to be 10.6 m^2 based on the overall height and width. The weight of the haul truck was approximately 50 tons empty and 150 tons fully loaded.

PM_{10} filter samples (47 mm Teflo™ Ringed Filter, 2 μm pore) were also collected on the SCAMPER trailer when it was attached to the haul truck using a Sierra Andersen model 241 inlet adapted to a 47 mm filter holder and sampled at 16.7 L m^{-1}. The inlets of these samples were collocated with the DustTrak™ inlets. A total of sixteen filter samples were collected. Each collection was conducted over one direction of the haul road. Filters were equilibrated to 25 °C and 40% RH and weighed before and after collection to the nearest microgram using a Cahn (Irvine, CA, USA) model C-25 electro-balance.

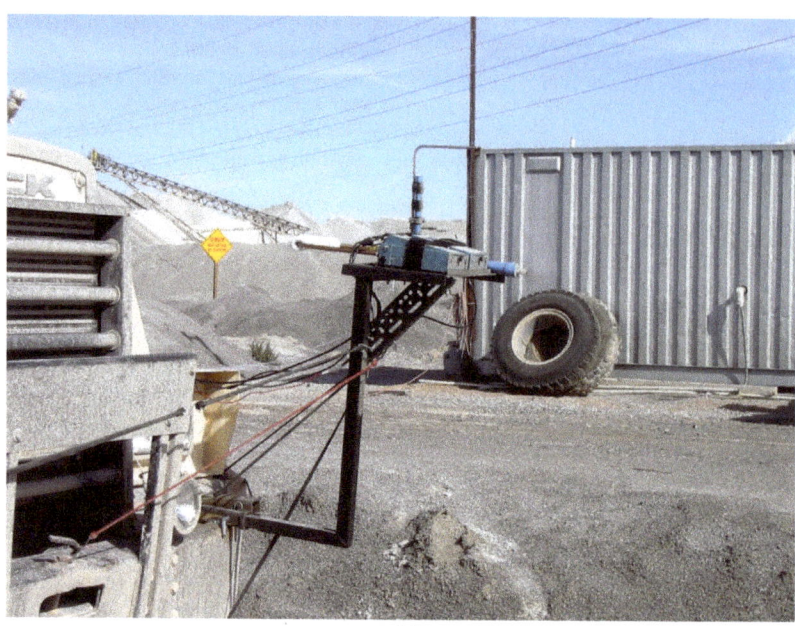

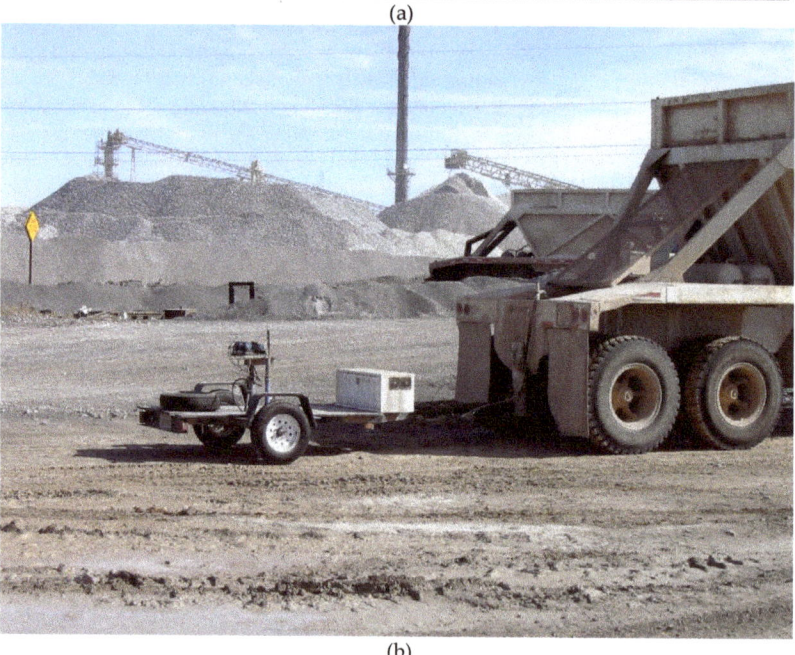

Figure 1. Photographs of the SCAMPER equipment outfitted on the front (**a**) and rear (**b**) of the mine haul vehicle.

3. Results

3.1. Arizona Public Roads

The zero of the DustTrak™ was determined before, after, and at least once during the test runs. The drift during the course of the each test day was less than a few μgm^{-3}, near the 1 μgm^{-3} detection limit of the instrument. The data for each test run was corrected for zero offset using the mean zero response for that day. The output of the rear DustTrak™ occasionally spiked, either positively or negatively. These spikes were probably due to physical shock from the rough unpaved roads. These spikes always showed up on two consecutive seconds. They were unlikely to be associated with an actual PM$_{10}$ concentration as concentrations rarely change to that degree in less than one second. The two-second characteristic of this noise spike was also expected from the internal averaging and output characteristics of the DustTrak™. On the time constant we selected (which is the shortest available) the DustTrak™ output was a two-second running average that updated every second. A large spike in a one-second period will therefore show up as two smaller spikes for two consecutive seconds. To filter this noise we tabulated the data as 5-second running medians. The two-second spikes therefore were removed from the data set. The net PM$_{10}$ concentration was determined by subtracting the concentration of the front DustTrak™ from that of the rear. The net value multiplied the net PM$_{10}$ concentration by the frontal area of the test vehicle, to obtain the PM$_{10}$ emission rate in units of mg m^{-1}.

3.1.1. SR 88

Figure 2 summarizes the data on a map. In this map the emission rates are represented as circles with the shading becoming darker as the emission rates become larger. Progressing from left to right, the emissions increase as the SCAMPER transverses paved, treated unpaved, and untreated unpaved roads. Figure 3 shows the time series of PM$_{10}$ emission rates calculated as a running ten-second average for periods when the running average speed was greater than 16 km h^{-1} (below this speed the wake may not be well formed). The units are in mg m^{-1}. The data from treated and untreated unpaved roads are highlighted, as are the paved road sections.

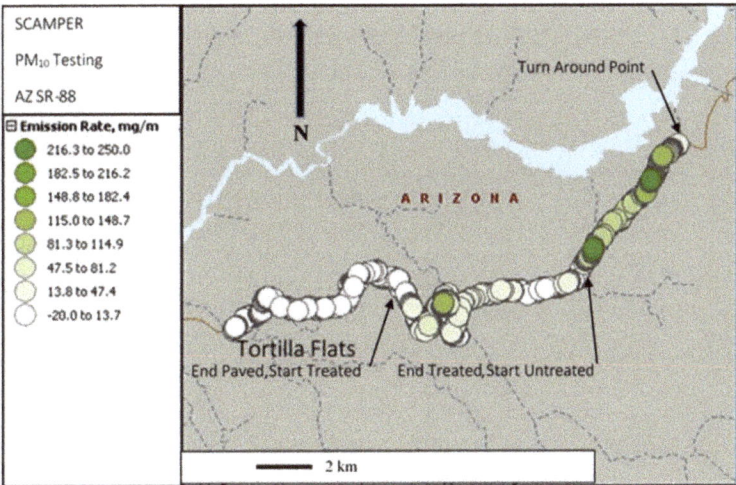

Figure 2. PM$_{10}$ emission rates in mg m^{-1} superimposed on the map of the test segments used on SR 88.

Table 1 summarizes the data for the three completed passes of the test route. The average emission rate of the treated gravel section was approximately five times lower than the untreated gravel section. In both cases the average speed was near 30 km h^{-1}. Spikes in the emission rate were observed at repeatable times for both treated and untreated sections, likely indicating road surfaces containing higher fractions of finer soil. Based on the reproducibility of the segment emission rate data, the precision of the measurements for both the treated and untreated sections was reasonable, especially considering the potential operational variability from run to run. In order to estimate the precision of the measurements the assumption was made that the east and west bound emission rates should be equivalent. The mean emission rate for each circuit are derived from a robust data set of hundreds of measurements conducted over 10 km. The relative standard deviation of the mean emission rates of the treated circuits was 15% while that of the untreated was 27%. This is in good agreement with the precision of approximately 20% for the much larger data set from paved roads [26].

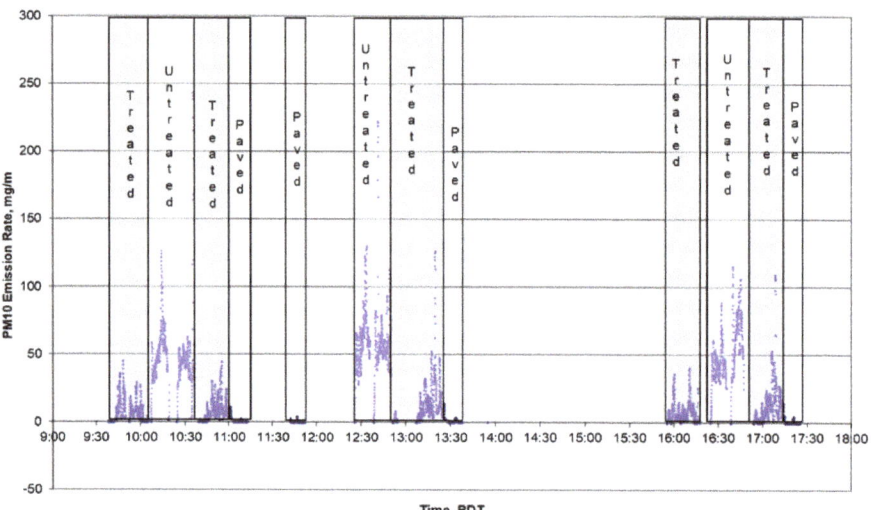

Figure 3. Time series plot of PM_{10} emission rates during the test conducted on SR88.

Table 1. Summary of mean PM_{10} emission rates (ER) for the test route on SR88.

Segment, Direction	Circuit1	Circuit2	Circuit3	Overall Means
Treated Time Eastbound	09:41–10:06		15:55–16:18	
Treated Mean ER Eastbound, mg/m	8.9		8.1	8.5
Treated Mean Speed Eastbound, km/h	31.7		32.1	31.9
Untreated Time Eastbound, MST	10:07–10:19	12:26–12:36	16:25–16:35	
Untreated Mean ER Eastbound, mg/m	51.6	60.5	42.8	51.6
Untreated Mean Speed Eastbound, km/h	27.3	30.0	31.3	29.5
Untreated Time Westbound, MST	1034–10:37	12:38–12:50	16:38–16:47	
Untreated Mean ER Westbound, mg/m	47.2	61.4	63.0	57.2
Untreated Mean Speed Westbound, km/h	28.0	26.6	33.5	29.3
Treated Time Westbound, MST	10:39–11:02	12:51–13:27	16:54–17:15	
Treated Mean ER Westbound, mg/m	8.5	13.8	13.3	11.9
Treated Mean Speed Westbound, km/h	30.4	30.2	33.3	31.3
Paved Road Westbound Time, MST	11:03–11:13	13:29–13:38	17:16–1725	
Paved ER Westbound to Tortilla Flats, mg/m	0.3	0.7	0.3	0.4
Paved Speed Westbound to Tortilla Flats, km/h	52.9	52.6	53.5	53.0
Paved Road Eastbound Time, MST	11:42–11:52			
Paved ER Eastbound from Tortilla Flats, mg/m	0.3			0.3
Paved Speed Eastbound from Tortilla Flats, km/h	50.9			50.9
Untreated Overall Mean Emission Rate, mg/m				54.4
Treated Overall Mean Emission Rate, mg/m				10.5
Paved Road Overall Mean Emission Rate, mg/m				0.4

While neither the silt nor the moisture content of the unpaved roadway was measured, we have typically measured silt content of 14% and moisture of less than 4% in soils from the desert southwestern United States. Using these values, a weight of 2.5 tons for the tow vehicle, and a mean speed of 30 km h^{-1} yields an emission rate of 700 mg m^{-1}. The AP-42 equation therefore appears to significantly overestimate the PM_{10} emissions from the unpaved road.

3.1.2. SR 288

Figure 4 summarizes the data on a map. The higher emissions at the top and bottom of the section are from the unpaved segments while the much lower ones are clearly seen in the middle. Figure 5 shows the time series of PM_{10} emission rates calculated as a running ten-second average for periods when the running average speed was greater than 16 km h^{-1}. The data from treated and untreated unpaved roads are highlighted.

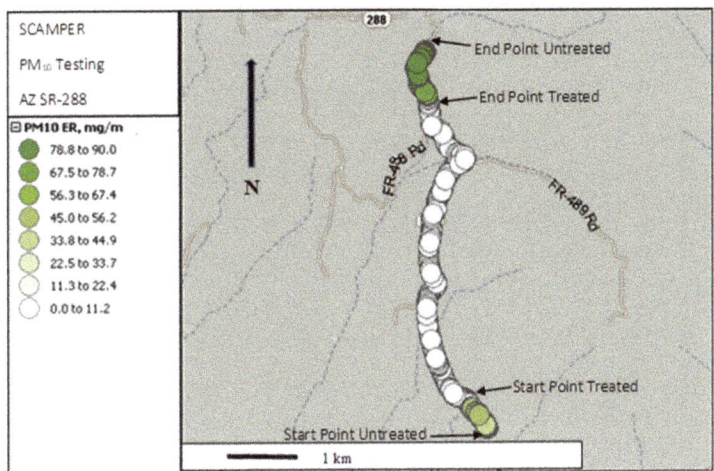

Figure 4. Map of the test segments used on SR288.

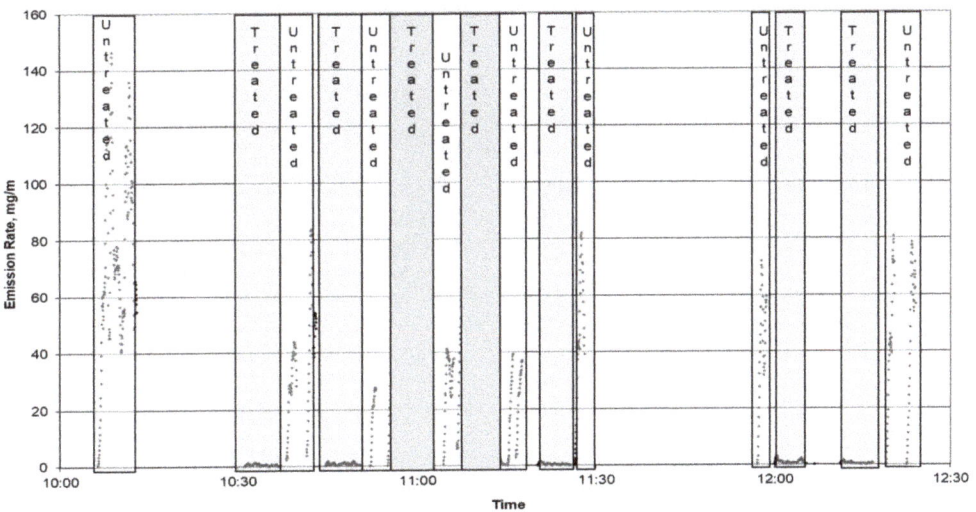

Figure 5. Time series plot of PM_{10} emissions during the test on SR288.

Table 2 summarizes the data. The PM_{10} emission rate from the untreated road was similar to that on the untreated section of SR 88 and much less than the AP-42 estimation of 700 mg m^{-1}. The average emission rate of the treated gravel section was approximately sixty times lower than the untreated gravel section. In addition, the average speed on the treated sections was nearly twice that of the untreated section (52 vs. 25 km h^{-1}), so higher emissions would be expected if the treatment was ineffective. Spikes in the emission rate were observed at repeatable times for only the untreated section, likely indicating road surfaces containing higher fractions of finer soil, which were not found on the treated section. The PM_{10} emission rate from the treated section was nearly as low as the asphalt paved portion of SR 88. Since SR 88 had a higher traffic density than SR 288, the emissions from its paved segment are expected to be lower than if a segment of SR 288 were paved. We therefore conclude that the PM_{10} emissions from the treated portion of SR 288 is what would be expected of asphalt pavement. Again assuming that both directions are equivalent, the relative standard deviation for all the untreated circuits was 43% while that of the treated was 32%. The higher value for the untreated segments was likely due to their relatively short lengths (0.4 km).

Table 2. Summary of mean PM_{10} emission rates for the test route on SR 288.

Direction, Segment	Circuit1	Circuit2	Circuit3	Circuit4	Circuit 5	Overall Means
South Untreated Time Northbound, MST	10:05–10:13	10:53–10:56	11:17–11:18	11:45–11:46	12:08–12:10	
South Untreated Mean ER Northbound, mg/m	74.4	29.4	22.7	ND*	ND	42.2
South Untreated Mean Speed Northbound, km/h	30.5	21.2	20.1	NA	NA	23.9
Treated Time Northbound, MST	10:31–10:37	10:57–11:03	11:20–11:26	11:40–11:52	12:11–12:17	
Treated Mean ER Northbound, mg/m	0.5	0.4	0.4	ND*	0.5	0.4
Treated Mean Speed Northbound, km/h	49.0	51.3	52.6	NA	53.6	51.0
North Untreated Time Northbound, MST	10:38–10:40	11:04–11:06	11:26–11:28	11:52–11:54	12:19–12:20	
North Untreated Mean ER Northbound, mg/m	26.8	28.7	40.2	ND*	39.3	31.9
North Untreated Mean Speed Northbound, km/h	21.7	42.6	22.5	NA	25.1	28.9
North Untreated Time Southbound, MST	10:40–10:43	11:07–11:08	11:35–11:36	11:57–11:59	12:23–12:24	
North Untreated Mean ER Southbound, mg/m	48.9	40.3	ND*	39.8	45.4	43.0
North Untreated Mean Speed Southbound, km/h	24.3	24.4	NA	24.3	25.1	24.3
Treated Time Southbound, MST	10:45–10:52	11:09–11:15	11:37–11:42	12:00–12:05	12:26–12:31	
Treated Mean ER Southbound, mg/m	0.7	0.7	ND*	0.9	ND	0.8
Treated Mean Speed Southbound, km/h	49.4	51.9	NA	55.8	NA	52.4
South Untreated Time Southbound, MST	10:52–10:53	11:15–11:16	11:43–11:44	12:07–12:08	12:32–12:33	
South Untreated ER Southbound, mg/m	16.4	18.0	ND*	ND	ND	17.2
South Untreated Speed Southbound, km/h	20.5	20.7	NA	NA	NA	20.6
Untreated Overall Mean Emission Rate, mg/m						36.2
Treated Overall Mean Emission Rate, mg/m						0.6
Untreated Overall Mean Speed, km/h						24.8
Treated Overall Mean Speed, km/h						51.9

ND* = No Data-filtered air control, ND = Rear DustTrak failed, NA = Not Available.

3.2. Mine Haul Road

Table 3 shows the average and standard deviation of the PM_{10} emission rate determined for each pass of the SCAMPER using the Ford Expedition as the test vehicle. The emission rate standard deviations of the individual test runs are higher than the mean value, indicating significant variation in emission rates along the roadway. The overall average emission rate in the northwest direction was 0.51 mg m^{-1}, while in the southeast direction it was 0.52 mg m^{-1}, values similar to the paved portion of SR 88. This shows that the PM_{10} emission potential for each direction is similar and that the measurement method is reproducible. The precision based on the relative standard deviation of the direction means was approximately 80% and may be due to the relatively low emission rates compared to unpaved roads.

Table 4 shows the average and standard deviation of the PM_{10} emission rate determined for each pass of the SCAMPER using the haul truck as the test vehicle. The values for the haul truck were, as expected, considerably higher than that obtained using the Ford Expedition. The average emission rate for the northeast direction (unloaded) was 4.0 mg m^{-1} while that for the southeast direction (loaded) was significantly higher at 7.3 mg m^{-1}. The overall precision based on the relative standard deviation was 80% in the unloaded direction and 70% in the loaded direction.

If one assumes 14% silt content, and applies the AP-42 equation for unpaved roads, the PM_{10} emission rate is calculated to be 450 mg m^{-1} for the Expedition, 1700 mg/m for an unloaded haul truck and 2800 mg/m for the loaded haul truck. It is clear that the AP-42 equation grossly over predicts the PM_{10} emission rate for this treated road. Taking the ratio of the AP-42 estimated emission rate to the mean measured rate gives 873 for the Expedition, 425 for the unloaded haul truck, and 383 for the loaded haul truck. Given the large differences between the weights of the Expedition compared to the haul truck, it is not surprising that ratios are quite different. The ratios for the unloaded and loaded haul truck, however, are similar, indicating the weight term in the AP-42 equation is valid.

Table 3. SCAMPER PM_{10} pass-averaged emission rate data for the Ford Expedition for each direction of each test run.

Time (Local)	Direction	Emission Rate mg m^{-1}	Std Dev Emission Rate mg m^{-1}	Mean Speed km h^{-1}
Day 1				
10:47	NW	0.22	0.82	67
11:05	NW	0.09	0.12	70
12:02	NW	0.08	0.78	73
12:19	NW	0.17	0.92	75
12:39	NW	0.63	0.63	75
10:57	SE	0.01	0.15	69
11:15	SE	0.15	0.35	76
12:11	SE	0.15	1.16	76
12:33	SE	0.46	0.67	75
12:51	SE	0.68	1.01	77
Day 2				
12:46	NW	0.91	2.37	67
13:05	NW	1.21	3.58	64
13:23	NW	0.76	1.38	71
12:55	SE	1.19	3.81	70
13:15	SE	0.88	2.84	72
13:33	SE	0.61	1.84	71
Mean	NW	0.51		70
Std Dev	NW	0.43		4
Mean	SE	0.52		73
Std Dev	SE	0.41		3

Table 4. SCAMPER PM_{10} pass-averaged emission rate data for the haul truck for each direction of each test run.

Date/Time (Local)	Direction	Emission Rate mg m^{-1}	Std Dev Emission Rate mg m^{-1}
Day 1			
8:26	NW	1.5	3.2
9:13	NW	3.9	11.8
10:00	NW	2.6	7.9
10:47	NW	4.6	7.1
13:18	NW	8.2	3.1
16:02	NW	4.4	8.4

Table 4. Cont.

Date/Time (Local)	Direction	Emission Rate mg m^{-1}	Std Dev Emission Rate mg m^{-1}
8:48	SE	4.9	13.7
9:35	SE	0.5	0.6
10:24	SE	1.4	3.1
13:41	SE	13.8	18.9
15:20	SE	12.9	8.2
16:26	SE	8.4	7.8
Day 2			
8:25	NW	0.1	0.3
10:49	NW	1.3	3.6
11:36	NW	3.9	7.0
13:54	NW	2.9	2.8
14:51	NW	3.5	3.6
11:13	SE	2.9	5.8
11:58	SE	10.7	7.1
14:23	SE	15.9	22.4
15:29	SE	11.2	14.2
Day 3			
7:22	NW	0.6	0.7
8:34	NW	1.6	2.1
9:36	NW	2.7	3.6
11:22	NW	4.7	4.0
12:21	NW	11.2	7.0
12:57	NW	10.7	5.9
8:04	SE	1.0	1.1
9:05	SE	2.1	2.0
10:07	SE	4.1	4.9
11:53	SE	13.3	22.6
12:40	SE	6.0	6.5
13:27	SE	7.3	7.7
Mean NW		4.0	
Std Dev		3.2	
Mean SE		7.3	
Std Dev		5.1	

Although the measured emission rates for the haul road were similar to those measured on paved roads, it is not clear that the AP-42 paved road equation would be appropriate to predict PM_{10} emission rates of the haul road. This would require vacuuming of the road surface to determine the surface silt loading, which may not be compatible with this treated surface. The AP-42 equation for estimating PM_{10} emissions from paved roads is as follows:

$$E = k(sL/)^{0.92} (W)^{1.01} \text{ g/VKT} \qquad (3)$$

where:

E = PM$_{10}$ emission factor in the units shown
k = A constant dependent on the aerodynamic size range of PM (0.62) for PM$_{10}$
sL = Road surface silt loading of material smaller than 75 μm in g/m^2
W = mean vehicle weight in tons
VKT = vehicle kilometer traveled

Based on the weight of the vehicles, it would be expected that the PM$_{10}$ emissions from the full haul truck would be 3 times that of the empty one and 65 times that of the Ford Expedition. The measured ratios were significantly lower, 1.8 and 14. As with the AP-42 values, the large difference in ratio between the haul truck and the Expedition are likely to be due to an over-extrapolation of the equation that was derived from lighter vehicles. The ratio between the unloaded and loaded haul trucks seems reasonable despite this potential over-extrapolation.

3.3. Comparison of DustTrak™ with Filter Samples

The DustTrak™ is calibrated at the factory using a standard NIST Arizona road dust. Figure 6 compares the PM$_{10}$ filter concentration data with the concentration data from the collocated DustTrak™ integrated over the period in which the collocated filter sampler was operated. The 0.41 R^2 value and slope of 2.5 is typical of what we have previously measured with SCAMPER [26], indicating that the DustTrak™ emission measurements presented here are low by this factor when compared to emission rates on a mass basis.

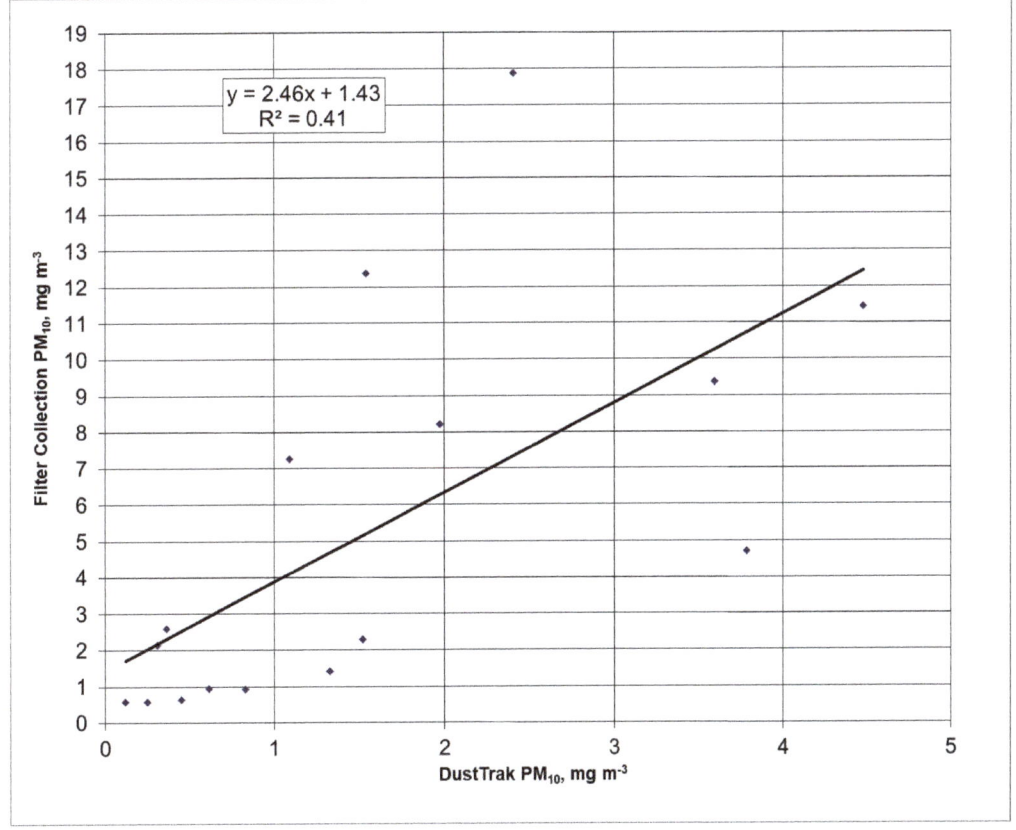

Figure 6. Comparison of PM$_{10}$ filter and DustTrak™ data.

4. Summary and Conclusions

The effectiveness of using dust suppressants to reduce PM_{10} reduction from unpaved roads was quantified for segments of SR 88 and 288. The suppressant applied to SR 88 five months ago reduced PM_{10} emissions by a factor of five. The suppressant applied to SR 288 a year ago reduced PM_{10} emissions by a factor of sixty. The SCAMPER has been shown to collect reliable emission rates from unpaved roads with a precision of approximately 20%. The measured emission rates, on a mass basis were approximately seven time higher than those predicted by the AP-42 unpaved road equation.

For the haul road measurements, the average PM_{10} emission rates were 4.0 and 7.3 mg m^{-1} for the unloaded and loaded haul trucks, respectively. The ratio of these emission rates are consistent with the weight variation predicted by the AP-42 equation for unpaved roads. The AP-42 PM_{10} equation for unpaved PM_{10} emission rates, however, over predicts the emission rates of this haul road by approximately a factor of approximately 170 on a mass basis for haul trucks. Based on the Expedition's measured emission rate on paved roads indicated that the emissions from this haul road are consistent with a paved road.

Author Contributions: Conceptualization, D.R.F.; Data curation, K.B.; Formal analysis, D.R.F.; Investigation, K.B.; Methodology, D.R.F.; Project administration, D.R.F.; Writing—original draft, D.R.F.; Writing—review & editing, D.R.F. All authors have read and agreed to the published version of the manuscript.

Funding: This research was directly funded by Sierra Research Inc. and Holland and Hart, LLP.

Institutional Review Board Statement: Not applicable.

Informed Consent Statement: Not applicable.

Data Availability Statement: The finalized data are contained within the article. The raw data do not reside in a publicly available data set, but are available from the corresponding author.

Acknowledgments: We thank Sierra Research Inc. and Holland and Hart LLP for providing the financial support to conduct this research.

Conflicts of Interest: The authors declare no conflict of interest.

References

1. Pope, C.A.; Thun, M.J.; Namboodiri, M.M.; Dockery, D.W.; Evans, J.S.; Speizer, F.E.; Heath, C.W. Particulate Air Pollution as a Predictor of Mortality in a Prospective Study of U.S. Adults. *Am. J. Respir. Crit. Care Med.* **1995**, *151*, 669–674. [CrossRef]
2. Chow, J.C.; Watson, J.; Lowenthal, D.H.; Solomon, P.A.; Magliano, K.L.; Ziman, S.D.; Richards, L.W. PM_{10} source apportionment in California's San Joaquin valley. *Atmos. Environ. Part A Gen. Top.* **1992**, *26*, 3335–3354. [CrossRef]
3. Venkatram, A.; Fitz, D.; Bumiller, K.; Du, S.; Boeck, M.; Ganguly, C. Using a dispersion model to estimate emission rates of particulate matter from paved roads. *Atmos. Environ.* **1999**, *33*, 1093–1102. [CrossRef]
4. Kauhaniemi, M.; Kukkonen, J.; Härkönen, J.; Nikmo, J.; Kangas, L.; Omstedt, G.; Ketzel, M.; Kousa, A.; Haakana, M.; Karppinen, A. Evaluation of a road dust suspension model for predicting the concentrations of PM_{10} in a street canyon. *Atmos. Environ.* **2011**, *45*, 3646–3654. [CrossRef]
5. Denby, B.; Sundvor, I.; Johansson, C.; Pirjola, L.; Ketzel, M.; Norman, M.; Kupiainen, K.; Gustafsson, M.; Blomqvist, G.; Omstedt, G. A coupled road dust and surface moisture model to predict non-exhaust road traffic induced particle emissions (NORTRIP). Part 1: Road dust loading and suspension modelling. *Atmos. Environ.* **2013**, *77*, 283–300. [CrossRef]
6. Abu-Allaban, M.; Gillies, J.A.; Gertler, A.W. Application of a multi-lag regression approach to determine on-road PM_{10} and $PM_{2.5}$ emission rates. *Atmos. Environ.* **2003**, *37*, 5157–5164. [CrossRef]
7. Abu-Allaban, M.; Gillies, J.A.; Gertler, A.W.; Clayton, R.; Proffitt, D. Tailpipe, resuspended road dust, and brake-wear emission factors from on-road vehicles. *Atmos. Environ.* **2003**, *37*, 5283–5293. [CrossRef]
8. Kumar, A.V.; Patil, R.; Nambi, K. A composite receptor and dispersion model approach for estimation of effective emission factors for vehicles. *Atmos. Environ.* **2004**, *38*, 7065–7072. [CrossRef]
9. Claiborn, C.; Mitra, A.; Adams, G.; Bamesberger, L.; Allwine, G.; Kantamaneni, R.; Lamb, B.; Westberg, H. Evaluation of PM_{10} emission rates from paved and unpaved roads using tracer techniques. *Atmos. Environ.* **1995**, *29*, 1075–1089. [CrossRef]
10. Kantamaneni, R.; Adams, G.; Bamesberger, L.; Allwine, E.; Westberg, H.; Lamb, B.; Claiborn, C. The measurement of roadway PM_{10} emission rates using atmospheric tracer ratio techniques. *Atmos. Environ.* **1996**, *30*, 4209–4223. [CrossRef]

11. Ferm, M.; Sjöberg, K. Concentrations and emission factors for $PM_{2.5}$ and PM_{10} from road traffic in Sweden. *Atmos. Environ.* **2015**, *119*, 211–219. [CrossRef]
12. Sehmel, G. Particle resuspension from an asphalt road caused by car and truck traffic. *Atmos. Environ.* **1973**, *7*, 291–309. [CrossRef]
13. Cowherd, C., Jr.; Englehart, P.J. *Paved Road Particulate Emissions*; U.S. Environmental Protection Agency Document EPA-600/7-84-077; U.S. Environmental Protection Agency: Washington, DC, USA, 1984.
14. Xueli, J.; Dahe, J.; Simei, F.; Hui, Y.; Pinjing, H.; Boming, Y.; Zhongliang, L.; Chang, F. Road dust emission inventory for the metropolitan area of Shanghai City. *Atmos. Environ. Part A Gen. Top.* **1993**, *27*, 1735–1741. [CrossRef]
15. Veranth, J.M.; Pardyjak, E.R.; Seshadri, G. Vehicle-generated fugitive dust transport: Analytic models and field study. *Atmos. Environ.* **2003**, *37*, 2295–2303. [CrossRef]
16. Gillies, J.; Etyemezian, V.; Kuhns, H.; Nikolic, D.; Gillette, D. Effect of vehicle characteristics on unpaved road dust emissions. *Atmos. Environ.* **2005**, *39*, 2341–2347. [CrossRef]
17. Qi, J.; Huang, Y.; Al-Ansari, N.; Knutsson, S. Dust Emission from unpaved roads in Luleå, Sweden. *J. Earth Sci. Geotech. Eng.* **2013**, *3*, 1–13.
18. Fitz, D.R. Measurements on PM_{10} and $PM_{2.5}$ Emission Factors from Paved Roads in California. Final Report to the California Air Resources Board under Contract No. 98-723. June 2001. Available online: https://ww2.arb.ca.gov/sites/default/files/classic/research/apr/reports/l819.pdf (accessed on 30 September 2021).
19. Kuhns, H.; Etyemezian, V.; Landwehr, D.; MacDougall, C.; Pitchford, M.; Green, M. Testing re-entrained aerosol kinetic emissions from roads (TRAKER): A new approach to infer silt loading on roadways. *Atmos. Environ.* **2001**, *35*, 2815–2825. [CrossRef]
20. Pirjola, L.; Johansson, C.; Kupiainen, K.; Stojiljkovic, A.; Karlsson, H.; Hussein, T. Road Dust Emissions from Paved Roads Measured Using Different Mobile Systems. *J. Air Waste Manag. Assoc.* **2010**, *60*, 1422–1433. [CrossRef]
21. Mathissen, M.; Scheer, V.; Kirchner, U.; Vogt, R.; Benter, T. Non-exhaust PM emission measurements of a light duty vehicle with a mobile trailer. *Atmos. Environ.* **2012**, *59*, 232–242. [CrossRef]
22. Kunz, B.K.; Green, N.S.; Albers, J.L.; Wildhaber, M.L.; Little, E.E. Use of Real-Time Dust Monitoring and Surface Condition to Evaluate Success of Unpaved Road Treatments. *Transp. Res. Rec. J. Transp. Res. Board* **2018**, *2672*, 195–204. [CrossRef]
23. U.S. Environmental Protection Agency. *AP-42 Compilation of Air Emission Factors, Section 13.2.2 Unpaved Roads*; U.S. Environmental Protection Agency: Washington, DC, USA, 2006.
24. U.S. Environmental Protection Agency. *AP-42 Compilation of Air Emission Factors, Section 13.2.1 Paved Roads*; U.S. Environmental Protection Agency: Washington, DC, USA, 2011.
25. Fitz, D.R.; Bumiller, K.; Bufalino, C.; James, D.E. Real-time PM_{10} emission rates from paved roads by measurement of concentrations in the vehicle's wake using on-board sensors. Part 1. SCAMPER method characterization. *Atmos. Environ.* **2020**, *230*, 117483. [CrossRef]
26. Fitz, D.R.; Bumiller, K.; Etyemesian, V.; Kuhns, H.D.; Gillies, J.A.; Nikolich, G.; James, D.E.; Langston, R.; Merle, R.S., Jr. Real-time PM_{10} emission rates from paved roads by measurement of concentrations in the vehicle's wake using on-board sensors. Part 2. Comparison of SCAMPER, TRAKER™, flux measurements, and AP-42 silt sampling under controlled conditions. *Atmos. Environ.* **2021**, *256*, 118453. [CrossRef]

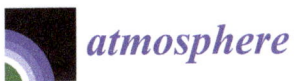

Article

Characterization of PM₁₀ Emission Rates from Roadways in a Metropolitan Area Using the SCAMPER Mobile Monitoring Approach

Dennis R. Fitz * and Kurt Bumiller

Center for Environmental Research and Technology, College of Engineering, University of California, 1084 Columbia Avenue, Riverside, CA 92507, USA; kurt@kurtbumiller.com
* Correspondence: dfitz@cert.ucr.edu

Abstract: The SCAMPER mobile system for measuring PM_{10} emission rates from paved roads was used to characterize emission rates from a wide variety of roads in the Phoenix, AZ metropolitan area. Week-long sampling episodes were conducted in March, June, September, and December. A 180 km-long route was utilized and traveled a total of 18 times. PM_{10} emission rate measurements were made at 5-s resolution for over 3200 km of roads with a precision of approximately 25%. The PM_{10} emission rates varied by over two orders of magnitude and were generally low unless the road was impacted with dust deposited by activities such as construction, sand and gravel operations, agriculture, and vehicles traveling on or near unpaved shoulders and roads. The data were tabulated into averages for each of 67 segments that the route was divided into. The segment-averaged PM_{10} emission rates ranged from zero to 2 mg m^{-1}, with an average of 0.079 mg m^{-1}. There was no significant difference in emission rates between seasons. There was a major drop in emission rates over a weekend, when dust generation activities such as construction are expected to be much reduced. By Monday, the PM_{10} emission rates had risen to the levels of the previous Friday. This indicates that roads quickly reach an equilibrium PM_{10} generating potential.

Keywords: PM_{10}; road dust; fugitive dust; particulate matter; paved roads; emission rates

Citation: Fitz, D.R.; Bumiller, K. Characterization of PM₁₀ Emission Rates from Roadways in a Metropolitan Area Using the SCAMPER Mobile Monitoring Approach. *Atmosphere* **2021**, *12*, 1332. https://doi.org/10.3390/atmos12101332

Academic Editors: Ashok Luhar, Omar Ramírez Hernández and Dmitry Vlasov

Received: 21 September 2021
Accepted: 5 October 2021
Published: 12 October 2021

Publisher's Note: MDPI stays neutral with regard to jurisdictional claims in published maps and institutional affiliations.

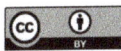

Copyright: © 2021 by the authors. Licensee MDPI, Basel, Switzerland. This article is an open access article distributed under the terms and conditions of the Creative Commons Attribution (CC BY) license (https://creativecommons.org/licenses/by/4.0/).

1. Introduction

Particulate matter (PM) has been shown by epidemiological studies to be responsible for premature deaths [1]. The U.S. Environmental Protection Agency has set air quality standards for particles both of less than 10 μm and 2.5 μm in aerodynamic diameter, PM_{10} and $PM_{2.5}$, respectively. Many government agencies have adopted these standards or have derived similar ones. Many of these standards are exceeded in urban areas and effective mitigation methods are necessary to meet these standards. In order to implement cost-effective control strategies, the sources of the PM must be determined as accurately as possible. Models have estimated that a significant amount of this material can originate from paved roadways [2–4].

Measurement of emission rates from fugitive sources such as PM from vehicles on roadways cannot be measured directly, but must be estimated. This has been done using dispersion modeling [5–7], receptor modeling [8] a combination of dispersion and receptor modeling [9,10], tracer studies [11–13], and measuring the flux of PM_{10} through a horizontal plane downwind of the source [14–17]. All of these methods require significant resources to characterize the emissions from actual roadways for inventory development in addition to presenting large uncertainties in the results.

The U.S. Environmental Protection Agency (EPA) used detailed measurements of PM flux through a plane for estimating the PM emissions from paved roads to derive an empirical equation using surface silt loading and vehicle weight as metrics [18]. This equation contains significant amounts of uncertainty and the EPA has revised it several times over the past decades based on reviews of the methods used. The current equation is as follows:

$$E = k(sL/)^{0.91} (W)^{1.02} \qquad (1)$$

where:

E = Particulate matter emission rate in the units of g/VKT
k = A constant dependent on the aerodynamic size range of PM (0.62 for PM_{10})
sL = Road surface silt loading of material smaller than 75 μm in g m^{-2}
W = mean vehicle weight in U.S. tons
VKT = vehicle kilometer traveled

Despite the uncertainties in this equation, it is widely used to estimate emission inventories in air basins. Compounding this, since the determination of silt loading is labor intensive and often dangerous, EPA default values for silt loading are often used to estimate emission rates for emission inventories. More recently, the direct measurement of PM emissions in real time using a moving vehicle have been reported. In one version, TRAKER™, the concentration of PM_{10} is measured in the wheel well of a moving vehicle [19]. This value is then related to an emission rate by calibrating with a downwind measurement of PM_{10} flux. Other investigators have used the TRAKER approach specialized for their own studies [20,21]. In another approach, SCAMPER (System for the Continuous Aerosol Measurement of Particulate Emissions from Roadways), the PM_{10} concentration is measured in front of a vehicle and a representative point in the wake behind it [22]. With this approach, as a first approximation the emission rate is determined by multiplying the net concentration difference by the frontal area of the vehicle. Both TRAKER and SCAMPER have been evaluated together using a dedicated roadway on which known amounts of soil were evenly deposited [23]. Measurements of PM_{10} emission rates were concurrently made using the flux method and measuring the silt loading. Reasonable agreement was found between all of these methods.

The objective of this study was to use the SCAMPER to:

1. Provide actual measurements of PM_{10} emission rates from roadways that could be used to construct a data-based emission inventory.
2. Evaluate the significance of construction activities on PM_{10} emission rates.
3. Determine if there are seasonal changes in the emission rates.
4. Evaluate the precision of the measured emission rates.

2. Materials and Methods

2.1. Test Route

The testing was conducted over streets in the greater Phoenix, AZ metropolitan area. This climate is typical of the Sonoran Desert with less than 13 cm of precipitation per year. No rain or other significant weather events occurred before or during the test periods. Except as noted, wind speeds were generally less than 10 km h^{-1}, similar to the conditions when the SCAMPER was operated under controlled conditions [23]. Temperatures, which were not expected to affect SCAMPER measurements, ranged from 13 °C in the winter to 33 °C in the summer. The route consisted of a mix of segments of different road types based on their Average Daily Traffic (ADT) or number of vehicles in both directions passing a point per day. Most segments were at least a half kilometer long so that time-integrated measurements could be collected with reasonable uncertainty. Five segment types were differentiated:

I: Less than 10,000 ADT: 43 km total
II: 10,000–19,999 ADT: 48 km total
III: 20,000–29,000 ADT: 12 km total
IV: Greater than 30,000 ADT: 7 km total
Limited Access: 70 km total

The route included representative lengths of all road classes (I–IV) and the limited access or freeway (Fwy). The total length was 180 km. Figure 1 is a map of the test route and Table 1 identifies each segment, what class of road it belongs to, and what type of land use area it was located in. The SCAMPER was driven at a speed corresponding to the general flow of traffic.

2.2. SCAMPER Description

The SCAMPER determines PM emission rates from roads by measuring the PM concentrations in front of (mounted on the hood) and behind the vehicle (mounted on a small open trailer) using optical sensors with a 1s time resolution. The system and its validation have previously been described [22,23]. Briefly, the SCAMPER, shown in Figure 2, includes five major components:

Tow vehicle and Trailer: A 1994 Chevrolet Suburban was used to tow a small (3.1 m wide by 2 m long) open flatbed trailer. The trailer was fitted with a 1 m hitch extension to place the rear sampling inlet 3 m behind the tow vehicle at a height of 0.8 m above the ground on the centerline of the trailer. This position was found to give PM_{10} concentrations that were representative of the mean concentration of PM_{10} in the wake of the tow vehicle [22].

PM_{10} Sensors: Thermo Systems Inc. (Shoreville, MN, USA) Model 8520 DustTrak™ optical PM sensors with PM_{10} inlets.

Isokinetic Sampling Inlets: A custom made inlet where the inlet speed is matched to the air speed by a laptop computer that monitors the static air pressure and adjusts the inlet pressure to match it by controlling a vacuum pump (mounted on the trailer). This condition creates a no-pressure-drop inlet; therefore, the sampled air stream has the same energy as the ambient air stream.

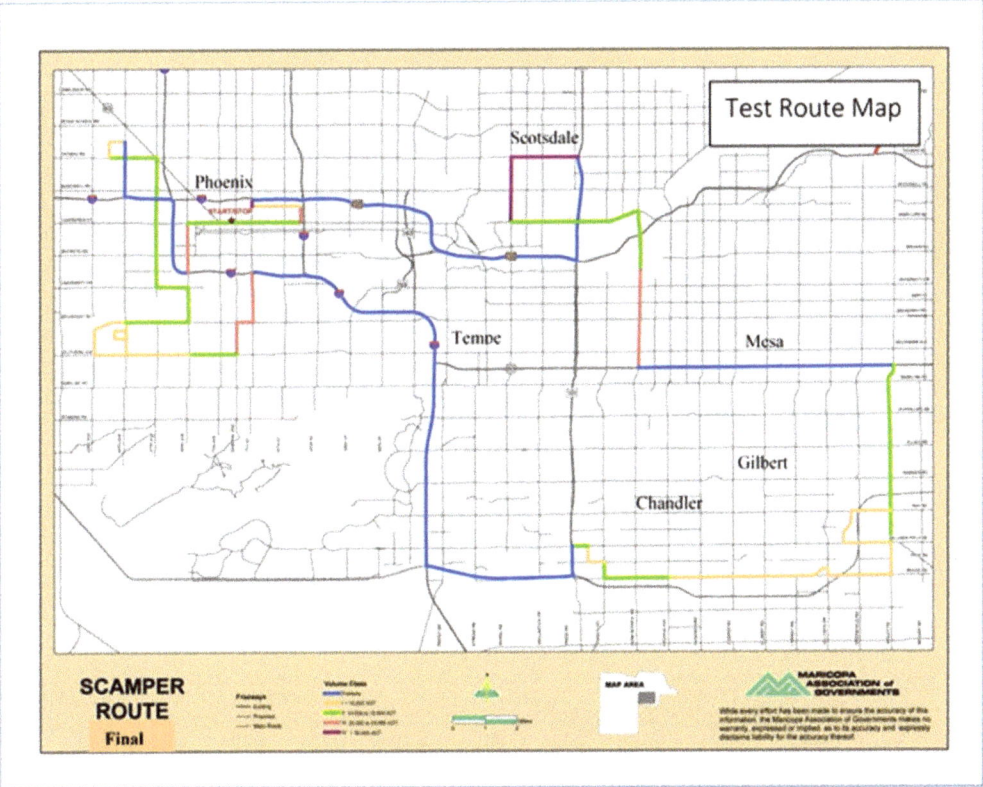

Figure 1. Map of the test route.

Table 1. List of test route segments and road classification type.

Seg #	Intersection	On Street	Dir	Length km	From Street	To Street	Vol Class	# of Lanes	Predominant Land Use
	Begin: 1st Ave/Van Buren	1st Ave	SB	—			II	3	Commercial
1	1st Ave/Van Buren	Van Buren St	EB	3.2	1st Ave	20th St	II	2	Commercial
2	Van Buren/20th St	20th St	NB	0.8	Van Buren St	Roosevelt St	III	5	Mixed
3	20th St/Roosevelt St	Roosevelt St	WB	2.4	20th St	7th St	I	1	Residential
4	Roosevelt/7th St	7th St	NB	0.8	Roosevelt	I-10E on-ramp	IV	3	Mixed
5	I-10 East/7th St	I-10 East	EB	1.6	7th St	SR 202	Fwy		Mixed
6	I-10 East/SR 202	SR 202	EB	14.4	SR 202	SR 101	Fwy		Mixed
7	SR 202/SR 101	SR 101	NB	2.4	SR 202	Thomas Rd	Fwy		Agricultural
8	SR 101/Thomas Rd	Thomas Rd	WB	3.2	SR 101	Scottsdale Rd	IV	2	Residential
9	Thomas/Scottsdale Rd	Scottsdale Rd	SB	3.2	Thomas Rd	McKellips Rd	IV	3	Comm/Res
10	Scottsdale/McKellips Rd	McKellips Rd	EB	6.7	Scottsdale Rd	Alma School Rd	II	2	Agricultural
11	McKellips/Alma School	Alma School Rd	SB	2.9	McKellips Rd	8th St	II	3	Industrial
12		Alma School Rd	SB	4.8	8th St	US 60	III	3	Commercial
13	Alma School/US 60	US 60	EB	12.6	Alma School Rd	Higley Rd	Fwy		Mixed
14	US 60/Higley	Higley Rd	SB	2.4	US 60	Guadalupe Rd	II	3	Agricultural/Res
15		Higley Rd	SB	1.6	Guadalupe Rd	Elliot Rd	II	3	Agricultural/Res
16		Higley Rd	SB	1.6	Elliot Rd	Warner Rd	II	1	Agricultural/Res
17		Higley Rd	SB	1.6	Warner Rd	Ray Rd	II	1	Agricultural/Res
18		Higley Rd	SB	1.6	Ray Rd	Williams Field Rd	II	1	Agricultural/Res
	Inner Loop #1								
19	Higley/Williams Field Rd	Williams Field Rd	WB	2.4	Higley Rd	Santan Valley Pky	I	1	Agricultural/Res
20	Williams Field/Santan Valley	Santan Valley Pky	NB	1.6	Williams Field Rd	Ray Rd	I	1	Agricultural/Res
21	Santan Valley/Ray Rd	Ray Rd	EB	2.4	Santan Valley Pky	Higley Rd	I	1	Agricultural/Res
18	Ray Rd/Higley Rd	Highley Rd	SB	1.6	Ray Rd	Williams Field Rd	I	1	Agricultural/Res
22		Higley Rd	SB	1.6	Williams Field Rd	Pecos Rd	I	1	Agricultural/Res
23	Higley/Pecos Rd	Pecos Rd	WB	1.6	Higley Rd	Greenfield Rd	I	3	Agricultural/Res
24		Pecos Rd	WB	1.8	Greenfield Rd	Val Vista Rd	I	3	Agricultural/Res
25		Pecos Rd	WB	1.8	Val Vista Rd	Lindsay Rd	I	2	Agricultural/Res
26		Pecos Rd	WB	1.4	Lindsay Rd	Gilbert Rd	I	1	Agricultural/Res
27		Pecos Rd	WB	1.6	Gilbert Rd	Cooper Rd	I	2	Agricultural/Res
28		Pecos Rd	WB	1.6	Cooper Rd	McQueen Rd	I	1	Agricultural/Res
29		Pecos Rd	WB	1.6	McQueen Rd	Arizona Ave	I	2	Agricultural/Res
30		Pecos Rd	WB	1.6	Arizona Ave	Alma School Rd	II	1	Agricultural/Res
31		Pecos Rd	WB	1.6	Alma School Rd	Dobson Rd	II	1	Agricultural/Res
32	Pecos Rd/Dobson	Dobson Rd	NB	0.6	Pecos Road	Frye Rd	II	1	Commercial
33	Dobson Rd/Frye Rd	Frye Rd	WB	0.8	Dobson Rd	Ellis Rd	I	1	Commercial
34	Frye Rd/Ellis Rd	Ellis Rd	SB	0.6	Frye Rd	Chandler Blvd	I	1	Commercial
35	Ellis/Chandler Blvd	Chandler Blvd	WB	0.8	Ellis Rd	Price Freeway	II	3	Commercial
36	Chandler Blvd/Price Fwy	Price Frontage Rd	SB	1.4	Chandler Blvd	Santan Freeway	Fwy		Commercial
37	Price Fwy/Santan Fwy	Santan Freeway	EB	8.2	Price Freeway	I-10 West	Fwy		Mixed
38	Santan Fwy/I-10 West	I-10 West	NB	17.6	Santan Freeway	I-17 West	Fwy		Mixed
39	I-10 West/I-17 West	I-17 West	WB	3.2	I-17W interchange	7th St off-ramp	Fwy		Mixed
40	I-17 West/7th Street	7th St	SB	2.4	7th St off-ramp	Broadway Rd	III	2	Mixed
41	7th St/Broadway Rd	Broadway Rd	WB	0.8	7th St	Central Ave	III	2	Mixed
42	Broadway/Central Ave	Central Ave	SB	1.6	Broadway Rd	Southern Ave	III	2	Mixed
43	Central/Southern Ave	Southern Ave	WB	2.4	Central Ave	19th Ave	II	1	Residential
44		Southern Ave	WB	1.6	19th Ave	27th Ave	I	1	Residential
45		Southern Ave	WB	1.6	27th Ave	35th Ave	I	1	Residential
46		Southern Ave	WB	1.6	35th Ave	43rd Ave	I	1	Industrial
47	Southern/43rd Ave	43rd Ave	NB	1.3	Southern Ave	Broadway Rd	I	1	Industrial
48	43rd Ave/Broadway Rd	Broadway Rd	EB	1.9	43rd Ave	35th Ave	I	1	Industrial
	Inner Loop #2								
49	Broadway/35th Ave	35th Ave	SB	1.6	Broadway Rd	Southern Ave	I	1	Industrial
50	35th Ave/Southern Ave	Southern Ave	WB	1.6	35th Ave	43rd Ave	I	1	Industrial
47	Southern/43rd Ave	43rd Ave	NB	1.3	Southern Ave	Broadway Rd	I	1	Industrial
48	43rd Ave/Broadway Rd	Broadway Rd	EB	1.9	43rd Ave	35th Ave	I	1	Industrial
51	Broadway/35th Ave	35th Ave	SB	0.5	Broadway Rd	Wier Ave	II	1	Commercial
52	35th Ave/Wier Ave	Wier Ave	WB	0.6	35th Ave	38th Ave	I	1	Residential
53	Wier Ave/38th Ave	38th Ave	SB	0.5	Wier Ave	Roeser Rd	I	1	Residential
54	38th Ave/Roeser Rd	Roeser Rd	EB	0.6	38th Ave	35th Ave	I	1	Residential
55	Roeser/35th Ave	35th Ave	NB	0.8	Roeser Rd	Broadway Rd	II	1	Agricultural/Res
56	35th Ave/Broadway	Broadway Rd	EB	3.2	35th Ave	19th Ave	II	1	Industrial
57	Broadway/19th Ave	19th Ave	NB	1.6	Broadway Rd	Lower Buckeye Rd	II	1	Industrial
58	19th Ave/Lower Buckeye	Lower Buckeye Rd	WB	1.6	19th Ave	27th Ave	II	1	Industrial
59	Lower Buckeye/27th Ave	27th Ave	NB	1.6	Lower Buckeye Rd	Buckeye Rd	II	2	Industrial
60		27th Ave	NB	1.6	Buckeye Rd	Van Buren St	II	2	Industrial
61		27th Ave	NB	1.6	Van Buren St	McDowell Rd	II	2	Industrial
62		27th Ave	NB	1.6	McDowell Rd	Thomas Rd	II	2	Industrial
63	27th Ave/Thomas Rd	Thomas Rd	WB	2.4	27th Ave	39th Ave	II	3	Commercial
64	Thomas/39th Ave	39th Ave	NB	0.8	Thomas Rd	Osborn Rd	I	1	Residential
65	39th Ave/Osborn Rd	Osborn Rd	EB	0.8	39th Ave	35th Ave	I	1	Residential
66	Osborn/35th Ave	35th Ave	SB	2.7	Osborn Rd	I-10E on-ramp	Fwy		Mixed
67	35th Ave/I-10 East	I-10 East	EB	2.7	35th Ave	I-17 E interchange	Fwy		Mixed
68	I-10 East/I-17 East	I-17 East	EB	3.7	I-10 East	19th Ave	Fwy		Industrial
69	I-17 East/19th Ave	19th Ave	NB	2.2	I-17 East	Van Buren St	III	2	Industrial
70	19th Ave/Van Buren	Van Buren St	EB	2.2	19th Ave	1st Ave	II	2	Commercial
	End: Van Buren/1st Ave	Total Length		180					

Global Positioning System (GPS): Garmin (Kansas City, MO, USA) Map76 GPS to determine vehicle speed and location.

Data Collection System: The laptop computer was used to collect GPS and DustTrak™ data at 1 s intervals in addition to controlling the inlet vacuum pumps.

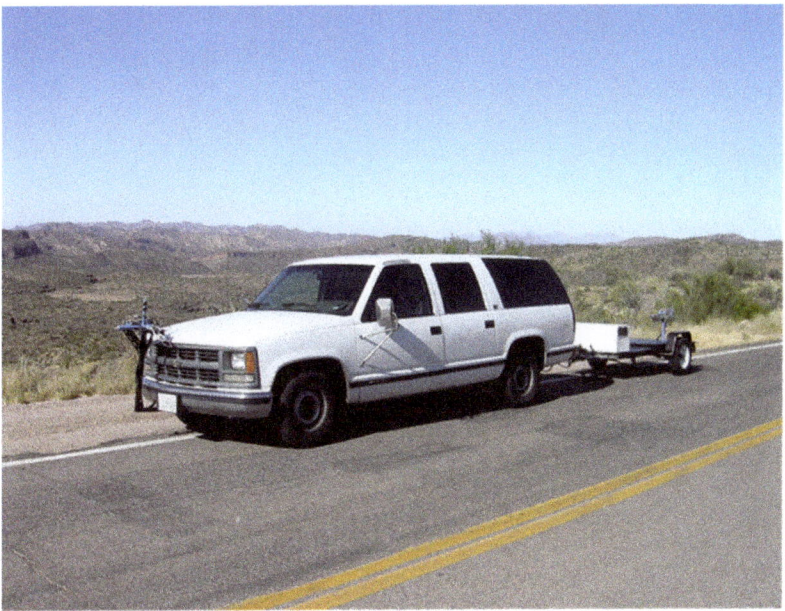

Figure 2. Photograph of the SCAMPER.

2.3. Data Quality Control and Quality Assurance

The data acquisition system recorded all data accurately. Data were downloaded from the laptop computer and entered into Excel worksheets where all of the calculations were made. Quality control data such as inlet pressure and various voltages were also entered into the master worksheet in addition to GPS location, time, speed, and DustTrak values. Data were validated from logbook entries, and by observing time series, to determine if the results made physical sense. The flow rate and zero of the DustTraks were determined before, after, and during test runs. The drift during the course of each test day was less than a few thousandths of a mg m^{-3}, near the 0.001 mg m^{-3} detection limit of the instrument. The instrument is temperature sensitive and therefore the zero drift may be different for moving and stationary modes. The data for each test run were corrected for zero offset using the mean zero response for that day. Two DustTraks were operated collocated at the rear during one test day to determine the precision of these instruments.

There were occasional periods when the GPS did not report data, most likely due to interferences in the sight path to a satellite. In these cases, the cell was filled with the average of the position before and the position after. The same was done for speed and PM. We found that the output of the rear DustTrak occasionally spiked, either positive or negative, most likely due to physical shock. These spikes always showed up for two consecutive seconds. These were unlikely to be associated with an actual PM concentration as concentrations rarely change to that degree in less than one second. This two-second characteristic of this noise spike is also expected from the internal averaging and output characteristics of the DustTrak. On the time constant we selected (which is the shortest available) the DustTrak output is a two-second running average that is updated every second. A large spike in a one-second period will therefore show up as two smaller spikes for two consecutive seconds. To filter this noise, we tabulated the data as five-second running medians. Two-second anomalous spikes therefore would be removed from the data set.

Figure 3 is a plot of the emission rates determined by operating two DustTraks collocated at the rear sampling position for one test day, June 19th. The values from the DustTraks are well-correlated with a slope near unity and an R^2 value of 0.96. Other days produced similar results.

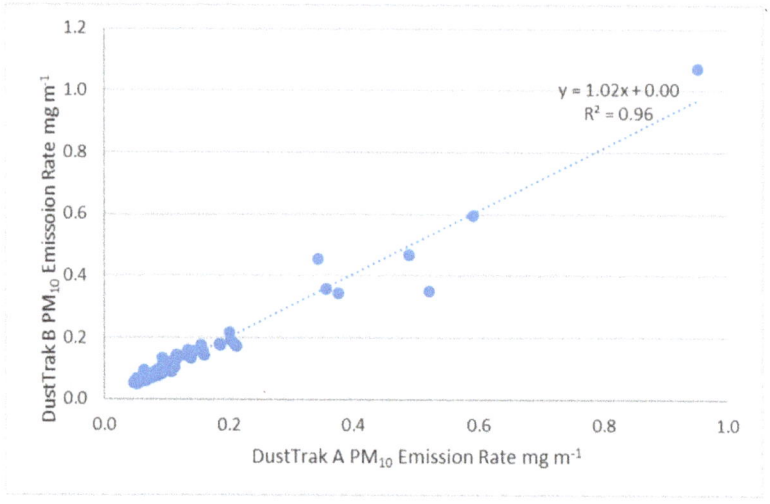

Figure 3. Scatter plot of PM_{10} emission rates determined from collocated rear DustTraks.

The differences between the front and rear DustTraks were calculated and the results were multiplied by the frontal area of the Suburban (3.66 m^2), to yield the emission rate in mg m^{-1}. The PM emission rates for speeds less than 16 km hr^{-1} were excluded from further analysis since they would be considered unreliable as the production of a well-mixed and defined plume behind the test vehicle was unlikely. This speed was determined visually by watching the test vehicle driven on an unpaved road as various speeds. The emission rate data were then sorted by segments of the route based on the GPS location at the time of data recording. Summary worksheets were prepared that included only time, location, speed, and PM_{10} emission rates.

During three of the test weeks, a short loop was run repeatedly when encountered during the test day. The 8 km long precision test loop was located at the southeast corner of the test route and consisted of segments 18–21. It was chosen to give relatively high emission rates due to the nearby construction activities. The precision of the measurement was determined from these test loops. Precision can also be determined by evaluating the day-to-day variability in the segment and loop-averaged PM emission rates. Since the PM-producing potential of the segments may vary daily due to activities, this evaluation may not fully represent measurement variability.

The response of the DustTraks were calibrated at the factory using Standard Reference Material 8632 from the U.S. National Institute of Standards and Technology. The mass-specific light-scattering response drops rapidly with increasing particle size for particles larger than 1 μm diameter, thus a small change in the particle-size distribution can change the response significantly. Since most PM_{10} regulations are based on collected mass, it was useful to relate the DustTrak output to a mass-based emission rate. A filter-based PM_{10} sampler was therefore operated collocated with the DustTrak mounted on the trailer. PM_{10} filter samples (47 mm Teflo™ Ringed Filter, 2 μm pore) were collected using a Sierra Andersen model 241 inlet adapted to a 47 mm filter holder and sampled at 16.7 l m^{-1}. Filters were equilibrated to 25 °C and 40% RH and weighed before and after collection to the nearest microgram using a Cahn (Irvine, CA, USA) model C-25 electro-balance. Filters were changed based on visual examination to ensure that sufficient material had been collected to allow for accurate mass determination and to facilitate a broad range of concentrations so that a linear correlation would be meaningful. The average PM_{10} concentration was determined from the DustTrak response during the entire sampling period.

3. Results

3.1. Precision Test Loop

Table 2 summarizes the results from 90 circuits of the test loops. While the mean PM_{10} emission rates were quite high in March, they dropped progressively during the year as construction activities changed. It should be noted that the relative standard deviation for one of the test days in March was four times higher than any of the other four days. Removing this single day results in a relative standard deviation of 18% for the March tests. These precision results are typical of those determined from the entire route as described in the following section.

Table 2. Summary of PM_{10} emission rates results from the precision test loop.

Date	# Circuits	Mean Emission Rate mg m^{-1}	Mean Standard Deviation mg m^{-1}	Relative Standard Deviation %
March	33	1.02	0.32	38
September	38	0.111	0.029	23
December	19	0.032	0.013	41

3.2. Summary of Emission Rate Data

The test route was traveled once per day, typically starting at approximately 8 a.m. Figures 4–7 are plots of the mean PM_{10} emission rates by segment for all of the test runs. Some segments are missing due to construction activities and detours that caused speed to be generally below 16 km h^{-1}. For the March testing, the overall PM_{10} emission rate was 0.094 mg m^{-1} with a relative standard deviation of 21%; these values are similar for the other three test periods.

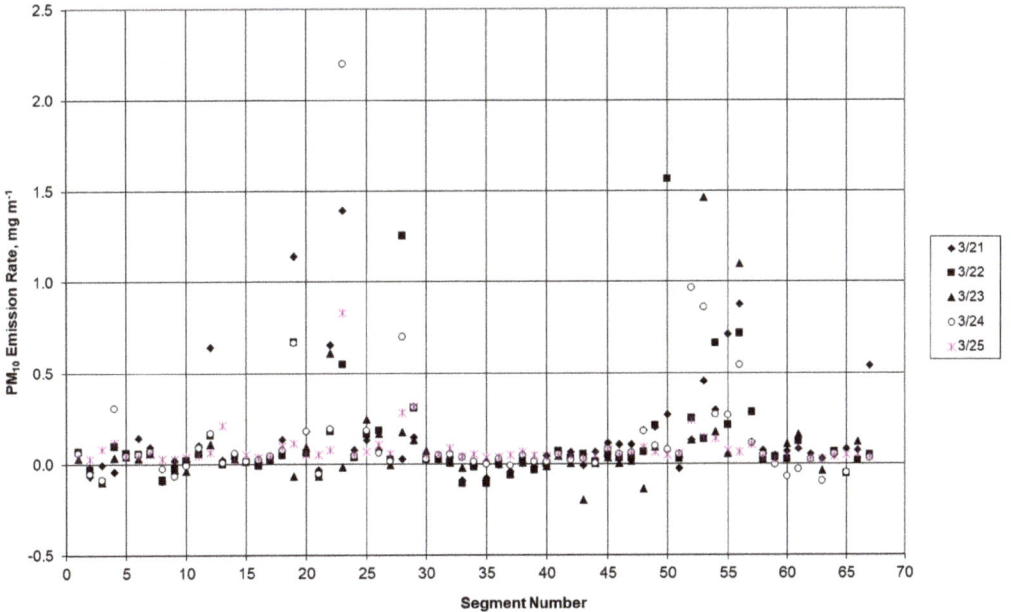

Figure 4. Plot of PM_{10} emission rate by segment number starting Tuesday, 21 March.

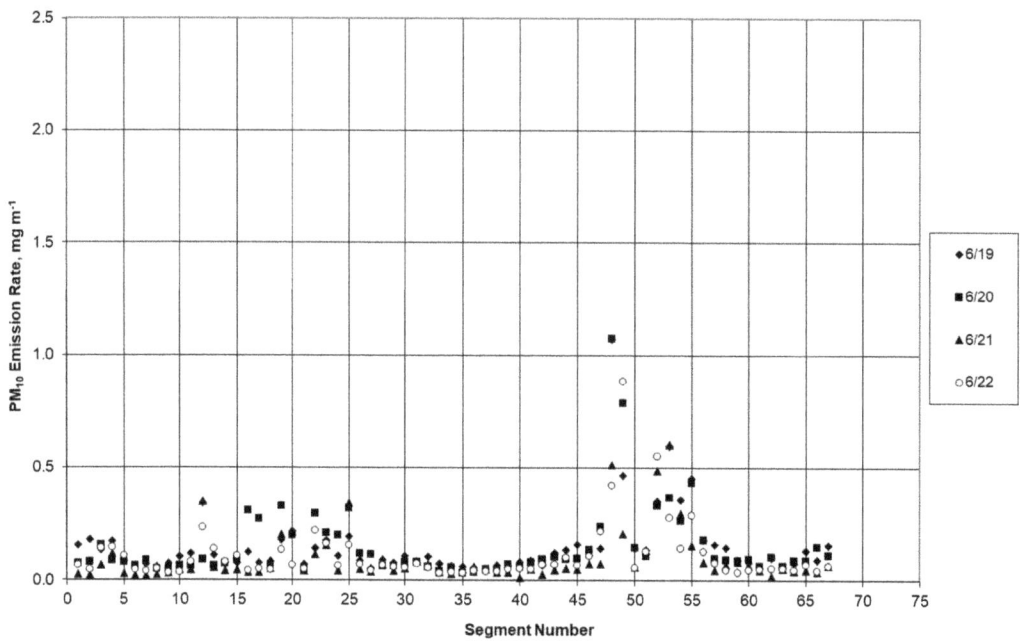

Figure 5. Plot of PM_{10} emission rate by segment number starting Monday, 19 June.

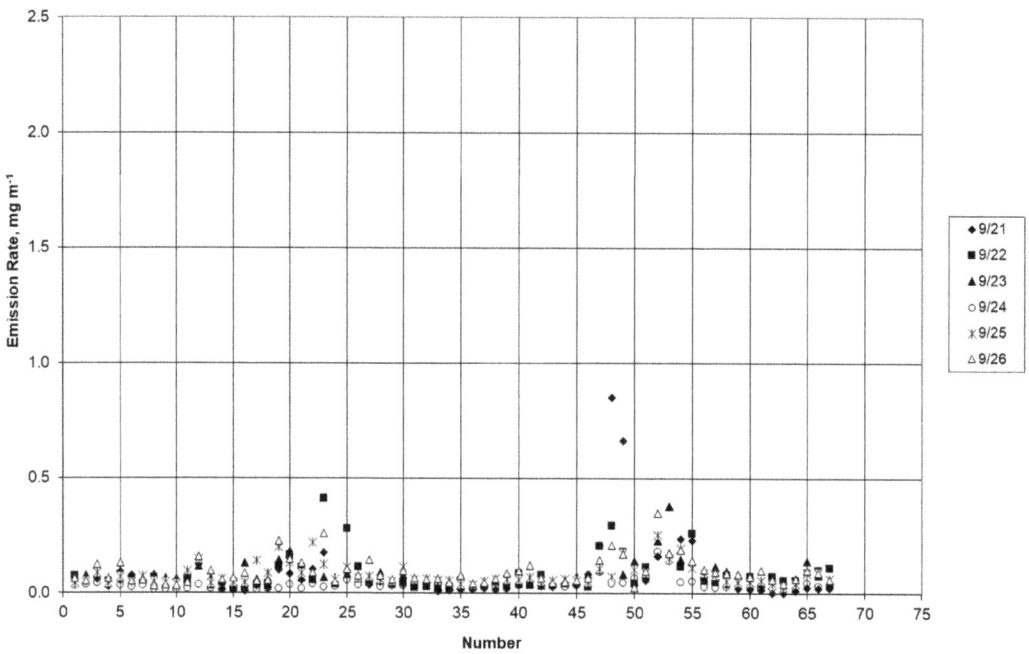

Figure 6. Plot of PM_{10} emission rate by segment number starting Thursday, 21 September.

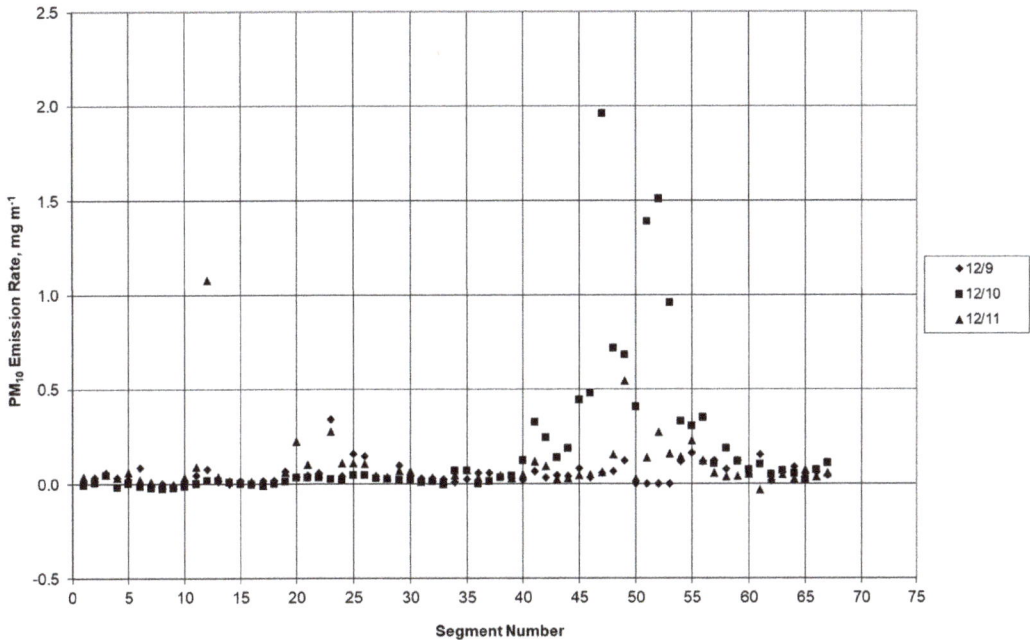

Figure 7. Plot of PM_{10} emission rate by segment number starting Saturday, 9 December.

It is clear that most of the PM_{10} emissions are due to a relatively small number of segments, and that these high values are generally repeated for the same segments and groups of segments for each day and for each season. The segments with high PM_{10} emissions were also highly variable in magnitude. This would be expected because of the sporadic nature of activities that deposit soil onto roadways. Note that during the first week of testing there were a number of negative emission rates. This was most likely due to SCAMPER following earth moving or other heavy duty diesel vehicles with noticeable exhaust smoke. These vehicles were avoided in the three remaining seasonal test sessions.

The drop in PM_{10} emission rates on Saturday 25 March is quite noticeable, with only segment #23 rising significantly above the other values. This may be due to a lowered amount of dust generation or deposition from construction activities on weekends. Excluding this anomalous day, the mean PM_{10} emission rate rises to 0.10 with a relative standard deviation of 16%.

In order to more fully examine this potential weekend effect, two study periods in September and December included weekends. Figure 4 shows a tendency for Saturday and Sunday (23 and 24 September) to have lower emission rates. Figure 8, shows a time-series plot of all valid data (not averaged by segment) for each day from Friday through Monday. It is clear that the PM_{10} emission rates drop from Friday to Saturday and drop further from Saturday to Sunday. By Monday the emission rates rise to nearly that of Friday and typical for weekdays. This weekday–weekend effect is very significant as it shows that the PM_{10}-producing potential of the roadway can change rapidly.

During the tests conducted in December, the Sunday test was compromised by high winds during the later portions of the test route, with gusts over 40 km h^{-1} which caused dust to be blown over the roadway. The high emission rates observed in Figure 5 are therefore not consistent with other test days.

The mean segment-averaged PM_{10} emission rates were sorted by the five roadway classes based on the ADT by test period. The results are shown in Table 3 along with the overall mean when all test periods were combined and when all classes were combined for a test period. The standard deviations are also included. As indicated by the standard deviations, there was an expected large amount of variability in emission rates. The class IV roadways (≥30,000 ADT) had the lowest emission rates followed by the freeways. The emission rate for the other classes went up as the ADT lowered. There was no significant variability between the seasons, although the December measurements were biased high due to high winds causing blowing dust in the later segments.

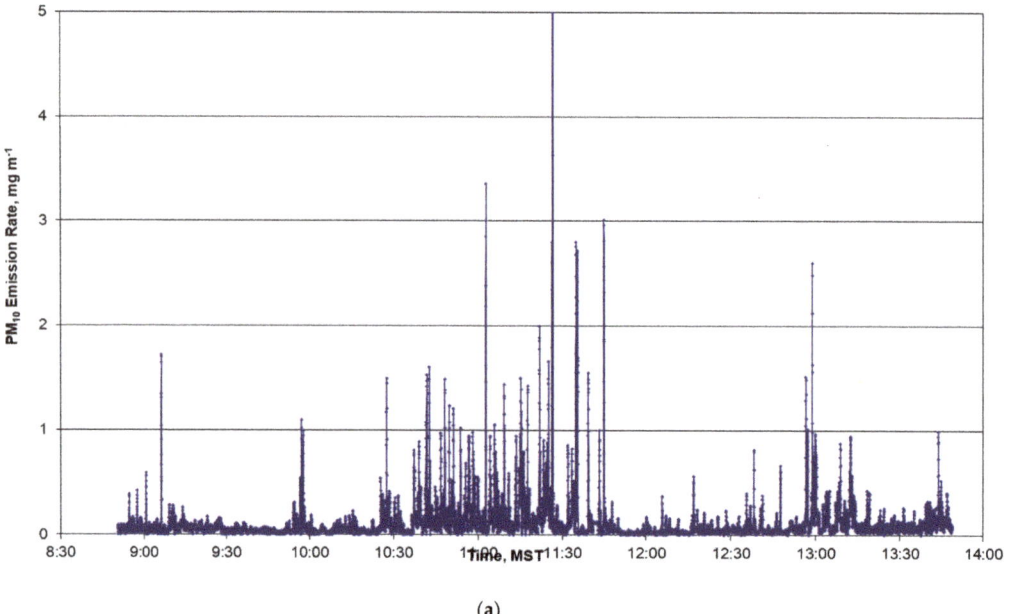

(a)

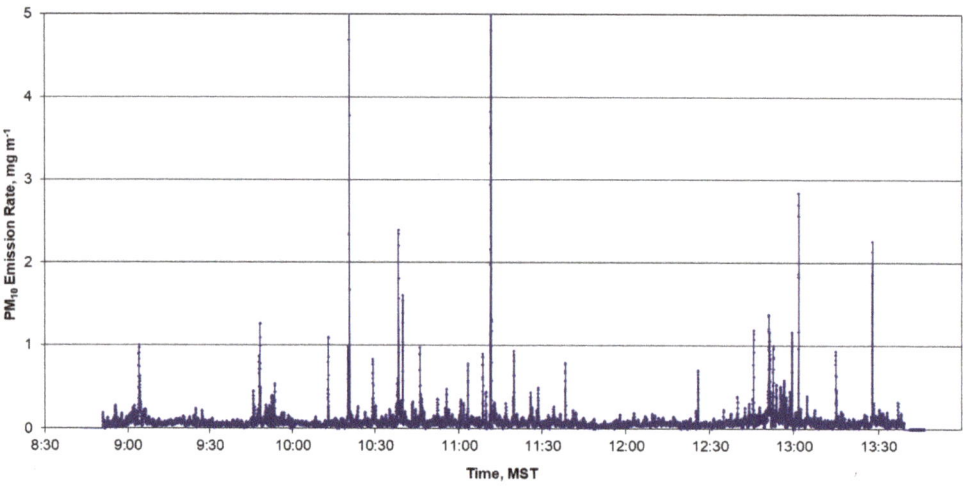

(b)

Figure 8. Cont.

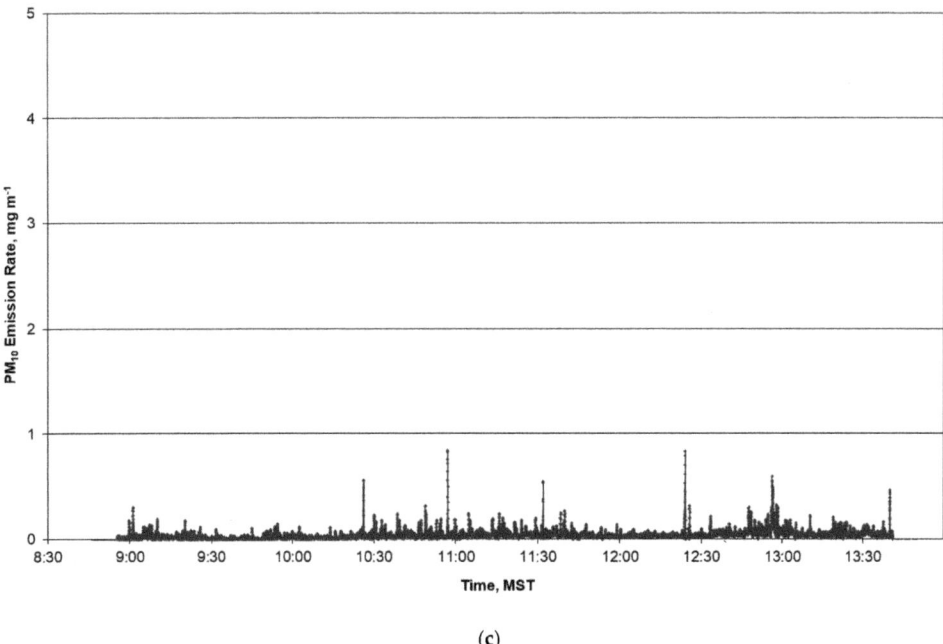

(c)

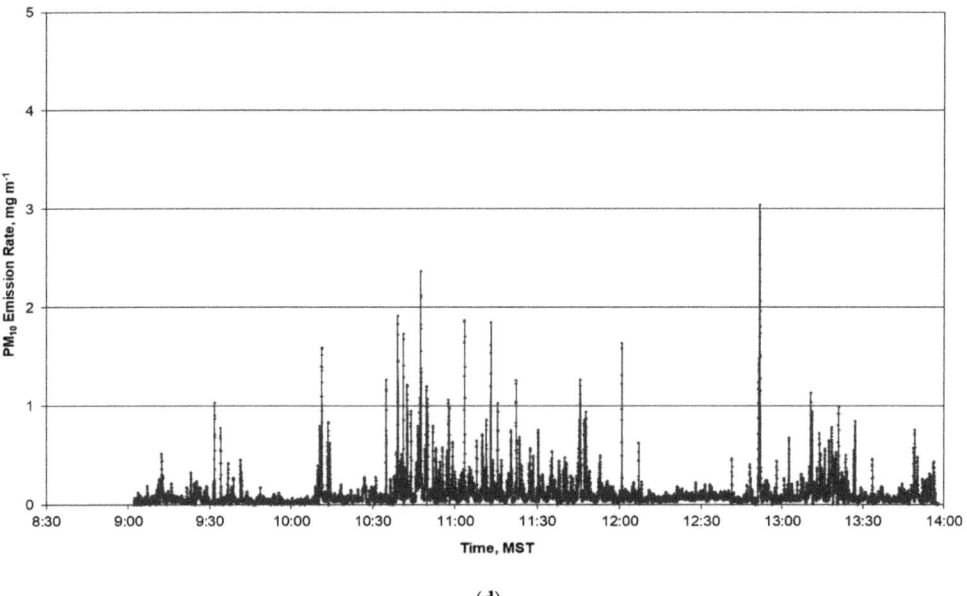

(d)

Figure 8. Time series plots of PM_{10} emission rates for Friday, 22 September (**a**), Saturday, 23 September (**b**) Sunday, 24 September (**c**), and Monday, 25 September (**d**).

Table 3. Summary of PM_{10} emission rates by season, all four seasons, and all five road types combined.

Road Type	Measurement	March	June	September	December	Combined
Freeway	Mean, mg m^{-1}	0.03	0.07	0.05	0.03	0.05
Freeway	Std Dev, mg m^{-1}	0.06	0.03	0.03	0.03	0.04
≥30,000 ADT	Mean, mg m^{-1}	0.00	0.05	0.04	0.00	0.02
≥30,000 ADT	Std Dev, mg m^{-1}	0.01	0.03	0.01	0.02	0.02
20,000–29,999 ADT	Mean, mg m^{-1}	0.06	0.08	0.05	0.08	0.07
20,000–29,999 ADT	Std Dev, mg m^{-1}	0.06	0.04	0.02	0.09	0.05
10,000–19,999 ADT	Mean, mg m^{-1}	0.13	0.12	0.07	0.08	0.10
10,000–19,999 ADT	Std Dev, mg m^{-1}	0.17	0.10	0.05	0.15	0.12
<10,000	Mean, mg m^{-1}	0.17	0.18	0.10	0.19	0.16
<10,000	Std Dev, mg m^{-1}	0.24	0.20	0.10	0.35	0.22
All Five Combined	Mean, mg m^{-1}	0.09	0.13	0.07	0.11	
All Five Combined	Std Dev, mg m^{-1}	0.02	0.05	0.02		

3.3. Comparison of DustTrak PM_{10} with Filter Samples

A large amount of scatter was observed when plotting the DustTrak measurements with filter-based ones. This is not unexpected since the relationship between the two is not linear with a changing particle-size distribution of the various PM_{10} emission sources encountered on the roadway. In addition, the cut-point of the filter sampler may vary with vehicle speed since the size-selective inlet was not designed for the range of speeds encountered on the test route. For this reason, all 46 pairs generated during the four seasonal test periods were plotted as shown in Figure 9. In the figure the least squares correlation line is forced through the origin since filter data precision would be significantly poorer with little collected material. There is considerable scatter, as expected, with an R^2 value of 0.46 showing a weak correlation. The slope indicates that the DustTrack data would need to be multiplied by 3.6 to be related to mass emission rates. This is consistent with a factor of 3.5 derived by comparing the mean concentrations.

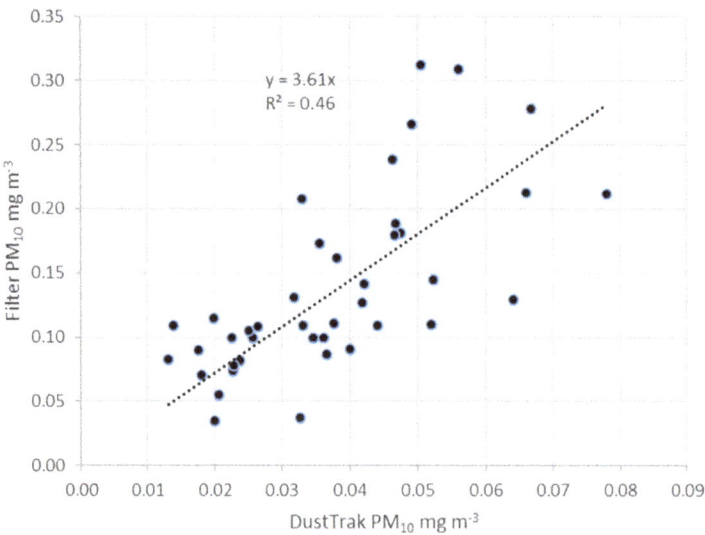

Figure 9. Comparison of filter-based and integrated DustTrak PM_{10} concentrations for all test periods.

4. Discussion and Conclusions

The SCAMPER mobile-based PM emission measurement approach has been used to fully characterize PM_{10} emissions from paved roads in Phoenix, AZ metropolitan area. PM_{10} emission rate measurements were made at 5-s resolution for over 3200 km of roads with a precision of approximately 25%. It would not be economically feasible to develop such a robust data set by performing silt measurements on the roads. The PM_{10} emission rates varied by over two orders of magnitude and were generally low unless the road was impacted with dust deposited by activities such as construction, sand and gravel operations, agriculture, and vehicles traveling on or near unpaved surfaces (e.g., dirt parking areas and shoulders). These impacted roads were clearly indicated in the data throughout the study, but would be difficult to determine without a mobile measurement system. It is unlikely that significant emissions are due to brake or tire wear from the tow vehicle since there were many periods where the measured emissions were near the detection limit despite high speeds on limited-access roads and braking maneuvers on the other roads. In addition, previous testing on damp roads showed no measurable PM0 emissions. There was no indication that the PM_{10} emission rate varied significantly with season. This is not unexpected since the Maricopa County climate leads to very dry conditions most of the time.

Of particular significance was the much lower PM_{10} emission rate on a weekend and especially Sunday, when dust generating activities such as construction are much reduced. This indicates that roads reach an equilibrium PM_{10} emission potential within a day. A rapid decline, within a few vehicle passes, of PM_{10} emissions have been reported using porous silica particles of various sizes impregnated with a fluorescent dye tracer [24]. By measuring the fluorescent intensity after each vehicle passes, it was reported that over half the particles greater than 10 µm were removed after the first two vehicles passed at 64 km h^{-1}. Further passes had little effect on the amount of deposit. Using mobile methods on a roadway with deposited soil, Fitz et al. [23] reported a similar rapid decrease after several vehicle passes followed by a slow decline in PM_{10} emission rates.

The sporadic nature of emissions near construction activities and the fairly rapid decrease when these activities lessen need to be taken into account when developing emission inventories and mitigation methods. The SCAMPER could be useful in identifying high emission episodes in real-time and verifying that the applied mitigation methods are effective.

The DustTrak most likely measures lower PM_{10} concentrations compared with weighed filter samples under these conditions because the larger particles found in suspended road dust scatter light much less efficiently than the particles used to calibrate the DustTraks. In our previous study it was found that the correction factor for the DustTrak was 2.8 when sampling next to a roadway with artificially-deposited material and 2.4 when the same material was re-suspended in a laboratory [23]. In another study using the SCAMPER in Las Vegas, NV on public streets the factor was found to be 1.25 [22]. All of these tests showed considerable scatter. If the SCAMPER results need to be related to regulatory-defined PM_{10} mass concentrations, then collocated filter sampling is recommended.

The EPA has a list of default silt loading values for normal baseline conditions which are widely used in emission inventories. Using equation 1 and assuming that $W^{1.02}$ is 2 results in the following emission rates in units of mg m^{-1}: <500: 0.78; 500–5000: 0.29; 5000–10,000: 0.095; >10,000: 0.051; limited access: 0.027. Since the ADT breakdowns are not consistent with the ones that we used, it is not possible to do a direct comparison. For the limited access freeway, the mean SCAMPER value was 0.05 mg m^{-1}. Applying the factor of 3.5 results in an emission rate of 0.18 mg m^{-1}, which is nearly 7 times higher than the EPA default value. A factor of 4 results if a Class II roadway is compared to the EPA's > 10,000. While these values are within an order of magnitude, one must consider that the route was chosen to include segments with significant construction activities and therefore high emission potential. In addition, the Phoenix metropolitan area, with an annual growth rate of approximately 3%, is one of the fastest growing in the United States and therefore has significantly higher construction activities than would be expected of a typical U.S. metropolitan area, for which the default values were presumably intended.

We conclude that the SCAMPER approach can easily and safely generate more appropriate PM_{10} emission rates from paved roads that are specific to a geographical area. The SCAMPER vehicle is representative of the vehicle mix in an urban area and can be driven at a speed typical of the traffic flow. The speed is important since the PM_{10} emission rate has been shown to be highly dependent on vehicle speed [23]. There is no need to barricade lanes and apply labor-intensive and sometimes dangerous silt loading measurements. Emission measurements can also be made on high-speed, limited access roadways for which silt loading measurements are simply not feasible. One of the limitations is that periods of high winds should be avoided since the SCAMPER has not been evaluated under these conditions and erratic results may be obtained that are not representative of normal weather conditions for a given location. Another limitation is that with wet pavement we have observed emission rates that were at or below the detection limit.

The real-time SCAMPER data could be used to improve the accuracy of PM_{10} emission inventories. SCAMPER is a relatively low-cost device to build and operate compared to other measurement approaches. A major advantage is that it has been shown to not require calibration by flux methods [23], which are labor- and equipment-intensive. In addition, activities that may cause high emissions of PM_{10} from roadways can be easily monitored for mitigation and enforcement purposes.

Author Contributions: D.R.F. was responsible for funding acquisition, project administration, conceptualization, methodology, formal analysis, and all writing. K.B. performed software integration, data collection, and data validation. All authors have read and agreed to the published version of the manuscript.

Funding: Funding was provided by Maricopa County Association of Governments contract # 284.

Institutional Review Board Statement: No human or animal studies were involved.

Informed Consent Statement: No humans were involved.

Data Availability Statement: The finalized data are contained within the article. The raw data do not reside in a publicly available data set, but are available from the corresponding author.

Acknowledgments: The authors thank the Maricopa County Association of Governments for funding this project and Cathy J. Arthur for providing the test route and many helpful suggestions.

Conflicts of Interest: The authors declare no conflict of interest.

References

1. Pope, C.A.; Thun, M.J.; Namboodiri, M.M.; Dockery, D.W.; Evans, J.S.; Speizer, F.E.; Heath, C.W. Particulate Air Pollution as a Predictor of Mortality in a Prospective Study of U.S. Adults. *Am. J. Respir. Crit. Care Med.* **1995**, *151*, 669–674. [CrossRef]
2. Chow, J.C.; Watson, J.G.; Lowenthal, D.H.; Solomon, P.A.; Magliano, K.; Ziman, S.; Richards, L.W. PM_{10} Source Apportionment in California's San Joaquin Valley. *Atmos. Environ.* **1992**, *26A*, 3335–3354. [CrossRef]
3. Harrison, R.H.; Stedman, J.; Derwent, D. New Directions: Why are PM_{10} concentrations in Europe not falling? Atmospheric science perspectives special series. *Atmos. Environ.* **2008**, *42*, 603–606. [CrossRef]
4. Amato, F.; Pandolfi, M.; Escrig, A.; Querol, X.; Alastuey, A.; Pey, J.; Perez, N.; Hopke, P.K. Quantifying road dust resuspension in urban environment by Multilinear Engine: A comparison with PMF2. *Atmos. Environ.* **2009**, *43*, 2770–2780. [CrossRef]
5. Venkatram, A.; Fitz, D.; Bumiller, K.; Du, S.; Boeck, M.; Ganguly, C. Using a dispersion model to estimate emission rates of particulate matter from paved roads. *Atmos. Environ.* **1999**, *33*, 1093–1102. [CrossRef]
6. Kauhaniemi, M.; Kukkonen, J.; Härkönen, J.; Nikmo, J.; Kangas, L.; Omstedt, G.; Ketzel, M.; Kousa, A.; Haakana, M.; Karppinen, A. Evaluation of a road dust suspension model for predicting the concentrations of PM_{10} in a street canyon. *Atmos. Environ.* **2011**, *45*, 3646–3654. [CrossRef]
7. Denby, B.; Sundvor, I.; Johansson, C.; Pirjola, L.; Ketzel, M.; Norman, M.; Kupiainen, K.; Gustafsson, M.; Blomqvist, G.; Omstedt, G. A coupled road dust and surface moisture model to predict non-exhaust road traffic induced particle emissions (NORTRIP). Part 1: Road dust loading and suspension modelling. *Atmos. Environ.* **2013**, *77*, 283–300. [CrossRef]
8. Abu-Allaban, M.; Gillies, J.A.; Gertler, A.W. Application of a multi-lag regression approach to determine on-road PM_{10} and $PM_{2.5}$ emission rates. *Atmos. Environ.* **2003**, *37*, 5157–5164. [CrossRef]

9. Abu-Allaban, M.; Gillies, J.A.; Gertler, A.W.; Clayton, R.; Proffitt, D. Tailpipe, resuspended road dust, and brake-wear emission factors from on-road vehicles. *Atmos. Environ.* **2003**, *37*, 5283–5293. [CrossRef]
10. Kumar, A.V.; Patil, R.; Nambi, K. A composite receptor and dispersion model approach for estimation of effective emission factors for vehicles. *Atmos. Environ.* **2004**, *38*, 7065–7072. [CrossRef]
11. Claiborn, C.; Mitra, A.; Adams, G.; Bamesberger, L.; Allwine, G.; Kantamaneni, R.; Lamb, B.; Westberg, H. Evaluation of PM_{10} emission rates from paved and unpaved roads using tracer techniques. *Atmos. Environ.* **1995**, *29*, 1075–1089. [CrossRef]
12. Kantamaneni, R.; Adams, G.; Bamesberger, L.; Allwine, E.; Westberg, H.; Lamb, B.; Claiborn, C. The measurement of roadway PM_{10} emission rates using atmospheric tracer ratio techniques. *Atmos. Environ.* **1996**, *30*, 4209–4223. [CrossRef]
13. Ferm, M.; Sjöberg, K. Concentrations and emission factors for $PM_{2.5}$ and PM_{10} from road traffic in Sweden. *Atmos. Environ.* **2015**, *119*, 211–219. [CrossRef]
14. Sehmel, G. Particle resuspension from an asphalt road caused by car and truck traffic. *Atmos. Environ.* **1973**, *7*, 291–309. [CrossRef]
15. Cowherd, C., Jr.; Englehart, P.J. *Paved Road Particulate Emissions*; U.S. Environmental Protection Agency Document EPA-600/7-84-077; U.S. Environmental Protection Agency: Washington, DC, USA, 1984.
16. Xueli, J.; Dahe, J.; Simei, F.; Hui, Y.; Pinjing, H.; Boming, Y.; Zhongliang, L.; Chang, F. Road dust emission inventory for the metropolitan area of Shanghai City. *Atmos. Environ. Part A Gen. Top.* **1993**, *27*, 1735–1741. [CrossRef]
17. Veranth, J.M.; Pardyjak, E.R.; Seshadri, G. Vehicle-generated fugitive dust transport: Analytic models and field study. *Atmos. Environ.* **2003**, *37*, 2295–2303. [CrossRef]
18. U.S. Environmental Protection Agency. AP-42 Compilation of Air Emission Factors, Section 13-2.1 Paved Roads, January 2011. Available online: https://www.epa.gov/sites/default/files/2020-10/documents/emission_factor_documentation_for_ap-42_section_13.2.1_paved_roads_.pdf (accessed on 20 September 2021).
19. Kuhns, H.; Etyemezian, V.; Landwehr, D.; MacDougall, C.; Pitchford, M.; Green, M. Testing re-entrained aerosol kinetic emissions from roads (TRAKER): A new approach to infer silt loading on roadways. *Atmos. Environ.* **2001**, *35*, 2815–2825. [CrossRef]
20. Pirjola, L.; Johansson, C.; Kupiainen, K.; Stojiljkovic, A.; Karlsson, H.; Hussein, T. Road Dust Emissions from Paved Roads Measured Using Different Mobile Systems. *J. Air Waste Manag. Assoc.* **2010**, *60*, 1422–1433. [CrossRef]
21. Mathissen, M.; Scheer, V.; Kirchner, U.; Vogt, R.; Benter, T. Non-exhaust PM emission measurements of a light duty vehicle with a mobile trailer. *Atmos. Environ.* **2012**, *59*, 232–242. [CrossRef]
22. Fitz, D.R.; Bumiller, K.; Bufalino, C.; James, D.E. Real-time PM_{10} emission rates from paved roads by measurement of concentrations in the vehicle's wake using on-board sensors. Part 1. SCAMPER method characterization. *Atmos. Environ.* **2020**, *230*, 117483. [CrossRef]
23. Fitz, D.R.; Bumiller, K.; Etyemesian, V.; Kuhns, H.D.; Gillies, J.A.; Nikolich, G.; James, D.E.; Langston, R.; Merle, R.S., Jr. Real-time PM_{10} emission rates from paved roads by measurement of concentrations in the vehicle's wake using on-board sensors. Part 2. Comparison of SCAMPER, TRAKER™, flux measurements, and AP-42 silt sampling under controlled conditions. *Atmos. Environ.* **2021**, *256*, 118453. [CrossRef]
24. Nicholson, K.W.; Branson, J.R.; Giess, P.; Cannell, R.J. The effects of vehicle activity on particle resuspension. *J. Aerosol Sci.* **1989**, *20*, 1425–1428. [CrossRef]

MDPI
St. Alban-Anlage 66
4052 Basel
Switzerland
Tel. +41 61 683 77 34
Fax +41 61 302 89 18
www.mdpi.com

Atmosphere Editorial Office
E-mail: atmosphere@mdpi.com
www.mdpi.com/journal/atmosphere

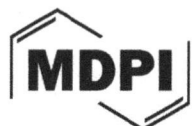

www.ingramcontent.com/pod-product-compliance
Lightning Source LLC
LaVergne TN
LVHW070151100526
838202LV00015B/1928